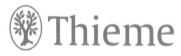

The Retina Illustrated

Justis P. Ehlers, MD
The Norman C. and Donna L. Harbert Endowed Chair for Ophthalmic Research
Director, The Tony and Leona Campane Center for Excellence in Image-Guided Surgery and
Advanced Imaging Research
Cole Eye Institute
Cleveland Clinic
Cleveland, Ohio

Assistant Editor
Thuy K. Le, BA
Project Lead, The Tony and Leona Campane Center for Excellence in Image-Guided Surgery
and Advanced Imaging Research
Cole Eye Institute
Cleveland Clinic
Cleveland, Ohio

407 illustrations

Thieme
New York • Stuttgart • Delhi • Rio de Janeiro

Library of Congress Cataloging-in-Publication Data

Names: Ehlers, Justis P., editor.

Title: The retina illustrated / [edited by] Justis P. Ehlers.

Description: New York : Thieme, [2020] | Includes bibliographical references and index.

Identifiers: LCCN 2019034798 (print) | LCCN 2019034799 (ebook) | ISBN 9781626238312 (paperback) | ISBN 9781626238336 (ebook)

Subjects: MESH: Retinal Diseases–diagnostic imaging | Retinal Diseases–surgery

Classification: LCC RE551 (print) | LCC RE551 (ebook) | NLM WW 270 | DDC 617.7/35–dc23

LC record available at https://lccn.loc.gov/2019034798

LC ebook record available at https://lccn.loc.gov/2019034799

Copyright © 2020 by Thieme Medical Publishers, Inc.

Thieme Publishers New York
333 Seventh Avenue, New York, NY 10001 USA
+1 800 782 3488, customerservice@thieme.com

Thieme Publishers Stuttgart
Rüdigerstrasse 14, 70469 Stuttgart, Germany
+49 [0]711 8931 421, customerservice@thieme.de

Thieme Publishers Delhi
A-12, Second Floor, Sector-2, Noida-201301
Uttar Pradesh, India
+91 120 45 566 00, customerservice@thieme.in

Thieme Revinter Publicações Ltda.
Rua do Matoso, 170 – Tijuca
Rio de Janeiro RJ 20270-135 - Brasil
+55 21 2563-9702
www.thiemerevinter.com.br

Cover design: Thieme Publishing Group
Typesetting by Thomson Digital, India

Printed in the United States of America
by King Printing Co., Inc.   5 4 3 2 1

ISBN 978-1-62623-831-2

Also available as an e-book:
eISBN 978-1-62623-833-6

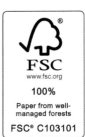

FSC
www.fsc.org
100%
Paper from well-managed forests
FSC® C103101

To my parents for showing me how to follow my dreams.

To my wonderful wife, Gina, and my two amazing children, Adelyn and Cooper,
for enabling me to live those dreams every day with each of you.

Contents

Part III Retinal Vascular Disease

Part IV Retinal Degenerations and Dystrophies

Part V Other Macular Disorders

Part VII Retinal Trauma and Other Conditions

Contents

Part X Pediatric Vitreoretinal Disease

Preface

For the last 15 years, I have been immersed in the world of ophthalmology and retinal disease. My journey began at Washington University in St. Louis where I found my passion for ophthalmology during medical school. My residency training took me to the Wills Eye Hospital where I developed a tremendous network of mentors and friends. At Wills, I had the unique privilege of serving under two inspirational leaders, Dr. William Tasman and Dr. Julia Haller. Through their generosity, I had my first opportunity to serve as one of the Co-Chief Editors for the *Wills Eye Manual, 5th Edition*. This project showed me the critical importance of a team-based approach to these comprehensive ophthalmic texts. After my time at Wills, I spent the next 2 years at the Duke Eye Center completing my vitreoretinal surgical fellowship. I was incredibly fortunate to work with an incredible group of mentors under the retina service leadership of Dr. Brooks McCuen and Dr. Glenn Jaffe. My journey then brought me to the Cole Eye Institute at the Cleveland Clinic where I have continued to develop knowledge in patient care, fellow/resident education, and research. Under the leadership of Dr. Dan Martin, our retina service had grown significantly over the last 10 years and I am surrounded by a wonderful team of partners and friends. It is through these amazing experiences that *The Retina Illustrated* emerges.

I hope that *The Retina Illustrated* will provide a rapid-fire yet thorough approach to the highly visual world of retinal disease. This book brings together authors from around the world to highlight the most common and critical retinal disorders encountered in eye care. My desire with this book is to provide a quick-reference guide that will provide easy access to key diagnostic imaging findings for the major retinal disorders that we manage as eye care providers.

This text includes over 100 chapters surveying a wide range of topics. Chapters in the book range from traditional common retinal diseases, such as age-related macular degeneration and diabetic retinopathy, to emerging retinal conditions, such as Zika and Ebola-related complications. In addition, *The Retina Illustrated* includes extensive examples of cutting-edge imaging technology, such as ultra-widefield angiography, intraoperative optical coherence tomography, and OCT angiography.

I believe that this text can be a critical reference for those providers serving on the front lines for presenting retinal disease, such as primary care physicians, emergency medicine physicians, optometrists, and comprehensive ophthalmologists. My hope is that this will provide an important educational tool for residents and fellows in the midst of their training. Finally, our team of authors were sure to make this text comprehensive enough to serve as an important quick reference for the retina specialist to be able to identify key imaging findings in a disorder of interest. Thank you for your interest in *The Retina Illustrated*.

Justis P. Ehlers, MD
The Norman C. and Donna L. Harbert Endowed Chair
for Ophthalmic Research
Director, The Tony and Leona Campane Center for Excellence
in Image-Guided Surgery and Advanced Imaging Research
Cole Eye Institute at the Cleveland Clinic
Cleveland, Ohio

Acknowledgments

This project would not have been possible without an outstanding team of individuals supporting it along the way. I want to thank all of the authors that contributed to this project. Your time and dedication are what ultimately brought this project together and elevated this book to a new level. The opportunity to work with such an amazing network of individuals of friends, residents, fellows, mentors, and colleagues made the project even more rewarding.

I want to thank my partners and friends at Cole Eye Institute who went above and beyond in their efforts for this book. I also want to acknowledge my Assistant Editor, Thuy Le, who truly brought this together. I want to thank the team at Thieme for the opportunity to create this book.

Finally, I want to thank my research program manager and my friend, Jamie L. Reese, for her tireless efforts in helping with this book, and I want to thank my family for supporting me through this process and tolerating my countless hours spent on this project.

Contributors

Aniruddha Agarwal, MD
Assistant Professor
Post Graduate Institute of Medical Education and
   Research (PGIMER)
Chandigarh, India

Daniel R. Agarwal, MD
Medical Retina Fellow
Cole Eye Institute
Cleveland Clinic
Cleveland, Ohio

Kanika Aggarwal, MS
Clinical Associate
Post Graduate Institute of Medical Education and
   Research (PGIMER)
Chandigarh, India

Thomas A. Albini, MD
Professor of Clinical Ophthalmology
Bascom Palmer Eye Institute
The Miller School of Medicine
The University of Miami
Miami, Florida

Mohsin H. Ali, MD
Clinical Associate
Duke University
Durham, North Carolina

Sarina Amin, MD
Ophthalmology Specialist
Private Practice
Los Angeles, California

Michael T. Andreoli, MD
Vitreoretinal Surgeon
Wheaton Eye Clinic
Wheaton, Illinois

Waseem H. Ansari, MD
Resident Physician
Cole Eye Institute
Cleveland Clinic
Cleveland, Ohio

Sruthi Arepalli, MD
Vitreoretinal Surgery Fellow
Cole Eye Institute
Cleveland Clinic
Cleveland, Ohio

Mary E. Aronow, MD
Assistant Professor of Ophthalmology
Retina Service
Massachusetts Eye and Ear
Harvard Medical School
Boston, Massachusetts

Jawad I. Arshad
4th Year Medical Student
Case Western Reserve University School of Medicine
Cleveland, Ohio

Malvika Arya, MID
OCT Research Fellow
New England Eye Center
Tufts Medical Center
Boston, Massachusetts

Amy S. Babiuch, MD
Staff Physician
Cole Eye Institute
Cleveland Clinic
Cleveland, Ohio

Sophie J. Bakri, MD
Professor of Ophthalmology
Mayo Clinic
Rochester, Minnesota

Alexander C. Barnes, MD
Fellow, Vitreoretinal Surgery
Emory Eye Center
Atlanta, Georgia

Claudine Bellerive, MD, MSc
Ocular Oncology Service
Centre Hospitalier Universitaire de Quebec
Professor of Ophthalmology
Faculte de Medecine
Universite Laval
Quebec, Canada

Nima Justin Bencohen
Student
University of California, Santa Barbara
Santa Barbara, California

Audina M. Berrocal, MD
Professor of Clinical Ophthalmology
Bascom Palmer Eye Institute
Miller School of Medicine
University of Miami
Miami, Florida

Angela P. Bessette, MD
Assistant Professor of Ophthalmology
University of Rochester
Flaum Eye Institute
Rochester, New York

Suruchi Bhardwaj Bhui, MD
Vitreoretinal Surgery Fellow
University of Virginia
Charlottesville, Virginia

Durga S. Borkar, MD
Assistant Professor of Ophthalmology
Vitreoretinal Surgery and Diseases
Duke University Eye Center
Durham, North Carolina

Enrico Borrelli, MD
Clinical Research Fellow
Doheny Eye Institute
Department of Ophthalmology
David Geffen School of Medicine at UCLA
Los Angeles, California

Joseph Daniel Boss, MD
Adult and Pediatric Vitreoretinal Specialist
Retina Specialists of Michigan
Grand Rapids, Michigan

Alexander R. Bottini, MD
Chief Resident
New York University Eye Center
New York, New York

Andrew W. Browne, MD, PhD
Assistant Professor
Gavin Herbert Eye Institute
University of California Irvine
Irvine, California

Linda A. Cernichiaro-Espinosa, MD
Retina and Vitreous
Pediatric Retina
Asociación para Evitar la Ceguera en México IAP
Mexico City, Mexico

Sai Chavala, MD
Professor
University of North Texas Health Science Center
North Texas Eye Research Institute
Fort Worth, Texas

Rachel C. Chen, MD
Ophthalmology Resident
Cole Eye Institute
Cleveland Clinic
Cleveland, Ohio

Daniel G. Cherfan, MD
Attending Physician
Beirut Eye and ENT Specialist Hospital
Mathaf Square, Beirut
Lebanon

Ijeoma S. Chinwuba, MD
Resident
NYU Langone Eye Center
Department of Ophthalmology
New York University School of Medicine
NYU Langone Health
New York, New York

Netan Choudhry, MD, FRCS(C)
Medical Director
Vitreous Retina Macula Specialists of Toronto
Toronto, Canada
Staff Ophthalmologist
Cleveland Clinic Canada
Ontario, Canada
Adjunct Faculty
Department of Ophthalmology & Visual Sciences
University of Toronto
Toronto, Canada

Michael N. Cohen, MD
Associate
NJ Retina
Teaneck, New Jersey

Robert J. Courtney, MD
Partner
Colorado Retina Associates
Denver, Colorado

Catherine A. Cukras, MD, PhD
Laker Scholar and Investigator
Head
Unit on Clinical Investigation of Retinal Disease
Director
Medical Retina Fellowship Program
National Eye Institute
National Institutes of Health
Bethesda, Maryland

Nathan E. Cutler, MD
Vitreoretinal Fellow
Cole Eye Institute
Cleveland Clinic
Cleveland, Ohio

Pouya Nachshon Dayani, MD
Partner
Vitreoretinal Surgery and Ocular Inflammation
Retina-Vitreous Associates Medical Group
Los Angeles, California

Meghan J. DeBenedictis, MS LGC, Med
Genetic Counselor
Cleveland Clinic
Cole Eye Institute
Cleveland, Ohio

Vaidehi S. Dedania, MD
Assistant Professor of Ophthalmology
New York University School of Medicine
New York, New York

Dilsher S. Dhoot, MD
Vitreoretinal Surgeon
California Retina Consultants
Santa Barbara, California

Kimberly A. Drenser, MD, PhD
Physician
Associated Retinal Consultants
Royal Oak, Missouri

Jay S. Duker, MD
Director
New England Eye Center
Professor and Chairman
Department of Ophthalmology
Tufts Medical Center
Tufts University School of Medicine
Boston, Massachusetts

Justis P. Ehlers, MD
The Norman C. and Donna L. Harbert Endowed Chair for
    Ophthalmic Research
Director, The Tony and Leona Campane Center for
    Excellence in Image-Guided Surgery and Advanced
    Imaging Research
Cole Eye Institute
Cleveland Clinic
Cleveland, Ohio

Sharon Fekrat, MD, FACS
Professor of Ophthalmology
Associate Professor of Surgery
Director,
Vitreoretinal Surgery Fellowship
Duke University School of Medicine
Associate Chief of Staff
Durham VA Medical Center
Durham, Virginia

Daniela Ferrara, MD, PhD
Assistant Professor of Ophthalmology
Tufts University School of Medicine
Boston, Massachusetts

Natalia Albuquerque Lucena Figueiredo, MD
Research Fellow
Cleveland Clinic
Cole Eye Institute
Cleveland, Ohio

Jorge Fortun, MD
Associate Professor of Clinical Ophthalmology
Medical Director
BPEI Palm Beach
Bascom Palmer Eye Institute
University of Miami Miller School of Medicine
Palm Beach Gardens, Florida

K. Bailey Freund, MD
Clinical Professor of Ophthalmology
Department of Ophthalmology
New York University School of Medicine
Vitreous Retina Macula Consultants of New York
New York, New York

Sunir J. Garg, MD, FACS
Professor of Ophthalmology
Co-Director Retina Research Unit
The Retina Service of Wills Eye Hospital
Editor in Chief, Retina Times
Thomas Jefferson University
Philadelphia, Pennsylvania

Robert B. Garoon, MD
Clinical Instructor
Bascom Palmer Eye Institute
Des Plaines, Illinois

Benjamin Kambiz Ghiam, MD
PGY-1
UCLA - Olive View Medical Center
Los Angeles, California

Dilraj Grewal, MD
Associate Professor of Ophthalmology
Duke Eye Center
Durham, North Carolina

Omesh P. Gupta, MD
Ophthalmologist
Mid-Atlantic Retina
Wills Eye Hospital
Philadelphia, Pennsylvania

James William Harbour, MD
Associate Director for Basic Research for Sylvester
   Comprehensive Cancer Center
Director of Ocular Oncology
Leader, Eye Cancer Site Disease Group
Mark J. Daily Chair in Ophthalmology
Vice Chairman for Translation Research
Bascom Palmer Eye Institute
Miami, Florida

Allen Ho, MD
Retina Specialist
Mid-Atlantic Retina
Wills Eye Hospital
Philadelphia, Pennsylvania

Jennifer C.W. Hu, MD, MS
Resident Physician
Internal Medicine - Preliminary
Mount Sinai Hospital
Department of Medicine
Resident Physician
Ophthalmology
Columbia University
Edward S. Harkness Eye Institute
New York, New York

Laryssa A. Huryn, MD
Medical Officer
Ophthalmic Genetics and Visual Function Branch
National Eye Institute, NIH
Bethesda, Maryland

S. Amal Hussnain, MD
Vitreoretinal Surgery Fellow
Columbia University, MRMNY, NY, MEETH
New York, New York

Makoto Inoue
Professor of Ophthalmology
Kyorin Eye Center
Kyorin University School of Medicine
Tokyo, Japan

Paul E. Israelsen, MD
Ophthalmology Resident
University of California, Irvine
Irvine, California

Yuji Itoh, MD, PhD
Assistant Professor
Faculty of Medicine
Department of Ophthalmology
Kyorin University
Tokyo, Japan

Glenn Jaffe, MD
Professor of Ophthalmology
Duke Eye Center
Durham, North Carolina

Ruben Jauregui, BS
Clinical Research Fellow
Edward S. Harkness Eye Institute
Columbia University Medical Center
New York, New York

Shangjun (Collier) Jiang, MD
Medical Student
Faculty of Medicine
University of Toronto
Ontario, Canada

Brett G. Jeffrey, MD
Staff Scientist
Ophthalmic Genetics and Visual Function Branch
National Eye Institute, NIH
Bethesda, Maryland

Mark W. Johnson, MD
Professor and Section Chief
Retina Section
Kellogg Eye Center
University of Michigan
Ann Arbor, Michigan

Talia R. Kaden, MD
Assistant Professor of Ophthalmology
Manhattan Eye, Ear, and Throat Hospital
Zucker School of Medicine
Hofstra University
New York, New York

Peter K. Kaiser, MD
Chaney Family Endowed Chair for Ophthalmic Research
Cole Eye Institute
Cleveland Clinic
Cleveland, Ohio

Rahul Kapoor, MD
Harkness Eye Institute
Columbia University Medical Center
New York, New York

Keiko Kataoka, MD, PhD
Assistant Professor
Department of Ophthalmology
Nagoya University Hospital
Nagoya, Japan

Rahul N. Khurana, MD
Associate Clinical Professor in Ophthalmology
University of California, San Francisco
San Francisco, California
Partner
Northern California Retina Vitreous Associates
Mountain View, California

Stephen J. Kim, MD
Vanderbilt Eye Institute
Nashville, Tennessee

Michael A. Klufas, MD
Assistant Professor of Ophthalmology
The Retina Service of Wills Eye Hospital
Thomas Jefferson University
Philadelphia, Pennsylvania

Jaya B. Kumar, MD
Associate
Florida Retina Institute
Orlando, Florida

Marisa K. Lau, MD
Vitreoretinal Surgery Fellow
University of Colorado
Aurora, Colorado

Jeremy A. Lavine, MD, PhD
Assistant Professor of Ophthalmology
Northwestern University
Chicago, Illinois

Thuy K. Le, BA
Project Lead, The Tony and Leona Campane Center for
   Excellence in Image-Guided Surgery and Advanced
   Imaging Research
Cole Eye Institute
Cleveland Clinic
Cleveland, Ohio

Belinda C.S. Leong, MD, FRANZCO
Medical Retina Specialist
Retina Associates
Sydney, New South Wales
Australia

Ashleigh Levison, MD
Consulting Physician and Surgeon for Vitreoretinal
   Disorders
Colorado Retina Associates
Denver, Colorado

Ang Li, MD
Resident
Cole Eye Institute
Cleveland, Ohio

Andrea Elizabeth Arriola-López, MD, MSc
Retina Specialist Innovación Ocular
Instituto de Innovación Cardiovascular GT
Guatemala City, Guatemala

Careen Lowder, MD, PhD
Attending Physician
Cole Eye Institute
Cleveland Clinic
Cleveland, Ohio

Ankur Mehra, MD
Resident Physician
University of Kentucky
Lexington, Kentucky

Nitish Mehta, MD
Resident
New York University
School of Medicine
New York, New York

Yasha S. Modi, MD
Assistant Professor
Department of Ophthalmology
New York University
New York, New York

Darius M. Moshfeghi, MD
Professor
Byers Eye Institute
Stanford University School of Medicine
Palo Alto, California

Prithvi Mruthyunjaya, MD
Associate Professor
Stanford University
Palo Alto, California

Timothy G. Murray, MD
Retina Specialist and Founding Director/CEO
Murray Ocular Oncology and Retina
South Miami, Florida

Rajinder S. Nirwan, MD
Fellow, Surgical Retina
University of Calgary
Calgary, Alberta, Canada

Quan Dong Nguyen, MD, MSc
Professor of Ophthalmology
Director
Uveitis and Ocular Inflammatory Service
Spencer Center for Vision Research
Byers Eye Institute
Member
Wu Tsai Neurosciences Institute
Stanford University School of Medicine
Palo Alto, California

Manuel Alejandro Paez-Escamilla, MD
Research Fellow
Bascom Palmer Eye Institute
Miami, Florida

Vishal S. Parikh, MD
Vitreoretinal Surgery Fellow
The Retina Institute
St. Louis, Missouri

Priya Patel, MD
Resident
Department of Ophthalmology
New York University
New York, New York

Paula Eem Pecen, MD
Assistant Professor
Department of Ophthalmology
University of Colorado
Aurora, Colorado

John D. Pitcher, III, MD
Retina Specialist
Medical Director
Vision Research Center
Eye Associates of New Mexico
Assistant Clinical Professor of Ophthalmology
University of New Mexico
Albuquerque, New Mexico

Omar S. Punjabi, MD
Ophthalmologist
Vitreo-retinal Diseases and Surgery
Charlotte, Eye, Ear, Nose, and Throat Associates (CEENTA)
Charlotte, North Carolina

Aleksandra Rachitskaya, MO
Assistant Professor of Ophthalmology
Cleveland Clinic
Cole Eye Institute
Cleveland, Ohio

Prethy Rao, MD, MPH
Assistant Professor
Adult and Pediatric Vitreoretinal Disease and Surgery
Emory Eye Center
Atlanta, Georgia

Carl D. Regillo, MD
Director, Retina Service
Wills Eye Hospital
Professor of Ophthalmology
Thomas Jefferson University
Philadelphia, Pennsylvania

Almyr S. Sabrosa, MD
Ophthalmologist
Ophthalmology Institute of Rio de Janeiro
Rio de Janeiro, Brazil

SriniVas Sadda, MD
President and Chief Scientific Officer
Stephen J. Ryan – Arnold and Mabel Beckman Endowed Chair
Doheny Eye Institue
Professor of Ophthalmology
Department of Ophthalmology
David Geffen School of Medicine at UCLA
Los Angeles, California

David Sarraf, MD
Clinical Professor of Ophthalmology
Stein Eye Institute, UCLA
Los Angeles, California

Matteo Scaramuzzi, MD
Pediatric Ophthalmology and Ophthalmic Genetic Fellow
Cole Eye Institute
Cleveland, Ohio
Ophthalmology Resident
University of Milan
Milan, Italy

Andrew P. Schachat, MD
Vice Chairman
Cole Eye Institute
Professor of Ophthalmology
Lerner College of Medicine
Cleveland, Ohio

Avery E. Sears
Medical Student
Case Western Reserve University MSTP
Cleveland, Ohio

Jonathan E. Sears, MD
Staff
Cole Eye Institute
Cleveland Clinic
Cleveland, Ohio

Anjali Shah, MD
Clinical Assistant Professor
Ophthalmology and Visual Sciences
University of Michigan
Ann Arbor, Michigan

Chirag Shah, MD, MPH
Assistant Professor of Ophthalmology
Tufts University School of Medicine
Lecturer
Harvard Medical School
Co-Director
Vitreoretinal Surgery Fellowship
Tufts/Ophthalmic Consultants of Bostom Vitreoretinal
  Surgery
Attending
Ophthalmic Consultants of Boston
Boston, Massachusetts

Gaurav K. Shah, MD
Partner
The Retina Institute
St. Louis, Missouri

Jessica G. Shantha, MD
Assistant Professor of Ophthalmology
National Institutes of Health Building Interdisciplinary
  Research Careers in Women's Health (BIRCWH) Scholar
Emory Eye Center
Emory University School of Medicine
Atlanta, Georgia

Priya Sharma, MD
Vitreoretinal Fellow
Ophthalmic Consultants of Boston
Boston, Massachusetts

Sumit Sharma, MD
Ophthalmologist
Cole Eye Institute
Cleveland Clinic
Cleveland, Ohio

Carol L. Shields, MD
Director
Ocular Oncology Service
Wills Eye Hospital
Professor of Ophthalmology
Thomas Jefferson University
Philadelphia, Pennsylvania

Jerry A. Shields, MD
Director Emeritus
Ocular Oncology Service
Wills Eye Hospital
Professor of Ophthalmology
Thomas Jefferson University
Philadelphia, Pennsylvania

Rishi P. Singh, MD
Staff Physician
Cole Eye Institute
Medical Director
Clinical Systems Office
Cleveland Clinic
Associate Professor of Ophthalmology
Case Western Reserve University
Cleveland, Ohio

Arun D. Singh, MD
Staff Physician
Cole Eye Institute
Cleveland Clinic
Cleveland, Ohio

Geraldine R. Slean, MD, MS
Associate Physician
Department of Ophthalmology
Kaiser Permanente
Greater Southern Alameda Area
Union City, California

Richard F. Spaide, MD
Partner
Vitreous, Retina, Macula Consultants of New York
New York, New York

Jayanth Sridhar, MD
Assistant Professor of Clinical Ophthalmology
Bascom Palmer Eye Institute
Miami, Florida

Sunil K. Srivastava, MD
Attending Physician
Cole Eye Institute
Cleveland Clinic
Cleveland, Ohio

Matthew R. Starr, MD
Resident
Mayo Clinic
Rochester, Minnesota

Nathan Steinle, MD
Ophthalmologist
California Retina Consultants
Santa Barbara, California

Maxwell S. Stem, MD
Clinical Assistant Professor of Ophthalmology
Mid Atlantic Retina
Wills Eye Hospital
Thomas Jefferson University
Philadelphia, Pennsylvania

Philip P. Storey, MD, MPH
Retina Fellow
Wills Eye Hospital
Philadelphia, Pennsylvania

Daniel Su, MD
Retina Fellow
Mid Atlantic Retina
Wills Eye Hospital
Philadelphia, Pennsylvania

Harris Sultan, MD
Retina Fellow
John F. Hardesty, MD Department of Ophthalmology and
   Visual Sciences
Washington University School of Medicine in St. Louis
St. Louis, Missouri

Katherine E. Talcott, MD
Attending Physician
Cole Eye Institute
Cleveland Clinic
Cleveland, Ohio

Heather M. Tamez, MD
Fellow in Vitreoretinal Diseases and Surgery
Vanderbilt Eye Institute
Nashville, Tennessee

Peter H. Tang, MD, PhD
Clinical Instructor
Byers Eye Institute
Stanford University School of Medicine
Palo Alto, California

Ramin Tadayoni, MD, PhD
Professor of Ophthalmology
Université de Paris
Hôpital Lariboisière
Paris, France

Hiroko Terasaki, MD, PhD
Professor and Chair
Department of Ophthalmology
Nagoya University Graduate School of Medicine
Nagoya, Japan

Akshay S. Thomas, MD, MS
Associate Physician
Vitreoretinal Surgery and Uveitis
Tennessee Retina
Nashville, Tennessee

Merina Thomas, MD
Assistant Professor
Retina Division
Casey Eye Institute
Oregon Health & Science University
Portland, Oregon

Atalie C. Thompson, MD, MPH
Ophthalmologist
Duke University
Department of Ophthalmology
Durham, North Carolina

Elias I. Traboulsi, MD, MEd
Professor of Ophthalmology
Director
The Center for Genetic Eye Diseases
Cole Eye Institute
Cleveland Clinic
Cleveland, Ohio

Stephen H. Tsang, MD, PhD
Lazlo T. Bito Associate Professor of Ophthalmology
Associate Professor of Pathology & Cell Biology
Edward S. Harkness Eye Institute
Columbia University Medical Center
New York, New York

Edmund Tsui
Uveitis Fellow
Francis I. Proctor Foundation
University of California
San Francisco, California

Atsuro Uchida, MD, PhD
Clinical Research Fellow
Cole Eye Institute
Cleveland Clinic
Cleveland, Ohio

Lejla Vajzovic, MD
Director
Duke Eye Center Continuing Medical Education
Co-Director
Duke Eye Center Continuing Medical Education
Director
Duke Center for Artificial and Regenerative Vision
Director
Duke fAVS and AVS Courses
Associate Professor of Ophthalmology
Adult and Pediatric Vitreoretinal Surgery and Diseases
Duke University Eye Center
Durham, North Carolina

Huber Martins Vasconcelos, Jr., MD
Retina/Genetics Fellow
Oregon Health & Science University
Casey Eye Institute
Portland, Oregon

Arthi Venkat, MD
Attending Physician
Cole Eye Institute
Cleveland Clinic
Cleveland, Ohio

Nandini Venkateswaran, MD
Resident Physician
Bascom Palmer Eye Instittue
Miami, Floria

Angela J. Verkade, MD
Resident
Baylor College of Medicine
Department of Ophthalmology
Cullen Eye Institute
Houston, Texas

Victor M. Villegas, MD
Resident
Associate Professor
Department of Ophthalmology
University of Puerto Rico
San Juan, Puerto Rico
Associate Professor
Department of Surgery
Ponce Health Sciences University School of Medicine
Ponce, Puerto Rico
Voluntary Assistant Professor in Clinical Ophthalmology
Bascom Palmer Eye Institute
University of Miami
Miami, Flordia

Nadia K. Waheed, MD, MPH
Associate Professor of Ophthalmology
New England Eye Center
Tufts Medical Center
Boston, Massachusetts

Kevin Wang, MD
Resident
Cole Eye Institute
Cleveland Clinic
Cleveland, Ohio

Christina Y. Weng, MD, MBA
Associate Professor
Department of Ophthalmology
Fellowship Program Director-Vitreoretinal Diseases
  & Surgery
Baylor College of Medicine
Medical Student Clinical Elective Director
Ben Taub General Hospital
Houston, Texas

Andre J. Witkin, MD
Assistant Professor
Tufts Medical Center
Department of Ophthalmology
Boston, Massachusetts

Edward H. Wood, MD
Assistant Professor of Ophthalmology
Byers Eye Institute
Department of Ophthalmology
Stanford University School of Medicine
Palo Alto, California

Jeremy D. Wolfe, MD, MS
Associate Professor
Associated Retinal Consultants
Oakland University William Beaumont School of Medicine
Royal Oak, Missouri

Charles C. Wykoff, MD, PhD
Director of Research
Retina Consultants of Houston
Deputy Chair for Ophthalmology
Blanton Eye Institute
Houston Methodist Hospital
Bellaire, Texas

David Xu, MD
Resident
Stein Eye Institute
University of California Los Angeles
Los Angeles, California

Lucy T. Xu, MD, PhD
Vitreoretinal Fellow
Emory University
Atlanta, Georgia

Paul Yang, MD, PhD
Assistant Professor of Ophthalmology
Ophthalmic Genetics and Ocular Immunology
Casey Eye Institute
Oregon Heath & Science University
Portland, Oregon

Steven Yeh, MD
M. Loise Simpson Associate Professor of Ophthalmology
Emory Eye Center
Emory University School of Medicine
Emory Global Health Institute
Atlanta, Georgia

Alex Yuan, MD
Assistant Professor in Ophthalmology
Cleveland Clinic Lerner College of Medicine
Cole Eye Institute
Cleveland, Ohio

Part I

Retinal Diagnostics

1 Optical Coherence Tomography

Rachel C. Chen and Peter K. Kaiser

Summary

Optical coherence tomography (OCT) is a noninvasive imaging technique that has become an invaluable tool in the diagnosis and treatment of retinal disease, including macular holes, age-related macular degeneration, diabetic macular edema, and central serous chorioretinopathy. OCT uses low-coherence interferometry to produce in vivo cross-sectional images of the retina and choroid. New advancements in OCT, including swept source OCT, OCT angiography, and intraoperative OCT, have found further use in imaging the choroid, the choroidal, and retinal vasculature and in surgical planning and execution, respectively.

Keywords: ellipsoid zone, intraretinal fluid, optical coherence tomography angiography, subretinal fluid

1.1 Diagnostic/Technology Overview

Optical coherence tomography (OCT) was first introduced in 1991 as a noninvasive technology that uses low-coherence interferometry to produce cross-sections of biological structures. OCT employs a light beam that travels to a beam splitter, which splits the beam into a sample and a reference beam (directed toward a mirror at a reference distance). The backscattered light from the sample then interferes with the reflected light from the reference mirror and is used to produce a reflectivity profile of the retina. Analogous to ultrasound, but using light instead of sound waves, OCT is able to obtain high-resolution images (ranging from 3 to 10 μm). The primary system currently used is spectral domain OCT, which uses Fourier transformation to obtain images faster and with higher resolution than time-domain OCT. Current OCT technology enables

visualization of the various retinal layers (▶ Fig. 1.1). Next-generation swept source OCT technology utilizes a longer wave length and a faster engine that enables greater tissue penetration (e.g., choroidal visualization) and scan sizes (▶ Fig. 1.2).

Since its introduction, OCT has become the primary diagnostic test for multiple diseases including macular holes, diabetic macular edema, age-related macular degeneration (AMD), vascular occlusion, and central serous chorioretinopathy (CSR).

1.2 Key Applications

1.2.1 Vitreoretinal Interface Disorders

OCT is the gold standard in diagnosis and evaluation of vitreoretinal interface disorders, including epiretinal membranes, vitreomacular traction, and macular holes (▶ Fig. 1.3).

1.2.2 Evaluation of Retinal Edema

Diabetic Macular Edema

OCT has become the standard of care for detecting diabetic macular edema (DME) and monitoring its response to treatment. The advantages of OCT include its ability to detect small amounts of intraretinal and subretinal fluid that are not visible by biomicroscopy and to precisely measure retinal thickness for treatment monitoring. In addition, OCT can characterize specific fluid patterns in DME that may prognosticate response to treatment (▶ Fig. 1.4).

Age-Related Macular Degeneration

AMD is initially characterized by drusen, proteinaceous deposits in Bruch's membrane, and changes in the retinal pigment epithelium (RPE). On OCT, drusen appear as convex RPE

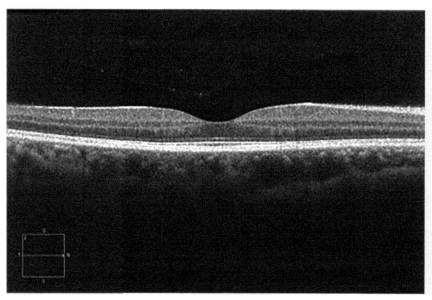

Fig. 1.1 Normal retinal anatomy. Optical coherence tomography demonstrating normal retinal anatomy. The layers of the retina (from inner to outer): nerve fiber layer, ganglion cell layer, inner plexiform layer, inner nuclear layer, outer plexiform layer, outer nuclear layer, external limiting membrane, ellipsoid zone, interdigitation zone, retina pigment epithelium, choroid.

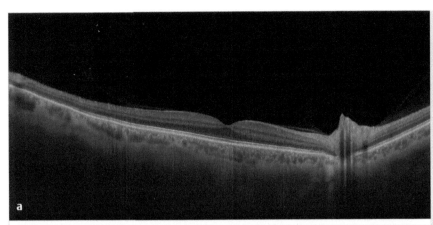

Fig. 1.2 Swept source optical coherence tomography (SS-OCT). Longer wavelength SS-OCT demonstrating outstanding visualization of the vitreous, retina, and choroid. Examples include **(a)** an eye without pathology and **(b)** an eye with neovascular age-related macular degeneration with extensive subfoveal hyperreflective material and subfoveal choroidal neovascularization.

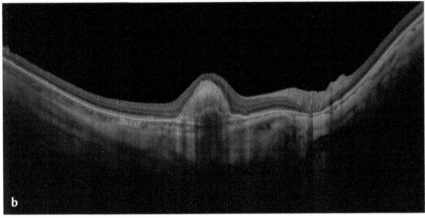

Fig. 1.3 Macular hole. Optical coherence tomography demonstrating a full thickness macular hole with overlying vitreous separation. Note the anvil-shaped deformity of the macula, the loss of photoreceptors, and the intraretinal fluid at the edges of the hole.

elevations of varying reflectivity. OCT may be used to monitor progression of drusen over time. Advanced nonneovascular AMD is characterized by geographic atrophy that appears on OCT as outer retinal thinning, loss of the RPE, and increased choroidal reflectivity due to hypertransmission. OCT is also a key tool in diagnosing and categorizing choroidal neovascularization that characterizes neovascular AMD (▶ Fig. 1.5, ▶ Fig. 1.2).

Retinal Arterial Occlusion

OCT can be used to confirm the presence of an acute or a chronic retinal arterial occlusion (RAO). Acute RAO may be characterized by increased inner retinal thickening and hyperreflectivity, corresponding with retinal whitening on biomicroscopy. Chronic RAO may manifest as an inner retinal thinning (▶ Fig. 1.6).

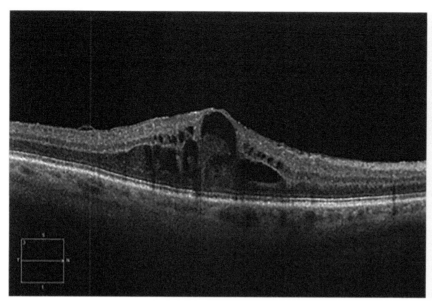

Fig. 1.4 Diabetic macular edema. Optical coherence tomography of a patient demonstrating diabetic cystoid macular edema. Note the multiple large ovoid areas of low reflectivity.

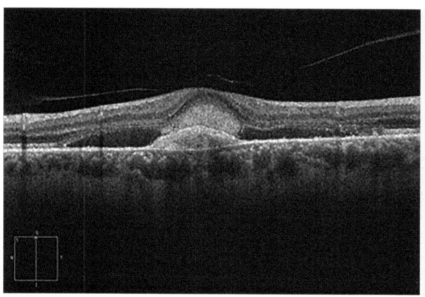

Fig. 1.5 Choroidal neovascular membrane (CNVM). Optical coherence tomography demonstrating CNVM. Note the subretinal pigment epithelium (sub-RPE) hyperreflective material (CNVM) with overlying subretinal fluid and subretinal hyperreflective material. Increased reflectivity is also noted in the outer retina.

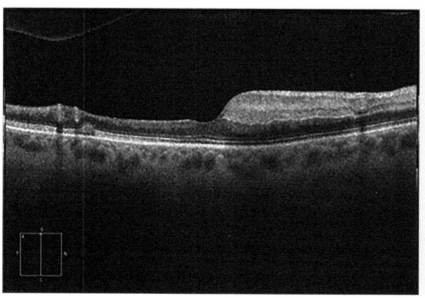

Fig. 1.6 Branch retinal artery occlusion (BRAO). Optical coherence tomography demonstrating chronic inferior BRAO with associated inner retinal atrophy. Superiorly, there is inner retinal hyperreflectivity, consistent with an acute ischemic process, likely representing a BRAO.

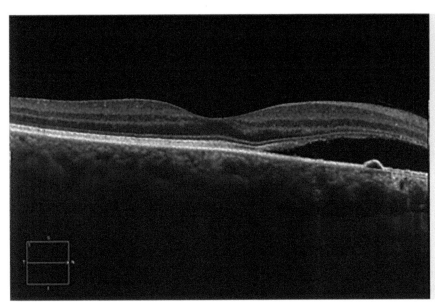

Fig. 1.7 Central serous chorioretinopathy (CSR). Enhanced-depth imaging optical coherence tomography demonstrating CSR. Note the thickened choroid, subretinal fluid, and pigment epithelial detachment.

1.2.3 Choroidal Visualization

Central Serous Chorioretinopathy

OCT, in particular enhanced-depth imaging OCT (EDI-OCT) or swept source OCT, can be used to characterize diseases that affect the choroid. EDI-OCT is a technique that focuses on the illumination at the choroid or inner sclera, producing a clearer image of the choroid. For example, EDI-OCT has shown significantly thickened choroid in CSR. Other OCT findings of CSR include serous retinal detachment and serous retinal pigment epithelial detachment (▶ Fig. 1.7).

Choroidal Tumors

EDI-OCT has also been used to characterize choroidal tumors, including choroidal nevus, melanoma, metastases, hemangioma, and lymphoma. In addition, swept source OCT provides better penetration into the choroid for enhanced visualization of choroidal anatomy and lesions (▶ Fig. 1.2).

Suggested Reading

[1] Adhi M, Duker JS. Optical coherence tomography—current and future applications. Curr Opin Ophthalmol. 2013; 24(3):213–221

[2] Kashani AH, Chen CL, Gahm JK, et al. Optical coherence tomography angiography: a comprehensive review of current methods and clinical applications. Prog Retin Eye Res. 2017; 60:66–100

2 Fluorescein Angiography

Jeremy A. Lavine and Justis P. Ehlers

Summary

Fluorescein angiography (FA) is a diagnostic test that utilizes fluorescein dye to image the retinal vasculature. Briefly, fluorescein is injected intravenously. Using blue and green filters, blue light excites fluorescein and green light is subsequently emitted and detected. Fluorescein is a small molecule and stays in the retinal arterioles and does not cross the retinal pigment epithelium if the blood–retinal barriers are intact. Images are acquired as the fluorescein dye flows through the eye to detect abnormalities in the choroidal circulation, retinal arteries, and retinal veins. Typical patterns of fluorescence include hypofluorescence from blockage and vascular filling defects, and hyperfluorescence caused by autofluorescence, staining, window defects, pooling, and leakage. Key applications of FA include the differentiation of macular edema etiology and diagnosis of retinal vascular disease. In addition, FA is helpful in the identification of choroidal neovascularization and the staging of diabetic retinopathy.

Keywords: blockage, fluorescein angiography, leakage, pooling, staining, vascular filling defects, window defects

2.1 Diagnostic/Technology Overview

Sodium fluorescein is an orange–red hydrocarbon molecule that circulates in the vasculature, 80% protein bound and 20% nonprotein bound. Nonprotein bound fluorescein will diffuse through fenestrated and leaky capillaries but will not move through the retinal pigment epithelium (RPE) or normal retinal capillaries. Nonprotein bound fluorescein will absorb and become excited by blue light (wavelength: 465–490 nm), causing fluorescent emission of green light (wavelength: 520–530 nm).

To perform fluorescein angiography (FA), white light passes through a blue filter, transmitting blue light to the retina (▶ Fig. 2.1). Fluorescein in the retina tissues and vasculature is excited by the blue light and emits green light. The green light is then detected by fundus photography using a green filter in a standard 30-degree (▶ Fig. 2.2), widefield 50-degree, or ultra-widefield camera (e.g., 200 degrees; ▶ Fig. 2.3).

Images are taken at multiple time points to assess retinal vascular dynamics. After the fluorescein dye is pushed through the intravenous catheter, images are taken in the pre-arterial phase before dye enters the retinal circulation, which occurs after 8 to 12 seconds. These images assess the lobular, patchy filling of the choroid. Next, arterial-phase imaging is performed (12–18 seconds) to evaluate the retinal arteriolar filling. Subsequently, images are obtained during the venous transit phase (15–25 seconds), including laminar venous filling (15–20 seconds) and complete venous filling (20–25 seconds). Finally, images are taken during the late or recirculation phase (5–10 minutes).

Fluorescein staining patterns include hypofluorescence and hyperfluorescence. Hypofluorescence is caused by either blockage or vascular filling defects. Blockage can occur from pigment hypertrophy (▶ Fig. 2.4) or hemorrhage (▶ Fig. 2.3). Vascular

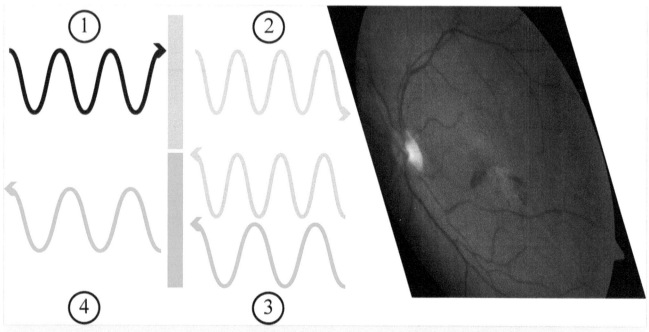

Fig. 2.1 Diagnostic overview of fluorescein angiography. (1) White unfiltered light passes through a blue filter, producing blue light (2) that will excite fluorescein in the retinal vasculature. (3) Blue light is reflected from the retina and green light is emitted from the excited fluorescein. After passing through a green filter, green light is transmitted (4) and detected by film or digital photography.

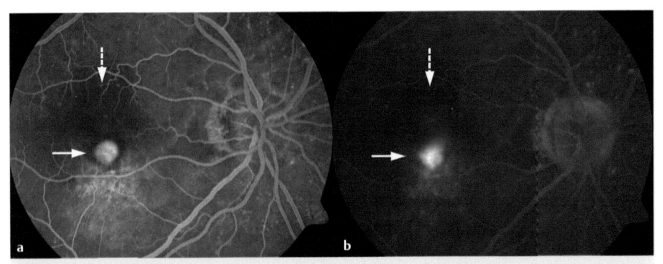

Fig. 2.2 Fluorescein angiography of neovascular age-related macular degeneration. **(a)** Venous phase angiogram showing numerous hyperfluorescent spots (*arrow*) and a larger hyperfluorescent lesion (*dashed arrow*). **(b)** Late phase angiogram showing hyperfluorescent spots without expanding borders (*arrow*), which correspond to staining of drusen. Additionally, the larger hyperfluorescent lesion (*dashed arrow*) now demonstrates expanding borders without discrete edges, demonstrating leakage from a choroidal neovascular membrane.

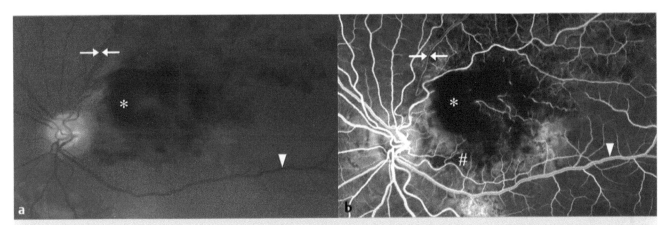

Fig. 2.3 Fluorescein angiography of a branch retinal vein occlusion (RVO). **(a)** Fundus photograph demonstrating retinal macular hemorrhage (*asterisk*), a dilated superior temporal retinal vein (between *arrows*), and a comparatively normal retinal vein (*arrowhead*). **(b)** Venous phase angiogram demonstrating complete venous filling in the normal retinal vein (*arrowhead*) compared to laminar venous filling in the superior temporal retinal vein (between *arrows*), demonstrating branch RVO. The macular hemorrhage shows blockage of retinal vasculature (*asterisk*) and blockage of underlying choroidal vasculature (*hashtag*), suggesting hemorrhage in multiple retinal layers.

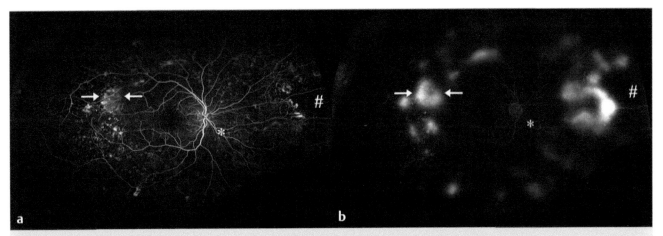

Fig. 2.4 Ultra-widefield fluorescein angiography of proliferative diabetic retinopathy. **(a)** Venous phase and **(b)** late phase angiogram demonstrating multiple areas of early hyperfluorescence from retinal neovascularization elsewhere with extensive late leakage (between *arrows*). Vascular filling defects from capillary nonperfusion (*hashtag*) are evident in both the venous and late phase angiograms. Additionally, there are numerous areas of alternating hypofluorescence, both venous and late phase, and hyperfluorescence with sharp borders that decrease in intensity in the late phase of the angiogram (*asterisk*). These areas are caused by pan-retinal photocoagulation scars, which display pigment hypertrophy causing blockage and window defects causing hyperfluorescence with discrete borders and fading intensity throughout the angiogram.

filling defects develop from large artery occlusions, including the ophthalmic artery, the central retinal artery, and the retinal arterioles. Vascular filling defects can also occur from capillary nonperfusion, as this occurs during the diabetic retinopathy (▶ Fig. 2.4). Hyperfluorescence occurs from autofluorescence, staining, window defects, pooling, and leakage. Staining is defined as hyperfluorescence that increases in intensity through the angiogram but maintains sharp borders (i.e., macular drusen; ▶ Fig. 2.2). Window defects occur from unmasking of the choroidal vasculature due to a defect in the RPE and demonstrate early hyperfluorescence that decreases in intensity throughout the angiogram (i.e., panretinal photocoagulation scars; ▶ Fig. 2.4). Pooling is when dye leaks into a defined space and maintains sharp borders in the late phase of the angiogram (i.e., retinal pigment epithelial detachment in central serous retinopathy). Leakage is defined as hyperfluorescence that grows in intensity with poorly defined borders. Examples of leakage include choroidal neovascularization (▶ Fig. 2.2) and retinal neovascularization (▶ Fig. 2.4).

2.2 Key Applications

2.2.1 Macular Disease

Age-Related Macular Degeneration

FA is most often used to discriminate between nonneovascular and neovascular macular degeneration, as well as to identify masquerade syndromes. Key findings include staining of drusen (▶ Fig. 2.2), leakage from choroidal neovascular membranes (▶ Fig. 2.2), blockage from hemorrhage, pooling into retinal pigment epithelial detachments, staining of disciform scars, and window defects from geographic atrophy.

Cystoid Macular Edema

FA assists in determining the cause of macular edema. Typical causes include age-related macular degeneration, retinal vein occlusion (RVO), diabetic retinopathy, and inflammatory cystoid macular edema. Irvine–Gass syndrome (pseudophakic cystoid

macular edema) and other inflammatory causes will typically show hyperfluorescence of the optic nerve with petaloid staining of the cystoid spaces in the outer plexiform layer around the fovea.

Central Serous Retinopathy

In central serous retinopathy, key findings include pinpoint areas of leakage, smokestack pattern leakage, stippled hyperfluorescence, and pooling into the subretinal pigment epithelial space.

2.2.2 Vascular Disease

Diabetic Retinopathy

FA can identify diabetes as the cause of macular edema, and differentiate between non-proliferative and early proliferative diabetic retinopathy. In non-proliferative disease, leakage from microaneurysms and blockage from hemorrhage are detected. In proliferative disease, neovascularization of the disc will be seen (▶ Fig. 2.4).

Retinal Vein Occlusion

Typical findings include delayed venous filling (▶ Fig. 2.3) with normal arterial filling, leakage into the macula, vascular filling defects from capillary nonperfusion, and blockage from hemorrhage (▶ Fig. 2.3).

Retinal Artery Occlusion

Typical findings include delayed filling of the central retinal artery or branch retinal arteriole with downstream vascular filling defects.

Suggested Reading

[1] Schachat AP, Ryan SJ, eds. Retina 4th Edition: Medical Retina, Vol. II. Philadelphia, PA: Elsevier; 2006

3 Indocyanine Green Angiography

Daniel R. Agarwal and Sumit Sharma

Summary

Indocyanine green angiography (ICG) is a vital tool in the comprehensive evaluation of chorioretinal diseases, aiding in the diagnosis and management of multiple potentially blinding conditions. Its ability to be performed in the setting of hemorrhage, cataract, pigment, and hazy vitreous media permits evaluation in challenging situations. Diseases such as central serous chorioretinopathy and polypoidal choroidal vasculopathy may be better delineated and monitored on ICG than fluorescein angiography (FA). ICG for uveitic diseases, including birdshot chorioretinopathy and serpiginous chorioretinopathy, can reveal lesions not well visualized on exam or FA. Choroidal hemangiomas will demonstrate intense hypercyanescence on ICG that can help distinguish them from other lesions. ICG is a specialized but useful test for evaluating complex choroidal disease processes.

Keywords: birdshot, central serous chorioretinopathy, hemangioma, indocyanine green angiography, uveitis

3.1 Diagnostic/Technology Overview

Indocyanine green (ICG) is a dye used for visualizing the choroidal circulation. During testing, 25 mg of ICG dye in 5 mL of water is injected intravenously with photographs taken starting shortly after injection, and late photographs taken 10 to 40 minutes after injection. An excitation filter (640–780 nm) should be used, along with a barrier filter (820–900 nm). Due to the transmission peak being near the infrared range, ICG angiography (ICGA, commonly referred to as simply ICG) has better penetration through hemorrhage, nuclear sclerotic cataracts, retinal pigment epithelium, cloudy vitreous fluid, and choroidal melanin pigment than fluorescein angiography (FA; ► Fig. 3.1). ICG dye is cleared quickly from the bloodstream, with only 4% remaining in plasma 20 minutes after injection. It is then excreted via the hepatic system.

Adverse reactions to ICG are uncommon. Nausea, vomiting, and itching occur in 0.2% of the patients. Rarely, ICG can result in severe reactions such as urticaria and syncope in 0.2% of the patients and anaphylaxis in 0.05% of the patients. Seafood allergies and liver disease are contraindications to ICG administration. In addition, dialysis patients have an increased risk of ICG-related complications.

3.2 Key Applications

3.2.1 Central Serous Chorioretinopathy

Central serous chorioretinopathy (CSR) will demonstrate areas of choroidal hyperpermeability that are more prominent in middle and late phases of the study (► Fig. 3.2). Dilated choroidal vessels with choroidal leakage can also be seen. These regions of choroidal hyperpermeability can remain in chronic and severe CSR cases. Occult serous pigment epithelial detachments, delays in choroidal arterial filling, and venous congestion may also be visible. Of note, ICG is useful in distinguishing CSR from occult choroidal neovascularization (CNV) in macular degeneration as well as polypoidal choroidal vasculopathy (PCV).

3.2.2 Polypoidal Choroidal Vasculopathy

PCV is characterized by an abnormal choroidal vascular network ending in an outpouching in the choroidal circulation that may be visible as a spherical polyp configuration. PCV can cause multiple serous and retinal pigment epithelial detachments from leakage of these vascular abnormalities. ICG can be used to identify the polyps seen in PCV, allowing for the potential of therapeutic treatments. Polyps often begin to appear approximately 6 minutes after injection of ICG. Choroidal vessels can be seen in a branching pattern with nodules that can correspond to orange subretinal nodules on exam. Early phase ICG will show a network of vessels with a hypercyanescent nodule that will gradually expand and leak slowly (► Fig. 3.3). Late phase ICG can reveal hypocyanescence of the lesion core with surrounding ring-shaped staining of the polyps. A pulsatile nodule on dynamic ICG is distinct to PCV.

3.2.3 Choroidal Neovascular Membrane

ICG can be useful in identifying CNV under unusual circumstances. In age-related macular degeneration, ICG can be used to identify recurrent or occult CNV lesions. It is especially helpful to find CNV lesions obscured by blood and when looking for feeder vessels to CNV lesions. In retinal angiomatous proliferation (RAP) type 3 CNV, ICG can more clearly highlight the vascular structure of the RAP lesion, aiding in earlier diagnosis. RAP lesions show dye filling a retinal arteriole as it travels into the deep retinal space to a vascular communication with the choroidal vasculature. This lesion filling can be better seen on dynamic ICG, further aiding diagnosis and treatment.

3.2.4 Uveitis/Vasculitis

Several features of posterior uveitis can be visualized using ICG imaging. Most commonly, choroidal inflammation on ICG will manifest as hypocyanescent spots appearing as dark dots. Hypercyanescence caused by leakage can be seen in various conditions such as Vogt–Koyanagi–Harada (VKH) disease, birdshot chorioretinopathy, toxoplasmosis, sarcoidosis, and Behçet disease. ICG can be especially useful in birdshot chorioretinopathy, as it can detect disease lesions, seen as round–oval, hypocyanescent lesions, better than FA (► Fig. 3.4). Serpiginous choroiditis on ICG shows blockage of fluorescence during active lesions with hypercyanescence along the lesion edge in the late phase of imaging. These lesions are larger than seen on exam or

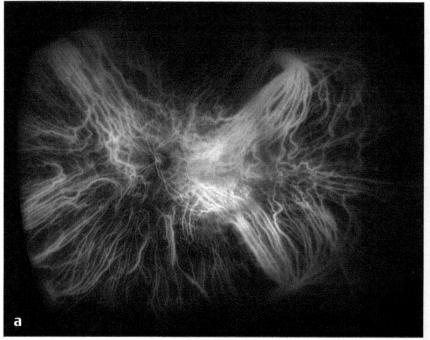

Fig. 3.1 (a) Normal ultra-widefield indocyanine green at approximately 30 seconds. (b) Normal ultra-widefield ICG at 7 minutes.

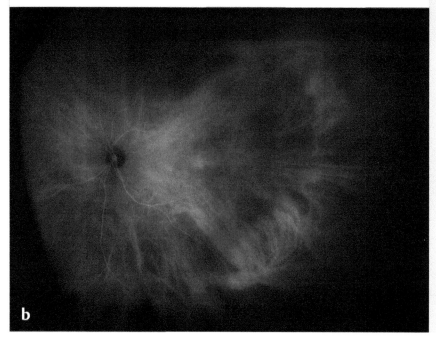

Fig. 3.2 Ultra-widefield indocyanine green in central serous retinopathy with multiple areas of hypercyanescence in the macula and near periphery with increased choroidal hyperpermeability. This image was taken at 5 minutes.

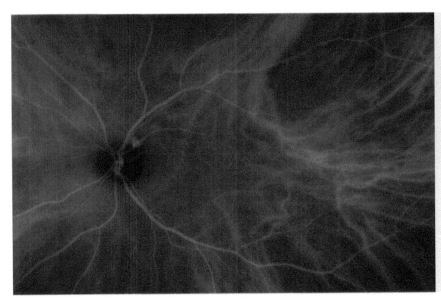

Fig. 3.3 Indocyanine green in polypoidal choroidal vasculopathy near the superotemporal margin of the optic disc with a polyp shaped area of hypercyanescence. This corresponded to an area of hyperfluorescence on fluorescein angiography. This image was taken at 5 minutes.

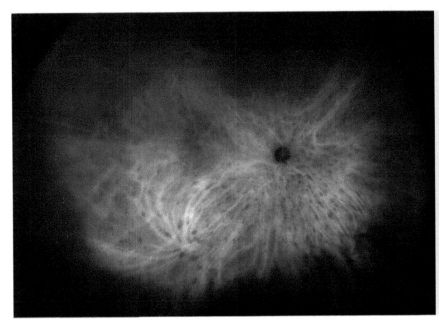

Fig. 3.4 Birdshot chorioretinopathy with numerous areas of hypocyanescence throughout the fundus. This image was taken approximately 12 minutes.

FA. Patients with acute posterior multifocal placoid pigment epitheliopathy will show marked choroidal hypocyanescence corresponding to the fundus placoid lesions throughout the ICG test into the late phase of the study (▶ Fig. 3.5). Multifocal choroiditis will show large hypocyanescence spots more numerous than seen on exam or FA. Presumed ocular histoplasmosis syndrome on ICG will demonstrate discrete spots that are hypercyanescent in early and hypocyanescent in intermediate and late phases of the study. Patients with multiple evanescent white dot syndrome are found to have multiple well-defined hypocyanescent spots in intermediate and late phases of the study, more numerous than seen on FA. VKH syndrome patients present on ICG with hypocyanescent spots spread throughout the fundus in the early stage of imaging. As the study progresses, pinpoint areas of hypercyanescence can be seen with leakage in later stages. Sarcoidosis can often have choroidal

granulomas that will present as areas of hypocyanescence on ICG imaging.

3.2.5 Choroidal Tumors

In choroidal hemangioma, ICG can be used to identify feeder vessels to the lesion as well as the vascular pattern of the tumor. Within 1 minute, choroidal hemangiomas show intense hypercyanescence with washout of the dye in later phases of the study (▶ Fig. 3.6). ICG may also demonstrate rapid dye clearance during the test along with choroidal ischemia away from the mass. Choroidal osteomas will show early hypocyanescence, followed by either late hypocyanescence if choriocapillaris loss is present or hypercyanescence if there is a CNV lesion. ICG is not commonly used to identify choroidal melanomas but can show abnormal vascular patterns and late leakage.

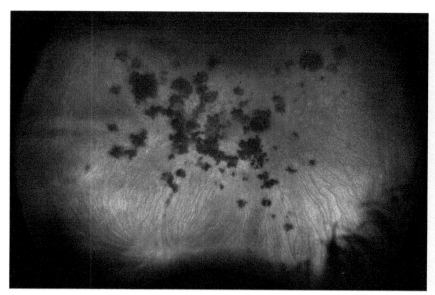

Fig. 3.5 Acute posterior multifocal placoid pigment epitheliopathy with hypocyanescent lesions diffusely in the macula and periphery visible approximately 11 minutes into the study.

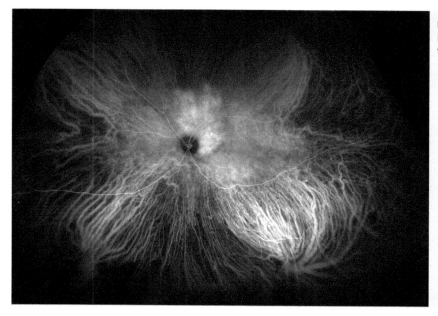

Fig. 3.6 Choroidal hemangioma with intense hypercyanescence early in the study superior to the optic disc. This image was taken at 1 minute.

Suggested Reading

[1] Staurenghi G, Bottoni F, Giani A. Clinical applications of diagnostic indocyanine green angiography. In: Schachat AP, Sadda SR, Hinton DR, Wilkinson CP, Wiedemann P, eds. Ryan's Retina. 6th ed. Philadelphia, PA: Elsevier; 2018:46–76

[2] Stanga PE, Lim JI, Hamilton P. Indocyanine green angiography in chorioretinal diseases: indications and interpretation: an evidence-based update. Ophthalmology. 2003; 110(1):15–21, quiz 22–23

[3] Agrawal RV, Biswas J, Gunasekaran D. Indocyanine green angiography in posterior uveitis. Indian J Ophthalmol. 2013; 61(4):148–159

[4] Koh AHC, Chen L-J, Chen S-J, et al. Expert PCV Panel. Polypoidal choroidal vasculopathy: evidence-based guidelines for clinical diagnosis and treatment. Retina. 2013; 33(4):686–716

4 Optical Coherence Tomography Angiography

Malvika Arya and Nadia K. Waheed

Summary

Optical coherence tomography angiography (OCTA) is a noninvasive imaging technique that provides depth-resolved images of retinal and choroidal vasculature. Angiographic data is coregistered with simultaneously acquired structural OCT data, creating a volumetric cube that can be scrolled through or segmented into layers. Despite its limitations, such as a small field of view and image susceptibility to degradation by artifacts, OCTA has potential utility in the diagnosis and management of several retinal vascular pathologies. This chapter briefly describes the clinical application of OCTA in diabetic retinopathy, choroidal neovascularization, macular telangiectasia, and retinal vein occlusion. Future improvements allowing for faster scan times, improved image resolution, artifact resolution, and imaging of a wider retinal field of view will allow OCTA to further revolutionize our understanding of retinal disease.

Keywords: age-related macular degeneration, choroidal neovascularization, diabetic retinopathy, angiography, macular telangiectasia, optical coherence tomography angiography, retinal vein occlusion, spectral-domain optical coherence tomography angiography, swept source optical coherence tomography

4.1 Diagnostic/Technology Overview

Optical coherence tomography angiography (OCTA) has recently emerged as a noninvasive technique for imaging the vasculature of the eye. OCTA relies on the rapid acquisition of multiple OCT scans at the same location on the retina. Because all of the structures in the back of the eye, except for the blood flowing through the vessels, are static, the only feature changing between the sequential scans would be blood flow. Utilizing unique computer algorithms to look for the difference between sequential, rapidly acquired B-scans (a process called decorrelation) results in a retinal vasculature map. Because the retina is transparent and OCT is a 3D imaging modality, point by point decorrelation can be applied in three dimensions, generating a depth-resolved map of the retinal vasculature. Depending on the penetration of the OCT beam past the retinal pigment epithelium, a map of the choriocapillaris may also be generated.

Two technologic advancements have been critical to the evolution of OCTA. The first is high scanning speeds to minimize interscan movement to enable decorrelation. The second is a resolution high enough to be able to visualize motion within the smaller blood vessels. Both of these conditions were met with the advent of spectral domain OCT (SD-OCT) machines and are also present in the next generation of swept source OCT (SS-OCT).

Moreover, since the angiographic data are acquired by decorrelation of structural OCT data, the OCTA comes coregistered with the structural OCT data. This allows for the overlay of the angiographic data with the simultaneously acquired structural OCT data, creating a volumetric cube that can be scrolled through or segmented into layers by automated or manual segmentation algorithms. Angiographic data is generated by analyzing changes in amplitude and/or phase of vascular flow, created by the movement of erythrocytes, which produce a decorrelation signal between consecutive scans. Numerous different algorithms can be used to do this: amplitude decorrelation, such as in the Split-Spectrum Amplitude-Decorrelation Angiography, or a combination of amplitude and phase based algorithms, such as OCT-based microangiography, which are used in commercially available OCTA devices.

There are two major ways of analyzing OCTA data. Volumetric data consisting of structural and angiographic images can be scrolled through to assess pathological changes at various retinal layers. While this method highlights pathology at various levels, it is often more time consuming and difficult to analyze. The other approach is segmentation of an area of interest to generate an en face image. Various automated algorithms have been employed to create segmentation slabs. However, accurate segmentation is always a challenge, especially in eyes with pathology where boundaries between layers may be difficult to delineate. Manual segmentation, although more time consuming, allows for changes in the slab thickness and repositioning of the segmentation lines for more accurate visualization and analysis of pathological lesions. Currently, most OCTA machines will present segmented data in two ways: an en face angiographic image that delineates the lesion, and a structural B-scan with flow overlay that allows for structure–vasculature association (▶ Fig. 4.1).

4.1.1 Artifacts

A major challenge of OCTA is its susceptibility to degradation by artifacts, predominantly projection and motion artifacts. Projection artifacts are created by the scattering of light by overlying blood vessels and subsequent reflection by the underlying layers, especially the highly reflective retinal pigment epithelium (RPE). This allows for the more superficial vessels to also be visualized in the deeper layers, hindering accurate analysis of the deeper layers. Projection artifact correction algorithms have been employed in commercial device software. While they do not completely remove projection artifacts, they are being improved upon.

Microsaccades, as well as patient and eye movement, may occur during image acquisition. These extraneous movements create motion artifacts that appear as white lines on an OCTA image. Nonvascular movement of reflective structures then generates a false decorrelation signal and gives the appearance of blood flow. Most devices employ some form of motion correction (software-based and/or eye-tracking-based). Motion-tracking software has significantly enhanced the quality of OCTA images but also increases scan time in patients with poor fixation.

Currently available OCTA scans have a field of view that is limited because of constraints on acquisition time; the eye can only hold still for so long. Thus, an increase in scanning area is

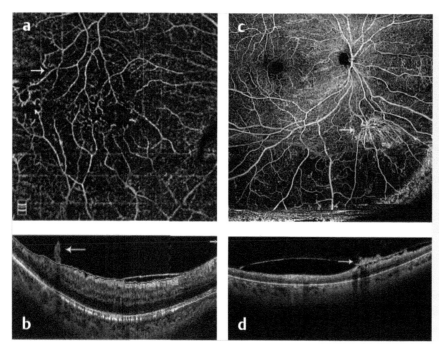

Fig. 4.1 **(a)** A 3 × 3 mm spectral domain optical coherence tomography angiography (SD-OCTA) scan centered at the fovea showing areas of nonperfusion, pruning of vessels (*arrow*), microaneurysms, and retinal neovascularization. **(b)** Extraretinal extension of the membrane on the corresponding coregistered B-scan (*arrow*) confirmed proliferative diabetic retinopathy. Note the presence of motion artifact in the lower portion of the en face image. **(c)** A swept source OCTA 12 × 12 mm scan centered at the parafoveal right lower quadrant showing areas of nonperfusion and retinal neovascularization. **(d)** The corresponding coregistered B-scan confirms proliferative diabetic retinopathy (*arrow*). Motion artifacts, while present in both, are more discernable in the SD-OCTA image.

likely to increase imaging time and compromise resolution. Since the principle application of OCTA is currently in macular and parafoveal pathologies, the 3 × 3 mm scan pattern helps visualize these areas with high resolution. However, 6 × 6 scans are also available on most SD-OCTA machines, and with higher speed SS-OCTA instruments larger scans can be visualized in a single acquisition.

4.2 Key Applications

Dye-based imaging modalities, such as fluorescein angiography (FA) and indocyanine green angiography (ICGA), have been the gold standard for the diagnosis of retinal and choroidal vascular pathologies. FA and ICGA offer certain advantages over OCTA, such as the ability to image a wider field, visualization of vessel leakage, and improved detection of aneurysms with slow flow. However, they also have disadvantages, including their invasive nature, which precludes frequent acquisition to follow pathology, and the fact that the angiographic scan does not come correlated to any structural scans, and therefore only approximate visual registration can be performed to compare structure (as seen on color photographs and OCT) to vasculature (as seen on the angiogram). Moreover, FA better visualizes larger and more superficial vessels. It has been shown not to visualize in any great detail the intermediate and deep capillary plexus of the retina. OCTA, on the other hand, is noninvasive, has minimal to no risk of complications, a shorter image acquisition time, and is independent of the circulation of dye. The 3D nature of the scan allows for independent visualization of the deeper retinal vasculature and the choriocapillaris. The resolution of vasculature seen on OCTA has been shown nearing the level of histological studies. Due to its noninvasive nature, discernible microvascular changes of the retina can be followed longitudinally by OCTA as often as clinically mandated.

4.2.1 Diabetic Retinopathy

OCTA is useful in identifying the characteristic lesions of diabetic retinopathy (e.g., capillary nonperfusion, retinal ischemia, neovascularization, and microaneurysms) and can be used to follow them longitudinally (▶ Fig. 4.2). Microvascular flow alterations such as capillary pruning, intraretinal microvascular abnormalities, and venous beading and looping may be detected at earlier stages with OCTA as compared to conventional clinical examination (▶ Fig. 4.1). Quantitative vessel density measurements may improve the staging of diabetic retinopathy.

4.2.2 Choroidal Neovascularization

The advent of OCTA has markedly facilitated the early recognition of choroidal neovascularization (CNV) in age-related macular degeneration (AMD). CNV can be identified, classified, and measured over time (▶ Fig. 4.3). OCTA has been shown to be able to detect CNV in patients with phenotypic dry AMD and has been linked to conversion risk for exudative AMD. From a research perspective, OCTA in AMD has shown a generalized decrease in choriocapillaris density with focal areas of nonperfusion and the upward displacement of larger choroidal vessels. These choroidal microvascular abnormalities have been shown to be proportional to drusen density.

4.2.3 Geographic Atrophy

OCTA has identified structural and flow abnormalities associated with geographic atrophy (GA). SS-OCTA imaging with variable interscan time analysis has demonstrated that choriocapillaris changes associated with GA demonstrate slow flow rather than complete attenuation. These alterations in

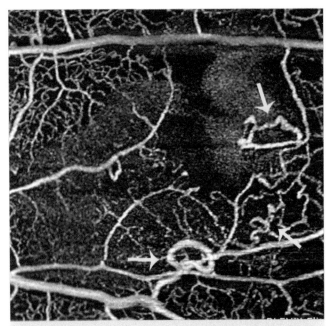

Fig. 4.2 Swept source optical coherence tomography angiography 3 × 3 mm scan of an eye with severe nonproliferative diabetic retinopathy. Visible are prominent venous looping (*arrow*), venous beading (*arrow*), and areas of capillary nonperfusion.

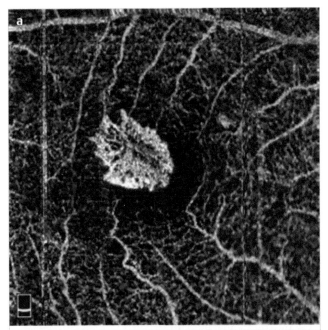

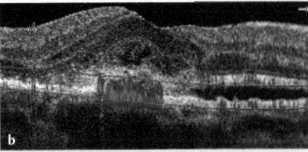

Fig. 4.3 (a) Spectral domain optical coherence tomography angiography 3 × 3 mm scan centered at the fovea of an eye with wet age-related macular degeneration depicting a choroidal neovascularization lesion. (b) The corresponding coregistered B-scan shows abnormal flow in the outer retina and choroid layers.

choroidal flow precede the development of GA and RPE atrophy and may extend beyond the boundaries of GA (▶ Fig. 4.4).

4.2.4 Macular Telangiectasias

OCTA can be useful for evaluation and follow up of the telangiectatic lesions and especially for the evaluation of neovascularization in the lesion. Initial telangiectatic vascular changes appear in the deep capillary plexus and extend to the superficial capillary plexus (▶ Fig. 4.5).

4.2.5 Venous Occlusions

OCTA demonstrated predominance of nonperfusion in the deep retinal capillary plexus and a decline in retinal vessel density with increasing severity of venous occlusion (▶ Fig. 4.6). Additionally, the foveal avascular zone increases in both central and branch retinal vein occlusions.

4.3 Future Developments

OCTA has advanced our understanding of various retinal vascular pathologies. Continuing improvements in hardware and software of OCTA will likely facilitate faster scan times, improved image resolution, improved choroidal imaging,

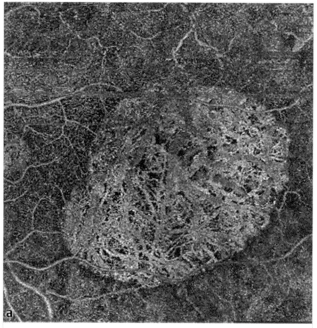

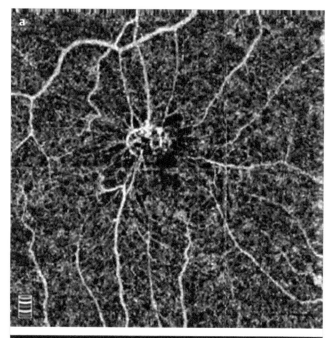

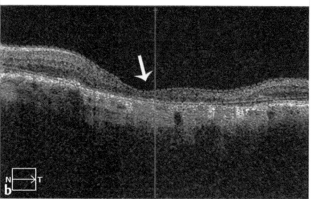

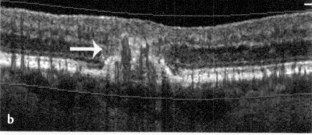

Fig. 4.5 (a) Spectral domain optical coherence tomography angiography 3 × 3 mm scan centered at the fovea from an eye with juxtafoveal telangiectasia. (b) Type 3 choroidal neovascularization (*arrow*) is evident on the corresponding B-scan through the lesion.

Fig. 4.4 (a) Spectral domain optical coherence tomography angiography (SD-OCTA) 6 × 6 mm scan centered at the fovea of an eye with geographic atrophy. Loss of architecture of a lobular region of the choriocapillaris and the inward displacement of larger choroidal vessels can be seen with preserved flow signal on the en face OCTA image. (b) The corresponding B-scan through the lesion demonstrates retinal thinning due to atrophy of the retinal pigment epithelium and outer retina (*arrow*).

resolution of artifacts, more accurate automated segmentation, and wider fields of view. Improved acquisition speeds offered by SS-OCTA may enable quantification of retinal and choroidal blood flow in the future.

Suggested Reading

[1] de Carlo TE, Romano A, Waheed NK, Duker JS. A review of optical coherence tomography angiography (OCTA). Int J Retina Vitreous. 2015; 1:5

[2] Spaide RF, Fujimoto JG, Waheed NK. Image artifacts in optical coherence tomography angiography. Retina. 2015; 35(11):2163–2180

[3] Louzada RN, de Carlo TE, Adhi M, et al. Optical coherence tomography angiography artifacts in retinal pigment epithelial detachment. Can J Ophthalmol. 2017; 52(4):419–424

[4] Zhang A, Zhang Q, Wang RK. Minimizing projection artifacts for accurate presentation of choroidal neovascularization in OCT micro-angiography. Biomed Opt Express. 2015; 6(10):4130–4143

[5] Kashani AH, Chen CL, Gahm JK, et al. Optical coherence tomography angiography: A comprehensive review of current methods and clinical applications. Prog Retin Eye Res. 2017; 60:66–100

[6] Ploner SB, Moult EM, Waheed NK, et al. Toward quantitative OCT angiography: visualizing flow impairment using variable interscan time analysis (VISTA). Seattle, WA: ARVO; 2016

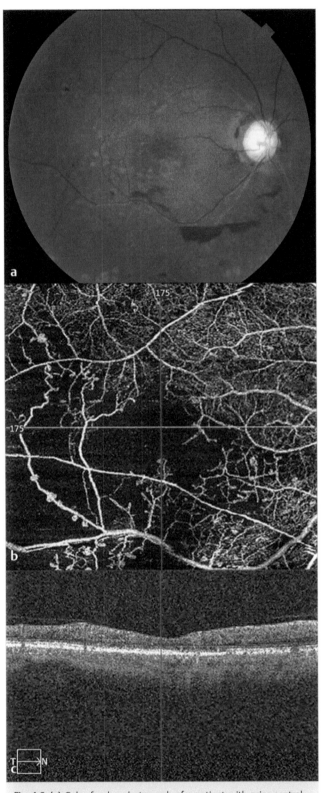

Fig. 4.6 **(a)** Color fundus photograph of a patient with prior central retinal vein occlusion. Characteristic features of sheathing of vessels, pre-retinal hemorrhages, and scattered laser scars are visible. **(b)** A 6 × 6 mm spectral domain optical coherence tomography angiography scan centered at the fovea obtained of the same eye showed decreased vascular flow, enlargement and disruption of the foveal avascular zone, venous tortuosity, and the formation of microaneurysms. **(c)** Corresponding B-scan with decorrelation overlay demonstrating reduction in flow.

5 Intraoperative Optical Coherence Tomography

Atsuro Uchida and Justis P. Ehlers

Summary

Intraoperative optical coherence tomography (OCT) allows the surgeon to view the surgical field from a different perspective using a standard ophthalmic microscope. Intraoperative OCT enables evaluation of vitreoretinal tissue microstructures and alterations that occur during a surgery. Utilization of this imaging modality significantly impacts clinical decision-making, may enhance surgical efficiency, and may reduce intraoperative complications. The current microscope-integrated OCT systems allow visualization of tissue–instrument interactions during surgical manipulation with real-time surgeon feedback. Applications for intraoperative OCT include membrane peeling procedures, repair of vitreoretinal interface abnormalities, retinal detachment repair, delivery of subretinal therapeutics, retinal prosthesis implant, and chorioretinal biopsy. Introduction of immersive 3D digital visualization system, faster OCT acquisition speed with improved image quality, automated tracking, integration of advanced ophthalmic diagnostics, and automated software analysis may further enhance surgeon feedback in the future generation of OCT-guided vitreoretinal surgery.

Keywords: intraoperative OCT, optical coherence tomography (OCT), microscope-integrated, spectral domain, swept source, vitreoretinal surgery

5.1 Diagnostic/Technology Overview

Intraoperative optical coherence tomography (OCT) allows the surgeon to view the surgical field from a different perspective than a standard ophthalmic microscope. Intraoperative OCT offers excellent resolution for vitreoretinal tissue structure and its alterations during vitreoretinal surgery (▶ Fig. 5.1). This added information significantly impacts surgical decision-making, may improve surgical efficiency, and help to reduce complications. Current commercial systems utilize spectral domain OCT technology within approximate wavelength of 840 to 860 nm, maximum axial resolution of 4 mm, and scanning speed up to 32,000-A scans per second. The microscope-integrated intraoperative OCT platform provides unique opportunities to visualize tissue–instrument interactions during vitreoretinal surgery with real-time surgeon feedback. In the commercial models, the OCT scanner is either fully integrated with the microscope (e.g., RESCAN 700; Zeiss), is attached to the microscope utilizing a camera port (e.g., iOCT; Haag-Streit), or is placed between the objective lens and microscope head (e.g., EnFocus system; Leica).

Another intraoperative OCT platform, the handheld or microscope-mounted portable spectral domain OCT (e.g., Envisu;

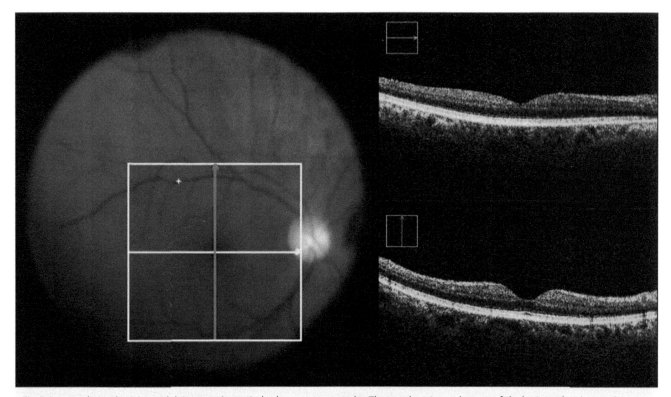

Fig. 5.1 Normal macula image with intraoperative optical coherence tomography. The scan location and extent of the horizontal and vertical B-scans are shown in blue and pink line on the surgical field.

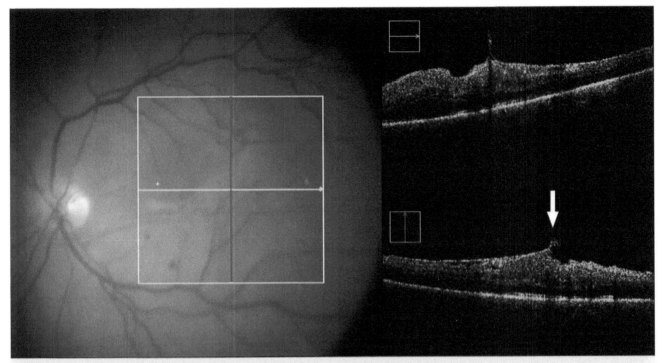

Fig. 5.2 Intraoperative optical coherence tomography of an epiretinal membrane. The extent of membrane peeling is clearly visualized on both horizontal and vertical B-scan, and the edge of the internal limiting membrane is observed (*arrow*).

Leica) allows manual tilting of the OCT scanner head and provides versatile usage in both the operating room and office, but does not have the advantages of a microscope-integrated system.

5.2 Key Applications

5.2.1 Membrane Peeling

Particularly useful during membrane peeling procedures to define the extent of membrane peeling, determine the edge of the membrane, and confirm completion of the membrane peeling (▶ Fig. 5.2).

5.2.2 Interface Abnormalities

Excellent for assessing the vitreoretinal interface abnormalities in various diseases including macular holes, epiretinal membrane, vitreomacular traction syndrome, proliferative diabetic retinopathy, proliferative vitreoretinopathy, myopic traction maculopathy, and pediatric vitreoretinopathies. Intraoperative OCT helps to identify posterior vitreous membrane causing vitreoretinal tractional force, locate residual membranes, understand the structure of fibrous/fibrovascular membrane complex, and verify the attainment of surgical goals (▶ Fig. 5.3).

5.2.3 Macula

Intraoperative assessment of the macula when preoperative fundus examination is not possible, for example, due to vitreous opacity or premacular hemorrhage. One example is an identification of occult full-thickness macular hole following hemorrhage removal, which enables optimal intraoperative management (▶ Fig. 5.4).

5.2.4 Microstructures

Evaluation of tissue microstructure alterations during vitreoretinal surgery, including expansion of ellipsoid zone and retinal pigment epithelium distance, tissue anomalies, and macular hole geometry. Clinical implications of these findings are not fully understood. However, some of the microstructure alterations have been linked to anatomical outcomes and visual prognosis.

5.2.5 Subretinal

Other described uses include identifying the presence and location of subretinal fluid and determining the optimal location for subretinal fluid drainage in retinal detachment repair. The identification of the extent of subretinal fibrosis can also be helpful in determining the necessity and location of retinotomy in complicated retinal detachment repair (▶ Fig. 5.5). Confirmatory imaging during the delivery of subretinal therapeutics (e.g., subretinal injection of virus vector for gene therapy or tissue plasminogen activator), placement of artificial visual prosthesis implant, and transretinal choroidal biopsy may also be an important application of intraoperative OCT.

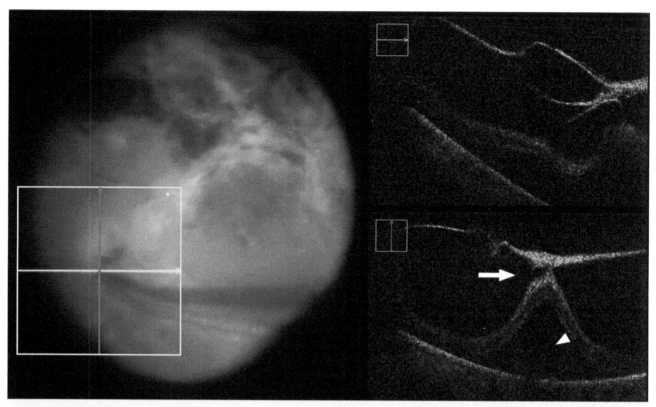

Fig. 5.3 Intraoperative optical coherence tomography of proliferative diabetic retinopathy. Cross-sectional scans visualize the cleavage plane between the fibrovascular tissue and the sensory retina. Vertical B-scan identifies the location of the epicenter (*arrow*) nasal to the optic disc and the presence of subretinal fluid (*arrowhead*).

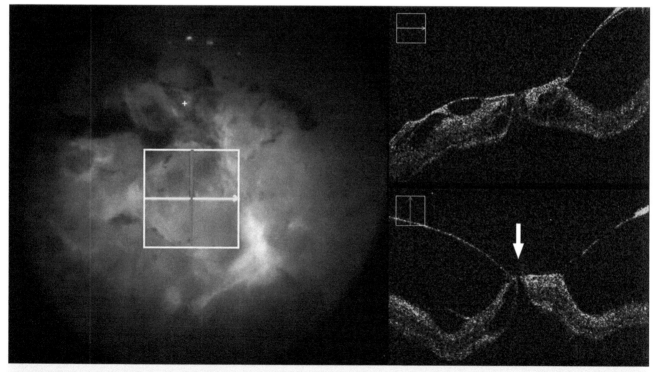

Fig. 5.4 Intraoperative optical coherence tomography of proliferative diabetic retinopathy. The horizontal B-scan of the macula reveals the existence of an occult full-thickness macular hole (*arrow*).

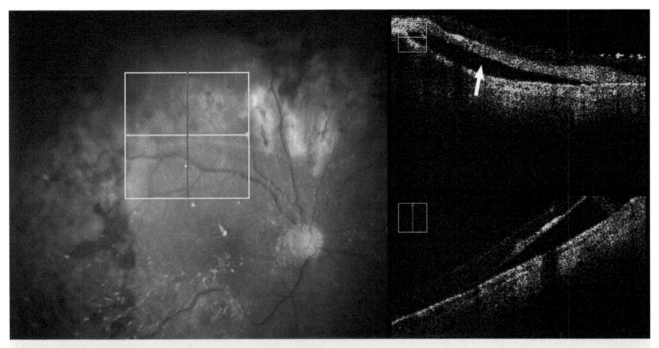

Fig. 5.5 Intraoperative optical coherence tomography of a recurrent retinal detachment. Cross-sectional scans clearly illustrate the presence and extent of thick subretinal fibrosis (*arrow*) preventing reattachment of the retina.

5.3 Future Developments

Prototype nonmetallic OCT compatible instruments with minimal shadowing may allow better visualization of tissue instrument interactions compared with metallic instruments. Research prototype, ultrahigh-speed swept source OCT offers real-time volumetric (3D) view of the surgical field. The integration of immersive 3D digital visualization systems (e.g., Ngenuity; Alcon) and intraoperative OCT may enhance opportunities for OCT-guided vitreoretinal surgery. Moreover, improved image quality, automated tracking, and integration of automated software analysis may further enhance surgeon feedback.

Suggested Reading

[1] Ehlers JP, Goshe J, Dupps WJ, et al. Determination of feasibility and utility of microscope-integrated optical coherence tomography during ophthalmic surgery: the DISCOVER Study RESCAN Results. JAMA Ophthalmol. 2015; 133 (10):1124–1132

[2] Carrasco-Zevallos OM, Keller B, Viehland C, et al. Live volumetric (4D) visualization and guidance of in vivo human ophthalmic surgery with intraoperative optical coherence tomography. Sci Rep. 2016; 6:31689

[3] Gregori NZ, Lam BL, Davis JL. Intraoperative use of microscope-integrated optical coherence tomography for subretinal gene therapy delivery. Retina. 2017

[4] Ehlers JP, Uchida A, Srivastava SK. Intraoperative optical coherence tomography-compatible surgical instruments for real-time image-guided ophthalmic surgery. Br J Ophthalmol. 2017; 101(10):1306–1308

6 Fundus Autofluorescence

SriniVas Sadda and Enrico Borrelli

Summary

Fundus autofluorescence (FAF) is a noninvasive retinal imaging technique which is used in clinical practice to provide a map of lipofuscin concentration. Lipofuscin is indeed the main ocular fluorophore and primarily accumulates in the retinal pigment epithelium. Several commercially available imaging systems are capable of FAF imaging, including flash fundus cameras, confocal scanning laser ophthalmoscopes, and the ultra-widefield imaging devices. Each system offers unique advantages for evaluating various retinal diseases.

The clinical applications of FAF are extensive and continue to increase. FAF is performed to assess age-related macular degeneration, macular dystrophies, retinitis pigmentosa, and various other retinal disorders. FAF may detect changes beyond those detected on funduscopic examination. Furthermore, FAF may be used to investigate disease pathogenesis to find genotype-phenotype correlations and to evaluate the effectiveness of novel therapies. This chapter summarizes common ocular fluorophores, imaging modalities, and FAF findings for a wide spectrum of retinal disorders.

Keywords: fundus autofluorescence, fluorophores, lipofuscin, retinopathy

6.1 Diagnostic/Technology Overview

Fundus autofluorescence (FAF) is a noninvasive imaging modality which is used to record the retinal and retinal pigment epithelial (RPE) autofluorescence (AF). Lipofuscin, which is a mixture of fluorophores, is considered to be the most intense source of AF in the posterior eye. Consequently, FAF is thought to be an effective surrogate for lipofuscin concentration in the RPE.

The RPE, which is composed of a single layer of hexagonal cells, separates the choroid from the neurosensory retina. An essential function of the RPE cells is the phagocytosis and degradation of shed photoreceptor outer segment discs with subsequent release of degraded material at the basal side of the cell. Lipofuscin, which forms in the RPE cells, is composed of several different molecules (the most important is A2E: N-retinyl-N-retinylidene ethanolamine) and derives primarily from phagocytized photoreceptor outer segments. Lipofuscin is not completely recognized by lysosomal enzymes and is thus incompletely removed and accumulates in the lysosomes. Strong evidence suggests that lipofuscin is not an inert by-product but that it may interfere with cell function, as well as may increase in quantity with age as well as in the setting of RPE dysfunction.

AF is the natural emission of light by biological molecules (fluorophores) following absorption of a higher energy shorter wavelength of light. FAF imaging uses the fluorescent properties of lipofuscin to generate a grayscale image, where dark pixel values correspond to relative low intensities of emission and bright pixel values correspond to high intensities of fluorescence emission. Commercially available FAF systems include flash fundus cameras, confocal scanning laser ophthalmoscopes (cSLO), and ultra-widefield imaging devices. Moreover, the AF of the retina and RPE can be excited across a broad range of wavelengths in the blue and green spectrum (blue- and green-light FAF, BAF, and GAF, respectively).

The naturally occurring AF of the ocular fundus is known to be of low intensity and to be characterized by a specific pattern: (i) the optic nerve head typically appears dark due to the absence of lipofuscin in this area; (ii) the areas with retinal vessels are characterized by a reduced FAF signal due to the absorption by blood; and (iii) FAF signal is also reduced in the central macular area, due to the absorption of blue light by the luteal pigment. In contrast to BAF imaging, GAF cSLO imaging is not as significantly affected by macular pigment due to a reduced amount of absorption (▸ Fig. 6.1). Causes for a reduced AF signal may include RPE loss, presence of intraretinal fluid or subretinal fibrosis, reduction in RPE lipofuscin density, or presence of luteal pigment. Causes for an increased AF signal may include loss of luteal or photopigment, increased RPE lipofuscin, or presence of subretinal AF material.

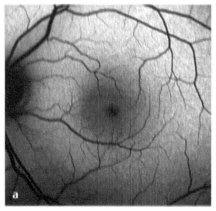
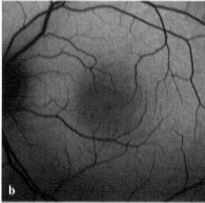

Fig. 6.1 (a) Blue-light fundus autofluorescence (FAF; Spectralis, Heidelberg Engineering, Heidelberg, Germany) from a healthy eye. The optic nerve head, retinal vessels, and macular area typically appear dark in the blue FAF (BAF) image. **(b)** In contrast to BAF imaging, green FAF (GAF) imaging is not significantly affected by macular pigment.

6.2 Key Applications

6.2.1 Age-Related Macular Degeneration

There is strong evidence that RPE cells play an important role in age-related macular degeneration (AMD) pathogenesis. This evidence is also supported by the fact that drusen composition includes incompletely degraded material from autophagy and phagocytosed shed photoreceptor outer segment discs.

Early/Intermediate Age-Related Macular Degeneration

The FAF signal may be normal, decreased, or increased in corresponding drusen areas (▶ Fig. 6.2). This may reflect the variable composition of drusen, including other fluorophores, as well as different reactive alterations in the overlying RPE cell monolayer. In 2005, the International FAF Classification Group defined eight phenotypic FAF patterns associated with early nonneovascular AMD: normal, minimal change, focal increase, patchy, linear, lace-like, reticular, and speckled. Patchy, linear, and reticular patterns are associated with an increased risk for choroidal neovascularization.

Geographic Atrophy

Geographic atrophy (GA) is the hallmark of advanced nonneovascular AMD. GA areas exhibit very low to extinguished AF signal as RPE cell death is accompanied by loss of lipofuscin (▶ Fig. 6.3). This leads to a high contrast between the atrophic and perilesional retina. Furthermore, the contrast is even further increased by perilesional areas that demonstrate hyper-AF. The latter finding is thought to be due to ongoing RPE cell dysfunction, vertically superimposed RPE cells, and variable progression to atrophy. These changes have been shown to have pathogenic relevance: areas of increased AF may be associated with variable degrees of retinal sensitivity loss and precede the development and enlargement of macular atrophy. Phenotypes of perilesional hyper-AF include none, focal, diffuse, banded, patchy, and trickling, with banded, diffuse, and especially trickling associated with more rapid enlargement of atrophy over time.

6.2.2 Pattern Dystrophies

Pattern dystrophies refer to a group of l macular dystrophies, which include adult-onset foveomacular vitelliform dystrophy, butterfly-shaped pigment dystrophy, reticular dystrophy, multifocal pattern dystrophy simulating fundus flavimaculatus, and fundus pulverulentus. Adult-onset foveomacular pigment epithelial dystrophy is characterized by bilateral yellowish (pseudovitelliform) lesions in the macula, which emit a well-circumscribed, homogeneous hyper-AF, while subsequent RPE atrophy results in a decreased AF. Multifocal pattern dystrophy simulating fundus flavimaculatus is characterized by yellow flecks, which are concentrated in the posterior pole and near the vascular arcades. On FAF, these flecks correspond to areas of increased AF. Classic "dot and halo" lesions with central hypo-AF and halo of hyper-AF are visible. The other pattern dystrophies may not show as characteristic FAF findings.

6.2.3 Central Serous Chorioretinopathy

Central serous chorioretinopathy (CSCR, CSC, or CSR) may show hypo-AF due to blockage by subretinal fluid in the acute phase. Furthermore, AF may be increased in active stages due to increased metabolic activity within the RPE. As the disease progresses, a granular hyper-AF may characterize CSCR, with hyper-AF dots that gravitate inferiorly and collect at the borders of the detachment. Over time in areas photoreceptor loss, there can be patches of hyper-AF due to lack of the blocking effect

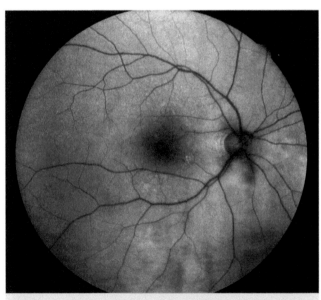

Fig. 6.2 Blue-light fundus autofluorescence (EIDON, Centervue, Padua, Italy) in intermediate age-related macular degeneration. FAF imaging shows several hyper-autofluorescence lesions throughout the macula.

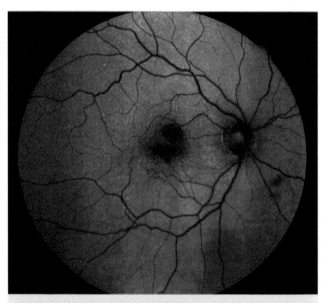

Fig. 6.3 Blue-light fundus autofluorescence (FAF; EIDON, Centervue, Padua, Italy) in geographic atrophy. The area of retinal pigment epithelium loss is characterized by well-demarcated reduced autofluorescence.

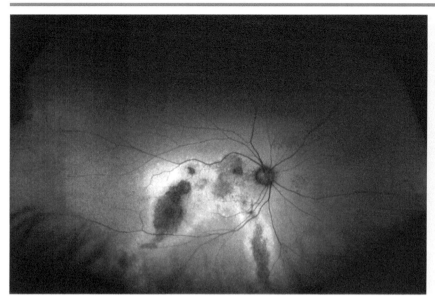

Fig. 6.4 Ultra-widefield green-light fundus autofluorescence (FAF; Optos, Marlborough, MA) in central serous chorioretinopathy. In the chronic stage, FAF reveals atrophic hypo-AF (autofluorescence) gravitational tracts with hyper-AF margins.

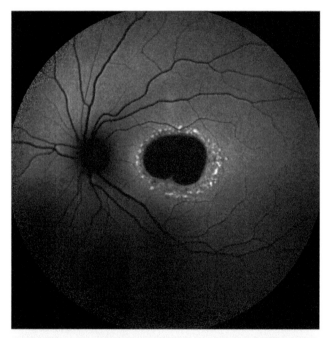

Fig. 6.5 Blue-light FAF (Spectralis; Heidelberg Engineering, Heidelberg, Germany) in Stargardt disease. FAF shows hyper-AF (autofluorescence) flecks surrounding a hypo-AF central macula corresponding to retinal atrophy.

from the photoreceptors and unmasking of the underlying RPE hyperfluorescence. In the chronic stage, FAF may show hypo-AF atrophic gravitational tracts that topographically correlate to resolved subretinal fluid (▶ Fig. 6.4).

6.2.4 Stargardt Disease

Stargardt macular degeneration is the most common hereditary juvenile macular dystrophy. This disorder most commonly results from an autosomal recessive mutation in ABCA4, leading to defective outer segment degradation, lipofuscin accumulation, and RPE and photoreceptor degeneration. FAF's character-

istics are dependent on the disease stage: (i) early stages are generally characterized by an increased AF; (ii) intermediate stages show a high variation in mean intensity and texture; and (iii) late disease shows macular hypo-AF from chorioretinal atrophy with hyper-AF flecks in the midperiphery (▶ Fig. 6.5).

6.2.5 Best Macular Dystrophy

Best disease leads to the accumulation of lipofuscin in the subretinal space, which results in bilateral yolk-like lesions in the macula. This disease may be separated into five stages, which are featured by different AF patterns: (i) the previtelliform stage is characterized by a normal AF or minimal hyper-AF changes; (ii) the vitelliform stage has macular well-circumscribed homogeneous hyper-AF lesions; (iii) the pseudohypopyon stage shows a gravitational layer of hyper-AF below iso-autofluorescent fluid; (iv) the vitelliruptive stage is characterized by a hypo-AF lesion with border of hyper-AF condensations; and (v) the atrophic stage with a diffuse hypo-AF due to chorioretinal atrophy.

6.2.6 Retinitis Pigmentosa

Retinitis pigmentosa (RP) refers to a genetically heterogeneous group of retinal dystrophies characterized by the degeneration of rod photoreceptors. Most RP eyes are characterized by a hyper-AF parafoveal ring that encroaches centrally with disease progression. This hyper-AF lesion is also known as "Robson Holder" ring, and corresponds to the border of ellipsoid zone disruption (▶ Fig. 6.6). FAF findings in RP eyes correlate well with visual function and can be useful in monitoring disease progression.

6.2.7 White Dot Syndromes

White dot syndromes refer to a wide spectrum of inflammatory chorioretinopathies featured by multifocal, small, yellow–white lesions located throughout the posterior pole and/or peripheral fundus. On FAF, these lesions may have variable AF signatures.

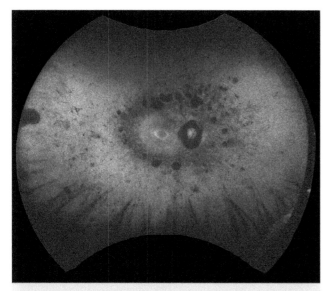

Fig. 6.6 Ultra-widefield green-light fundus autofluorescence (FAF; Optos, Marlborough, MA) in retinitis pigmentosa. FAF shows an area of normal preserved retina at the posterior fundus bordered by a hyper-AF (autofluorescence) "Robson Holder" ring. Mottled hypo-AF outside the ring corresponds to areas of photoreceptor degeneration.

6.3 Future Developments

FAF has been thought to be an effective surrogate for lipofuscin concentration in the RPE; however, other minor fluorophores contribute to the fluorescence intensity. These minor fluorophores may emit in the shorter wavelength end of the spectrum, and thus can be distinguished from lipofuscin. Recently, the fluorescence emitted from these minor fluorophores has been isolated in atrophic AMD eyes; however, its predictive and prognostic value is uncertain at this time.

Suggested Reading

[1] Bindewald A, Bird AC, Dandekar SS, et al. Classification of fundus autofluorescence patterns in early age-related macular disease. Invest Ophthalmol Vis Sci. 2005; 46(9):3309–3314

[2] Hariri AH, Nittala MG, Sadda SR. Quantitative characteristics of spectral-domain optical coherence tomography in corresponding areas of increased autofluorescence at the margin of geographic atrophy in patients with age-related macular degeneration. Ophthalmic Surg Lasers Imaging Retina. 2016; 47(6):523–527

[3] Hariri AH, Tepelus TC, Akil H, Nittala MG, Sadda SR. Retinal sensitivity at the junctional zone of eyes with geographic atrophy due to age-related macular degeneration. Am J Ophthalmol. 2016; 168:122–128

[4] Borrelli E, Lei J, Balasubramanian S, et al. Green emission fluorophores in eyes with atrophic age-related macular degeneration: a color fundus autofluorescence pilot study. Br J Ophthalmol. 2018 Jun; 102(6):827–832

Part II

Macular and Peripheral Vitreoretinal Interface Disorders

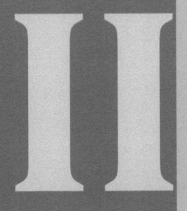

7 Posterior Vitreous Detachment

Natalia Albuquerque Lucena Figueiredo and Justis P. Ehlers

Summary

Posterior vitreous detachment (PVD) is the dehiscence of the posterior vitreous cortex from the retina, usually in patients aged 50 and over, as a result of the weakening of the vitreoretinal adhesion in conjunction with vitreous liquefaction (synchysis senilis). PVD typically begins in the perifoveal macula and extends slowly over months or years until complete vitreous separation occurs. PVD manifestations are usually benign, but in some cases vitreous liquefaction occurs without concurrent weakening of vitreoretinal adherence, which may induce numerous pathologic events at the vitreoretinal interface. The most known PVD complications usually occur in the retinal periphery, following the complete PVD, such as retinal tear and rhegmatogenous retinal detachment. Visual symptoms related to PVD include floaters and photopsias, which tend to improve over time. The conventional method for diagnosing PVD is slit-lamp biomicroscopy or indirect ophthalmoscopy by the presence of Weiss ring attached to the posterior hyaloid membrane. Ultrasonography and optical coherence tomography may also have value. No active treatment is usually needed; however, in cases of PVD complications, laser or pars plana vitrectomy surgery may be required.

Keywords: posterior vitreous detachment, synchysis senilis, vitreous, vitreoretinal, posterior hyaloid membrane, retinal detachment

7.1 Features

Posterior vitreous detachment (PVD) is the separation between the posterior vitreous cortex and the internal limiting membrane of the retina. Usually it occurs after the fifth decade of life, with a prevalence of 53% after 50 years with increasing occurrence with age. PVD is part of natural aging and represents the result of two progressive vitreous alterations: the weakening of the vitreoretinal adhesion and vitreous liquefaction (synchysis senilis). PVD typically begins in the perifoveal macula as a shallow separation from the perifoveal retina and slowly extends until vitreous separation from the optic disc margin is complete (▶ Fig. 7.1). In the absence of PVD-related complications, the early stages of PVD are asymptomatic. However, if vitreous liquefaction occurs before adequate weakening of the vitreoretinal adhesion, the traction forces may lead to several pathologic events at the vitreoretinal interface. These complications may occur throughout the retinal surface, including in the retinal periphery (e.g., retinal tears and vitreous hemorrhage retinal detachment; ▶ Fig. 7.2a) and also in the posterior pole (e.g., epiretinal membrane, macular hole, and vitreomacular traction; ▶ Fig. 7.3).

7.1.1 Common Symptoms

Asymptomatic in its early stages. In a subset of patients, the liquefied vitreous may lead to the appearance of floaters, which

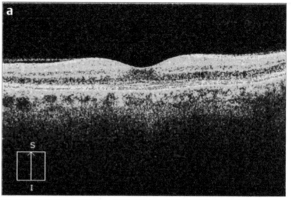

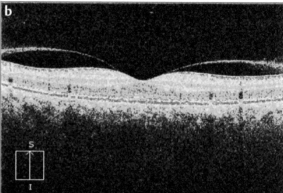

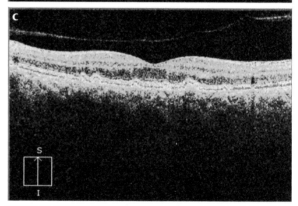

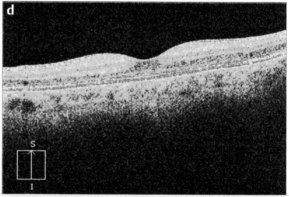

Fig. 7.1 Optical coherence tomography images of posterior vitreous detachment (PVD) stages. **(a)** Early-stage PVD with shallow vitreous separation from the perifoveal retina. **(b)** Perifoveal PVD with vitreofoveal adhesion. **(c)** PVD progression through the fovea. **(d)** Complete PVD.

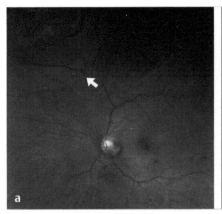
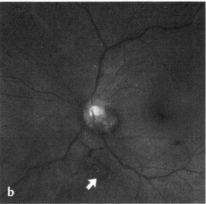

Fig. 7.2 Fundus photograph of a complete posterior vitreous detachment (PVD). **(a)** Fundus photograph showing peripheral retinal tear associated with rhegmatogenous retinal detachment (*arrow*), 2 weeks after PVD symptoms. **(b)** Zoom demonstrating Weiss ring (*arrow*).

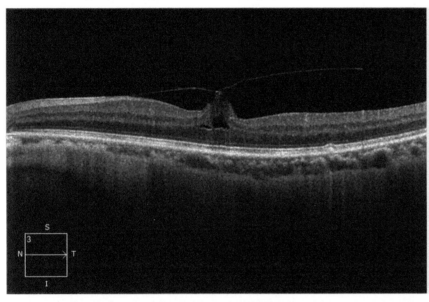

Fig. 7.3 Optical coherence tomography scan of symptomatic patient (visual acuity 20/40), presenting vitreofoveal traction syndrome; note vitreofoveal adhesion with anterior traction of the macula causing foveal thickening.

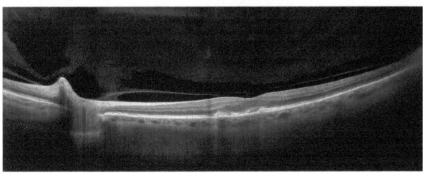

Fig. 7.4 Optical coherence tomographic scan of an asymptomatic 75-year-old woman showing premacular liquefied vitreous lacuna and vitreous separation from the perifoveal macula with residual vitreofoveal adhesion.

tend to improve over time. Complications of late-stage PVD are responsible for the sudden onset of photopsias and significant floaters. Anomalous separation at the posterior pole may also lead to macula-related symptoms such as metamorphopsia or blurred vision.

7.1.2 Exam Findings

PVD is identified via a slit-lamp biomicroscopy or an indirect ophthalmoscopy by the presence of a glial tissue ring (Weiss ring) attached to the posterior hyaloid membrane (▶ Fig. 7.2b). In some cases, it is possible to visualize the detached posterior hyaloid, retinal hemorrhages, vitreous opacities, vitreous

hemorrhage, and vitreous pigmented cells (i.e., tobacco dust). The finding of vitreous hemorrhage or pigmented cells in the vitreous is strongly suggestive of a retinal break.

7.2 Key Diagnostic Tests and Findings

7.2.1 Optical Coherence Tomography

Optical coherence tomography (OCT; e.g., spectral domain and swept source) offers noninvasive high-resolution cross-sectional imaging of vitreoretinal relationships (▶ Fig. 7.4). OCT enables visualization of early hyaloid separation, which would be otherwise undetectable. In addition, it is the diagnostic of choice to evaluate the macula and fovea for tractional-related complications. Once a PVD has occurred, the posterior hyaloid is usually no longer visible on the OCT.

7.2.2 Ultrasonography

Ultrasonography is often used in cases of significant media opacity and may also enable visualization of PVD-related complications, such as retinal tear or retinal detachment.

7.3 Critical Work-up

A patient who reports symptoms of PVD should undergo a comprehensive fundus examination through a fully dilated pupil with scleral depression to rule out associated retinal holes/tears or detachments.

7.4 Management

7.4.1 Treatment Options

Careful observation is appropriate for PVD. Treatment for the tractional-related complications may be required. In a small subset of patients, floaters and vitreous debris may be visually disabling and may require treatment. Pars plana vitrectomy and YAG laser vitreolysis have both been utilized in these cases. It is important to balance risks of both procedures with the severity of the patient's symptoms.

7.4.2 Follow-up

Depending on exam findings and symptoms, follow-up exam should be considered for repeat depressed peripheral exam, following presentation with acute PVD. Patients should be instructed about the warning signs of tractional-related complications, such as retinal tear or detachment (e.g., increased photopsias, increasing number of floaters, or changes in peripheral vision) and the importance of urgent follow-up if these symptoms occur.

Suggested Reading

[1] Johnson MW. Posterior vitreous detachment: evolution and complications of its early stages. Am J Ophthalmol. 2010; 149(3):371–82.e1

[2] Johnson MW. Posterior vitreous detachment: evolution and role in macular disease. Retina. 2012; 32 Suppl 2:S174–S178

[3] American Academy of Ophthalmology. Section 12: retina and vitreous. In: Basic and Clinical Science Course. San Francisco, CA: American Academy of Ophthalmology; 2013

[4] Shah CP, Heier JS. YAG laser vitreolysis vs sham YAG vitreolysis for symptomatic vitreous floaters: a randomized clinical trial. JAMA Ophthalmol. 2017; 135(9):918–923

8 Epiretinal Membrane

Ramin Tadayoni

Summary

Epiretinal membranes are essentially cellular proliferations on the surface of the macula and often appear after posterior vitreous detachment. They may be asymptomatic and are discovered incidentally or due to presenting symptoms of metamorphopsia and visual acuity impairment. Fundus examination and optical coherence tomography facilitate diagnosis. In cases with visual impairment, surgery can be proposed after a risk–benefit evaluation. Visual recovery is variable but visual acuity following surgery can be excellent.

Keywords: macula, membrane, OCT, retina, vitreous, vitrectomy

8.1 Features

Epiretinal membranes (ERMs) are essentially cellular proliferations on the surface of the macula and often appear after posterior vitreous detachment (PVD). They may be asymptomatic and are discovered incidentally or due to presenting symptoms of metamorphopsia and visual acuity impairment. Epiretinal membranes may result in anatomic distortion of the retinal tissue and foveal architecture. These distortions can result in retinal dysfunction and subsequent visual symptoms. Fundus examination and optical coherence tomography (OCT) facilitate diagnosis and evaluation of anatomic changes.

8.1.1 Common Symptoms

Commonly asymptomatic and discovered incidentally during a fundus examination or imaging (often OCT) performed for other reasons. Patients may discover symptomatic change when they close the fellow eye. Patients can complain of various visual symptoms predominantly progressive vision loss, blurred vision, aniseikonia (macropsia), metamorphopsia, and much less frequently monocular diplopia. Moderate foveal displacement due to the ERM can explain vision loss and metamorphopsia. Metamorphopsia is also assumed to be related to inner nuclear layer changes. Macropsia is assumed to be due to central photoreceptor contraction in a smaller area and may be responsible for aniseikonia.

8.1.2 Exam Findings

Cellophane glistening reflex of ERM on fundus biomicroscopy is the main examination finding. A careful examination may also notice a thickening of the macula or in some cases cystic changes. Contraction of the ERM may also result in a "macular pseudohole" appearance (a round reddish foveal image that looks like a hole but is not a full thickness macular hole) in about 15% of cases. In some cases, ERM contraction is so severe that it results in deep retinal folds, resulting in an impairment of the axoplasmic transport, appearing as long cotton wool spots. In addition, centripetal contraction of the membrane results in an elevation of central photoreceptors and subsequently a subfoveal yellow spot on funduscopy. In the majority of cases, ERMs are related to PVD which can be noted. Rarely, ERMs complicate the course of other diseases, including diabetic retinopathy, posterior and intermediate uveitis, and retinal detachment. A careful fundus examination should exclude any of these causal diseases.

8.2 Key Diagnostic Tests and Findings

8.2.1 Optical Coherence Tomography

OCT is the gold standard diagnostic test for ERM. It can show the presence of the ERM as a hyperreflective structure of variable thickness lining the inner retinal surface, more visible when it bridges inner retinal folds. The coronal scans (C-scans) segmented at the vitreoretinal interface provide very suggestive images of the ERM and induced retinal folds. OCT also has the advantage of showing and quantifying the macular thickening induced by ERM contraction. Another common finding caused by the constriction of the ERM is the disappearance of the foveal depression. The anterior profile of the macula may be flat, irregular, or often convex (▶ Fig. 8.1). Conversely, in other

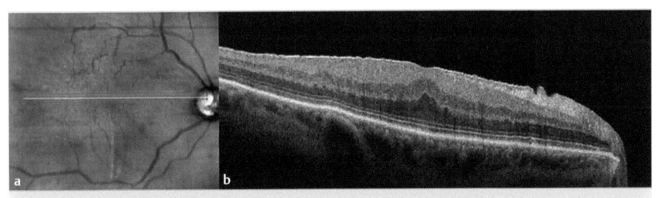

Fig. 8.1 (a,b) Typical appearance of an epiretinal membrane (ERM) on a horizontal optical coherence tomography scan of a right eye. The ERM appears as a hyperreflective line on the surface of the retina. The macula is thickened. The scan passes through the foveal center as confirmed by the thickening of the outer nuclear hyporeflective zone due to the elevation of the foveal pit and disappearance of foveal depression.

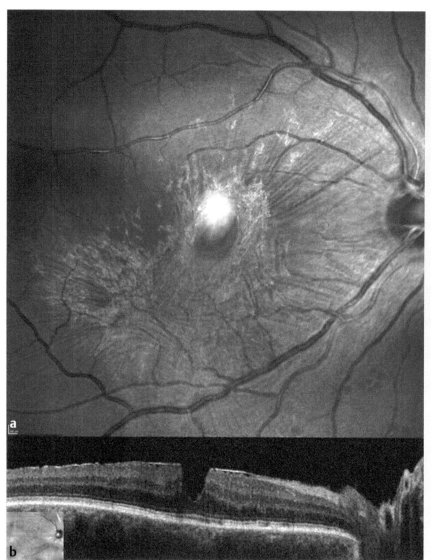

Fig. 8.2 (a) Blue reflectance scanning laser ophthalmoscope image of an epiretinal membrane in the right eye which delineates the membrane and its extent well. **(b)** The optical coherence tomography scan shows the membrane and its contraction causing a steepened foveal pit and thickened foveal that often results in the clinical appearance of a macular pseudohole.

cases OCT may show an atypical foveal profile of macular pseudohole with a steepened foveal pit combined with thickened foveal edges and a small foveal pit diameter (▶ Fig. 8.2). Sometimes some degree of intraretinal stretching or cleavage in the foveal edge is also associated (▶ Fig. 8.3). Cystic changes can also be noted on OCT (▶ Fig. 8.4). A subfoveal hyperreflective deposit can be found in about 20% of cases on OCT.

8.2.2 Fluorescein Angiography or Ultra-Widefield Fluorescein Angiography

Fluorescein angiography (FA) is rarely needed in the evaluation of ERM. In cases with significant intraretinal fluid, FA may be utilized to evaluate for concurrent disorders that may be the primary cause of the fluid.

8.2.3 Fundus Photography and Angiography

Color and red-free images may also be used for documenting clinical appearance and for patient education. Blue reflectance photography better displays the retinal surface and abnormal reflectivity of the ERM (▶ Fig. 8.2).

8.3 Critical Work-up

Besides for a clinical history, comprehensive ophthalmic exam, and OCT, no additional work-up is often needed. Clinical evaluation for secondary causes of ERM is important.

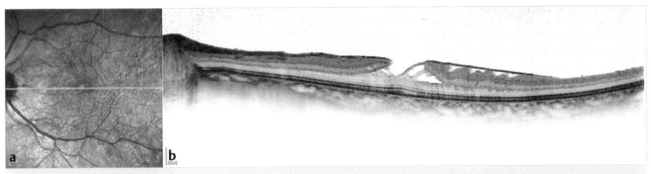

Fig. 8.3 Horizontal optical coherence tomography (OCT) scan of a left eye with an epiretinal membrane. **(a)** Contraction of the membrane can be seen on infrared scanning laser ophthalmoscope image of the fundus as folds mainly on the temporal side of the fovea. **(b)** The tangential traction causes a schisis of the edges of the fovea associated to superficial folds easily noticeable on the temporal side of the OCT scan.

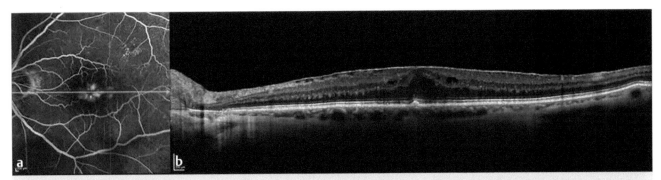

Fig. 8.4 (a) An epiretinal membrane in a left eye exhibiting hyperfluorescent petaloid leakage consistent with cystoid macular edema on fluorescein angiogram. **(b)** The optical coherence tomography demonstrates hyporeflective cystic spaces, an overlying hyperreflective epiretinal membrane, elevation of the foveal center caused by traction and a subfoveal hyperreflective deposit.

8.4 Management

8.4.1 Treatment Options

Observation

In eyes with good vision and minimal symptoms at the time of diagnosis observation can be proposed. The visual acuity remains stable in many cases.

Surgery

For eyes with significant symptoms, surgery should be considered. While patients with significant preoperative disturbance often benefit more from surgery, patients with a better initial visual acuity achieve better visual outcomes. Pars plana vitrectomy with membrane peeling is the typical approach. Staining the ERM is often used to facilitate dissection; different dyes are used in different countries based on approvals and availability. Many instruments have been developed to facilitate ERM peeling including forceps, membrane loops, and membrane scrapers. The dissection is started remote from the fovea. Internal limiting membrane (ILM) peeling may be performed simultaneously to ERM removal or with a secondary peel. The need for

ILM removal is controversial. Studies have suggested ILM removal reduces recurrence rate but may carry other risks (e.g., delaying visual recovery). Intraoperative OCT has been shown to aid the surgery in particular by avoiding restaining in case of doubt of complete removal of the ERM. Risks with surgery include retinal detachment and endophthalmitis.

8.4.2 Follow-up

Eyes that are being observed are often followed every 3 to 6 months initially to watch for progression and worsening symptoms. Following vitrectomy, typical postoperative follow-up is carried out. Visual recovery may takes months and even years. Patients frequently recover some visual acuity, but those with shorter duration of symptoms and better initial vision often achieve the best outcomes. OCT remains the key imaging for evaluating the macular changes. The macular thickness usually significantly decreases after surgery, although it rarely returns to normal, and the foveal pit reappears only in some cases. This does not prevent visual improvement. The presence of a dissociated optic nerve fiber layer on the OCT C-scan or on blue reflectance images may reflect the extent of ILM peeling (► Fig. 8.5).

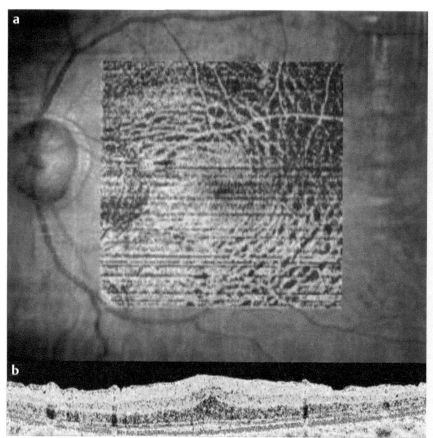

Fig. 8.5 Postoperative optical coherence tomography (OCT) following epiretinal membrane removal. **(a)** "Dimples" on the surface of the retina visible particularly on the *en face* image representing dissociated optic nerve fiber layer (DONFL). These are oval areas of retinal thinning alongside optic nerve fibers (dark area, **a**), typically in the area of internal limiting membrane peeling. **(b)** Despite good visual recovery, the OCT demonstrates typical residual thickening of the macula.

Suggested Reading

[1] Wilkins JR, Puliafito CA, Hee MR, et al. Characterization of epiretinal membranes using optical coherence tomography. Ophthalmology. 1996; 103(12): 2142–2151

[2] Haouchine B, Massin P, Tadayoni R, Erginay A, Gaudric A. Diagnosis of macular pseudoholes and lamellar macular holes by optical coherence tomography. Am J Ophthalmol. 2004; 138(5):732–739

[3] Pison A, Dupas B, Couturier A, Rothschild PR, Tadayoni R. Evolution of subfoveal detachments secondary to idiopathic epiretinal membranes after surgery. Ophthalmology. 2016; 123(3):583–589

[4] Tadayoni R, Paques M, Massin P, Mouki-Benani S, Mikol J, Gaudric A. Dissociated optic nerve fiber layer appearance of the fundus after idiopathic epiretinal membrane removal. Ophthalmology. 2001; 108(12):2279–2283

9 Macular Holes

Philip P. Storey and Carl D. Regillo

Summary

Macular holes are a group of vitreoretinal interface disorders that are characterized by an abnormality in the foveal architecture, ranging from a full-thickness hole to a partial hole with minimal tissue disruption. This chapter provides an overview of the concepts, classification, and pathophysiology surrounding macular holes. Risk factors and common features are reviewed. The gold standard for diagnostic testing is optical coherence tomography. Finally, the critical work-up and management options including include surgical intervention are discussed.

Keywords: macular holes, management, optical coherence tomography, vitrectomy

9.1 Features

A full-thickness macular hole (FTMH) is a complete retinal defect that results in the separation of retinal layers and typically occurs in the fovea. FTMH prevalence has been reported to be 0.2 to 2.9 per 1,000 people. In patients with unilateral macular holes, studies have shown that the risk of developing a hole in the other eye within 5 years ranges from approximately 10 to 20% if the posterior hyaloid is still attached to the fovea. The risk is significantly reduced if a posterior vitreous detachment (PVD) is already present (i.e., < 1%). Conversely, if vitreofoveal traction is present, the risk is quite high (i.e., ~ 50%). Women are at higher risk for primary FTMH development than men. Older age, generally defined as over 65 years, is also associated with increased risk of primary FTMH.

Vitreomacular traction (VMT) during anomalous posterior vitreous separation plays a key role in the formation of primary FTMH. If vitreous liquefaction and contraction outpace the release of the vitreofoveal interface, an FTMH may develop. Secondary FTMH may be due to a number of etiologies including trauma, high myopia, intraocular surgery, macular edema, neovascular age-related macular degeneration following intravitreal injection, and lightning strikes.

Differential diagnosis includes macular pseudohole, VMT, and lamellar macular hole. A pseudohole is a clinical diagnosis based on the fundus appearance that mimics an FTMH. Optical coherence tomography (OCT) confirms no loss of foveal tissue. An epiretinal membrane is typically responsible for the pseudohole appearance. VMT without FTMH may also appear similar on clinical exam. Lamellar macular holes are partial-thickness retinal defects that may exhibit splitting of the inner retinal layers and disruption of the outer retinal layers. Hyporeflective preretinal tissue is often identified on OCT in these lamellar holes.

9.1.1 Common Symptoms

Decreased vision, central scotoma, and/or visual distortion (i.e., metamorphopsia).

9.1.2 Exam Findings

Examination of the macula reveals a round or oval red spot in the central macula often surrounded by a gray halo, representing a cuff of subretinal fluid and/or retinal edema (▶ Fig. 9.1). A

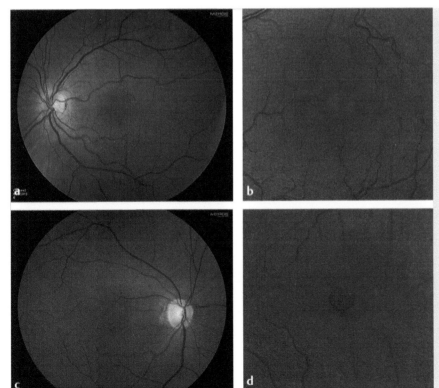

Fig. 9.1 **(a)** Fundus image demonstrating small full-thickness macular hole (FTMH) with **(b)** high magnification view demonstrating full-thickness defect and surrounding cystic changes (*arrow*). **(c,d)** Larger FTMH with gray surrounding cuff of subretinal fluid (*arrow*).

cyst at the hole margin or operculum above the hole may be present. Yellowish deposits on the surface of the RPE may be present in the base of the FTMH. A lamellar hole (i.e., not full-thickness) will often be less red and lack a gray halo. A glistening from an epiretinal membrane may be present.

9.2 Key Diagnostic Tests and Findings

9.2.1 Optical Coherence Tomography

OCT is the gold standard imaging modality for FTMH and vitreoretinal interface abnormalities (▶ Fig. 9.2, ▶ Fig. 9.3, ▶ Fig. 9.4, ▶ Fig. 9.5). OCT facilitates staging, prognostication, and treatment decision-making OCT imaging will demonstrate full-thickness disruption of all retinal layers in FTMH and also enables visualization of hole size, the presence of VMT, and concurrent macular disease. OCT of the fellow eye also helps to stratify risk for FTMH development through visualizing the vitreoretinal interface. In pseudoholes, OCT will confirm intact foveal tissue, often with an associated epiretinal membrane with alterations to the foveal architecture (▶ Fig. 9.6a). In lamellar macular holes, foveal tissue is often missing or disrupted on OCT. In addition, preretinal thickened epiretinal membrane

with hyporeflective material is often seen on OCT in lamellar macular holes (▶ Fig. 9.6).

9.2.2 Fluorescein Angiography or Ultra-Widefield Fluorescein Angiography

Fluorescein angiography (FA) is not routinely used to diagnosis FTMH, but exhibit a characteristic appearance on FA with early hyperfluorescence without evidence of late leakage. FA may be helpful in cases of significant concurrent disease to better evaluate overall management strategy.

9.2.3 Ultrasonography

In the hands of a skilled echographer, ultrasonography may show large full-thickness FTMH but is of little clinical value to detect small holes.

9.3 Critical Work-up

Patient history should include the review of prior trauma, surgery, family history, and complete ophthalmic examination, including slit-lamp biomicroscopy examination and indirect examination of the peripheral fundus.

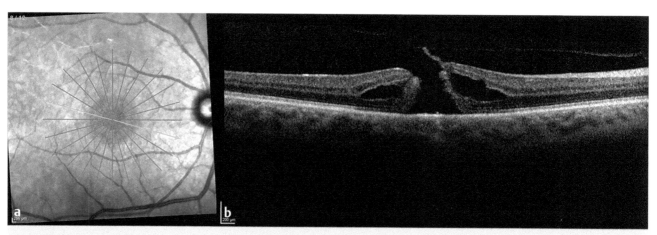

Fig. 9.2 (a,b) Optical coherence tomography showing full thickness macular hole with vitreomacular traction on one edge of the hole.

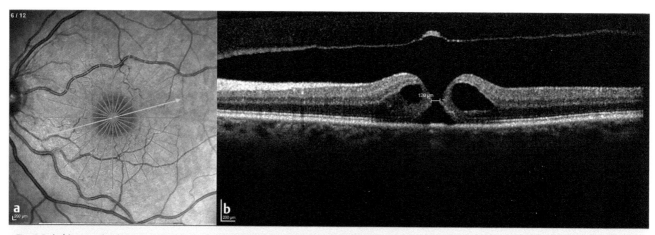

Fig. 9.3 (a,b) Optical coherence tomography with full thickness macular hole with vitreous separation from the macular surface and an operculum.

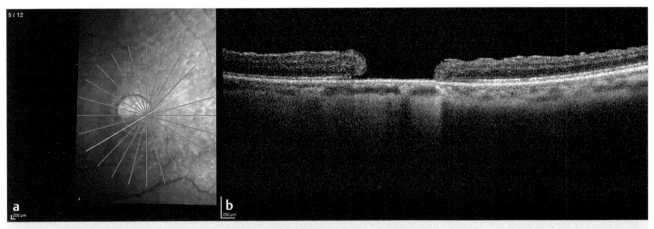

Fig. 9.4 (a,b) Optical coherence tomography of a chronic, large, full thickness macular hole.

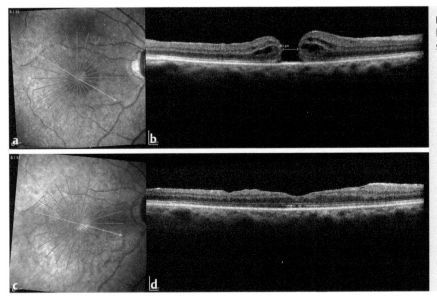

Fig. 9.5 Medium-sized full-thickness macular hole (a,b) prior to and (c,d) 6 months following surgical repair.

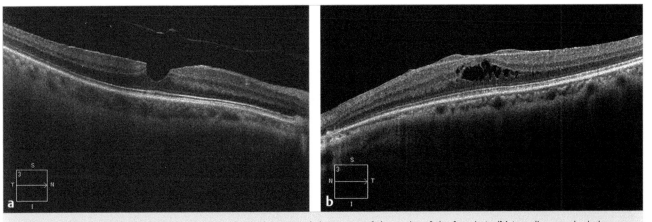

Fig. 9.6 (a) Macular pseudohole with preservation of retinal tissue and sharpening of the angles of the foveal pit. (b) Lamellar macular hole demonstrating hyporeflective preretinal tissue.

Table 9.1 OCT-based international VMT classification system and commonly used clinical macular hole stages

OCT-based international VMT classification system	Historical staging of macular holes—Stages 1–4 Gass Classification
Vitreomacular adhesion	Stage 0: partial perifoveal detachment in eye where the fellow eye has experienced an FTMH
VMT	Stage 1: impending macular hole
Small FTMH with VMT	Stage 2: small hole
Medium or large FTMH with VMT	Stage 3: large hole
FTMH with complete PVD	Stage 4: hole with complete PVD

Abbreviations: FTMH, full-thickness macular hole; OCT, optical coherence tomography; PVD, posterior vitreous detachment; VMT, vitreomacular traction.

OCT is typically performed to confirm the diagnosis and better visualization of the vitreoretinal interface. Various staging systems have been described, including the Gass classification and a more recent OCT-based classification (▶ Table 9.1). The size of macular holes, as evaluated by OCT, has been shown to predict success rates of both surgical and pharmacologic interventions. Small FTMH are defined as less than 250 mm wide and have very high rates of closure with surgical intervention (>95%). These small holes may be amenable to office-based pharmacologic or pneumatic treatment. Medium holes are between 250 and 400 mm and have high rates of closure with vitrectomy and may be successfully treated with intravitreal pharcovitreolysis or pneumatic vitreolysis, although with lower success rates than small holes (▶ Fig. 9.3). Large holes are defined as having an aperture great than 400 mm (▶ Fig. 9.4). Surgical success rates of large hole closure have been reported in the 90 to 95% range, but declines as the hole gets larger.

9.4 Management

9.4.1 Treatment Options

Observation

Spontaneous resolution of FTMH is rare and observation is typically only considered for a short period of time. Treatment for lamellar holes remains controversial as visual results have been highly variable with surgery. These are often observed. Macular pseudoholes are often observed if they are minimally symptomatic, but may be treated with vitrectomy and membrane peeling when significant symptoms develop.

Pharmacologic and Pneumatic Vitreolysis

Ocriplasmin is a truncated form of the human protease plasmin and may be injected into the vitreous to create vitreous separation in the macula. Overall success rates for closing small to medium FTMH (i.e., <400 mm) with associated VMT on OCT using ocriplasmin is approximately 40%. Pharmacologic vitreolysis has not been shown to successfully close large macular holes. Potential complications of pharmacologic vitreolysis may include failure to close the hole, floaters, photopsias, vision loss, and ellipsoid zone loss. Although these complications in most cases are transient, safety concerns for prolonged decreased visual acuity have impacted its use. Pneumatic vitreolysis through the office-based intravitreal injection of expansile gas offers an additional nonsurgical alternative, which may have comparable or better hole closure rates. Potential complications include failure to close the hole, floaters, and retinal tear/detachment.

Surgery

Success rates of macular hole surgery have increased to over 90 to 95% with improvements in surgical technology and technique. During surgical repair, a pars plana vitrectomy with posterior hyaloid elevation is performed to release any residual VMT (▶ Fig. 9.2). Epiretinal membrane and internal limiting membrane peeling is frequently performed and improves hole closure, particularly for larger FTMH. Gas tamponades including air, C_3F_8, and SF_6 are used to facilitate hole closure. Though controversial, facedown positioning for several days is frequently recommended to position the gas against the FTMH and facilitate closure. Complications of surgery may include retinal tear/detachment, cataract formation, and visual field defects along with other, rare complications associated with vitrectomy such as infection.

9.4.2 Follow-up

The frequency of follow-up will vary depending on the specific clinical scenario and the management strategy selected. Ongoing surveillance for the fellow eye may also be required based on the status of the posterior hyaloid.

Suggested Reading

[1] Gass JD. Idiopathic senile macular hole. Its early stages and pathogenesis. Arch Ophthalmol. 1988; 106(5):629–639

[2] Duker JS, Kaiser PK, Binder S, et al. The International Vitreomacular Traction Study Group classification of vitreomacular adhesion, traction, and macular hole. Ophthalmology. 2013; 120(12):2611–2619

[3] Stalmans P, Benz MS, Gandorfer A, et al. MIVI-TRUST Study Group. Enzymatic vitreolysis with ocriplasmin for vitreomacular traction and macular holes. N Engl J Med. 2012; 367(7):606–615

[4] Yu G, Duguay J, Marra KV, et al. Efficacy and safety of treatment options for vitreomacular traction: a case series and meta-analysis. Retina. 2016; 36(7): 1260–1270

10 Vitreomacular Traction

Almyr S. Sabrosa, Daniela Ferrara, and Jay S. Duker

Summary

Vitreomacular traction is an abnormality of the vitreoretinal interface, characterized by incomplete posterior vitreous detachment and persistent adherence between the posterior hyaloid and the retinal surface causing architectural changes of the neurosensory retina and often secondary visual disturbance. Symptoms may include metamorphopsia, aniseikonia, photopsia, micropsia, central scotoma, or significant decrease of central vision. Optical coherence tomography (OCT) is sufficient and often necessary to confirm the diagnosis. In addition, OCT can reveal associated macular abnormalities such as loss of foveal depression, intraretinal cystic changes, macular schisis, and subfoveal serous retinal detachment. Therapeutic intervention can be considered in cases with significant visual disturbance and anatomic alteration. Pars plana vitrectomy with removal of the adherent hyaloid and associated epiretinal membrane is the surgery most commonly performed. Use of an in-office pneumatic vitreolysis (i.e., intraocular gas injection [e.g., perfluoropropane, C_3F_8]) attempting to induce posterior vitreous detachment may be beneficial in select cases. Pharmacologic vitreolysis (e.g., ocriplasmin [Jetrea]) may be another therapeutic option for selected cases.

Keywords: epiretinal membrane, metamorphopsia, optical coherence tomography, vitreomacular adhesion, vitreoretinal interface, vitreomacular traction

10.1 Features

Vitreomacular traction (VMT) is characterized by an incomplete posterior vitreous detachment and persistent adherence between the posterior hyaloid and the retinal surface causing architectural changes of the neurosensory retina and secondary visual disturbance. Optical coherence tomography (OCT) is sufficient and, in some cases, necessary to confirm the diagnosis. Therapeutic intervention can be considered in cases with significant visual disturbance and anatomic change.

10.1.1 Common Symptoms

It may be asymptomatic. Visual symptoms may include metamorphopsia, aniseikonia, photopsia, micropsia, central scotoma, or significant decrease of central vision. Natural history is difficult to predict from presenting symptomatology or anatomic appearance.

10.1.2 Exam Findings

The diagnosis of VMT can be difficult by clinical examination alone as the findings are often subtle. Slit-lamp biomicroscopy may reveal an abnormal foveal reflex and elevated fovea with a partially detached vitreous cortex. On ophthalmoscopy, VMT may be difficult to distinguish from idiopathic epiretinal membrane or cases of cystoid macular edema. Severe cases of VMT can result in retinal pigment epithelium changes from persistent traction. Significant traction may result in schisis-like changes or even localized tractional retinal detachment.

10.2 Key Diagnostic Tests and Findings

10.2.1 Optical Coherence Tomography

OCT is the critical ancillary test to confirm the diagnosis of VMT and to rule out concurrent and/or mimicking conditions. In addition, OCT can also show associated macular architecture changes resulting from the traction such as loss of foveal depression, intraretinal cystic changes, macular schisis, epiretinal membrane, and subfoveal serous retinal detachment (▶ Fig. 10.1). An OCT-based International Classification System defined VMT and subclassified it based on the diameter of the vitreomacular adhesion (VMA) on cross-sectional OCT B-scan (e.g., focal VMT [< 1,500 μm]; diffuse VMT [≥ 1,500 μm]). When associated with other macular disease such as retinal vein occlusion or diabetes, VMT is classified as "concurrent." Otherwise, it is considered to be "primary."

10.2.2 Fluorescein Angiography

Fluorescein angiography is not a key imaging modality for the diagnosis or management of VMT but may show mild leakage in the macular area.

10.2.3 Ultrasonography

B-scan ultrasonography can demonstrate movable membranes of medium reflectivity that adhere to some anatomical aspects of the fundus such as the macula and optic disc, correspondent to posterior vitreous detachment. However, due to its lower image definition, ultrasonography is not routinely performed for VMT.

10.3 Critical Work-up

Dilated fundus exam is important to evaluate the macula and peripheral retinal status, but OCT is the key tool to diagnose, monitor, and guide treatment decisions for VMT. Cross-sectional OCT can document the anatomic effects and extent of vitreoretinal adhesions, which is particularly relevant in those cases with central visual symptoms secondary to VMT. VMT should be differentiated from VMA. VMA does not cause architectural changes of the neurosensory retina nor secondary visual impairment and represents the normal "aging" process of the vitreous (i.e., not pathologic). OCT can easily discern the two entities as VMA OCTs are characterized by incomplete separation between the posterior hyaloid and the retinal surface, but with no architectural changes of the neurosensory retina

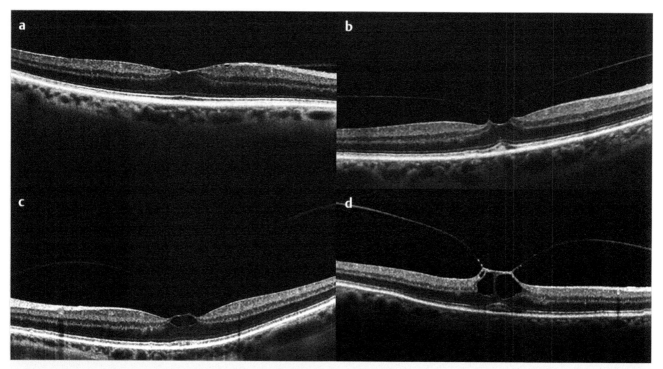

Fig. 10.1 Vitreomacular traction is characterized by an incomplete posterior vitreous detachment and persistent adherence between the posterior hyaloid and the retinal surface, which causes architectural changes of the neurosensory retina and secondary visual disturbance. **(a)** Optical coherence tomography shows associated macular changes, including minimal traction, **(b)** mild traction with outer retinal changes, **(c)** inner cystic changes with traction, and **(d)** significant traction with inner retinal cystic changes and subretinal fluid.

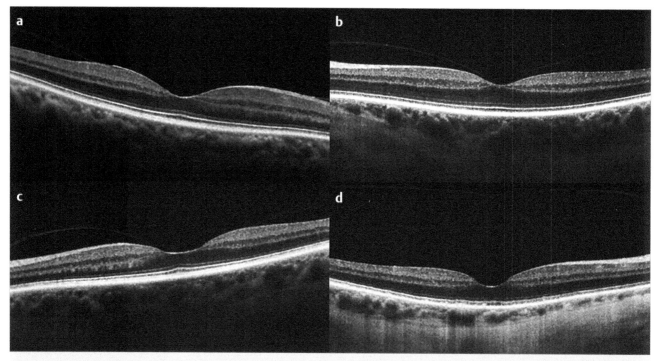

Fig. 10.2 (a–d) Vitreomacular adhesion is a finding on optical coherence tomography characterized by incomplete separation between the posterior hyaloid and the retinal surface without architectural changes of the neurosensory retina or secondary visual symptoms.

(▶ Fig. 10.2). Other vitreomacular interface abnormalities that can be associated with VMT include epiretinal membrane, lamellar macular hole, or full-thickness macular hole. VMA can have variable length of adhesion and is not pathologic, but rather a normal finding of the natural evolution of vitreous separation. Other entities in the differential diagnosis for VMT include cystoid macular edema, full-thickness macular hole, diabetic macular edema, and epiretinal membrane (▶ Fig. 10.3).

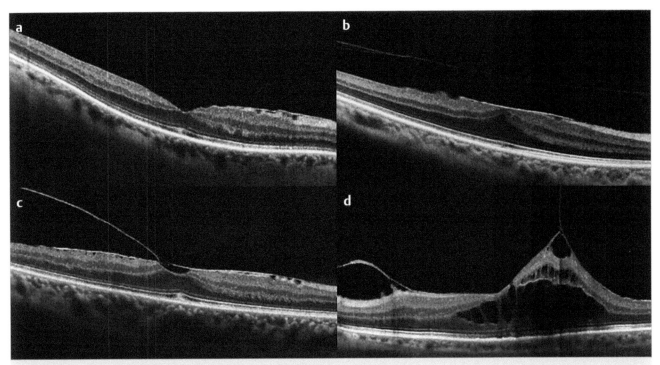

Fig. 10.3 Epiretinal membrane is visible on optical coherence tomography as a hyperreflective tissue on the inner retinal surface. **(a,b)** It must be considered as a differential diagnosis of vitreomacular traction (VMT) or **(c,d)** it can be associated with VMT (i.e., the VMT syndrome).

10.4 Management

10.4.1 Treatment Options

Observation

As spontaneous separation of the posterior hyaloid occurs not infrequently, conservative management with observation is frequently considered initially, especially with relatively good visual acuity. Treatment for VMT should be considered according to the visual symptoms, as well as anatomic appearance on OCT, particularly in cases with progressive visual impairment.

Pars Plana Vitrectomy

The primary intervention for VMT is pars plana vitrectomy with or without removal of the internal limiting membrane and/or epiretinal membrane. Several surgical series with posterior pars plana vitrectomy report acceptably low complication rates. Better results may be achieved with earlier surgical intervention.

Pneumatic Vitreolysis

Intravitreal injection of perfluoropropane (C_3F_8) or sulfur hexafluoride (SF_6) is a more conservative alternative to surgery to attempt to induce posterior vitreous detachment. The success rate of this procedure has been reported to be fairly high (i.e., > 80%). Adverse events are uncommon, but may include increased intraocular pressure, cataract formation, endophthalmitis retinal tears, retinal detachment, and vitreous hemorrhages.

Pharmacologic Vitreolysis

Intravitreal injection of ocriplasmin (Jetrea) is approved for the treatment of VMT (▶ Fig. 10.4). Ocriplasmin acts on laminin, fibronectin, and collagen type 4 resulting in vitreous liquefaction and separation of the posterior cortex of the retinal vitreous. Favorable VMT characteristics for ocriplasmin success include focal VMT (adhesion < 1,500 µm) and lack of associated epiretinal membrane. However, the success rates are limited with the phase 3 clinical trials demonstrating a 30% VMT resolution rate versus 8% in placebo group. The safety profile of ocriplasmin is controversial with select patients demonstrating ellipsoid zone changes on OCT and electroretinogram changes, suggesting panretinal dysfunction. However, these findings are usually transitory.

10.4.2 Follow-up

OCT should be used to monitor patients with VMT over time. Both eyes should be followed, particularly if the fellow eye still has an attached vitreous since the rate of bilateral vitreomacular

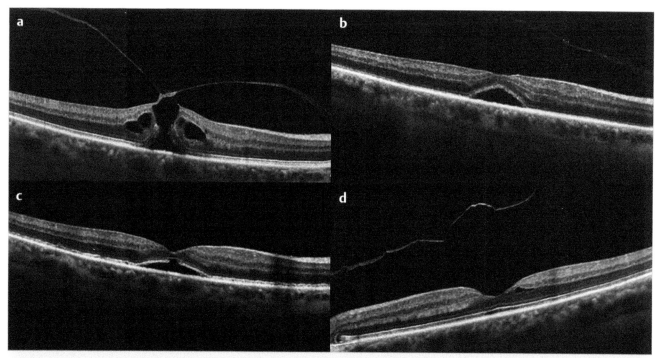

Fig. 10.4 **(a)** Optical coherence tomography demonstrating vitreomacular traction and associated small macular hole. **(b)** One week following treatment with ocriplasmin, the adherence between the posterior hyaloid and the retinal surface has been released, but subretinal fluid is still present with ellipsoid zone attenuation. **(c)** One month later, the foveal contour is improving despite residual subretinal fluid. Early ellipsoid zone restoration is visible. **(d)** Four months later, the appearance of the neurosensory retina is almost normal with complete ellipsoid zone reconstitution, with only small intraretinal cystic spaces still present.

interface disease approaches 50%. Progressive vision loss and/or worsening symptoms are indications for treatment and should be monitored.

Suggested Reading

[1] Duker JS, Kaiser PK, Binder S, et al. The International Vitreomacular Traction Study Group classification of vitreomacular adhesion, traction, and macular hole. Ophthalmology. 2013; 120(12):2611–2619

[2] Bottós JM, Elizalde J, Rodrigues EB, Maia M. Current concepts in vitreomacular traction syndrome. Curr Opin Ophthalmol. 2012; 23(3):195–201

[3] Barak Y, Ihnen MA, Schaal S. Spectral domain optical coherence tomography in the diagnosis and management of vitreoretinal interface pathologies. J Ophthalmol. 2012; 2012:876472

[4] Jackson TL, Nicod E, Angelis A, et al. Pars plana vitrectomy for vitreomacular traction syndrome: a systematic review and metaanalysis of safety and efficacy. Retina. 2013; 33(10):2012–2017

[5] Steinle NC, Dhoot DS, Quezada Ruiz C, et al. Treatment of vitreomacular traction with intravitreal perfluoropropane (C3F8) injection. Retina. 2017; 37(4): 643–650

11 Retinal Tears and Holes

Vishal S. Parikh, Anjali Shah, and Gaurav K. Shah

Summary

Retinal breaks are any full-thickness disruption in the sensory retina providing a conduit for fluid to enter the potential space between the sensory retina and retinal pigment epithelium. Sometimes retinal holes and tears are asymptomatic; however, the sudden appearance of flashes and floaters may indicate a hole or tear. Goldmann three-mirror lens viewing can aid in examination of anterior periphery to find retinal breaks, a scleral depressed exam allows for examination out to the ora serrata, and B-scan ultrasonography may enable identification of retinal breaks through dense vitreous hemorrhage.

Keywords: retinopexy, subretinal fluid vitreous hemorrhage

11.1 Features

Retinal breaks are any full thickness disruption in the sensory retina providing a conduit for fluid to enter the potential space between the sensory retina and retinal pigment epithelium (RPE). Sometimes retinal holes and tears are asymptomatic; however, the sudden appearance of flashes and floaters may indicate a hole or tear. The most common cause of retinal tears is vitreous detachment/separation from the retinal surface.

11.1.1 Common Symptoms

Photopsias, floaters, and shade/curtain over central vision if progression to retinal detachment.

11.1.2 Exam Findings

Pigment in the anterior vitreous, also known as tobacco dust or Shafer's sign, is a strong indicator of a potential retinal break

(i.e., approximately 90%, ▶ Fig. 11.1). Posterior vitreous detachment with or without vitreous hemorrhage (VH) is often present and is generally identified by the presence of a Weiss ring. Bridging vessel involvement at the area of the tear can result in VH (▶ Fig. 11.2a). Horseshoe/flap retinal tears have a base toward vitreous base and apex of flap points toward posterior pole (▶ Fig. 11.2a). For round holes with operculum, traction with or without subretinal fluid (SRF) may remain on the edges of the hole despite operculum (▶ Fig. 11.2b). An increase in pigmentation suggests chronicity. Atrophic breaks with/without lattice may have minimal traction (▶ Fig. 11.2c). Retinal dialysis is associated with retinal trauma and represents the separation of the sensory retina from the RPE occurs at the ora serrata, most commonly inferior temporal in the eye (▶ Fig. 11.2d).

11.2 Key Diagnostic Tests and Findings

11.2.1 Goldmann Three-Mirror Lens

Can aid in examination of anterior periphery to find retinal breaks.

11.2.2 Scleral Depressed Exam

Allows for examination out to the ora serrata; can assist with mobilizing the retinal tear or hole for improved visualization.

11.2.3 Ultrasonography

Retinal break may be identified through dense VH on B-scan (▶ Fig. 11.2e).

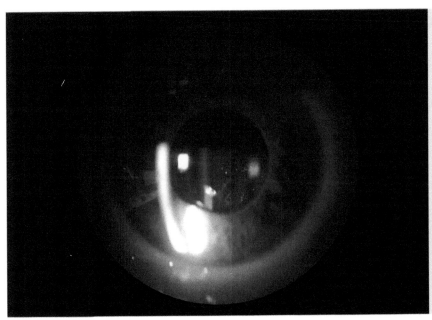

Fig. 11.1 Slit-lamp photograph demonstrating Shafer sign with pigment in anterior vitreous noted with the slit beam focused behind the intraocular lens.

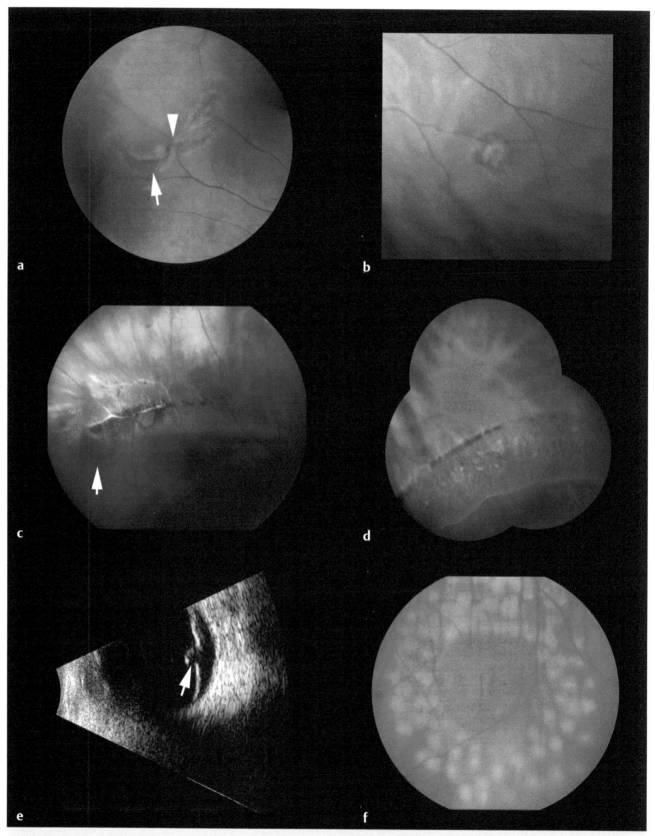

Fig. 11.2 (a) Fundus photography of horseshoe tear (*arrow*) with bridging vessel (*arrowhead*). (b) Pigmented retinal hole with operculum. (c) Atrophic hole (*arrow*) in lattice. (d) Retinal dialysis. (e) B-scan ultrasound demonstrating retinal break (*arrow*). (f) Horseshoe tear after laser retinopexy.

11.2.4 Widefield Optical Coherence Tomography

Many retinal breaks may be too peripheral for identification on OCT, but newer techniques and systems may enable visualization/confirmation of retinal tears/holes utilizing OCT.

11.3 Management

11.3.1 Treatment Options

Symptomatic Retinal Breaks or Retinal Breaks with Presence of SRF

Goal of treatment is to prevent further migration of SRF into a retinal detachment. Retinopexy is performed via laser photocoagulation or cryotherapy (▶ Fig. 11.2f). Laser photocoagulation is often first-line treatment. Cryotherapy is often used when there is significant VH and/or debris reducing visualization. Pars plana vitrectomy is used if unable to treat completely with above treatments.

Asymptomatic or Atrophic Retinal Breaks

Observation may be considered if hyperpigmentation is present and/or there is absence of traction/SRF. Less than 2% of atrophic holes in lattice progress to retinal detachment. Retinopexy can be considered if symptomatic, progressive traction, or fellow eye history of retinal detachment.

11.3.2 Follow-up

Patient education is critical so that patients understand the signs and symptoms of retinal detachment (i.e., increase in floaters, flashes, or a shade/curtain) for sooner follow-up.

Symptomatic Retinal Break

Close follow-up (e.g., 1–4 weeks) after treatment of a symptomatic retinal break to monitor for progression of SRF, followed by spacing out of follow-ups.

Asymptomatic Retinal Breaks without Fluid

Follow-up is frequently based on overall clinical picture (e.g., tear may be followed more closely than atrophic hole). At a minimum, an annual dilated exam is recommended.

Suggested Reading

[1] Tanner V, Harle D, Tan J, Foote B, Williamson TH, Chignell AH. Acute posterior vitreous detachment: the predictive value of vitreous pigment and symptomatology. Br J Ophthalmol. 2000; 84(11):1264–1268

[2] American Academy of Ophthalmology Retina/Vitreous Panel. Preferred Practice Pattern Guidelines. Posterior Vitreous Detachment, Retinal Breaks, and Lattice Degeneration. San Francisco, CA: American Academy of Ophthalmology; 2014

12 Primary Rhegmatogenous Retinal Detachment

Priya Sharma and Chirag Shah

Summary

Rhegmatogenous retinal detachment is a condition that can lead to vision loss due to separation of the neurosensory retina from the retinal pigment epithelium (RPE). The diagnosis is made by clinical exam with the use of additional ancillary testing, as needed. Management can include laser retinopexy, pneumatic retinopexy, pars plana vitrectomy, scleral buckling, or combined pars plana vitrectomy with scleral buckle. This chapter summarizes clinical features, diagnostic testing, and management options of rhegmatogenous retinal detachment.

Keywords: laser, pneumatic, retinal detachment, retinopexy, scleral buckle, tear, vitrectomy

12.1 Features

Retinal tears most frequently develop from vitreous traction, often during a posterior vitreous detachment (PVD). Such tears are typically horseshoe in configuration, with an anterior retinal "flap" that is tightly adherent to the posterior hyaloid. Liquefied vitreous can travel through the tear and underneath the neurosensory retina, leading to subretinal fluid accumulation and creating a rhegmatogenous retinal detachment. Customarily, rhegmatogenous retinal detachments are described by their clock hours of involvement, and whether or not the macula is affected. Macula-involving retinal detachments are at higher risk for some level of persistent visual compromise once repaired. Risk factors for rhegmatogenous retinal detachment include acute PVD, lattice degeneration, ocular trauma, high myopia (defined as a spherical equivalent of –6.0 diopters or more, or an axial length of at least 26 mm), cataract surgery (especially in the setting of vitreous loss) and certain genetic syndromes (e.g., Stickler, Marfan, Ehlers Danlos, or Wagner syndrome). The incidence of primary rhegmatogenous retinal detachment is estimated to be around 12 in 10,000 people per year (0.01% annual risk). With appropriate surgical intervention, the single surgery anatomic success rate approaches 90%, but the visual prognosis varies.

12.1.1 Common Symptoms

Common symptoms include rapid, monocular photopsias that occur for a few seconds, floaters, the abrupt appearance of floaters, loss of peripheral vision (often noticed as a "curtain" or "shade" over vision), and potentially central vision loss. Flashes and floaters will often precede the onset of vision loss, and most often reflect the initial development of a retinal tear prior to the subsequent retinal detachment.

12.1.2 Exam Findings

Clinical examination reveals subretinal fluid with an associated retinal break(s) (although the retinal break[s] may not always be readily identifiable). Additional potential findings include pigmented cell in the anterior vitreous (Shaffer's sign or tobacco dust), low intraocular pressure (due to drainage of subretinal fluid via sclerochoroidal drainage), one or more retinal breaks, areas of retinal thinning (lattice degeneration), and vitreous hemorrhage (often due to traction on a retinal vessel). Patients with chronic rhegmatogenous retinal detachments may exhibit proliferative vitreoretinopathy (PVR; due to unregulated proliferative of retinal pigment epithelial and glial cells, manifesting as starfolds, retinal contraction, retinal folds, or preretinal fibrosis), intraretinal cysts, retinal macrocysts, pigmented demarcation lines (reflecting RPE cells at the edge of slowly advancing subretinal fluid), and high intraocular pressure (due to Schwartz Matsuo syndrome where RPE cells block the trabecular meshwork).

12.2 Key Diagnostic Tests and Findings

12.2.1 Optical Coherence Tomography

Optical coherence tomography (OCT) may be helpful in diagnosis and is especially helpful to assess macular involvement. OCT can identify areas of shallow macular subretinal fluid and show its proximity to the fovea which may guide urgency of repair (▶ Fig. 12.1). Another potential finding with OCT includes the presence of a PVD, depending on the position of the posterior hyaloid. OCT can also show preexisting conditions such as epiretinal membrane, macular edema, macular degeneration, or myopic degeneration, which can be helpful to know preoperatively for visual prognosis. Postoperatively, OCT can be used to confirm resolution of subretinal fluid and evaluate the anatomic status of the fovea, including ellipsoid zone integrity and presence of cystoid macular edema.

12.2.2 Fundus Photography

With the advent of wide-angle imaging techniques, fundus photography is now being used increasingly to visualize/diagnose retinal detachments. Nonmydriatic widefield imaging may be particularly helpful for patients with poorly dilating pupils or nystagmus (▶ Fig. 12.2).

12.2.3 Ultrasonography

Occasionally, a retinal detachment is obscured by dense vitreous hemorrhage or other media opacity (e.g., cataract). For these cases, B-scan ultrasonography is necessary to identify retinal detachments. B-scan ultrasonography can help identify the location of a retinal tear in the absence of a retinal detachment, although tears are often subtle and easy to miss. In the setting of a spontaneous vitreous hemorrhage without retinal tear or detachment, the eye can be monitored with serial ultrasonography; if the eye develops a retinal detachment, intervention is imperative (▶ Fig. 12.3).

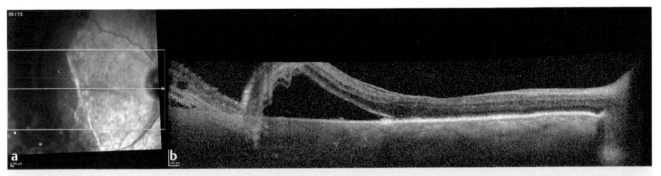

Fig. 12.1 Optical coherence tomography in retinal detachment. **(a)** En face imaging reveals temporal subretinal fluid in the macula, **(b)** while the cross-sectional B-scan shows fluid underneath the temporal macula, encroaching the fovea.

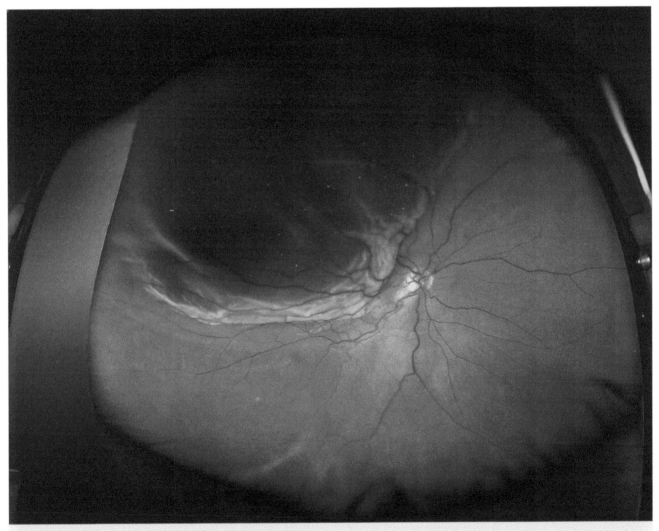

Fig. 12.2 Ultra-widefield fundus photograph of a macula-off retinal detachment. Fundus photography was used as an ancillary imaging tool due to a poorly dilating pupil and identified the superior retinal detachment.

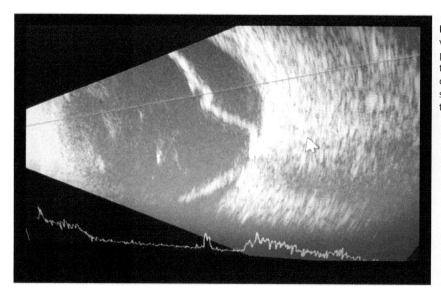

Fig. 12.3 B-scan ultrasonography for a dense vitreous hemorrhage without a view to the posterior pole. B-scan ultrasonography showed a total macula-off retinal detachment, with a corresponding A-scan cross vector overlay showing a spike of high reflectivity corresponding to the retinal detachment.

12.3 Critical Work-up

Primary diagnosis of retinal detachments relies on clinical examination, including a careful indirect ophthalmoscopic examination. Scleral depression can be helpful to visualize the ora serrata and identify all retinal breaks. Occasionally, additional imaging tests can be helpful for diagnosis. Rarely, there can be certain genetic conditions that can lead to a higher incidence of rhegmatogenous retinal detachment, such as Stickler, Marfan, Ehlers Danlos, or Wagner syndrome. If there is a strong family history of retinal detachment and any associated features of the above syndromes, genetic testing may be warranted.

12.4 Management

12.4.1 Treatment Options

Prevention

In phakic patients with retinal detachment, prophylactic laser retinopexy to lattice degeneration in the fellow eye can decrease the risk of retinal detachment in the fellow eye. Laser retinopexy should also be considered in eyes with acute symptoms and newly diagnosed retinal tears.

Laser Retinopexy

Localized retinal detachments that are asymptomatic (without noticeable peripheral visual loss) are often amenable to laser retinopexy. Typically, several rows of laser are applied with minimal spacing, encircling the retinal detachment to the ora serrata (▶ Fig. 12.4).

Pneumatic Retinopexy

Pneumatic retinopexy is an office-based procedure that can be used to repair certain retinal detachments. Patient selection is a key factor to achieving successful repair. Characteristics that increase likelihood of anatomic success after pneumatic retinopexy include the following:

- Isolated superior retinal breaks from 9 o'clock to 3 o'clock.
- Retinal breaks within 1 clock hour of each other.
- Phakic status.
- Presence of a PVD.
- Ability of patient to position.
- Absence of other peripheral retinal pathology, such as lattice degeneration.

Pneumatic retinopexy involves localizing the retinal break(s) and applying judicious cryotherapy to the edges of the retinal break(s) and then injecting an intravitreal gas bubble. Alternatively, gas can be injected initially to tamponade the break and flatten the retina, followed by laser photocoagulation to the flat break (▶ Fig. 12.5). Success of pneumatic retinopexy is not as high as traditional surgical interventions, but optimal patient selection can achieve high rates of success, up to 70 to 80%. Potential complications of pneumatic retinopexy include development of new tears requiring laser retinopexy or cryotherapy, failure to achieve anatomic success, or development of a new retinal detachment necessitating more invasive surgery.

Scleral Buckle

This operating room-based procedure involves an external approach, in which a thin silicone band is threaded underneath the rectus muscles for 360 degrees and placed underneath areas of retinal thinning and breaks. After tightening the band, vitreous traction is relieved, and the band is able to support the breaks, allowing for resorption of subretinal fluid. Cryotherapy of the retinal breaks and possible external drainage of fluid are often used in conjunction to achieve anatomic success. Good candidates for primary scleral buckling with or without radial elements involve the following:
- Younger individuals with clear lens.
- Extensive peripheral retinal pathology, such as lattice degeneration or retinal dialysis.
- Absence of significant media opacity, such as a dense cataract or vitreous hemorrhage.

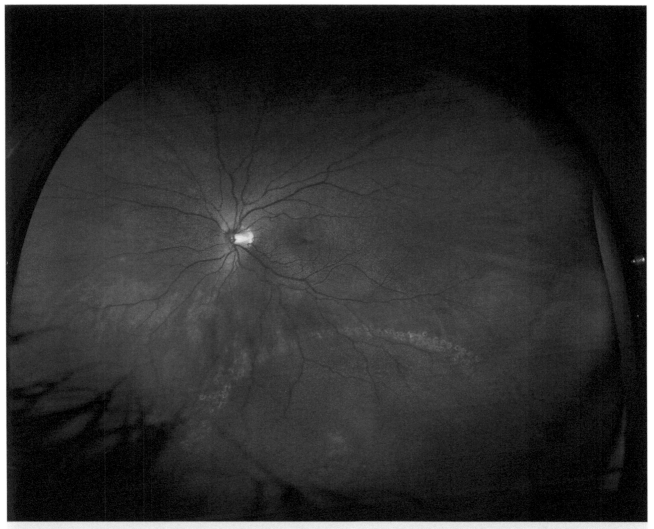

Fig. 12.4 Ultra-widefield fundus photograph of a highly myopic eye one month after laser retinopexy for an asymptomatic inferior retinal detachment from atrophic holes. The retinal detachment remains well barricaded by laser.

Induced myopia often occurs due to mechanical elongation of the globe. Anatomical success has been reported at around 90%. Potential complications of scleral buckle include failure to achieve anatomic success, transient diplopia, transient ptosis, and transient pain. Rarely, postoperative diplopia and ptosis can persist, and rarely buckle extrusion or infection can occur.

Pars Plana Vitrectomy

With the advent of smaller gauge vitrectomy systems and improved fluidics, pars plana vitrectomy is increasingly becoming the surgery of choice for retinal detachments. Vitrectomy involves an internal approach by creating three sclerotomies to access and visualize the internal structures of the eye, mechanically removing the vitreous gel, draining subretinal fluid, applying endolaser, and tamponading the retina with a complete gas bubble. Good candidates for vitrectomy involve the following:

- Presence of a PVD.
- Posterior break(s).
- Pseudophakic retinal detachments (▶ Fig. 12.2).

- Patients with vitreous hemorrhage obscuring retinal details.

After vitrectomy, postoperative cataract develops at high frequency. Success rates of vitrectomy have been reported from 82 to 95%. Potential complications include failure to achieve anatomic success, cataract formation, and transient intraocular pressure rise. Rare complications include infection, hypotony, glaucoma, choroidal detachments, and vitreous hemorrhage.

Combined Pars Plana Vitrectomy and Scleral Buckle

In certain circumstances, combined pars plana vitrectomy and scleral buckling procedures are used to achieve optimal single surgery success. Good candidates for a combined procedure include the following:

- Extensive pathology (e.g., numerous breaks, vitreous hemorrhage).
- Concerns for PVR.
- Patients with retinal detachments overlying retinoschisis (▶ Fig. 12.6).

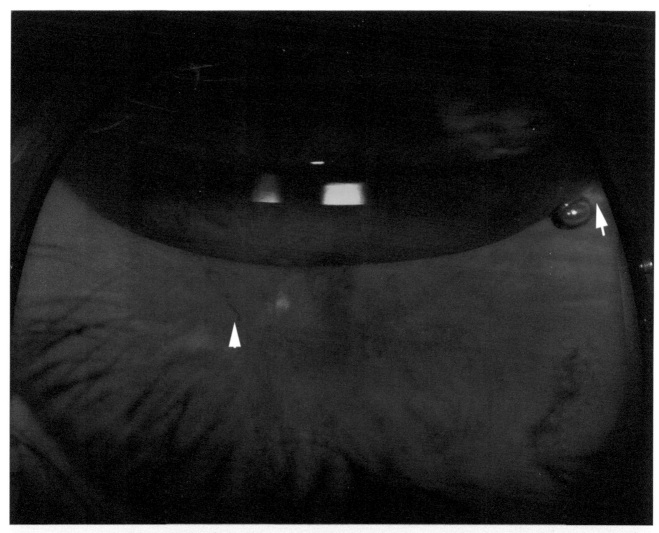

Fig. 12.5 Ultra-widefield fundus photograph one day after pneumatic retinopexy for a superior macula-off retinal detachment with a superotemporal tear. A large SF6 gas bubble can be seen in the vitreous cavity, with a small adjacent bubble. Early cryotherapy is visible in the superotemporal quadrant (*arrow*). Mild vitreous debris/hemorrhage is also noted (*arrowhead*).

Combined surgery has similar single-surgery success to primary pars plana vitrectomy, although some clinicians feel that that the scleral buckle can be helpful to prevent redetachments in these more complex detachments. Potential complications are similar to those for scleral buckle and vitrectomy.

12.4.2 Follow-up

Postoperative positioning is often needed to tamponade the retinal breaks while the retinopexy matures. The presence of the gas bubble in an eye precludes flying in an airplane or traveling to high altitudes to intraocular gas expansion at low atmospheric pressure and subsequent rise in intraocular pressure. Regardless of the type of intervention for retinal detachment, careful patient monitoring in the postoperative period is critical to ensure that subretinal fluid is resolving, to monitor for new retinal tears or detachments. While retinal redetachments are not common, swift recognition and management is critical to optimizing visual outcomes. Patients should be followed carefully during the first several months after intervention, and based on their progress, extended to longer intervals. Rarely, patients can develop postoperative cystoid macular edema, epiretinal membrane, cataract, or PVR, all of which may necessitate further treatment. Thereafter, all patients with a history of retinal detachment should have a biannual or annual exam, and should have a low threshold to call for any new symptoms of flashes, floaters, or changes in vision.

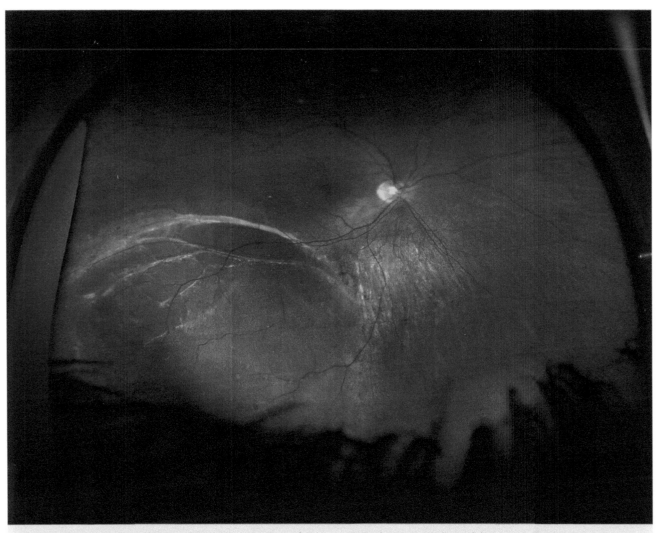

Fig. 12.6 Ultra-widefield fundus photograph of acute worsening of a chronic retinoschisis-associated retinal detachment. Multiple demarcation lines and subretinal proliferative vitreoretinopathy bands are present confirming chronicity.

Suggested Reading

[1] Sodhi A, Leung LS, Do DV, Gower EW, Schein OD, Handa JT. Recent trends in the management of rhegmatogenous retinal detachment. Surv Ophthalmol. 2008; 53(1):50–67

[2] Yoon YH, Marmor MF. Rapid enhancement of retinal adhesion by laser photo-coagulation. Ophthalmology. 1988; 95(10):1385–1388

[3] Goldman DR, Shah CP, Heier JS. Expanded criteria for pneumatic retinopexy and potential cost savings. Ophthalmology. 2014; 121(1):318–326

[4] Noori J, Bilonick RA, Eller AW. Scleral buckle surgery for primary retinal detachment without posterior vitreous detachment. Retina. 2016; 36(11): 2066–2071

[5] Orlin A, Hewing NJ, Nissen M, et al. Pars plana vitrectomy compared with pars plana vitrectomy combined with scleral buckle in the primary management of noncomplex rhegmatogenous retinal detachment. Retina. 2014; 34(6): 1069–1075

13 Giant Retinal Tear

Daniel Su and Allen Ho

Summary

Giant retinal tears (GRTs) are full-thickness breaks in the retina extending for more than 3 clock hours. They occur due to dynamic vitreous traction where there are areas of retinal abnormality. Currently, the main surgical approach to management of GRT associated retinal detachments is pars plana vitrectomy with or without a scleral buckle. Due to the reported incidence of a retinal tear in the fellow eyes of GRTs being relatively high, especially in patients with inherited vitreoretinal degenerations, prophylactic treatment of any peripheral breaks or lattice degeneration in the fellow eye should be considered.

Keywords: giant retinal tear, posterior vitreous detachment, proliferative vitreoretinopathy

13.1 Features

Giant retinal tears (GRTs) are full-thickness breaks in the retina extending for more than 3 clock hours (▶ Fig. 13.1). Patients with a GRT present with symptoms associated with the corresponding retinal detachment. GRTs can be quite large and may even extend for 360 degrees. The risk of proliferative vitreoretinopathy (PVR) is increased in the setting of GRT due to greater access of retinal pigment epithelial cells to the vitreous cavity; extensive membranes can form on both sides of the retina. Diffuse proliferation may result in a closed-funnel configuration because of unrestrained contraction of the large retinal flaps.

13.1.1 Common Symptoms

Floaters, photopsia, and peripheral visual field cuts that can progress to central vision loss.

13.1.2 Exam Findings

It is important to differentiate GRTs from retinal dialyses due to differences in pathogenesis with implications for surgical management. The posterior flap of the tear in a GRT has a tendency to fold over in a "taco formation" because of the associated posterior vitreous detachment (PVD), especially if the GRT extends near 180 degrees in circumference. Retinal tissue is present anterior to the GRT location. A retinal dialysis, on the other hand, is most often associated with blunt trauma and the retinal break occurs at the ora serrata with an avulsed vitreous base. The posterior flap in a dialysis does not typically fold over and may be relatively immobile due to the overlying vitreous base. There is no retinal tissue anterior to the retinal break in a dialysis due to its location at the ora.

The configuration of GRTs and extent of the associated retinal detachments vary widely. Larger tears result in more rapidly spreading retinal detachments due to easier access of fluid to the subretinal space. Radial extensions (horns) can occur at the edges of the GRT, and the resulting retinal flap may have a higher tendency to fold over. Radial tears are more likely to be associated with vitreous hemorrhage due to larger retinal vessels in their path.

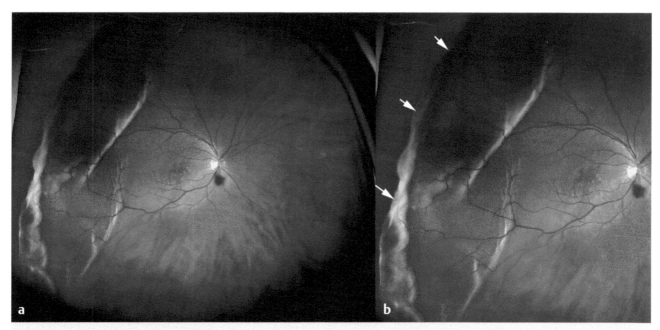

Fig. 13.1 (a) Ultra-widefield photograph demonstrating giant retinal tear (GRT) with macula involving retinal detachment and **(b)** high-magnification view of the edge (*arrows*) of the GRT extending for approximately 5 to 6 clock hours.

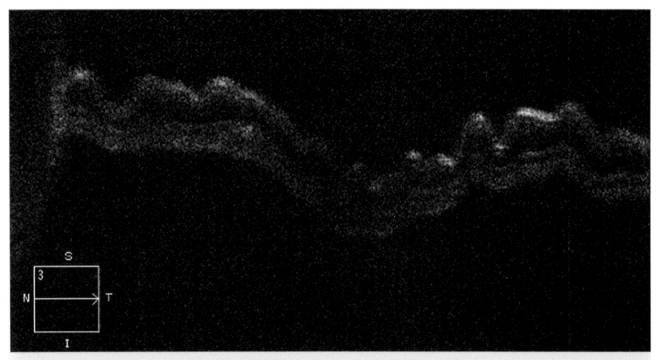

Fig. 13.2 Optical coherence tomography of a giant retinal tear folded over (i.e., inverted) showing the photoreceptor layers toward the top of the image and the inner retinal layers at the bottom of the image due to the inverted retinal flap.

13.2 Key Diagnostic Tests and Findings

13.2.1 Optical Coherence Tomography

Optical coherence tomography (OCT) is generally not necessary but may provide information regarding macular status. OCT may also facilitate identification of retinal inversion in cases of significant retinal folding (▶ Fig. 13.2).

13.2.2 Fundus Photography

Preoperative documentation of extent of retinal detachment is now feasible with ultra-widefield imaging.

13.2.3 Ultrasonography

B-scan ultrasonography may be useful in cases of vitreous hemorrhage or media opacity with limited visibility. Double linear echoes may be seen in cases of a rolled over flap of retina from the GRT.

13.3 Critical Work-up

Perform careful indirect ophthalmoscopy with scleral depression and a thorough examination of both the anterior and posterior segments including cornea and lens status.

13.4 Management

13.4.1 Treatment Options

Surgical Technique

Currently, the main surgical approach to management of GRT-associated retinal detachments is pars plana vitrectomy with or without a scleral buckle (▶ Fig. 13.3). Perfluorocarbon liquids is particularly useful in cases of retinal folding. Endolaser photocoagulation is applied to the areas of pathology. A major concern during surgical repair of GRT retinal detachments is slippage of the posterior flap during air-fluid exchange. Silicone oil and a long-acting gas such as C_3F_8 are the most common tamponade agents in GRT retinal detachments. In the presence of PVR or an inferior GRT, silicone oil may be more appropriate. Short-acting gases such as SF_6 provide inadequate support for GRT detachments and have been associated with higher re-detachment rates. The placement of a scleral buckle in addition to vitrectomy in the setting of a GRT is still a topic of debate. In the presence of PVR, most surgeons would consider adding a scleral buckle to counteract against the contraction forces of PVR.

Fellow Eye Management

The incidence of a retinal tear in the fellow eyes of GRTs is relatively high. Many surgeons advocate for prophylactic treatment of any peripheral breaks or lattice degeneration in the fellow eye.

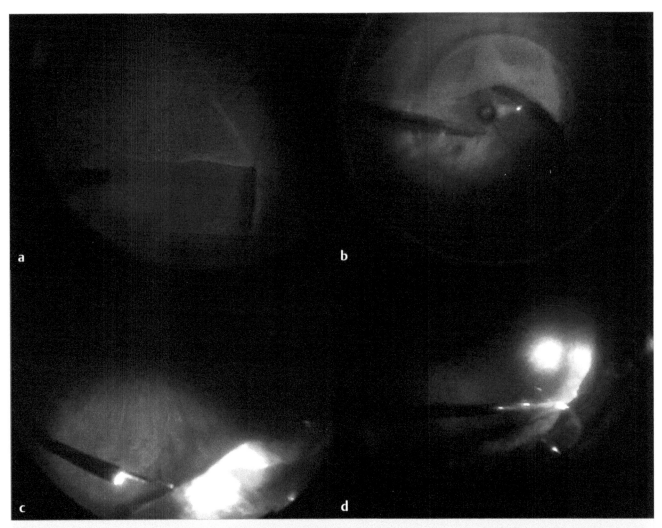

Fig. 13.3 Intraoperative photograph of a giant retinal tear (GRT) extending for 5 clock hours with the posterior flap folded over. **(a)** The vitreous cutter is visualized in the image. **(b)** Intraoperative photograph of a near 180-degree GRT being unfolded with the instillation of perfluorocarbon liquid under the posterior flap. **(c)** Intraoperative photograph of endolaser being applied to the edge of a GRT under perfluorocarbon liquid tamponade. **(d)** Intraoperative photograph of an air-fluid exchange being performed with the extrusion cannula at the edge of the GRT.

Suggested Reading

[1] Ryan SJ. Retina. 3rd ed. St. Louis, MO: Mosby; 2001

[2] Pitcher JD, III, Khan MA, Storey PP, et al. Contemporary management of rhegmatogenous retinal detachment due to giant retinal tears: a consecutive case series. Ophthalmic Surg Lasers Imaging Retina. 2015; 46(5):566–570

[3] Gonzalez MA, Flynn HW, Jr, Smiddy WE, Albini TA, Tenzel P. Surgery for retinal detachment in patients with giant retinal tear: etiologies, management strategies, and outcomes. Ophthalmic Surg Lasers Imaging Retina. 2013; 44 (3):232–237

[4] Berrocal MH, Chenworth ML, Acaba LA. Management of giant retinal tear detachments. J Ophthalmic Vis Res. 2017; 12(1):93–97

14 Retinal Dialysis

Maxwell S. Stem and Jeremy D. Wolfe

Summary

A retinal dialysis may occur following ocular trauma and is defined as a separation between the retina and the pars plana at the ora serrata. A dialysis may or may not be associated with a retinal detachment. Care must be taken to distinguish a dialysis from a giant retinal tear, as the natural history and treatments are different for the two conditions. The prognosis for retinal reattachment for patients with a retinal dialysis is excellent; such patients are typically treated with laser retinopexy or scleral buckling and the final anatomic success rate is more than 95%.

Keywords: retinal dialysis, retinal detachment, scleral buckle, trauma, ora serrata, pars plana

14.1 Features

A retinal dialysis is defined histologically and clinically as a separation between the neurosensory retina and the nonpigmented pars plana epithelium at the ora serrata (► Fig. 14.1). While idiopathic and familial causes of retinal dialysis have been reported, the most common etiology is ocular trauma. Young adult men comprise the majority of retinal dialysis patients, and the most common location for a dialysis to occur is the inferotemporal quadrant of the retina.

The natural history of untreated retinal dialyses is evolution to a retinal detachment, which can occur coinciding with or years after the initial injury that caused the retinal dialysis. There is often an interval of several months or even years between an initial eye injury/retinal dialysis and the onset of a symptomatic retinal detachment. This is likely because retinal dialyses tend to occur in younger patients with a formed vitreous, which helps guard against the occurrence of a coexistent retinal detachment. However, as the vitreous liquefies with age and gains entrance to the subretinal space, patients may progress to a symptomatic retinal detachment.

14.1.1 Common Symptoms

Patients with a retinal dialysis who lack other ocular pathology may be totally asymptomatic; if the dialysis is associated with a retinal detachment or avulsion of the vitreous base, the patient may complain of floaters or a blind spot in their vision (► Fig. 14.2). Patients may have symptoms, such as decreased vision, unrelated to the dialysis but are due instead to coincident ocular pathology secondary to the trauma (e.g., commotio retinae, traumatic optic neuropathy, macular hole, vitreous hemorrhage, and hyphema).

14.1.2 Exam Findings

Indirect ophthalmoscopy with scleral depression can provide a definitive diagnosis of a retinal dialysis. The dialysis is seen as a slit or broad separation between the retina and the pars plana at the level of the ora serrata. There may be subretinal fluid associated with the dialysis, especially if the vitreous base has avulsed (which can be seen as a thick, tortuous rope-like structure overlying the area of dialysis) or part of the vitreous is liquefied (as in older patients).

At times it may be difficult to differentiate a giant retinal tear (GRT) from a retinal dialysis, but it is important to make this distinction due to differences in the natural history and management of each condition. A GRT is defined as a retinal tear that extends for 3 or more clock hours. GRTs occur in association with a posterior vitreous detachment and are found at the posterior edge of the vitreous base. Thus, in GRTs, there is always a strip of retina anterior to the tear, and the junction between the retina and the pars plana remains intact (unlike in a retinal dialysis). Furthermore, since the retina posterior to the tear in a GRT is no longer affixed to any vitreous scaffolding, it may fold over on itself and obscure other areas of the fundus. In contrast, the vitreous often remains attached to the retina in a retinal dialysis, which prevents the retina from folding over on itself.

14.2 Key Diagnostic Tests and Findings

14.2.1 Optical Coherence Tomography

Optical coherence tomography is not utilized for the diagnosis for retinal dialysis, but may be useful for evaluation of concurrent pathology associated with trauma and to assess macular status/anatomy prior to proceeding with surgery.

14.2.2 Ultra-Widefield Fundus Photography

Ultra-widefield photography may be utilized to document the presence of a dialysis and/or retinal detachment.

14.3 Critical Work-up

Patients suspected of having a retinal dialysis require a careful history and complete examination of both eyes. The history should focus on whether there was ever any trauma to the globe or orbit, and a complete family ocular history should be obtained. A thorough eye examination should be performed, and in cases of suspected trauma, it is imperative to rule out a ruptured globe. In cases of acute trauma with evidence of motility deficits, suspected ruptured globe, or potential foreign body, an orbital CT scan is an indispensable part of the work-up to search for potential foreign bodies and orbital fractures.

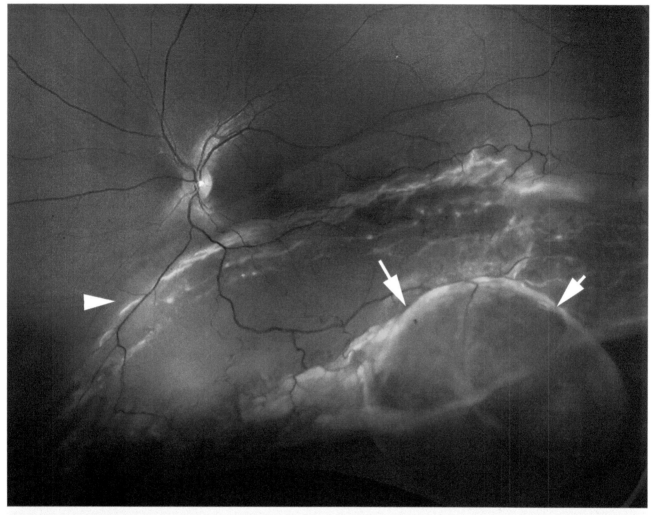

Fig. 14.1 Ultra-widefield photograph of a chronic retinal detachment secondary to a retinal dialysis with subretinal fluid extending posteriorly (*arrowhead*) and retinal microcyst (*arrows*).

14.4 Management

14.4.1 Treatment Options

Retinopexy

Generally, small, isolated retinal dialyses with no or very minimal subretinal fluid can be successfully treated with laser demarcation. Cryotherapy can be used as an alternative, particularly when there is slightly more subretinal fluid present, but is generally less favored due to its potential to increase intraocular inflammation.

Surgical

Patients who have a retinal dialysis with associated retinal detachment typically require surgery with cryotherapy and placement of a segmental or encircling scleral buckle (▶ Fig. 14.3). External drainage of subretinal fluid is may be performed if significant subretinal fluid remains despite support

from the buckle. In younger patients, the vitreous base often acts as a tamponade minimizing the need for an intraocular gas bubble. The prognosis for patients with retinal dialysis is excellent with regard to anatomic success (i.e., reattachment of the retina), with most series reporting a success rate more than 95%. Proliferative vitreoretinopathy rarely complicates retinal detachment associated with retinal dialysis, but when it does occur the success rate following surgery is predictably reduced.

14.5 Follow-up

Patients are followed up closely following initial trauma for ongoing surveillance for retinal dialysis visualization, particularly in patients with media opacity at the time of trauma. Following retinopexy or surgical repair, patients are also followed up closely to confirm successful healing and repair. Once stabilized, follow-up interval can be extended. Patients should be counseled on the warning signs of retinal detachment formation (e.g., floaters, flashes, and peripheral vision loss).

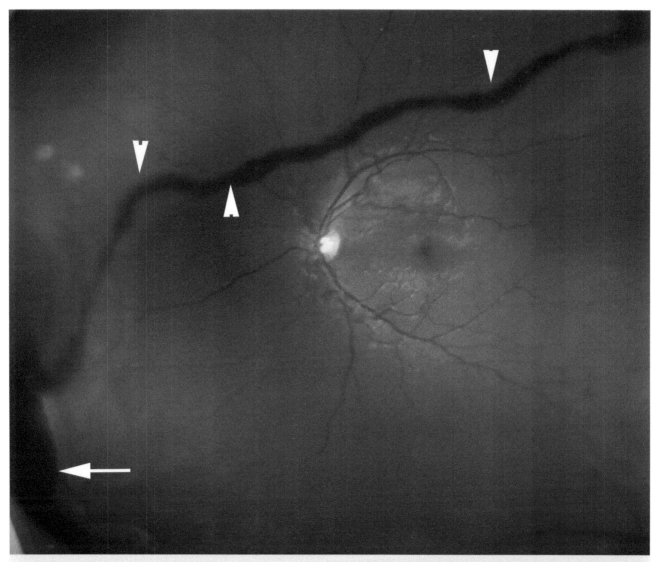

Fig. 14.2 Ultra-widefield fundus photograph of a traumatic retinal dialysis with avulsion of the vitreous base. The free edge of retina can be seen nasally (*arrow*), and the avulsed vitreous base is represented by the dark, rope-like structure in the superior portion of the photograph (*arrowheads*).

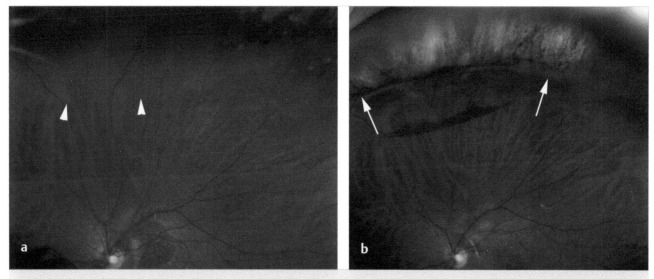

Fig. 14.3 Ultra-widefield fundus photographs of a traumatic retinal dialysis with retinal detachment (*arrowheads*) (**a**) before and (**b**) after surgery with segmental scleral buckle (*arrows*) and cryotherapy.

Suggested Reading

[1] Kennedy CJ, Parker CE, McAllister IL. Retinal detachment caused by retinal dialysis. Aust N Z J Ophthalmol. 1997; 25(1):25–30

[2] Ross WH. Traumatic retinal dialyses. Arch Ophthalmol. 1981; 99(8):1371–1374

15 Proliferative Vitreoretinopathy

Jeremy A. Lavine and Justis P. Ehlers

Summary

Proliferative vitreoretinopathy (PVR) is the most common cause for failure of retinal detachment (RD) repair surgery. In patients with PVR, the retina detaches due to epiretinal proliferation of scar tissue, which contracts over time, causing tractional retinal detachment or stretch holes, resulting in combined tractional and rhegmatogenous RD. Patients experience painless visual field loss that may progress to central vision with or without flashes of light and floaters in the vision. Examination often identifies vitreous haze or pigment, epiretinal proliferation, retinal breaks, retinal detachment, and/or subretinal bands. Ancillary testing includes optical coherence tomography to identify epiretinal membranes and B-scan ultrasonography to evaluate retinal stiffness and mobility. Treatment options include careful observation for patients with asymptomatic small peripheral tractional changes or surgical repair. Surgical repair of PVR-associated RD typically includes removal of the crystalline lens (if present), scleral buckling (if not previously performed), and pars plana vitrectomy. During pars plana vitrectomy, key steps include separation and removal of the posterior hyaloid (if still present), core vitrectomy, shaving of the vitreous base, removal of epiretinal proliferative tissue, relaxing retinectomy if necessary to flatten the retina, laser photocoagulation, and tamponade with silicone oil or perfluoropropane.

Keywords: retinal pigment epithelium, retinal detachment, star folds, epiretinal proliferation, subretinal strands

15.1 Features

Proliferative vitreoretinopathy (PVR) is a disease where epiretinal membranes form on the surface of the retina, creating traction and ultimately retinal detachment (RD). PVR is the most common cause of failed primary rhegmatogenous RD repair, causing recurrent tractional or combined tractional and rhegmatogenous RD. The molecular pathophysiology is poorly understood. Surgical histopathology studies identify retinal pigment epithelial (RPE) cells, glial cells, and macrophages within the epiretinal membranes. The current hypothesis is that RPE cells undergo transdifferentiation into glial or fibroblast-like cells on the surface of the retina, proliferate, and ultimately contract, causing tractional RD or creating retinal stretch holes, leading to combined tractional and rhegmatogenous RD.

15.1.1 Common Symptoms

Painless vision loss, sometimes associated with flashing lights or floaters in the vision. In the setting of chronic RD with PVR, symptoms include peripheral visual field loss that may progress centrally. Due to the predilection for inferior pathology, superior visual field loss may be a presenting symptom. The most frequent time of presentation is 1 to 3 months after primary RD surgery.

15.1.2 Exam Findings

Examination begins with assessment of the lens. Due to the need to maximize vitreous base shaving and peripheral membrane peeling, phakic individuals are typically made pseudophakic. Next, the vitreous is assessed, identifying haze and pigment clumps in the vitreous or on the retina surface (▶ Fig. 15.1, *white circle*), which are defining features of grade A PVR (Table 15-1). In patients with recurrent RD, identification of residual vitreous strands/traction and evaluation of the vitreous base for contracture or anterior displacement define grade CA PVR (Table 15-1). Careful scrutiny of the retinal surface in patients with grade B PVR will identify wrinkling of the retinal surface (▶ Fig. 15.2a, *white arrowhead*), retinal stiffness, vessel tortuosity (▶ Fig. 15.2a, *white arrow*), and rolled or irregular edges (▶ Fig. 15.1; ▶ Fig. 15.2a, *white arrows*) of the retinal break(s) (Table 15-1). In patients with grade C PVR, full-thickness retinal folds often called star folds (▶ Fig. 15.1, *white arrowhead*) and subretinal strands (▶ Fig. 15.3c) can be identified. Assessment of the location of star folds, will classify grade C PVR as anterior (grade CA) or posterior (grade CP) to the equator (Table 15-1).

15.2 Key Diagnostic Tests and Findings

15.2.1 Optical Coherence Tomography

Hyperreflectivities in the vitreous (grade A PVR), wrinkling of the inner retinal surface (grade B PVR), and membranes on the retinal surface (▶ Fig. 15.3d) or in the subretinal (▶ Fig. 15.3c) space (grade C PVR). Optical coherence tomography can be helpful to delineate location of bands and possible location of dissection planes. In addition, the macular status and retinal anatomic integrity can be potentially evaluated.

15.2.2 Fundus Photography

Can function as a useful adjunct to the examination and for preoperative planning. Ultra-widefield fundus photography can be particularly useful to follow progression of PVR and identify features that may be less apparent on examination.

15.2.3 Ultrasonography

In patients with poor media clarity, B-scan ultrasonography can be essential to the diagnosis of PVR. On kinetic ultrasonography, retinal stiffness (▶ Fig. 15.2b) can be identified, suggesting the presence of PVR. Other features suggestive of PVR include a funnel-shaped RD with apposition of posterior retina or anterior membranes which bridge the mouth of the funnel.

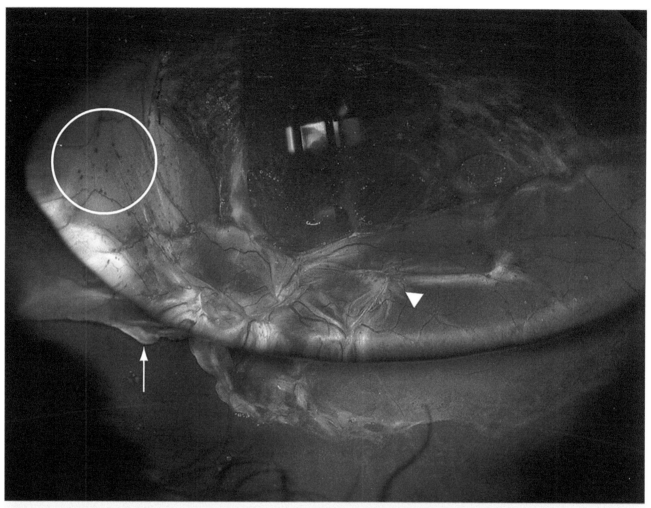

Fig. 15.1 Ultra-widefield fundus photograph of a postvitrectomy eye with partial silicone oil fill with the arcuate meniscus visible across the middle of the image. Areas of grade A proliferative vitreoretinopathy (PVR) are highlighted by the white circle with pigment clumps on the retina surface. Areas of grade B PVR are shown by the white arrow, demonstrating rolled edges of the inferior retinal break. An area of grade CP PVR with a full-thickness star fold is identified by the arrowhead.

15.3 Management

15.3.1 Treatment Options

There are currently no medical therapies for PVR. Multiple clinical trials have evaluated adjunctive treatments to RD surgical repair to prevent PVR in primary surgical cases or prevent recurrent PVR in complex RD repairs. To date, intravitreal steroids, daunorubicin, and heparin with 5-fluorouracil have been ineffective to prevent or reduce PVR recurrence.

The only current treatment options for PVR include careful observation (e.g., for grade B-CP PVR without RD or asymptomatic peripheral tractional RD) and surgical treatment for PVR with significant recurrent RD. The surgical approach begins with addressing the crystalline lens, if present. It is recommended to proceed with lens extraction with intraocular lens implantation to improve visualization of the retina and aid dissection of the vitreous base. If not already present, a scleral buckle should be considered to reduce peripheral retinal traction and support the vitreous base. Next, pars plana vitrectomy is performed with separation and removal of the posterior hyaloid (if still present), core vitrectomy, and shaving of the vitreous base. Subsequently, dissection of epiretinal membranes should be accomplished to remove all retinal traction. If large breaks are created or epiretinal membranes are too extensive for removal, peripheral relaxing retinectomy (► Fig. 15.3b) should be completed to enable flattening of the retina. Once the retina is flat, laser photocoagulation is applied to the retinal breaks and/or retinectomy edges. Based upon the results of the silicone oil study, perfluoropropane (C_3F_8) or silicone oil should be used for tamponade, and not sulfur hexafluoride (SF_6) due to its inferior outcomes.

15.3.2 Follow-up

Patients with PVR without RD should be closely followed up at short intervals to identify progression and possible need for surgery. Patients with grade C PVR will typically require surgical repair and are then followed up in the standard postoperative manner.

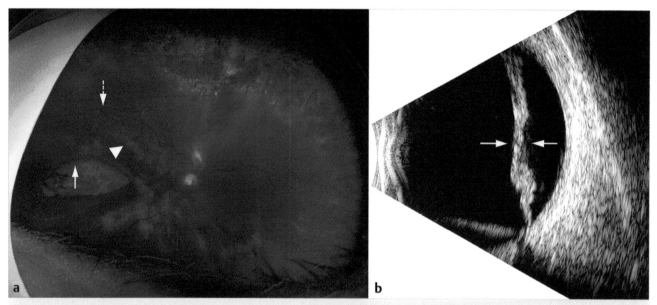

Fig. 15.2 (a) Ultra-widefield fundus photograph of a post-vitrectomy eye with a large temporal retinal break with rolled edges (*arrow*), retinal wrinkling (*arrowhead*), and vessel tortuosity (*dashed arrow*). (b) B-scan ultrasonography shows thickened retina (*between white arrows*) and stiffness of this area on kinetic ultrasound.

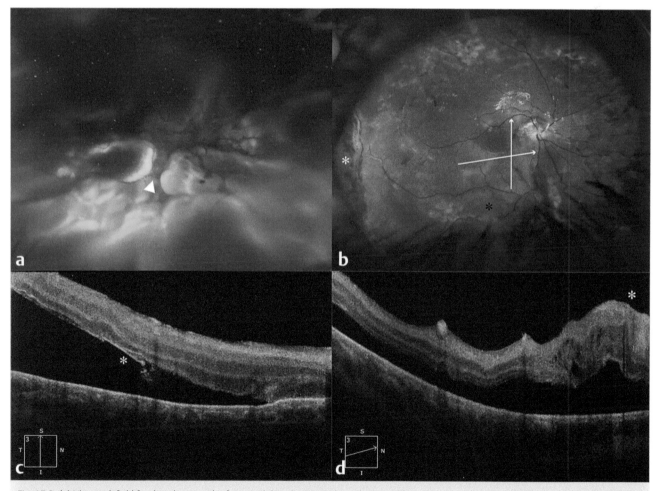

Fig. 15.3 (a) Ultra-widefield fundus photograph of a retinal detachment with grade CP proliferative vitreoretinopathy (PVR) (*star folds, arrowhead*). (b) Ultra-widefield fundus photograph post-vitrectomy with a silicone oil-filled vitreous cavity, temporal retinectomy (*white asterisk*), inferior subretinal fluid (*black asterisk*), and (c,d) recurrent PVR. The *white arrows* demonstrate the location of the optical coherence tomography (OCT). (c) Vertical OCT showing subretinal membranes (*asterisk*) and subretinal fluid. (d) Horizontal OCT identifying epiretinal membranes (*asterisk*) and subretinal fluid.

Table 15.1 Classification system for PVR

Grade	Features
A	Vitreous haze, vitreous pigment clumps, pigment clusters on inferior retina
B	Wrinkling of inner retinal surface, retinal stiffness, vessel tortuosity, rolled and irregular edge of retinal break, decreased mobility of vitreous
CP (1–12)	Posterior to equator: focal, diffuse, or circumferential full-thickness retinal folds or subretinal strands expressed in total numbers of clock hours involved
CA (1–12)	Anterior to equator: focal, diffuse, or circumferential full-thickness retinal folds, subretinal strands, or anterior displacement of the vitreous base expressed in total numbers of clock hours involved. Condensed vitreous strands

Abbreviation: PVR, proliferative vitreoretinopathy.

Suggested Reading

[1] Banerjee PJ, Quartilho A, Bunce C, et al. Slow-release dexamethasone in proliferative vitreoretinopathy: a prospective, randomized controlled clinical trial. Ophthalmology. 2017; 124(6):757–767

[2] Wiedemann P, Hilgers RD, Bauer P, Heimann K, Daunomycin Study Group. Adjunctive daunorubicin in the treatment of proliferative vitreoretinopathy: results of a multicenter clinical trial. Am J Ophthalmol. 1998; 126(4):550–559

[3] Wickham L, Bunce C, Wong D, McGurn D, Charteris DG. Randomized controlled trial of combined 5-Fluorouracil and low-molecular-weight heparin in the management of unselected rhegmatogenous retinal detachments undergoing primary vitrectomy. Ophthalmology. 2007; 114(4):698–704

[4] Group TSS. Vitrectomy with silicone oil or sulfur hexafluoride gas in eyes with severe proliferative vitreoretinopathy: results of a randomized clinical trial. Silicone Study Report 1. Arch Ophthalmol. 1992; 110(6):770–779

[5] Machemer R, Aaberg TM, Freeman HM, Irvine AR, Lean JS, Michels RM. An updated classification of retinal detachment with proliferative vitreoretinopathy. Am J Ophthalmol. 1991; 112(2):159–165

16 Retinoschisis

Yuji Itoh

Summary

Retinoschisis is the splitting within the layers of the retina. There are many pathophysiological conditions that cause retinoschisis, such as X-linked retinoschisis, myopic retinoschisis, optic disc anomalies (e.g., optic pit), and degenerative retinoschisis. Multiple elements may be helpful for diagnosis including family history, fundus findings, optical coherence tomography image, electroretinogram, fluorescein angiography. Initial management is often observation, but may involve surgical intervention depending on the clinical features.

Keywords: degenerative retinoschisis, optic disc pit, retinoschisis, X-linked retinoschisis

16.1 Features

Retinoschisis is a pathological retinal condition characterized by abnormal splitting of the neural retina. There are many categories and pathophysiological conditions that cause retinoschisis. General classification of retinoschisis can be considered as degenerative, hereditary, tractional, and exudative. The location of schisis also varies from foveal to peripheral. Retinoschisis may also be a finding (rather than the primary disorder) in various conditions including tractional changes in proliferative diabetic retinopathy and exudative changes in severe neovascular age-related macular degeneration. X-linked retinoschisis is associated with the mutations of RS1 gene, characterized by macular retinoschisis, peripheral schisis, and electroretinogram changes including negative pattern.

The macular retinoschisis is also characterized by foveal microcysts in a spoke–wheel pattern and the spoke–wheel-like appearance in the inner retina is found in all cases of X-linked retinoschisis. Peripheral retinoschisis is present in around half of the cases of X-linked retinoschisis. This chapter will focus on degenerative and hereditary X-linked retinoschisis.

16.1.1 Common Symptoms

May be asymptomatic. Visual acuity loss and visual field loss may be present. Absolute scotoma in the area of the schisis.

16.1.2 Exam Findings

Degenerative Retinoschisis

Peripheral retinal exam demonstrates inner retinal elevation that may be low-lying or bullous. The elevation tends to be smooth without corrugations, in contrast to retinal detachment. This can occur anywhere in the retinal periphery but is most common in the inferotemporal quadrant. Scleral depressed exam does not result in apposition of the retina to the retinal pigment epithelium (RPE) and decreased height of the elevation. Outer retinal holes may be present. Pigmentary changes are uncommon. Yellow–white surface dots may be present in the area of the schisis (▶ Fig. 16.1; ▶ Fig. 16.2).

Hereditary X-Linked Retinoschisis

Nearly all patients have foveal schisis that is seen as a spoke–wheel pattern emanating from the fovea (▶ Fig. 16.3). Extension of the schisis out into the retinal periphery may be present. Other findings include subretinal fibrosis, vascular attenuation, and retinal flecks.

16.2 Key Diagnostic Tests and Findings

16.2.1 Optical Coherence Tomography

Degenerative Retinoschisis

Peripheral optical coherence tomography (OCT) can be a critical diagnostic test to identify retinal splitting and confirming the diagnosis of retinoschisis with persistent apposition of the outer retina to the RPE (▶ Fig. 16.2). OCT helps to definitively distinguish between retinal detachment and retinoschisis. OCT may also demonstrate outer retinal breaks and conversion to a schisis detachment (▶ Fig. 16.4).

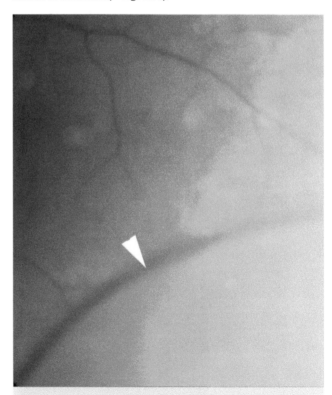

Fig. 16.1 Fundus photograph of bullous degenerative retinoschisis (*arrowhead*) in the inferotemporal periphery.

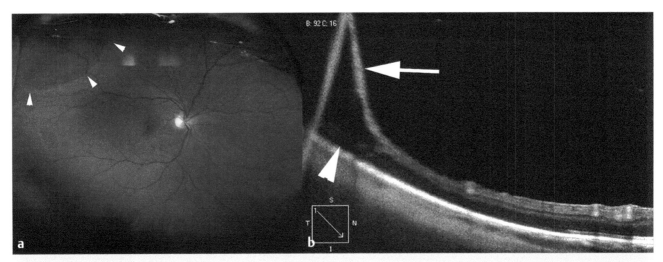

Fig. 16.2 (a) Ultra-widefield fundus photograph of superotemporal bullous degenerative retinoschisis (*arrowhead*). (b) Peripheral optical coherence tomography demonstrating peripheral retinal splitting with elevation of the inner retina (*arrow*) and stable attachment of the outer retina to the retinal pigment epithelium (*arrowhead*).

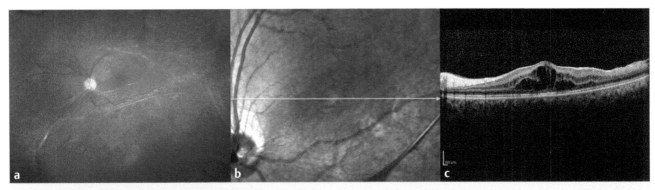

Fig. 16.3 (a) Ultra-widefield fundus photograph (left) in X-linked juvenile retinoschisis with macular and peripheral changes with fibrosis and multiple areas of retinoschisis. (b) Near-infrared and (c) spectral domain optical coherence tomography of the same eye demonstrating foveal cystic changes.

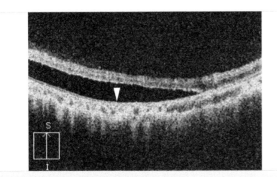

Fig. 16.4 Peripheral optical coherence tomography demonstrating conversion to retinal detachment with definitive subretinal fluid (*arrowhead*) rather than retinal splitting.

Hereditary X-Linked Retinoschisis

OCT demonstrates inner retinal schisis and splitting with cystic hyporeflective spaces in the fovea (▶ Fig. 16.3). Peripheral retinal splitting may also be identified.

16.2.2 Fluorescein Angiography or Ultra-Widefield Fluorescein Angiography

Hereditary X-Linked Retinoschisis

Fluorescein angiography characteristically demonstrates non-leaking cystoid macular edema.

16.2.3 Electroretinography

Typically shows electronegative waveform (reduced b-wave amplitude with a relatively preserved a-wave amplitude) in mixed rod and cone electroretinography in X-linked retinoschisis.

16.2.4 Fundus Photography

Fundus photography can be useful for documenting location and extent of retinoschisis for monitoring for progression.

16.2.5 Goldmann Perimetry

The visual field defect associated with peripheral retinoschisis is absolute scotoma in the field corresponding to the location of peripheral retinoschisis (more precipitous compared to retinal detachment).

16.3 Critical Work-up

Multiple elements are helpful to diagnosis including family history, fundus findings, OCT image, electroretinogram, fluorescein angiography. Genetic testing may be considered for the RS1 (retinoschisin) gene for X-linked retinoschisis.

16.4 Management

16.4.1 Treatment Options

Degenerative Retinoschisis

The vast majority of cases remain stable and are able to just be observed. The development of a progressive rhegmatogenous retinal detachment is uncommon. If a progressive retinal detachment develops, surgical repair is indicated. Surgical repair may include scleral buckle and/or vitrectomy.

Hereditary X-Linked Retinoschisis

Medical therapy with topical or systemic carbonic anhydrase inhibitors may be considered for the management of foveal cystic changes. Gene therapy is currently being evaluated as a potential future therapy. Surgical intervention is indicated for development of retinal detachment or vitreous hemorrhage.

Suggested Reading

[1] Zimmerman LE, Spencer WH. The pathologic anatomy of retinoschisis with a report of two cases diagnosed clinically as malignant melanoma. Arch Ophthalmol. 1960; 63:10–19

[2] Strupaitė R, Ambrozaitytė L, Cimbalistienė L, Ašoklis R, Utkus A. X-linked juvenile retinoschisis: phenotypic and genetic characterization. Int J Ophthalmol. 2018; 11(11):1875–1878

[3] Molday RS, Kellner U, Weber BH. X-linked juvenile retinoschisis: clinical diagnosis, genetic analysis, and molecular mechanisms. Prog Retin Eye Res. 2012; 31(3):195–212

17 Lattice Degeneration

Jennifer C.W. Hu and Justis P. Ehlers

Summary

Lattice degeneration is a peripheral retinal finding with associated retinal thinning, hyalinization of retinal vessels, and increased vitreous adherence at the margins of degenerative changes. It is an important risk factor in the development of retinal tears and retinal detachment. Lattice degeneration is asymptomatic, but it may be associated with conditions that cause floaters or photopsias. Widefield/peripheral optical coherence tomography can reveal anterior and posterior vitreous separation over areas of lattice as well as the irregular nature of the retinal thinning. Regular follow-up and examination of the fellow eye is recommended.

Keywords: lattice degeneration, posterior vitreous detachment, retinal tear, rhegmatogenous retinal detachment, vitreoretinal traction

17.1 Features

Lattice degeneration is a peripheral retinal condition in which there is retinal thinning, possible hyalinization of retinal vessels creating a "lattice" appearance, and increased vitreoretinal adhesion. Patients with lattice degeneration are at an increased risk for retinal tears and rhegmatogenous retinal detachment. Lattice degeneration can be associated with two types of retinal breaks: round atrophic holes (full-thickness breaks with no associated free operculum and no posterior vitreous detachment, PVD) and those associated with tractional tears (usually located at the border of lattice lesions).

17.1.1 Common Symptoms

Asymptomatic but associated with conditions such as PVD, retinal tears, detachments, or vitreoretinal traction, which may cause floaters or photopsias.

17.1.2 Exam Findings

Morphology can be quite varied. The shape of the lattice degeneration can be round, oval, or linear and it tends to be located near the equator of the retina or between the equator and the vitreous base. It tends to be oriented parallel to the ora serrata (in a circumferentially oriented pattern). Lattice degeneration derives its name from the whitish lines which represent hyalinized retinal vessels, though this is not always present. Other features include superficial whitish yellow flecks, patches of varying degrees of pigmentation, and small atrophic round holes.

17.2 Key Diagnostic Tests and Findings

17.2.1 Optical Coherence Tomography

Optical coherence tomography (OCT) is not typically performed or necessary for diagnosis. However, OCT may identify focal areas of traction, retinal thinning, and disruption of retinal tissue in areas of retinal breaks. This may be visualized with widefield/peripheral OCT or intraoperative OCT (▶ Fig. 17.1).

17.2.2 Ultra-Widefield Fundus Photography

Peripheral photography may be utilized to document extent of lattice and associated retinal holes (▶ Fig. 17.2).

17.3 Critical Work-up

It is important that when lattice degeneration is identified in one eye, the fellow eye is also examined as this is often bilateral in nature. Careful peripheral retinal exam is important to rule out retinal tears or retinal detachments, particularly in symptomatic individuals.

17.4 Management

17.4.1 Treatment Options

Laser retinopexy is controversial. Laser is more commonly considered in patients who have new onset symptoms of vitreoretinal tractions, associated retinal tears, atrophic retinal holes with associated subretinal fluid, and when the fellow eye has experienced a retinal detachment.

17.4.2 Follow-up

Regular follow-up with dilated exam of both eyes. Patients are counseled on the symptoms related to retinal tears and retinal detachments with instructions for urgent follow-up if any new symptoms develop.

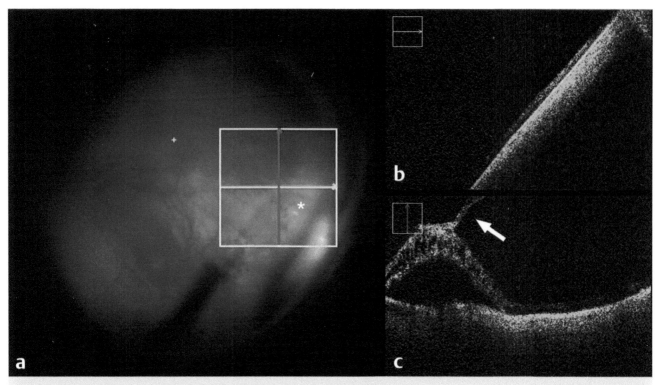

Fig. 17.1 (a) Intraoperative optical coherence tomography (OCT) of lattice degeneration. Intraoperative photograph with OCT cross-hairs over area of lattice degeneration (*asterisk*). **(b)** Horizontal OCT (*green arrow* in **[a]**) demonstrates flat retina in area adjacent to lattice degeneration. **(c)** Vertical OCT (*pink arrow* in **[a]**) through the lattice degeneration demonstrates significant vitreoretinal traction (*white arrow*) and subretinal fluid with associated cystic changes.

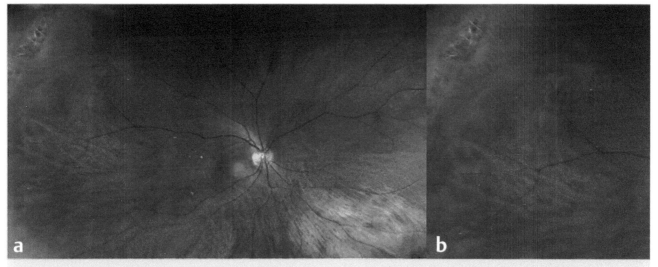

Fig. 17.2 (a) Ultra-widefield photograph of superotemporal lattice degeneration with associated retinal holes. **(b)** High-magnification view.

Suggested Reading

[1] Wilkinson CP. Prevention of retinal detachment. In: Ryan's Retina. 6th ed. Philadelphia, PA: Elsevier; 2018:2017–2030

[2] Freund KB, Sarraf D, Mieler WF, Yannuzzi LA. Peripheral retinal degenerations and rhegmatogenous retinal detachment. In: The Retinal Atlas. 2nd ed. Philadelphia, PA: Elsevier; 2017:969–1001

[3] Tasman W. Peripheral retinal lesions. In: Ophthalmology. 4th ed. Philadelphia, PA: Elsevier; 2014:638–641.e1

[4] Choudhry N, Golding J, Manry MW, Rao RC. Ultra-widefield steering-based spectral-domain optical coherence tomography imaging of the retinal periphery. Ophthalmology. 2016; 123(6):1368–1374

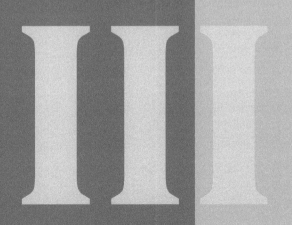

Part III

Retinal Vascular Disease

III

18 Diabetic Retinopathy and Diabetic Macular Edema

Natalia Albuquerque Lucena Figueiredo and Justis P. Ehlers

Summary

Diabetic retinopathy (DR) and diabetic macular edema (DME) are leading causes of blindness in the working age population worldwide. DR is more common and severe in patients with long-standing or poorly controlled diabetes mellitus. Hypertension and dyslipidemia are also modifiable risk factors for developing DR. Early detection of retinopathy in diabetic patients is critical as the early stages are often asymptomatic. DR/DME can lead to visual loss through a variety of mechanisms, including macular edema, macular ischemia, vitreous hemorrhage and traction retinal detachment. Fundus biomicroscopy and photography are the current mainstays determining the severity of retinopathy, while optical coherence tomography represents the gold standard technology in cases of macular edema. Multiple clinical trials have reported significant advances in intravitreal pharmacotherapy for diabetic eye disease, including anti-vascular endothelial growth factor and steroid agents. Panretinal photocoagulation remains a frequently used therapy for reducing progression risk for proliferative DR, whereas intravitreal pharmacotherapy is now the first line treatment for DME. In cases of more advanced disease, such as persistent vitreous hemorrhage, traction retinal detachment, and posterior hyaloidal traction, pars plana vitrectomy should be considered.

Keywords: anti-VEGF, diabetes mellitus, diabetic macular edema, diabetic retinopathy, fluorescein angiography, optical coherence tomography, photocoagulation, risk factors, steroids, vitrectomy

18.1 Features

Diabetic retinopathy (DR) represents a retinal microvascular complication of diabetes mellitus (DM) and is the foremost cause of preventable vision loss in working age adults; its prevalence has been estimated at nearly 35% of all diabetic adults aged 40 and over. DR is more common and severe in patients with long-standing or poorly controlled diabetes mellitus. Early detection of retinopathy in diabetic patients is critical since the first stages are asymptomatic. The risk of developing DR increases with patient age and the duration of diabetes. Control of blood glucose, blood pressure, and blood lipids are also modifiable risk factors. Hemoglobin A1c level in most patients should be 7% or lower. Diabetic eye disease can lead to visual loss through a variety of mechanisms, including DME, macular ischemia, vitreous hemorrhage, and traction retinal detachment.

The clinical presentation of DR subdivide it into two stages: (1) nonproliferative diabetic retinopathy (NPDR), which represents microvascular abnormalities without neovascularization/fibrovascular tissue and (2) proliferative diabetic retinopathy (PDR), the most advanced stage of DR characterized by the development neovascularization. Each of these two stages can also be subdivided into various levels of severity (e.g., mild, moderate, severe for NPDR; ▸ Fig. 18.1, ▸ Fig. 18.2, ▸ Fig. 18.3).

PDR may also be described by the presence or absence of high-risk features (e.g., vitreous hemorrhage, size/location of neovascularization, traction retinal detachment; ▸ Fig. 18.4, ▸ Fig. 18.5). DME is classified separately from the stages of DR as it can be found in both nonproliferative and proliferative groups (▸ Fig. 18.6, ▸ Fig. 18.7). DME represents the breakdown of the inner blood/retinal barrier leading to capillary leakage and macular swelling.

18.1.1 Common Symptoms

Asymptomatic in early stages. Symptoms can vary widely based on the disease presentation, but may include floaters (e.g., vitreous hemorrhage), vision loss (e.g., DME, traction retinal detachment, vitreous hemorrhage), and metamorphopsia (e.g., DME). Symptoms usually affect both eyes asymmetrically.

18.1.2 Exam Findings

Nonproliferative Diabetic Retinopathy

Clinically, microaneurysms are often the earliest manifestation of NPDR. Other classic retinal lesions include intraretinal hemorrhages, hard exudates, cotton wool spots, intraretinal microvascular abnormalities (IRMA, i.e., dilated capillaries between an arteriole and venule), and venous beading (i.e., alternating areas of venous dilation and constriction). As defined by the Early Treatment Diabetic Retinopathy Study (ETDRS), severe NPDR is characterized by any of the following (4:2:1 rule): intraretinal hemorrhages in four quadrants, venous beading in two quadrants, or IRMA in one quadrant (▸ Fig. 18.2).

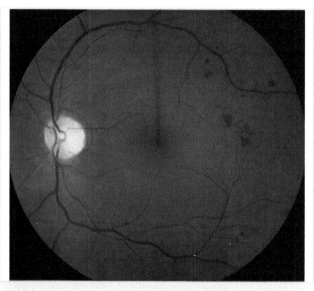
Fig. 18.1 Fundus photograph of moderate nonproliferative diabetic retinopathy.

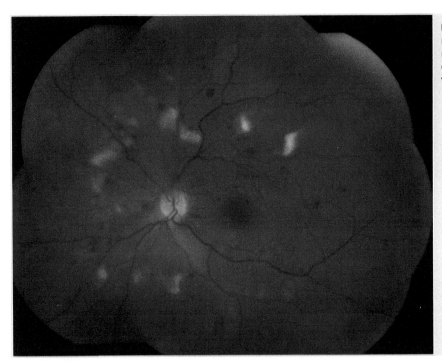

Fig. 18.2 Fundus photograph montage of severe nonproliferative diabetic retinopathy with microaneurysms, intraretinal hemorrhages, cotton wool spots, and venous beading of arcade vessels.

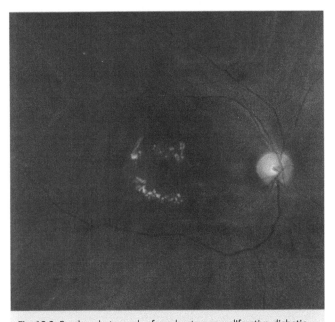

Fig. 18.3 Fundus photograph of moderate nonproliferative diabetic retinopathy associated with diabetic macular edema demonstrating a circinate ring of hard exudates surrounding a group of microaneurysms.

Diabetic Macular Edema

DME is represented by intraretinal fluid accumulation and macular thickening. It may be defined as focal or diffuse macular edema based on the leakage pattern; focal macular edema is caused by foci of capillary abnormalities such as microaneurysms usually associated with a circinate ring of hard exudates (▶ Fig. 18.3); diffuse macular edema is caused by extensive leakage and may be associated with large cystoid spaces. Currently, DME is also described based on location on optical

coherence tomography (OCT), including noncentral DME or central-involving DME. Historically, clinically significant macular edema (CSME) is defined when one of the following conditions occur: retinal thickening at or within 500 µm of the center of the macula, hard exudate at or within 500 µm of the center of the macula with adjacent thickening, or retinal thickening larger than 1 disc area located within 1 disc diameter of the center of the macula (▶ Fig. 18.3, ▶ Fig. 18.6, ▶ Fig. 18.7). However, with the advent of OCT, the clinical entity of CSME is less commonly used as a treatment criteria compared to DME location.

Proliferative Diabetic Retinopathy

PDR is characterized by the onset of neovascularization resulting from retinal ischemia. The new vessels, located at the disc (NVD) or elsewhere in the retina (NVE), may cause preretinal and vitreous hemorrhages (▶ Fig. 18.4). Neovascularization may also fibrose and contract (fibrovascular proliferation) resulting in epiretinal membrane formation, vitreoretinal traction and/or traction retinal detachments (TRD; ▶ Fig. 18.5). According to the Diabetic Retinopathy Study (DRS), high-risk PDR is defined when NVD is accompanied by vitreous hemorrhage, when NVD occupies greater than one-quarter to one-third disc area, or when NVE is larger than one-half disc area with vitreous hemorrhage.

18.2 Key Diagnostic Tests and Findings

18.2.1 Optical Coherence Tomography

Gold standard for evaluating for the presence of macular edema and vitreoretinal interface abnormalities. Allows for quantitative retinal thickness analysis and is the most common method for evaluating need for treatment for DME and assessing treatment response to therapy (▶ Fig. 18.6, ▶ Fig. 18.7).

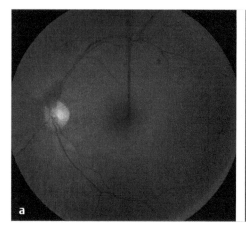

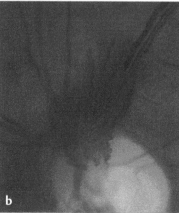

Fig. 18.4 (a,b) Fundus photograph of proliferative diabetic retinopathy demonstrating neovascularization of the disc.

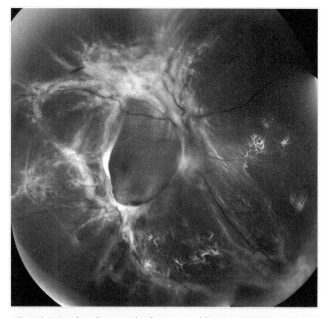

Fig. 18.5 Fundus photograph of severe proliferative diabetic retinopathy with associated fibrovascular proliferation and extensive traction retinal detachment.

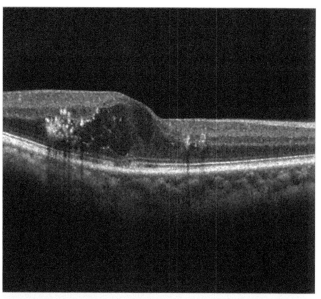

Fig. 18.6 Optical coherence tomography of diabetic macular edema, note hard exudates located mainly in the outer plexiform and some in the outer nuclear layer of the retina.

18.2.2 Fluorescein Angiography

Fluorescein angiography (FA) provides an important evaluation for retinal vascular dynamics, including microaneurysms, leakage, nonperfusion, and neovascularization. Ultra-widefield fluorescein angiography (UWFA) provides panretinal assessment of retinal vascular abnormalities and enables greater visualization of the retinal periphery compared to conventional FA (▶ Fig. 18.8). UWFA appears to be more sensitive for detection of neovascularization and other peripheral lesions. FA may be used as a guide for targeting laser photocoagulation, both for focal laser treatment and panretinal photocoagulation (▶ Fig. 18.9).

18.2.3 Ultrasonography

An important tool to evaluate for significant vitreoretinal interface abnormalities such as significant traction and the presence

of retinal detachment in cases of vitreous hemorrhage or other media opacity.

18.2.4 Color Fundus Photography

The main test to classify and document the severity of DR.

18.2.5 Optical Coherence Tomography Angiography

Optical coherence tomography angiography (OCTA) is an emerging diagnostic test that uses OCT technology with a high-speed engine that enables identification and reconstruction of depth-encoded retinal vascular flow maps. This diagnostic provides unique structural assessment of vascular perfusion and abnormalities, providing opportunities for quantifying foveal avascular zone and perfusion density. Newer systems are now enabling widefield assessment with OCTA (▶ Fig. 18.10).

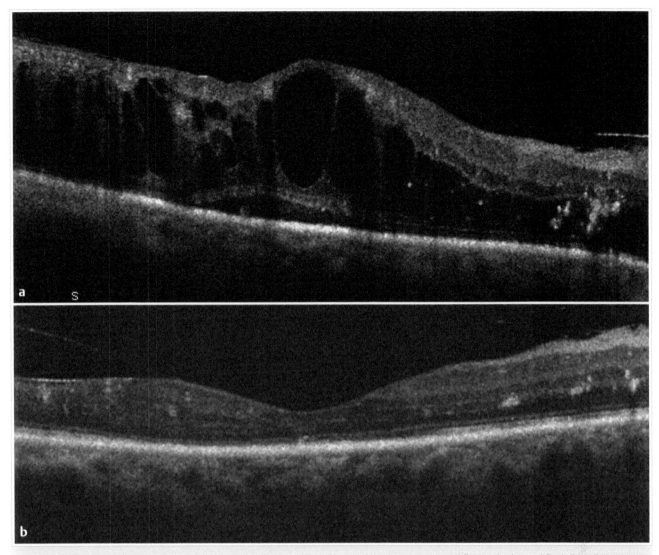

Fig. 18.7 (a) Optical coherence tomography of severe diabetic macular edema with extensive intraretinal fluid and subretinal fluid. (b) Following anti-vascular endothelial growth factor therapy, dramatic improvement with near resolution of fluid with residual ellipsoid zone attenuation and dissociated inner retinal layers.

18.3 Critical Work-up

The most important lab tests for DR patients include fasting blood glucose and hemoglobin A1c. Systemic history should be investigated, particularly regarding renal disease, serum lipid levels and blood pressure control. Close follow-up with a primary care physician and/or endocrinologist should be encouraged.

18.4 Management

18.4.1 Treatment Options for Diabetic Macular Edema

Laser Photocoagulation

Focal/grid laser photocoagulation has been the historical gold standard for the treatment of CSME since the ETDRS results.

However, focal/grid has largely been supplanted by intravitreal pharmacotherapy as the first line treatment for DME/CSME. Focal may still be considered for focal leaking microaneurysms away from the fovea.

Anti-Vascular Endothelial Growth Factor

Currently, intravitreal injection of anti-vascular endothelial growth factor (anti-VEGF) is the first-line treatment for center-involving macular edema. Multiple clinical trials have demonstrated efficacy and safety of anti-VEGF agents for the treatment of DME.

Steroids

Intravitreal steroids have also demonstrated positive results in the treatment of DME, particularly in pseudophakic patients.

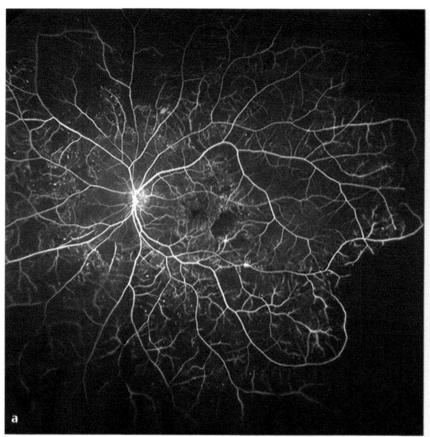

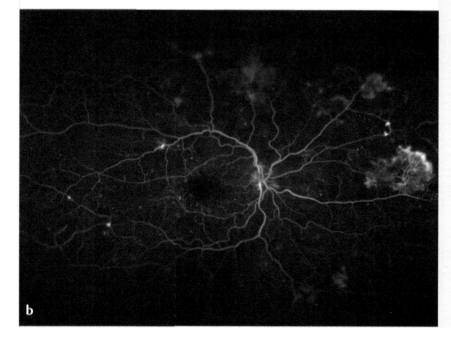

Fig. 18.8 **(a)** Ultra-widefield fluorescein angiography (UWFA) with proliferative diabetic retinopathy (PDR) showing microaneurysms and severe peripheral nonperfusion with areas of vascular leakage and minimal neovascularization. **(b)** UWFA in PDR demonstrating extensive neovascularization throughout the retinal periphery, nonperfusion, microaneurysms.

Potential adverse effects, such as cataracts and intraocular pressure rise, should be considered.

Pars Plana Vitrectomy

In eyes with tractional macular edema or significant vitreoretinal interface abnormalities that are contributing to the macular edema, pars plana vitrectomy with membrane peeling should be considered.

18.4.2 Treatment Options for Diabetic Retinopathy

Laser Photocoagulation

Panretinal photocoagulation (PRP) has been a mainstay for preventing the progression of PDR, especially in cases of high-risk

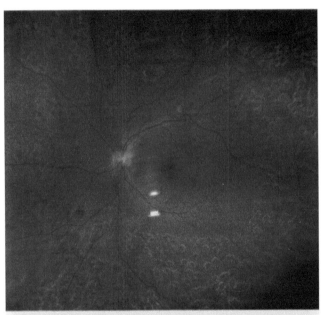

Fig. 18.9 Fundus photograph of proliferative diabetic retinopathy patient treated with panretinal photocoagulation showing scars surrounding the macular region, note fibrovascular membranes in the superior temporal vascular arcade.

PDR (▶ Fig. 18.7). PRP should also be strongly considered for patients with rubeosis and/or neovascular glaucoma. PRP is also considered for very severe NPDR (i.e., preproliferative) and particularly for patients with poor adherence to follow-up with high-risk retinopathy. Potential side effects related to PRP include reduction of peripheral vision, development of DME, and difficulty with night vision.

Anti-Vascular Endothelial Growth Factor

Intravitreal anti-VEGF therapy has been demonstrated in multiple clinical trials to be effective at reducing DR severity with fewer adverse effects than PRP. However, the transient effect of anti-VEGF therapy make patient adherence critical. Optimal dosing strategies and intervals are currently under investigation.

Pars Plana Vitrectomy

Consider surgery in patients with nonclearing vitreous hemorrhage of 1- to 3-month duration, active PDR despite complete PRP, epiretinal membrane, traction retinal detachment involving macula or combined with rhegmatogenous component. The use of anti-VEGF drugs as an adjunct to vitrectomy surgery may be helpful to reduce intraoperative/postoperative bleeding and facilitate membrane peeling.

18.4.3 Follow-up

Patients with mild to moderate NPDR should typically be examined within 6 to 12 months. Patients presenting DME, severe NPDR, or PDR should be observed closely (e.g., every 1–4 months). The frequency depends on treatment regimen, impact on visual acuity and overall severity.

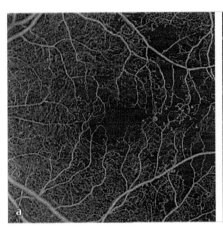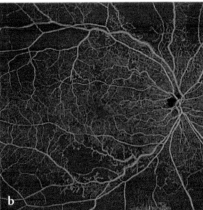

Fig. 18.10 (a) Optical coherence tomography (OCT) angiography of macula demonstrating multiple microaneurysms, vascular remodeling, and areas of flow voids corresponding to capillary nonperfusion. Widefield OCT angiography with visualization past the arcades using swept source OCT technology. **(b)** Extensive nonperfusion is present.

Suggested Reading

[1] Emptage NP, Kealey S, Lum FC, Garratt S. Preferred practice pattern: diabetic retinopathy. Am J Ophthalmol. 2014

[2] American Association of Ophthalmology. Retina and vitreous surgery. In: Basic and Clinical Science Course. San Francisco, CA: American Association of Ophthalmology; 2013

[3] International Council of Ophthalmology. ICO guidelines for diabetic eye care. http://www.icoph.org/downloads/ICOGui-delinesforDiabeticEyeCare.pdf. Accessed September 1, 2017

[4] Wells JA, Glassman AR, Ayala AR, et al. Diabetic Retinopathy Clinical Research Network. Aflibercept, bevacizumab, or ranibizumab for diabetic macular edema: two-year results from a comparative effectiveness randomized clinical trial. Ophthalmology. 2016; 123(6):1351–1359

19 Retinal Vein Occlusion

Sharon Fekrat and Mohsin H. Ali

Summary

Retinal vein occlusion (RVO) is a major cause of ocular morbidity and represents the second most common etiology of retinal vascular disease after diabetic retinopathy. Left untreated, RVOs are often vision-threatening. It is characterized by intraretinal hemorrhages primarily in the inner retina that are typically accompanied by engorged and tortuous retinal veins. The distribution depends on the type of RVO. Diagnostic tests include optical coherence tomography and fluorescein angiography. Treatment is dependent on the presence of macular edema and/or the presence of neovascularization.

Keywords: branch vein occlusion, central retinal vein occlusion, hemiretinal vein occlusion, macular edema, retinal vein occlusion

19.1 Features

Retinal vein occlusions (RVO) vary considerably based on distribution of the venous occlusive event, perfusion status of the affected retina, duration of untreated disease, and presence or absence of cystoid macular edema or retinal neovascularization and its sequelae. Because these factors result in myriad disease manifestations, clinicians must identify the correspondingly variable symptoms and examination findings.

A "typical" RVO presents at an older age (typically older than 50 years, with over 50% of affected patients being older than 60 years) and with known systemic vasculopathic risk factors (e.g., history of cigarette smoking, hypertension, hyperlipidemia, diabetes mellitus, peripheral vascular disease, renal disease, cerebrovascular accident, transient ischemic attacks, myocardial infarction, or thromboembolism). An "atypical" RVO may present at a younger age (i.e., younger than 50 years) without known systemic vasculopathic risk factors.

19.1.1 Common Symptoms

Vary from asymptomatic to acute, unilateral, painless vision loss. More widespread vision loss is typically present with central retinal vein occlusion (CRVO), compared to segmental visual field loss in patients with branch or hemiretinal vein occlusions (BRVO or HRVO).

19.1.2 Exam Findings

RVO is characterized by intraretinal hemorrhages confined primarily to the inner retina with accompanying engorged and tortuous retinal veins. The retinal distribution of findings depends on the type of RVO. Cystoid macular edema is common. There may be cotton wool spots and yellowish intraretinal exudates in the affected regions. Optic disc edema may be present. In later stages with more severe underlying ischemia, neovascularization of the retina or optic nerve head may occur resulting in vitreous hemorrhage, fibrovascular proliferation and traction, and/or neovascularization of the angle and iris with resulting neovascular glaucoma (▶ Fig. 19.1, ▶ Fig. 19.2,

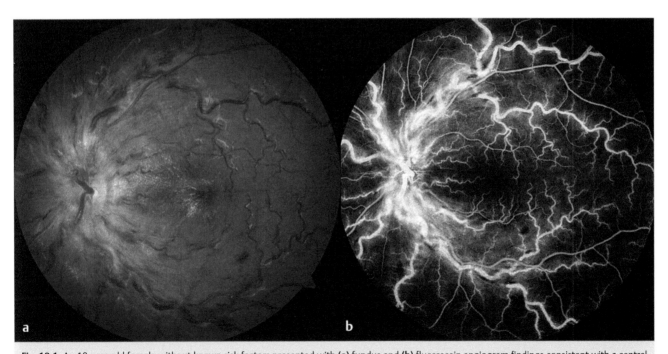

Fig. 19.1 An 18-year-old female without known risk factors presented with **(a)** fundus and **(b)** fluorescein angiogram findings consistent with a central retinal vein occlusion. A hypercoagulable work-up suggested the possibility of a protein S deficiency. **(a)** The classic fundus findings of optic disc edema and hyperemia, blurring of the disc margins, engorged and tortuous retinal veins, intraretinal hemorrhage, and macular lipid exudates are seen. **(b)** Fluorescein angiography revealed dilated and tortuous retinal veins and blockage from intraretinal hemorrhage.

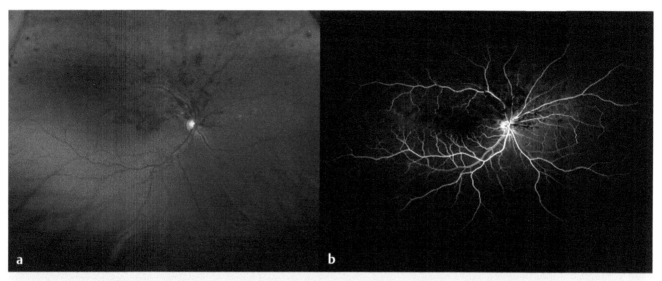

Fig. 19.2 (a) Ultra-widefield fundus imaging of a hemiretinal vein occlusion. There are intraretinal hemorrhages in the superotemporal and superonasal quadrants (superior hemisphere) respecting the horizontal raphe along with an engorged and tortuous superior retinal vein. (b) Ultra-widefield fluorescein angiography in the laminar venous filling phase shows delayed venous filling of the superior retinal vein in addition to blockage from superior intraretinal hemorrhage.

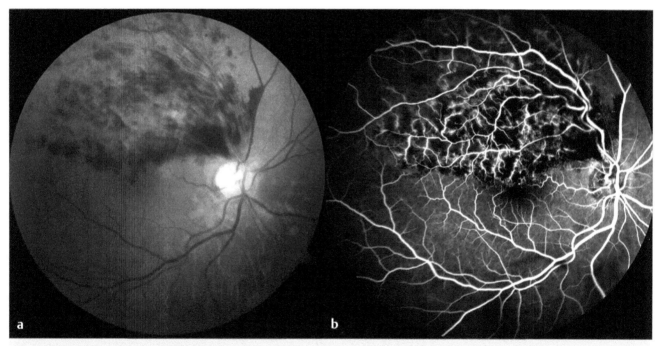

Fig. 19.3 (a) Fundus photograph and (b) fluorescein angiography showing superotemporal intraretinal hemorrhage respecting the horizontal raphe consistent with a branch retinal vein occlusion.

▶ Fig. 19.3). Other findings in chronic RVO may include macular retinal pigment epithelium alterations due to long-standing edema, epiretinal membrane, and optociliary shunt vessels. In chronic RVO, many of the findings mentioned may be absent and diagnosis may require ancillary diagnostic testing (e.g., fluorescein angiography [FA], optical coherence tomography [OCT], OCT angiography [OCTA]). The subtypes of RVO are as follows:

Central Retinal Vein Occlusion

All four quadrants will be affected and elevated intraocular pressures and glaucoma may be independently associated with CRVO development.

Hemiretinal Vein Occlusion

The superior or inferior hemisphere will be affected.

Branch Retinal Vein Occlusion

One quadrant or less will be affected, with the superotemporal quadrant being more commonly affected (66%) than the inferotemporal quadrant (29%); the occlusion almost always occurs at the site of an arteriovenous crossing and the artery is commonly located anterior to the vein at this site.

19.2 Key Diagnostic Tests and Findings

19.2.1 Optical Coherence Tomography

May demonstrate intraretinal fluid, subretinal fluid, hyperreflective foci secondary to intraretinal exudates, or hemorrhage. In addition, disruption of the ellipsoid zone and/or external limiting membrane and/or inner retinal atrophy may be present secondary to chronic macular edema or macular ischemia (▶ Fig. 19.4).

19.2.2 Fluorescein Angiography or Ultra-Widefield Fluorescein Angiography

May reveal normal choroidal and arteriolar filling with delayed retinal venous filling, blockage from intraretinal hemorrhage, arteriovenous collateral vessels, leakage from the optic nerve if optic disc edema is present, and leakage from neovascularization of the optic disc or retina. The macular region may exhibit leakage if macular edema is present or capillary nonperfusion if macular ischemia is present (▶ Fig. 19.1, ▶ Fig. 19.2, ▶ Fig. 19.3). FA is used to determine the extent of nonperfusion in RVO. Greater than 5 disc areas of nonperfusion in BRVO and greater than 10 disc areas of nonperfusion in CRVO (i.e., ischemic CRVO)

portend a poorer prognosis. More novel methods to accurately assess the extent of retinal capillary nonperfusion and its implication on neovascularization risk imaged on ultra-widefield angiography are being evaluated.

19.2.3 Optical Coherence Tomography Angiography

OCTA may demonstrate panmacular flow voids in cases of CRVO with macular ischemia or segmental flow deficits in BRVO or HRVO (▶ Fig. 19.5). Widefield OCTA may also be useful in the future for evaluating overall ischemic burden or identifying neovascularization.

19.3 Critical Work-up

19.3.1 Known Vasculopathic Risk Factors

Systemic work-up is often of low yield in patients older than 50 with known vasculopathic risk factors as the systemic associations are already known. Work-up may include screening for the most common risk factors: hypertension, diabetes mellitus, dyslipidemia, and cardiovascular disease.

Some evidence suggests the possibility that certain hypercoagulable conditions may increase the risk of RVO. These include leukemia, polycythemia vera, hyperhomocysteinemia, factor 5 Leiden mutation, prothrombin gene mutation, protein C or S deficiency, antithrombin III gene mutation, and presence of anticardiolipin antibody or lupus anticoagulant, among others. Low levels of vitamin B6 and folic acid have also been suggested as independent risk factors for RVO. However, these are not usually tested for unless unique circumstances are present.

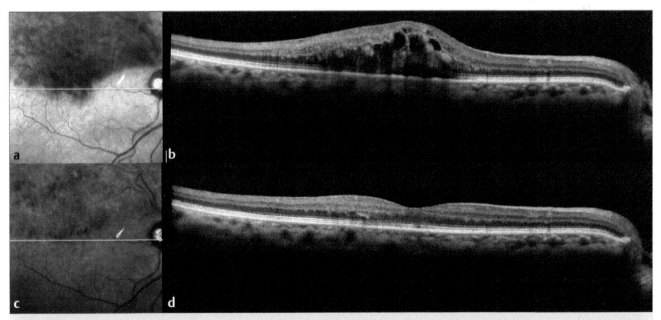

Fig. 19.4 (a,b) Optical coherence tomography of the eye in ▶ Fig. 19.3 with branch retinal vein occlusion and cystoid macular edema and **(c,d)** after three intravitreal anti-vascular endothelial growth factor injections. Visual acuity improved from 20/64 to 20/40 in the treated eye.

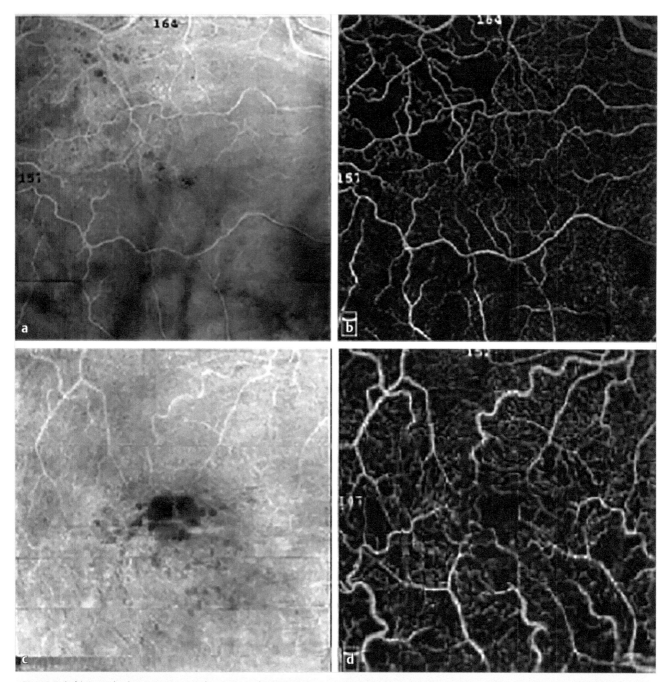

Fig. 19.5 (a,b) Optical coherence tomography angiography (OCTA) demonstrating mild vascular tortuosity, vascular remodeling, and multi-focal areas of nonperfusion. (c,d) OCTA with significant vascular tortuosity and mild focal areas of nonperfusion.

19.3.2 No Known Vasculopathic Risk Factors

When no known systemic vasculopathic risk factors are present, particularly in younger patients, a diagnostic work-up may reveal a contributory etiology. Consider obtaining or recommending some or all of the following: blood pressure testing, complete blood count, metabolic profile, glycated hemoglobin, lipid profile, and a hypercoagulable work-up (such as polymerase chain reaction assay for factor 5 Leiden mutation and serum levels of homocysteine, vitamin B6, folic acid, antithrombin III, protein C and S, lupus anticoagulant, and anticardiolipin antibody). Review the patient's current medications to identify medications potentially associated with RVO such as oral contraceptives and diuretics. Smoking should be discouraged.

19.4 Management

19.4.1 Treatment Options

Management of RVOs is influenced by three main factors: (1) the presence or absence of cystoid macular edema; (2) the presence or absence of neovascularization; and (3) the likelihood that the patient will be able to follow up as advised. Multiple clinical trials have evaluated observation, grid-pattern laser photocoagulation, intravitreal corticosteroids, panretinal photocoagulation, and intravitreal anti-vascular endothelial growth factor (i.e., anti-VEGF) agents. Intravitreal pharmacotherapy has become first-line therapy for RVO with macular edema. Typically, anti-VEGF agents are used initially with intravitreal steroids as an alternative option. Grid laser has been shown to be effective in BRVO but is less effective than intravitreal pharmacotherapy. When neovascularization is present, anti-VEGF agents are frequently used in combination with panretinal photocoagulation. Eyes without macular edema or neovascularization are usually closely observed.

19.4.2 Follow-up

Follow-up monthly for the first 4 to 6 months to observe for the development of sequelae requiring treatment. In eyes with sequelae undergoing treatment, follow-up intervals are dictated by disease response and required treatment frequency. In eyes with severe ischemia undergoing anti-VEGF therapy, close monitoring should be continued after anti-VEGF cessation to evaluate for rebound neovascularization.

Suggested Reading

[1] Wong TY, Scott IU. Clinical practice. Retinal-vein occlusion. N Engl J Med. 2010; 363(22):2135–2144

[2] Rogers SL, McIntosh RL, Lim L, et al. Natural history of branch retinal vein occlusion: an evidence-based systematic review. Ophthalmology. 2010; 117 (6):1094–1101.e5

[3] McIntosh RL, Rogers SL, Lim L, et al. Natural history of central retinal vein occlusion: an evidence-based systematic review. Ophthalmology. 2010; 117 (6):1113–1123.e15

[4] Ehlers JP, Fekrat S. Retinal vein occlusion: beyond the acute event. Surv Ophthalmol. 2011; 56(4):281–299

20 Retinal Artery Occlusion

Rishi P. Singh and Ang Li

Summary

Retinal artery occlusion (RAO) may be due to embolism or thrombosis, resulting in either branch retinal artery occlusion (BRAO), or central retinal artery occlusion (CRAO). RAO typically causes sudden, painless, vision loss or visual field defect, usually unilaterally. Patients need routine eye screening for neovascularization following the inciting event and often evaluation for underlying risk factors. There are no proven treatments to reverse either BRAO or CRAO.

Keywords: branch retinal artery occlusion, central retinal artery occlusion, neovascularization

20.1 Features

Retinal artery occlusion (RAO) typically occurs due to embolism or thrombosis, resulting in either branch retinal artery occlusion (BRAO) or central retinal artery occlusion (CRAO). Vision loss is often severe in the areas impacted by the RAO. Central visual acuity can be maintained if the fovea is not involved.

20.1.1 Common Symptoms

Branch Retinal Artery Occlusion

Occasionally asymptomatic. Symptoms include sudden, acute, unilateral, painless, and partial vision loss. Possible prior history of amaurosis fugax (transient vision loss). Visual acuity varies widely.

Central Retinal Artery Occlusion

Sudden, painless, and typically profound unilateral vision loss. Possible prior history of amaurosis fugax. Vision loss typically involves entire visual field. Associated symptoms of jaw claudication, scalp hyperalgesia, and temporal headaches are concerning for concurrent giant cell arteritis (GCA).

20.1.2 Exam Findings

Branch Retinal Artery Occlusion

Fundus findings if examined at time of symptom onset may be absent. Within hours classic findings appear, including retinal whitening in the distribution of occluded arteriole (▶ Fig. 20.1), arteriolar attenuation, and possible Hollenhorst plaque (i.e., platelet–fibrin–cholesterol intravascular emboli). Relative afferent pupillary defect may be present.

Central Retinal Artery Occlusion

Findings include retinal whitening, cherry red spot, arteriolar attenuation, boxcarring (segmental stagnant blood flow), and Hollenhorst plaque. About 15 to 25% of eyes have cilioretinal artery that perfuses part of the macula, which preserves central

vision (▶ Fig. 20.2). For the majority of cases, however, presenting visual acuity ranges from 20/200 to counting fingers. Relative afferent pupillary defect frequently presents.

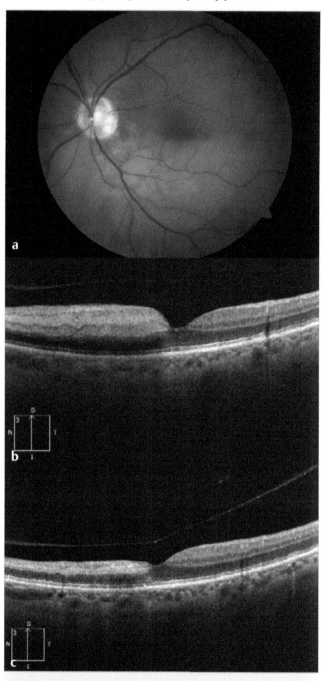

Fig. 20.1 **(a)** Fundus photograph demonstrating inferior branch retinal artery occlusion (BRAO). **(b)** Optical coherence tomography demonstrating increased inner retinal thickening with associated increased hyperreflectivity consistent with acute BRAO. A follow-up after four weeks demonstrates persistent though less hyperreflectivity and early inner retinal atrophy consistent with previous BRAO. **(c)** The regional atrophy is consistent with a BRAO.

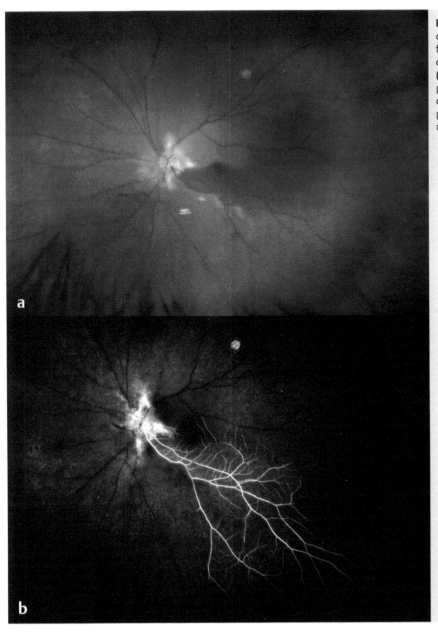

Fig. 20.2 (a) Ultra-widefield fundus photo shows disc pallor, macular whitening with sparing of fovea, and temporal wedge supplied by cilioretinal artery. No visible plaques are present. (b) Ultra-widefield fluorescein angiography shows patchy and delayed choroidal filling, delayed central retinal artery filling, and profound peripheral nonperfusion. Cilioretinal artery to the macula and inferotemporal arcade was spared.

20.2 Key Diagnostic Tests and Findings

20.2.1 Optical Coherence Tomography

Branch Retinal Artery Occlusion

Acute BRAO has inner retina thickening and hyperreflectivity; chronic has inner retina thinning and atrophy (► Fig. 20.1).

Central Retinal Artery Occlusion

Acute CRAO has inner retina thickening and hyperreflectivity (► Fig. 20.3); chronic has inner retina thinning and atrophy. Rarely, may be associated with intraretinal fluid that may reflect combined vein occlusion (► Fig. 20.3). Some cases show

patchy areas of increased reflectivity from deep capillary bed ischemia, referred to as paracentral acute middle maculopathy.

20.2.2 Fluorescein Angiography or Ultra-Widefield Fluorescein Angiography

Branch Retinal Artery Occlusion

Reveals delayed filling in area of obstruction and nonperfusion.

Central Retinal Artery Occlusion

Delayed or absent filling of central retinal artery; 15% have preservation of cilioretinal filling (► Fig. 20.2). A dark ring or triangular area of both choroidal and retinal nonperfusion

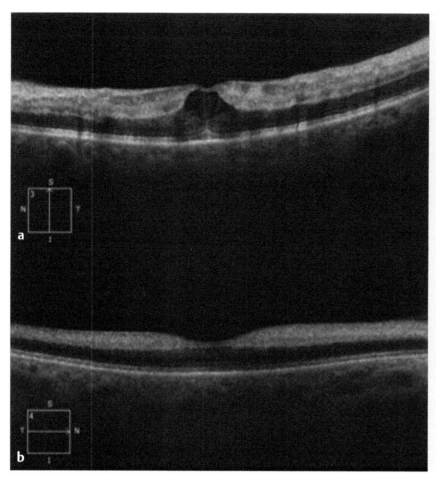

Fig. 20.3 Optical coherence tomography (OCT) demonstrating scattered multifocal hyperreflective inner retinal paracentral middle maculopathy–like lesions consistent with inner retinal ischemia in a retinal artery occlusion (RAO). **(a)** Mild cystic changes are also present. **(b)** OCT with diffuse inner retinal hyperreflectivity consistent with central RAO.

around the optic nerve is indicative of cilioretinal artery occlusion from GCA.

20.2.3 Indocyanine Green Angiography

Branch Retinal Artery Occlusion and Central Retinal Artery Occlusion

Patchy and delayed choroidal filling is pathognomonic for posterior ciliary artery occlusion and is highly suggestive of GCA.

20.2.4 Optical Coherence Tomography Angiography

Branch Retinal Artery Occlusion

Prominent flow voids present in retinal circulation in distribution of affected artery.

Central Retinal Artery Occlusion

Prominent flow voids present throughout retinal circulation typically visualized.

20.3 Critical Work-up

20.3.1 Branch Retinal Artery Occlusion

Acute and symptomatic BRAO warrants prompt evaluation for vascular occlusive disease and for risk of a subsequent stroke. Patients should be evaluated for causes of embolic disease including carotid stenosis and cardiac valve disease which require carotid imaging (e.g., carotid Doppler, CT angiography, MR angiography), electrocardiogram, and echocardiography. For patients younger than 50, evaluation for hypercoagulable state should also be considered.

20.3.2 Central Retinal Artery Occlusion

Acute CRAO from an embolic etiology requires timely assessment as risk for ischemic stroke is particularly high within one week of visual symptom onset. CRAO in patients over 50 years of age are most frequently due to vascular occlusive disease or cardiac valve disorder. For patients 50 or younger, consider work-up for hypercoagulable states. It is important to rule out GCA with erythrocyte sedimentation rate, C-reactive protein, and platelets in patients over 50 years old, particularly with associated symptoms of jaw claudication, scalp paresthesia, and temporal headache. Temporal artery biopsy should be considered in patients with symptoms of GCA even with normal lab values.

20.4 Management

20.4.1 Treatment Options

Branch Retinal Artery Occlusion

There is no proven treatment to reverse BRAO, but systemic work-up and management should be initiated to evaluate for the root cause of occlusion (embolic, inflammatory, infectious, or autoimmune).

Central Retinal Artery Occlusion

There are no proven treatments to reverse CRAO. If inflammatory markers are elevated or clinical symptoms suggestive, systemic high-dose steroids are immediately indicated for presumed GCA to reduce risk to the fellow eye. Current evidence for thrombolytic or interventional treatment other than steroids for CRAO is still controversial. Despite a multitude of treatments options, there is no proven efficacy for medical therapies such as antiglaucoma medications, digital massage, inhalation of carbogen, intravenous or intra-arterial recombinant tissue plasminogen activator, and vasodilation with pentoxifylline or sublingual isosorbide dinitrate. Surgical treatment options (e.g., anterior chamber paracentesis, Nd:YAG laser embolysis, pars plana vitrectomy with embolectomy) also have no definitive evidence.

20.4.2 Follow-up

RAO patients need regular follow-up evaluation for neovascularization in the months following the inciting event. Neovascular sequelae are typically treated with panretinal/sectoral photocoagulation and/or intravitreal anti-vascular endothelial growth factor if patient develops iris or retinal neovascularization or neovascular glaucoma. For anterior segment neovascularization with profound retinal ischemia, a complete panretinal photocoagulation is warranted. Results of examination should be communicated to patient's primary care physician for continued work-up and management of systematic risk factors.

Central Retinal Artery Occlusion

If GCA is suspected, start systemic steroids immediately.

Suggested Reading

[1] Olsen TW, Pulido JS, Folk JC, Hyman L, Flaxel CJ, Adelman RA. Retinal and ophthalmic artery occlusions preferred practice pattern. Ophthalmology. 2017; 124(2):120–P143

[2] Sim S, Ting DSW. Diagnosis and management of central retinal artery occlusion. EyeNet Magazine 2017:33–34

[3] Miller A, Green M, Robinson D. Simple rule for calculating normal erythrocyte sedimentation rate. Br Med J (Clin Res Ed). 1983; 286(6361):266

[4] Wener MH, Daum PR, McQuillan GM. The influence of age, sex, and race on the upper reference limit of serum C-reactive protein concentration. J Rheumatol. 2000; 27(10):2351–2359

21 Ocular Ischemic Syndrome

Talia R. Kaden and Yasha S. Modi

Summary

Ocular ischemic syndrome (OIS) is a rare but serious disease caused by a reduction of blood flow to the eye. It may manifest with both anterior and posterior segment changes and in severe forms may be associated with a reduction in vision. Treatment options for the eye are limited, but it is essential that patients with suspected OIS be evaluated for possible carotid or other vascular disease in order to reduce the patient's risk of mortality and morbidity.

Keywords: carotid ultrasound, mid-peripheral dot-blot hemorrhages, ocular ischemic syndrome

21.1 Features

Ocular ischemic syndrome (OIS) is a rare but serious disease. While our understanding of this entity has improved, OIS is still often misdiagnosed or missed on initial clinical exam. OIS is an ischemic state caused by a reduction of blood flow to the eye. It is frequently associated with ipsilateral carotid stenosis, yet not all patients with OIS have stenotic carotids. It is important to consider evaluation for other vascular stenosis/occlusions, including within the aortic arch, the ophthalmic artery, central retinal artery, or ciliary arteries, as patients with OIS have a 40% mortality rate at 5 years, often from ischemic cardiac disease.

OIS is more prevalent in individuals over the age of 50 and the incidence rises with increasing age. The rates of OIS in men are twice than those in women. OIS is more common in patients with diabetes, which can confound the diagnosis if there is underlying diabetic retinopathy. Thus recognition of asymmetric diabetic retinopathy should prompt an evaluation for OIS.

While typically unilateral, rates of OIS in the fellow eye have been reported to be anywhere between 20 and 50%.

21.1.1 Common Symptoms

May present with a history of transient visual loss (~ 15%) or complain of a dull ache (~ 40%). The etiology of the discomfort may be related to ischemia of the ciliary body (manifested as flare in the eye from breakdown of the blood–aqueous barrier) or frank pain, which may be secondary to neovascularization of the iris (NVI) and secondary neovascular glaucoma (NVG). Patients may also report worsening of the pain when upright, as the reduced blood flow in that position can result in increased ischemia.

21.1.2 Exam Findings

In the anterior segment NVI is frequently present (▶ Fig. 21.1), and many will go on to develop NVG. Patients may also manifest flare in excess of cell in the anterior chamber or a fixed, sluggishly reactive pupil. Rarely, patients may present with bullous keratopathy and Descemet's folds.

In the posterior segment, classic findings include narrowed arteries and dilated, but not tortuous veins, which can help differentiate OIS from a central retinal vein occlusion (where the veins are generally both dilated and tortuous). Midperipheral hemorrhages are frequently present (~ 80%) and usually deep (dot/blot, ▶ Fig. 21.2). The presence of posterior segment neovascularization, both at the disc and elsewhere, may be seen in severe cases. Occasionally, severe OIS may manifest with a central retinal artery occlusion. This can be associated with NVG, as an increased intraocular pressure can overwhelm the low perfusion pressure of the central retinal artery.

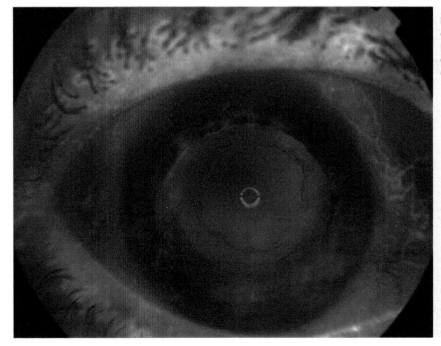

Fig. 21.1 Fluorescein angiography demonstrating neovascularization of the iris in a patient with ocular ischemic syndrome. There is early leakage of the iris vessels visible, even in a dilated eye.

21.2 Key Diagnostic Tests and Findings

21.2.1 Fluorescein Angiography or Ultra-Widefield Fluorescein Angiography

Fluorescein angiography (FA) is an essential tool for diagnosis. The hallmark feature is delayed choroidal and retinal filling (▶ Fig. 21.3). Normal choroidal filling time is approximately 5 seconds after the first visualization of dye in the choroidal arteries. In OIS, patchy or significantly delayed choroidal filling is common, in some cases extending past 1 minute. Retinal vascular filling may also be delayed, but while very sensitive for OIS, the delay in retinal circulation is less specific, as it can be seen in central retinal artery and vein occlusions. However, because of the sensitivity of the FA, it is imperative that the timing of dye injection be carefully recorded in order to make this diagnosis. FA can also be used to differentiate OIS from diabetic

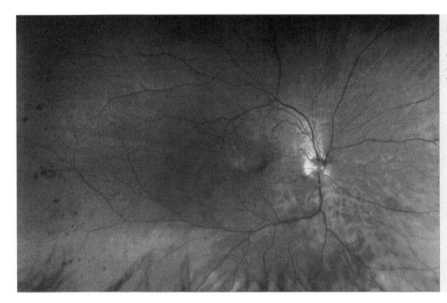

Fig. 21.2 Scattered dot–blot hemorrhages in the midperiphery of a patient who had 99% stenosis of the carotid artery. There is narrowing of the arteries and dilation of the veins, with minimal tortuosity.

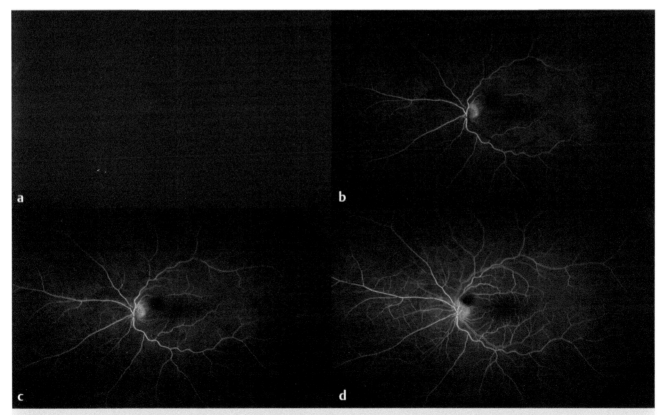

Fig. 21.3 Ultra-widefield fluorescein angiography of the posterior segment in ocular ischemic syndrome. (a) There is significant delay in arm to eye circulation time (>40 seconds) as well as in (b–d) arteriovenous circulation. (d) There is a persistent delay (>90 seconds) in filling time of the retinal veins with no dye present in some veins.

retinopathy, as the latter would demonstrate retinal capillary non-perfusion (an uncommon finding in OIS). FA is also helpful to identify associated neovascularization.

21.2.2 Red Free

Red free images highlight hemorrhages in the fundus with greater contrast relative to traditional fundus photography. This can help identify the pattern of dot-blot hemorrhages in the midperiphery that is characteristically seen in OIS. Additionally, the red free image highlights venous-to-venous collaterals, which would identify the pathology as more consistent with chronic retinal vein occlusion, rather than OIS.

21.3 Critical Work-up

If OIS is suspected, it is imperative that carotid imaging be performed (e.g., ultrasound, MR angiography, and CT angiography), as over 90% of patients will have some occlusion of the common or internal carotid artery. Referral for evaluation for carotid endarterectomy should be conducted if significant stenosis is detected, although endarterectomy is only an option in near, rather than complete, internal carotid occlusion.

21.4 Management
21.4.1 Treatment Options
Vascular Surgery

Most OIS patients will present with chronic carotid stenosis and their management is not always straightforward. If partially occluded, a carotid endarterectomy is usually considered. Endovascular carotid artery stenting can also be used, though generally it is reserved for situations in which surgery is deemed too high risk (e.g., patients with medical comorbidities or with difficult anatomy secondary to prior neck irradiation or surgery). If the carotid artery is completely occluded, the data is more inconclusive.

Laser

In cases with neovascularization and retinal ischemia on FA, panretinal photocoagulation (PRP) may be used alone. However, regression of iris neovascularization is frequently incomplete if treated with laser alone. For this reason, combination intravitreal pharmacotherapy with anti-vascular endothelial growth factor (anti-VEGF) therapy is frequently employed.

Anti-Vascular Endothelial Growth Factor Therapy

Anti-VEGF therapy has become first-line therapy for neovascularization, often in combination with PRP as outlined above.

Other Therapies

Cycloplegics can decrease pain by stabilizing the blood aqueous barrier and minimizing the formation of posterior synechiae. In addition to the retinal therapy required, medical and surgical therapy, including glaucoma drainage implants, may be needed to control secondary NVG with protracted intraocular pressure elevation after anti-VEGF therapy.

21.4.2 Follow-up

While there are no established guidelines of follow-up intervals for patients with OIS, patients should be followed regularly for any secondary NVI or NVG. During active treatment and early monitoring, patients are often seen every 4 to 8 weeks. Once stable, patients may be followed less frequently. Care should be taken to ensure that patients have appropriate follow-up with their primary care physician or a vascular surgeon.

Suggested Reading

[1] Kim YH, Sung MS, Park SW. Clinical features of ocular ischemic syndrome and risk factors for neovascular glaucoma. Korean J Ophthalmol. 2017; 31(4): 343–350
[2] Mendrinos E, Machinis TG, Pournaras CJ. Ocular ischemic syndrome. Surv Ophthalmol. 2010; 55(1):2–34
[3] Mizener JB, Podhajsky P, Hayreh SS. Ocular ischemic syndrome. Ophthalmology. 1997; 104(5):859–864
[4] Powers WJ, Clarke WR, Grubb RL, Jr, Videen TO, Adams HP, Jr, Derdeyn CP, COSS Investigators. Extracranial-intracranial bypass surgery for stroke prevention in hemodynamic cerebral ischemia: the Carotid Occlusion Surgery Study randomized trial. JAMA. 2011; 306(18):1983–1992
[5] Thanvi B, Robinson T. Complete occlusion of extracranial internal carotid artery: clinical features, pathophysiology, diagnosis and management. Postgrad Med J. 2007; 83(976):95–99

22 Retinal Arterial Macroaneurysm

Kevin Wang and Justis P. Ehlers

Summary

Retinal arterial macroaneurysms (RAMs) are acquired, saccular or fusiform dilatations of large retinal arterioles, usually within the first three orders of bifurcation. They are most commonly seen in women older than 60 years with hypertension (~75%) and dyslipidemia. They are frequently asymptomatic, but patients may develop significant vision loss due to exudation or hemorrhage. Management strategies are based on RAM location and associated sequelae.

Keywords: retinal arterial macroaneurysms, macular edema, retinal hemorrhage

22.1 Features

Retinal arterial macroaneurysms (RAMs) are acquired, saccular or fusiform dilatations of large retinal arterioles, usually within the first three orders of bifurcation. The diameter of dilatation is typically within 100 to 250 μm. This is most commonly seen in women older than 60 years with hypertension (~75%) and dyslipidemia.

22.1.1 Common Symptoms

Commonly asymptomatic. Sudden painless vision loss may occur due to vitreous, retinal, or subretinal hemorrhage. More slowly developing vision loss may occur secondary to edema and exudation.

22.1.2 Exam Findings

Focal saccular dilatation of retinal arterioles. Intravitreal, preretinal, intraretinal, and subretinal hemorrhages are possible from RAM rupture. Macular edema and surrounding circinate exudates are common (▸ Fig. 22.1).

22.2 Diagnostic Tests and Findings

22.2.1 Fluorescein Angiography or Ultra-Widefield Fluorescein Angiography

Early images display focal macroaneurysm filling with possible leakage in late images.

22.2.2 Indocyanine Green Angiography or Ultra-Widefield Indocyanine Green Angiography

Images display focal macroaneurysm filling. Useful for diagnosis in presence of preretinal, intraretinal, and subretinal hemorrhages.

22.2.3 Optical Coherence Tomography and OCT Angiography

Optical coherence tomography (OCT) is useful for evaluating structural alterations associated with exudation, including intraretinal fluid and subretinal fluid. In addition, OCT can be helpful to delineate hemorrhage location. Occasionally, the vascular dilation may be visualized on the OCT. OCT angiography (OCTA) can readily visualize the saccular dilation of the retinal vessel flow abnormality if the structural change is within the field of the OCTA. Widefield OCTA may be useful for identifying more peripheral RAM.

22.3 Critical Work-up

Evaluation for hypertension and dyslipidemia.

22.4 Management

22.4.1 Treatment

Observation with close follow-up and management of hypertension and/or dyslipidemia. Most RAMs do not require treatment as most regress spontaneously, particularly after hemorrhage (▸ Fig. 22.2). Cases of significant subretinal hemorrhage or vitreous hemorrhage call for pars plana vitrectomy with subretinal tissue plasminogen activator (in cases of subretinal hemorrhage). Focal laser photocoagulation directly to the RAM is considered for visually significant exudation. Downstream vascular occlusion may complicate laser photocoagulation so caution should be exercised if the RAM is located upstream to the fovea.

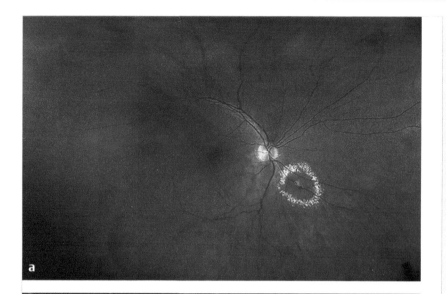

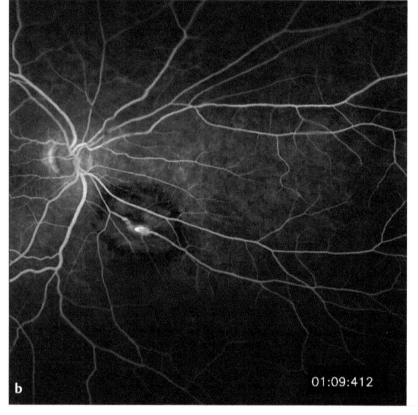

Fig. 22.1 Retinal arterial macroaneurysm with circinate lipid exudate as seen on (a) fundus photo and (b) fluorescein angiography.

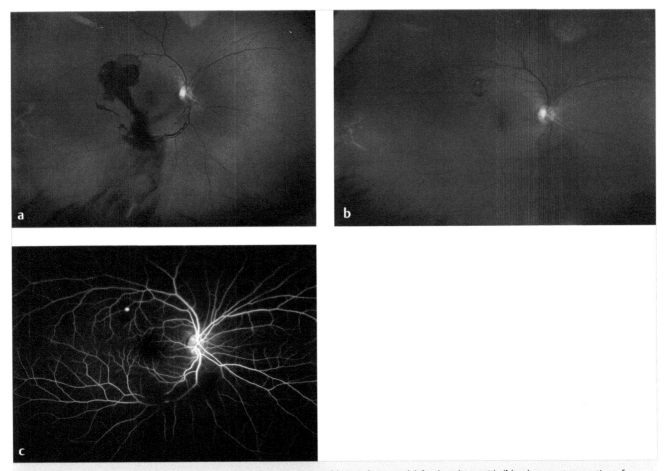

Fig. 22.2 Ruptured retinal arterial macroaneurysm (RAM) with subretinal hemorrhage on **(a)** fundus photo with **(b)** subsequent resorption of hemorrhage at 3 month follow-up visit. **(c)** Ultra-widefield fluorescein angiography demonstrates clear RAM at site of hemorrhage.

22.4.2 Follow-up

Close follow-up following recent hemorrhage or active exudation is recommended until clinically stable. Asymptomatic/inactive RAMs may typically be observed every 6 to 12 months.

Suggested Reading

[1] Pitkänen L, Tommila P, Kaarniranta K, Jääskeläinen JE, Kinnunen K. Retinal arterial macroaneurysms. Acta Ophthalmol. 2014; 92(2):101–104

[2] Townsend-Pico WA, Meyers SM, Lewis H. Indocyanine green angiography in the diagnosis of retinal arterial macroaneurysms associated with submacular and preretinal hemorrhages: a case series. Am J Ophthalmol. 2000; 129(1):33–37

[3] Abdel-Khalek MN, Richardson J. Retinal macroaneurysm: natural history and guidelines for treatment. Br J Ophthalmol. 1986; 70(1):2–11

23 Radiation Retinopathy

Peter H. Tang and Prithvi Mruthyunjaya

Summary

Radiation retinopathy is a potential visually significant adverse effect of ocular exposure to therapeutic radiation for malignancies of the eye, orbit, and surrounding head and neck structures. Aside from changes within the retina, this term is also used to encompass sequela occurring within the choroid (radiation choroidopathy) and the pigment epithelium (radiation retinal pigment epitheliopathy). Common methods of radiation therapy that induce radiation retinopathy include plaque radiotherapy (brachytherapy), proton beam radiotherapy, external beam radiotherapy, and Cyberknife radiosurgery. With the increasing trend toward globe-salvaging therapeutic strategies for uveal melanoma and therapeutic efficacy in retinoblastoma and ocular metastasis, the more routine use of radiation therapy and improved detection with multi-modal imaging has increased the reported incidence of radiation retinopathy.

Keywords: brachytherapy, external beam, metastasis, radiation, radiation retinopathy, tumors

23.1 Features

While clinical findings of radiation retinopathy and diabetic retinopathy (DR) overlap considerably, a discussion of the initiating insults can provide a better understanding of the disease process. Ionizing radiation induces killing of tumor cells through two general mechanisms: (1) DNA disruption in rapidly proliferating cells and (2) oxidative damage by reactive oxygen species (ROS). A secondary consequence of this process is the collateral damage sustained by local healthy tissue, creating the foundation for the development of radiation retinopathy. In brachytherapy, the dose prescription target volume is defined by the apex of the tumor and a small margin of retina (~ 2 mm) surrounding the tumor base to account for any undetectable tumor extension and imprecision with plaque placement. Retinal regions that fall outside of this area typically have very minimal radiation exposure. Proton beam radiotherapy (PBT) has theoretical advantages over brachytherapy for treating difficult-to-reach posterior tumors as well as minimizing radiation exposure beyond the treatment zone, a phenomenon termed the Bragg peak. External beam radiotherapy (EBT) exposes the entire fundus to radiation, thus this modality can produce radiation retinopathy over a greater area of retina if radiation dosage is not adjusted appropriately. DNA disruption induces degeneration of both endothelial cells and neuroglia, a cell that is critical to support retinal neurons through myelination, homeostasis, and nutrition. Endothelial cells are particularly susceptible to ROS damage from their exposure to high amounts of oxygen and iron within the blood. Furthermore, arteries are affected more than veins due to the higher oxygen tension of arterial circulation. This is in direct contrast to DR, which initially affects pericytes instead of endothelial cells. Patients with concurrent diabetes mellitus are at a higher risk for developing aggressive radiation retinopathy from increased susceptibility given the underlying vascular damage.

23.1.1 Common Symptoms

Early or mild retinopathy may be asymptomatic; more advanced disease can present with decreased vision or floaters.

23.1.2 Exam Findings

Initially microaneurysms, intraretinal hemorrhages, lipid exudation, and leakage of serous fluid into the surrounding tissues maybe seen (▶ Fig. 23.1). Larger retinal vessels become affected later in the disease course and occlude, leading to a progressive vasculopathy with detrimental effects on numerous fundus structures. Susceptibility to developing radiation retinopathy and subsequent response to various treatment modalities varies greatly among patients.

Similar to DR, radiation retinopathy can be further differentiated into subtypes: nonproliferative radiation retinopathy (NPRR), proliferative radiation retinopathy (PRR), and radiation macular edema (RME). Common findings of NPRR include peripheral retinal vascular changes, intraretinal hemorrhages, retinal telangiectasia, retinal exudates, and cotton wool spots. PRR arises from advanced disease inducing large areas of retinal capillary nonperfusion and neovascularization of the retina and optic disc (▶ Fig. 23.2). Uncontrolled PRR can eventually lead to neovascular glaucoma, vitreous hemorrhage, and traction retinal detachment.

23.2 Key Diagnostic Tests and Findings

23.2.1 Optical Coherence Tomography

Essential for detecting the development of RME through identification intraretinal fluid and subretinal fluid. Optical coherence tomography (OCT) is indispensable to help guide treatment strategy and evaluate treatment response.

23.2.2 Fluorescein Angiography or Ultra-Widefield Fluorescein Angiography

Fluorescein angiography can provide invaluable information such as areas of retinal nonperfusion, retinal and optic disc neovascularization, and microvascular changes (▶ Fig. 23.3). Ultra-widefield fluorescein angiography may have particular utility to assess panretinal disease burden.

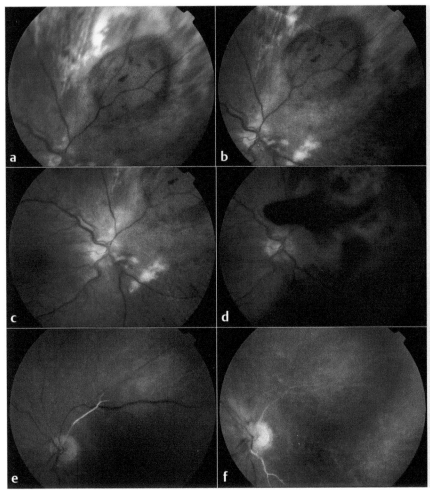

Fig. 23.1 Progression of radiation retinopathy after treatment of choroidal melanoma. **(a–c)** Early on in the disease course, there is extensive lipid exudation surrounding the tumor lesion as well as mild vascular attenuation and peripapillary cotton wool spots. **(d)** As disease progresses, proliferative retinopathy results in vitreous hemorrhage due to neovascularization. **(e–f)** Advanced stages of the disease include sclerosis of retinal vessels leading to vascular nonperfusion and contributing to proliferative disease elsewhere in the retina.

23.2.3 Optical Coherence Tomography Angiography

Emerging noninvasive modality that provides information on vascular flow and capillary nonperfusion (▶ Fig. 23.4). Wide-field OCT angiography has the potential to provide information related to the retinal periphery perfusion.

23.3 Critical Work-up

The hallmark of diagnosing radiation retinopathy is to elicit from the history of prior radiation therapy with a focus to the eye, head/neck regions, and brain tumors that were close to the orbit since onset of radiation retinopathy can range from 1 month to over a decade afterwards. In addition, comprehensive ophthalmic exam and imaging assessment make up the cornerstone of surveillance for radiation retinopathy.

23.4 Management

23.4.1 Treatment

Radiation Retinopathy

Treatments mirror similar principles that are applied for DR. Sectoral retinal photocoagulation has been shown to have mixed success in inducing the regression of neovascularization in PRR. Intravitreal anti-vascular endothelial growth factor (anti-VEGF) therapies have been used successfully in treating neovascularization of PRR and subsequent sequelae including neovascular glaucoma.

Radiation Macular Edema

RME is a significant cause of vision loss in patients with radiation retinopathy. Intravitreal anti-VEGF medications are the current first line therapy and have been shown to be very effective; however, it usually requires ongoing therapy. Intravitreal steroids have also been utilized with some success in cases that are refractory to anti-VEGF therapies, suggesting inflammation to be a likely component of radiation retinopathy.

23.4.2 Prevention

Mediating the balance between successful treatment of the tumor and minimizing ocular exposure to radiation is the foundation for preventing radiation retinopathy. This requires a customized approach for each patient. Extensive studies have been conducted to evaluate minimal radiation dosage needed for effective tumor treatment while minimizing complications.

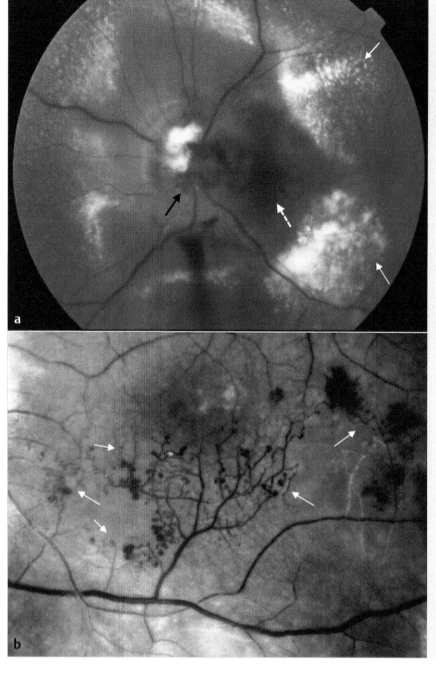

Fig. 23.2 Proliferative radiation retinopathy. **(a)** Fundus image of peripapillary choroidal melanoma treated with radiation resulting in lipid exudation (*white arrows*), intraretinal hemorrhaging (*dashed white arrow*), and choroidal neovascularization of the optic disc (*black arrow*). **(b)** Red free fundus imaging highlights macular retinal neovascularization (*white arrows*).

Dosage

The risk for developing radiation retinopathy after brachytherapy is related to the total radiation dosage, size of the plaque used for treatment, and implantation site based on the tumor location. Studies have shown that the incidence of radiation retinopathy increase substantially when radiation dosage exceeds 45 Gy or more than 60% of the retina is exposed. Radiation retinopathy is more often found after treatment of posterior uveal melanomas due to the need for radiation dosages ranging from 80 to 100 Gy to the tumor apex, compared to brachytherapy treatment for retinoblastoma (30–45 Gy) and choroidal metastasis (25–50 Gy).

External Beam Radiotherapy

In EBT, shaped radiation beams are aimed from several angles to intersect at the tumor, providing a much larger absorbed dose at that region than in the surrounding healthy tissue. One method to combat the risk for developing radiation retinopathy is fractionated radiotherapy whereby the total radiation dosage is divided into smaller quantities to be given over numerous treatments.

Anti-Vascular Endothelial Growth Factor

Long-term intravitreal anti-VEGF therapies have been shown to be effective for treating and preventing radiation retinopathy

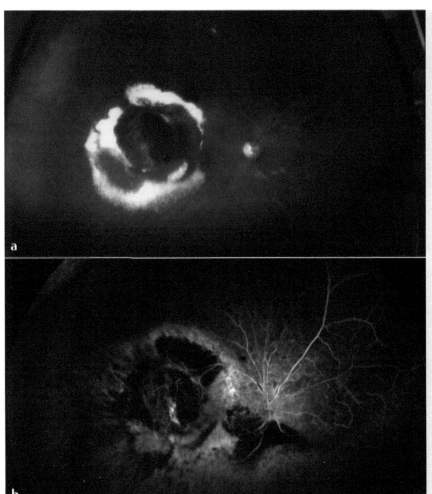

Fig. 23.3 Proliferative radiation retinopathy. **(a)** Ultra-widefield fundus photo demonstrating extensive lipid exudation and vascular attenuation with intraretinal and subretinal hemorrhage. **(b)** Ultra-widefield fluorescein angiography images demonstrating vascular nonperfusion and vascular leakage.

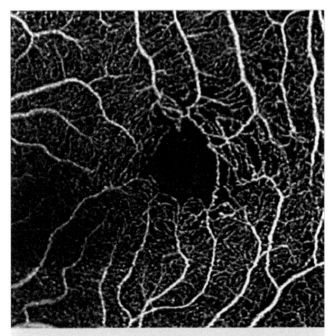

Fig. 23.4 Radiation retinopathy and optical coherence tomography angiography (OCTA). OCTA demonstrates foveal avascular zone enlargement, vascular remodeling and areas of flow voids consistent with capillary nonperfusion.

associated with brachytherapy and PBT. While the exact mechanism remains unknown, periodic treatment with bevacizumab or ranibizumab appear to disrupt the natural pathway for the development of radiation retinopathy. Factors such as dosing of the anti-VEGF agent, frequency of treatments necessary, and long-term complications require further studies for clarification.

Suggested Reading

[1] Finger PT, Chin K. Anti-vascular endothelial growth factor bevacizumab (Avastin) for radiation retinopathy. Arch Ophthalmol. 2007; 125(6):751–756

[2] Finger PT, Chin KJ, Semenova EA. Intravitreal anti-VEGF therapy for macular radiation retinopathy: a 10-year study. Eur J Ophthalmol. 2016; 26 (1):60–66

[3] Perez BA, Mettu P, Vajzovic L, et al. Uveal melanoma treated with iodine-125 episcleral plaque: an analysis of dose on disease control and visual outcomes. Int J Radiat Oncol Biol Phys. 2014; 89(1):127–136

[4] Shah SU, Shields CL, Bianciotto CG, et al. Intravitreal bevacizumab at 4-month intervals for prevention of macular edema after plaque radiotherapy of uveal melanoma. Ophthalmology. 2014; 121(1):269–275

[5] Kim IK, Lane AM, Jain P, Awh C, Gragoudas ES. Ranibizumab for the prevention of radiation complications in patients treated with proton beam irradiation for choroidal melanoma. Trans Am Ophthalmol Soc. 2016; 114:T2

24 Sickle Cell Retinopathy

Paul E. Israelsen and Andrew W. Browne

Summary

The ocular manifestations of sickle cell disease (SCD) result from vascular occlusion, which may occur in the conjunctiva, iris, retina, and choroid. Occlusion of retinal arterioles leads to downstream capillary nonperfusion, neovascularization, and the subsequent complications. Patients with early sickle cell retinopathy are usually asymptomatic, although temporary or permanent vision loss is possible. Because the ocular changes produced by SCD can be seen in other diseases, it is important to rule out other causes of occlusion.

Keywords: neovascularization, sickle cell retinopathy, blood viscosity

24.1 Features

Sickle cell retinopathy (SR) is more common among patients who have the SC or SThal genotype than those with the SS genotype. One study estimated the lifetime incidence of proliferative sickle cell retinopathy (PSR) to be 33, 14, and 3% in Hemoglobin SC, SThal, and SS, respectively. Patients with any of those hemoglobinopathies are prone to red blood cell (RBC) sickling due to polymerization of the abnormal hemoglobin molecules after deoxygenation. These sickled cells increase blood viscosity and hypercoagulability, predisposing patients to occlusive thrombosis in organs throughout the body, including the eye. Occlusion of retinal arterioles leads to downstream capillary nonperfusion and subsequent neovascularization (NV).

24.1.1 Common Symptoms

SR patients are frequently asymptomatic. As the disease progresses, patients may become symptomatic with floaters, photopsias, or dark "curtains" in visual fields. Significant vision loss is possible but uncommon.

24.1.2 Exam Findings

The Goldberg classification system outlines the pathophysiological progression of SR and the exam findings that are associated with each stage (► Fig. 24.1). The findings of SR are generally divided into those associated with non-PSR and PSR. Each of the descriptive stages can overlap.

Nonproliferative Sickle Cell Retinopathy

Stage 1: peripheral arterial occlusion (► Fig. 24.2).
• Caused by high viscosity of blood in patients with sickled RBCs.
• Most easily seen on angiography, but "silver wiring" of permanently occluded peripheral arterioles may be visualized.

Stage 2: peripheral arteriovenous anastomoses (► Fig. 24.2).
• Represent dilated preexisting capillaries.
• Usually follow the border of nonperfusion.

Proliferative Sickle Cell Retinopathy

Stage 3: NV and fibrous proliferation (► Fig. 24.2).
• Classically in a "sea-fan" configuration.
• NV usually forms at the border of nonperfusion and grows toward the ora serrata.
• Most common location for NV is superotemporal periphery, followed by inferotemporal, and then nasal.
• Often NV will autoinfarct due to upstream vascular occlusion, leading to change in their color from red to white.

Stage 4: vitreous hemorrhage.
• Caused by traction on newly formed vessels.

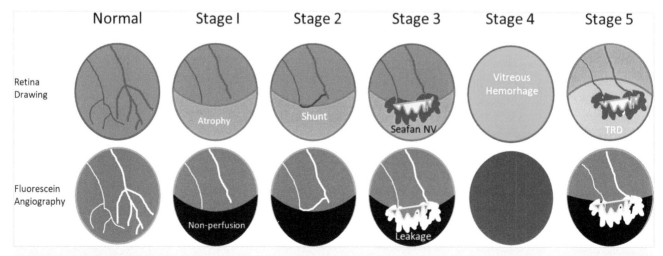

Fig. 24.1 Schematic illustrations of pathologic findings seen in sickle cell retinopathy according to the Goldberg classification system. The top row of images corresponds to retina drawings, while the bottom row of images corresponds to typical fluorescein angiography findings.

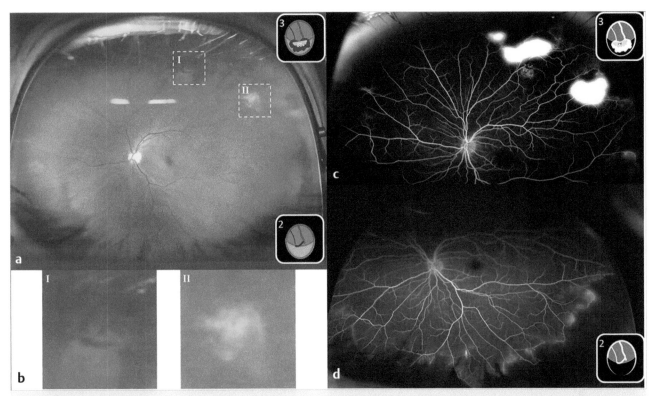

Fig. 24.2 (a) Ultra-widefield color fundus photograph of a left eye demonstrating (b) a black sunburst lesion (c) and a focus of superotemporal fibrovascular tissue likely representing a regressed sea-fan. (c) Late-phase ultra-widefield fluorescein angiogram of the same eye demonstrating peripheral nonperfusion and leakage from areas of neovascularization in the superotemporal peripheral retina. (d) Late-phase ultra-widefield fluorescein angiogram of the same eye demonstrating mild leakage from inferotemporal arteriovenous fistulas, formed to bypass ischemic capillary beds.

Stage 5: tractional retinal detachment (▶ Fig. 24.3).
• Usually forms in periphery in areas of NV.
• Traction may also result in retinal tears and rhegmatogenous retinal detachment.

Additional Potential Exam Findings

Anterior segment: "comma-shaped" conjunctival blood vessels, most commonly seen in the inferior bulbar conjunctiva; anterior segment ischemia with secondary segmental iris atrophy, corectopia, and iris NV.

Posterior segment: small red dots representing arteriolar occlusions in optic nerve head. The "macular depression sign" is an oval shaped blunting of the foveal reflex due to ischemic atrophy of the inner retina and rarely macular hole, epiretinal membrane, or macular schisis may be seen. Vessels may display tortuosity, choroidal infarction from posterior ciliary artery occlusion, and rarely central retinal artery occlusion and choroidal NV. Additional findings include salmon patch hemorrhage (i.e., pinkish–orange hemorrhage that occurs between the nerve fiber layer and internal limiting membrane representing a "blowout" of an occluded arteriole; ▶ Fig. 24.4), iridescent (refractile) spots representing hemosiderin-filled macrophages within a previous area of intraretinal hemorrhage, black sunburst lesion (i.e., a stellate or round area of retinal pigment epithelial (RPE) hyperpigmentation, hypertrophy, or hyperplasia;

▶ Fig. 24.2a inset), and angioid streaks seen in 1 to 2% of SS patients (▶ Fig. 24.5 inset).

24.2 Key Diagnostic Tests and Findings

24.2.1 Optical Coherence Tomography

Optical coherence tomography (OCT) often reveals foveal and parafoveal retinal thinning (primarily of the inner retina) and blunting of foveal contour.

24.2.2 Fluorescein Angiography or Ultra-Widefield Fluorescein Angiography

Fluorescein angiography may demonstrate enlarged foveal avascular zone, nonperfusion beyond areas of vascular occlusion, arteriovenous anastomoses seen most often at border of perfused and nonperfused areas, pooling and leaking in salmon patches, leakage in areas of NV, and slow leakage from arteriovenous anastomoses. Ultra-widefield fluorescein angiography (UWFA) may be particularly useful for visualizing the peripheral vascular abnormalities.

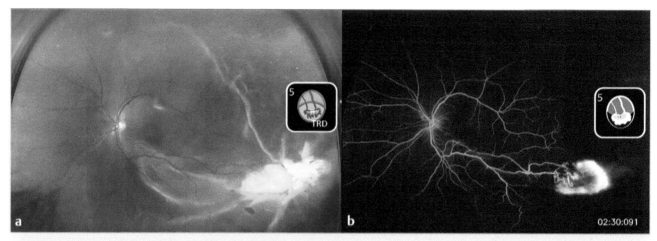

Fig. 24.3 (a) Ultra-widefield color fundus photograph of a left eye demonstrating a combined tractional and rhegmatogenous detachment involving all but the nasal retina. Exudate and tractional bands are seen inferotemporally near multiple retinal breaks. Another small break is seen in the periphery superior to the optic disc. (b) Late-phase ultra-widefield fluorescein angiography of the same eye demonstrating leakage from a neovascularization sea-fan lesion inferotemporally which corresponds to the area of exudate and tractional bands in (a).

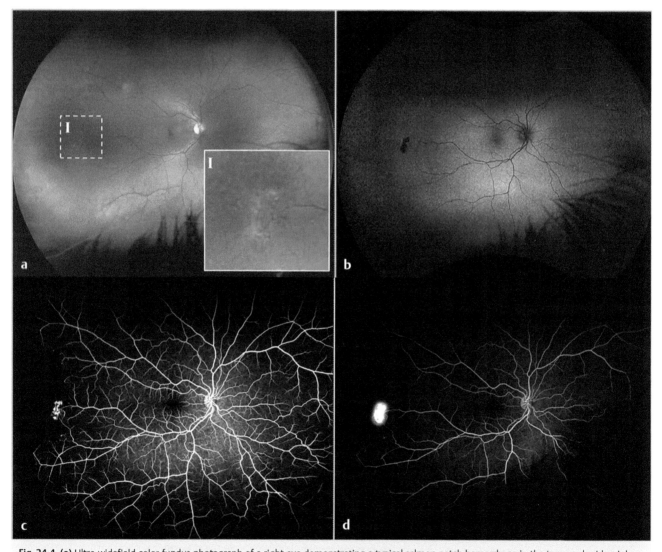

Fig. 24.4 (a) Ultra-widefield color fundus photograph of a right eye demonstrating a typical salmon patch hemorrhage in the temporal midperiphery (inset). (b) Fundus autofluorescence image of the same eye demonstrating hypo-autofluorescence in the area corresponding to the salmon patch hemorrhage. (c) Arteriovenous phase ultra-widefield fluorescein angiography image of the same eye demonstrating stippled staining in the area of the salmon patch hemorrhage. (d) Late-phase angiogram with leakage in the same area corresponding to neovascularization.

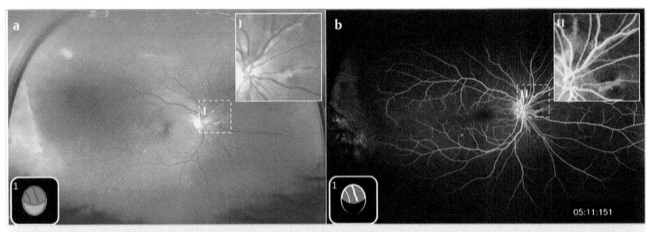

Fig. 24.5 (a) Ultra-widefield color fundus photograph of a right eye demonstrating retinal atrophy and pallor in the far temporal periphery as well as angioid streaks radiating from the optic nerve head (inset). (b) Ultra-widefield fluorescein angiography of the same eye demonstrating peripheral nonperfusion in the far temporal periphery, and redemonstrating angioid streaks (inset).

24.2.3 Fundus Autofluorescence

Proliferation of RPE in black sunburst lesions yielding mixed hyper- and hypo-autofluorescence.

24.2.4 Optical Coherence Tomography Angiography

Vascular remodeling and nonperfusion in the superficial and deep retinal capillary plexi.

24.3 Critical Work-up

Work-up typically includes UWFA, OCT, and serum hemoglobin electrophoresis (if not done previously). Ensure the patient has follow-up with primary care physician and hematologist. Differential diagnoses to consider include diabetic retinopathy, hypertensive retinopathy, retinal vascular occlusion, and ocular ischemic syndrome. Less common entities to consider include hyperviscosity conditions (leukemia), inflammatory vasculopathies (sarcoid, tuberculosis, syphilis), retinopathy of prematurity, familial exudative vitreoretinopathy, and Coat's disease.

24.4 Management

24.4.1 Treatment Options

Asymptomatic

Conservative observation with close follow-up. Most neovascular lesions will autoinfarct.

Proliferative Disease

Scatter laser photocoagulation to peripheral ischemic retina may be considered but should be used with caution because retinal holes and rhegmatogenous detachment is of greater concern after treatment in PSR than in proliferative diabetic retinopathy. Intravitreal anti-VEGF injection appears to be effective in causing regression of NV but optimal long-term management is unknown.

Vitreous Hemorrhage or Retinal Detachment

Pars plana vitrectomy (PPV) is typically performed for nonclearing vitreous hemorrhage and PPV retinal detachment. Scleral buckle should be used with caution due to risk of anterior segment ischemia.

Hyphema

Hyphemas often cause an increase in intraocular pressure (IOP) in sickle cell patients, likely due to clogging of the trabecular meshwork with sickled RBCs. Even a small increase in IOP in sickle cell disease can lead to complications such as central or branch retinal artery occlusion, so aggressive IOP-lowering treatment is indicated. Do not use carbonic anhydrase inhibitors (e.g., topical dorzolamide or brinzolamide, and oral acetazolamide) as these lower the pH of the blood and aqueous, causing further sickling. Consider early surgical management such as anterior chamber washout for patient with IOP more than 25 for more than 24 hours.

24.4.2 Follow-up

Asymptomatic, quiescent disease can typically be followed every 6 to 12 months. Active SR should be followed based on clinical scenario.

Suggested Reading

[1] Goldberg MF. Natural history of untreated proliferative sickle retinopathy. Arch Ophthalmol. 1971; 85(4):428–437

[2] Scott AW, Lutty GA, Goldberg MF. Hemoglobinopathies. Retinal Vascular Disease. Retina. 2013:1071–1082

[3] Cantor LB, Rapuano CJ, Cioffi GA, et al. Other retinal vascular diseases. In: Basic and Clinical Sciences Course, Section 12: Retina and Vitreous. 2016:137–41

[4] Myint KT, Sahoo S, Thein AW, Moe S, Ni H. Laser therapy for retinopathy in sickle cell disease. Cochrane Database Syst Rev. 2015(10):CD010790

[5] Moshiri A, Ha NK, Ko FS, Scott AW. Bevacizumab presurgical treatment for proliferative sickle-cell retinopathy-related retinal detachment. Retin Cases Brief Rep. 2013; 7(3):204–205

25 Hypertensive Retinopathy

Marisa K. Lau and Paula Eem Pecen

Summary

Systemic hypertension can produce visual symptoms, and findings on funduscopic exam and advanced imaging can be critical in the diagnosis and management of systemic and ocular manifestations of the disease. Acute hypertension typically produces vasospastic changes related to autoregulation for perfusion while chronic, persistent systemic hypertension causes atherosclerotic vascular changes, which predisposes patients to vaso-occlusive events. Mild hypertensive retinopathy can have minimal visual impact while severe hypertensive retinopathy can have significant visual changes with varying duration. Multiple imaging modalities including optical coherence tomography, fluorescein angiography and indocyanine green angiography can aid in the diagnosis of the disease.

Keywords: choroidopathy, hypertension, retinopathy

25.1 Features

25.1.1 Common Symptoms

Ocular

Range from asymptomatic to decreased visual acuity and scotoma typically related to the location and extent of hypertensive retinopathy changes.

Systemic

Headache, neurologic deficits, chest pain, respiratory distress, mental status change, nausea, and/or vomiting warrant expedited treatment to reduce mortality and morbidity of hypertensive emergency and other end organ damage.

25.1.2 Exam Findings

Findings on ophthalmoscopy of hypertensive retinopathy in the early phase can include focal intraretinal periarteriolar transudates, cotton wool spots, exudates, retinal hemorrhages, and macular edema (▶ Fig. 25.1). Later and more chronic hypertensive changes include hard exudates, arteriolar attenuation, arteriovenous nicking (▶ Fig. 25.2), arteriolar copper-wiring or silver-wiring (▶ Fig. 25.2), microaneurysms, intraretinal microvascular abnormalities, and macroaneurysms. Rarely, more severe findings may include retinal neovascularization and multilayered retinal hemorrhages (▶ Fig. 25.3). There may be superimposed hypertensive choroidopathy (▶ Fig. 25.4) which can manifest as serous retinal detachments or pigmented lesions along choroidal vessels indicative of fibrinoid necrosis (Siegrist streaks). Evidence of prior acute hypertensive retinopathy episodes includes atrophy from focal choroidal infarcts (i.e., Elschnig spots, ▶ Fig. 25.4). Hypertensive optic neuropathy can manifest acutely as optic disc edema and chronically as optic atrophy.

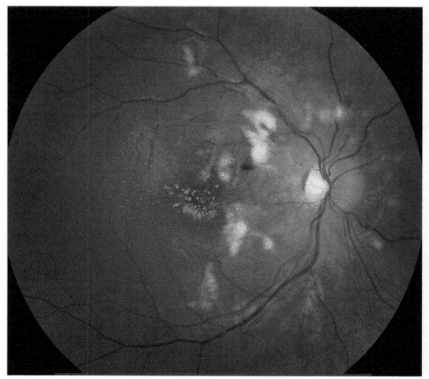

Fig. 25.1 Acute hypertensive emergency demonstrating extensive cotton wool spots, retinal exudates/macular star formation, optic disc edema, macular edema, optic disc pallor, and retinal hemorrhages. (Courtesy of Ang Li, Alex Yuan and Jonathan Sears.)

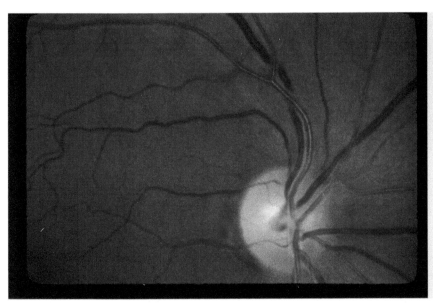

Fig. 25.2 Chronic hypertensive retinopathy demonstrating arteriovenous nicking and early copper wiring.

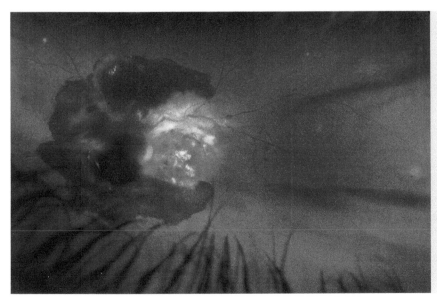

Fig. 25.3 Severe acute hypertensive emergency with underlying severe chronic retinal vascular changes including neovascularization. Extensive preretinal and subretinal hemorrhage is present. Cotton wool spots and macular exudates are present.

25.2 Key Diagnostic Tests and Findings

25.2.1 Optical Coherence Tomography

Intraretinal fluid and subretinal fluid, inner retinal hyperreflectivity due to nerve fiber layer infarcts, and intraretinal hyperreflective material corresponding to exudates (▶ Fig. 25.5). Chronically, atrophy may be noted.

25.2.2 Fluorescein Angiography or Ultra-Widefield Fluorescein Angiography

Early or mild hypertensive retinopathy may appear normal, but more severe hypertensive retinopathy may demonstrate retinal capillary nonperfusion, micro- and macroaneurysms, and reti-

nal vascular leakage. Rarely retinal neovascularization may be seen. If there is choroidal involvement, there can be patchy choroidal filling. In addition, in the acute phase there can be focal deep areas of hyperfluorescence and leakage associated with choroidal involvement (▶ Fig. 25.6). If there is optic nerve involvement, there can be optic disc hyperfluorescence or leakage.

25.2.3 Indocyanine Green Angiography

Patchy choroidal filling possible if there is concurrent hypertensive choroidopathy.

25.3 Critical Work-up

Work-up should include vital signs and dilated fundus exam, especially noting evidence of acute versus chronic hypertensive changes. The patient's history should be carefully vetted for vasculopathic risk factors, prior diagnosis of hypertension,

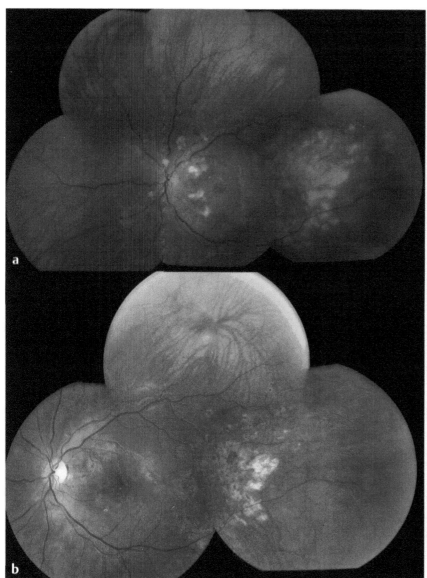

Fig. 25.4 (a) Acute hypertensive retinopathy and choroidopathy in setting of acute hypertensive emergency. The posterior pole demonstrates optic nerve pallor and edema. Extensive cotton wool spots with and few retinal hemorrhages are noted. A serous macular detachment is present. In the temporal mid-periphery, numerous whitish choroidal lesions are present consistent with choroidal infarcts and Siegrist streaks. (b) Following resolution of hypertensive episode, chronic sequelae are noted with optic nerve pallor and extensive pigmentary changes (Elshnig spots) particularly in the temporal macula and mid-periphery from previous choroidal infarcts. (Courtesy of Ang Li, Alex Yuan and Jonathan Sears.)

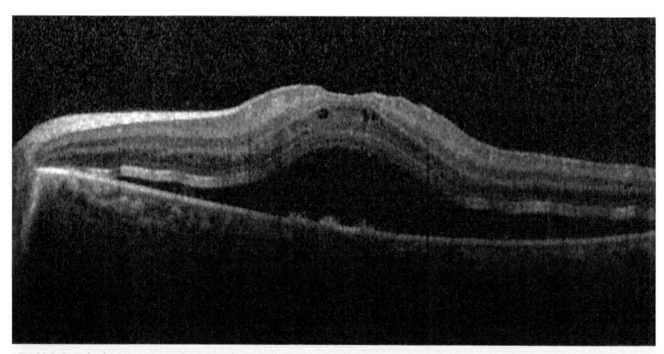

Fig. 25.5 Optical coherence tomography in acute hypertensive retinopathy/choroidopathy demonstrating subretinal fluid and intraretinal fluid confirming the presence of an exudative retinal detachment.

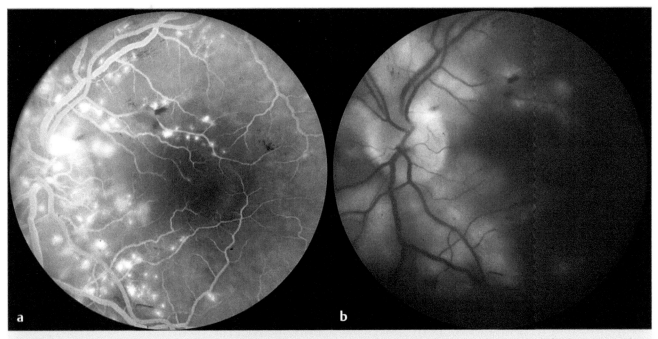

Fig. 25.6 Fluorescein venous phase angiogram in acute hypertensive retinopathy and choroidopathy demonstrating multiple focal deep areas of leakage consistent with choroidal involvement. **(a)** Blockage from retinal hemorrhage is present and areas of vascular nonperfusion are also visible. **(b)** Late phase angiogram demonstrates extensive deep leakage consistent with choroidal involvement.

diabetes, or prior regional radiation. Concurrent symptoms of other organ system damage should be carefully elicited (e.g., neurologic symptoms, chest pain, and shortness of breath). Based on clinical suspicion and urgency of work-up results, the patient can be referred to their primary care physician or the emergency department for systemic evaluation, stabilization, and blood pressure management.

25.4 Management

25.4.1 Treatment Options

Reduction in blood pressure by a primary care physician is sometimes necessitating hospital admission for emergent and regulated blood pressure reduction to prevent end organ nonperfusion. Management of the ischemic sequelae may occasionally be treated by panretinal photocoagulation or anti-vascular endothelial growth factor therapy. Secondary causes of malignant hypertension should be ruled out.

25.4.2 Follow-up

Depending on the severity of visual symptoms and stability funduscopic findings, the patient can be followed up yearly. However, in acute setting of malignant hypertension, more frequent follow-up is usually needed. Long-term follow-up is recommended to monitor for signs of neovascularization.

Suggested Reading

[1] DellaCroce JT, Vitale AT. Hypertension and the eye. Curr Opin Ophthalmol. 2008; 19(6):493–498
[2] Hayreh SS. Classification of hypertensive fundus changes and their order of appearance. Ophthalmologica. 1989; 198(4):247–260
[3] Hayreh SS, Servais GE, Virdi PS, Marcus ML, Rojas P, Woolson RF. Fundus lesions in malignant hypertension. III. Arterial blood pressure, biochemical, and fundus changes. Ophthalmology. 1986; 93(1):45–59
[4] Wong TY, Mitchell P. The eye in hypertension. Lancet. 2007; 369(9559):425–435

Part IV

Retinal Degenerations and Dystrophies

IV

26 Dry Age-Related Macular Degeneration

Sruthi Arepalli and Andrew P. Schachat

Summary

Age-related macular degeneration (AMD) is the most common cause of new blindness in the United States in those over the age of 50 years. The majority of AMD cases fall under the dry category. Dry AMD may cause gradual vision loss and is characterized by drusen, retinal pigment epithelial pigmentary changes, geographic atrophy, and thinning of the underlying choroid. The presence of hemorrhage, lipid or fluid signifies the conversion to neovascular or wet AMD. Dry AMD is classified as early, intermediate, or late/advanced, and ancillary testing such as optical coherence tomography, fluorescein angiography, and fundus autofluorescence are instrumental in monitoring disease progression. While there is no proven cure for AMD, Age-Related Eye Disease Study (AREDS) has shown that multivitamins may slow the progression to advanced disease in certain individuals.

Keywords: atrophic, age-related macular degeneration, Age-Related Eye Disease Study, basal linear/laminar, drusen, geographic atrophy

26.1 Features

Age-related macular degeneration (AMD) is a degenerative disorder of the choroid and outer retina, and the most common cause of blindness in those over the age of 50 in developed countries. AMD falls into two categories: atrophic (dry) and neovascular (wet). It is estimated that 15 million North Americans have some degree of dry AMD (accounting for 85–90% of AMD patients in North America). The most agreed upon risk factor is age, with studies demonstrating an increased prevalence in those 65 years or older. To a lesser degree, other factors include family history, race, female sex, light iris color, cigarette smoking, and medical conditions such as hypertension, hypercholesteremia, and cardiovascular disease. Furthermore, multiple genes involving collagen matrix production, the complement cascade, and lipid metabolism and transport are implicated.

In AMD, a lipid material, rich in apolipoprotein B, accumulates anterior to Bruch's membrane. These lipid aggregations fall into two broad categories: drusen and basal deposits. Drusen are subdivided into typical and subretinal drusen/pseudodrusen. Basal deposits are further categorized as basal linear and basal laminar deposits. Typical drusen are focal collections between the retinal pigmented epithelial (RPE) basal lamina and inner collagenous layer of Bruch's membrane. Subretinal drusen exist in the subretinal space, above the RPE. Neither basal linear nor laminar deposits are visible on fundus examination.

There are several changes in the RPE associated with AMD, including focal areas of hypopigmentation, hyperpigmentation, and atrophy that are visible on examination. Pigmentary changes of the RPE are considered secondary to RPE migration, with hyperpigmentary changes generally preceding hypopigmentary changes. Atrophy appears late in the disease process and is thought to occur where drusen regress with corresponding areas of death of the overlying RPE and retina and thinning of the underlying choriocapillaris.

Dry AMD can be classified as early, intermediate, or advanced. Early dry AMD consists of small or a few medium-sized drusen. Intermediate AMD is defined by more than 20 intermediate indistinct drusen, or 50 distinct drusen, or at least one large drusen, and/or the presence of nonfoveal involving atrophy (▶ Fig. 26.1, ▶ Fig. 26.2). Advanced AMD consists of foveal involving atrophy, or in the case of neovascular AMD, a choroidal neovascular membrane (▶ Fig. 26.3). Atrophy commonly spares the fovea until the later stages of the diseases.

26.1.1 Common Symptoms

Dry AMD is often asymptomatic; when present vision loss is gradual. Symptoms may include mild central vision changes, greater light requirements, slower dark/light adaptation, and mild metamorphopsia. When subfoveal atrophy is present, vision loss can be severe.

26.1.2 Exam Findings

Drusen are yellow deposits and fall into three size categories: small (< 63 μm), intermediate (between 63 and 124 μm), and large (> 125 μm) and can be hard or soft, depending on the sharpness of the borders. Hyperpigmentation and/or hypopigmentation of the RPE may be present. Geographic atrophy results from thinning of the overlying retina and RPE, with sharply demarcated window defects exposing the underlying choroidal circulation.

26.2 Key Diagnostic Tests and Findings

26.2.1 Optical Coherence Tomography

Optical coherence tomography (OCT) has become instrumental in determining the location of drusen in dry AMD and surveillance for subclinical wet AMD (▶ Fig. 26.3c). Additional findings, such as drusen features and hyperreflective outer retinal foci may have prognostic significance. Early atrophy may be best visualized with OCT. Atrophic features include outer retinal thinning, ellipsoid zone loss, RPE loss, and increased reflectivity of the choroid due to hypertransmission of the OCT beam.

26.2.2 Fluorescein Angiography or Ultra-Widefield Fluorescein Angiography

Fluorescein angiography and ultra-widefield fluorescein angiography are less frequently used in dry AMD and may demonstrate variable staining of the drusen and possible window defects associated with atrophy.

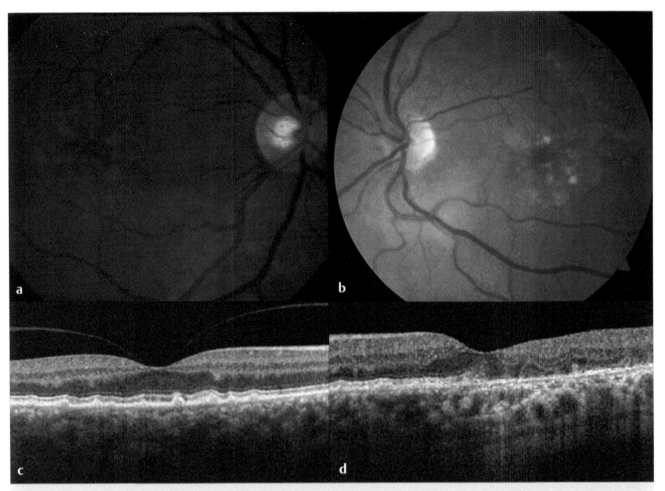

Fig. 26.1 (a) Fundus photograph of the right eye depicting intermediate age-related macular degeneration (AMD), with many intermediate and large drusen without geographic atrophy. (b) Fundus photograph of the left eye depicting advanced AMD, with many intermediate and large drusen with geographic atrophy. (c) Optical coherence tomography (OCT) through the areas of drusen showing subretinal pigment epithelium collections without fluid or atrophy. (d) OCT through the areas of drusen showing subretinal pigment epithelium collections with additional areas of RPE atrophy and outer retinal atrophy.

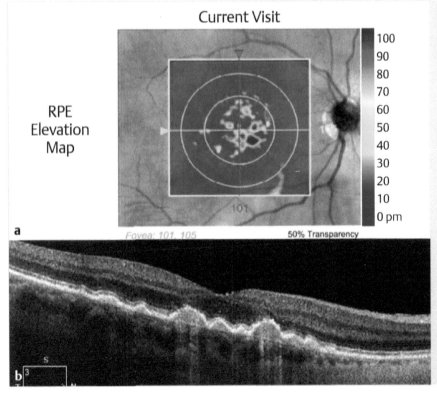

Fig. 26.2 (a) Retinal pigment epithelium map showing elevations corresponding to drusen location and height. (b) Corresponding optical coherence tomography demonstrating significant drusen burden without evidence of fluid.

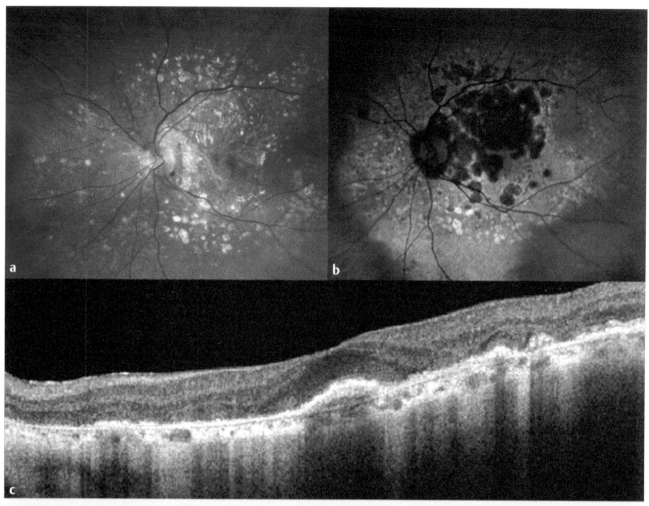

Fig. 26.3 (a) Fundus photograph of a left eye showing multiple, widespread drusen and geographic atrophy. (b) Fundus autofluorescence showing corresponding areas of drusen as hyper-autofluorescent and atrophy as hypo-autofluorescent. (c) Optical coherence tomography through the atrophy shows thinning of the outer retina, loss of the ellipsoid zone in the fovea, and thinning of the underlying choriocapillaris with increased signal transmission into the choroid.

26.2.3 Fundus Autofluorescence

Fundus autofluorescence can be used for monitoring geographic atrophy size, which appears densely hypo-autofluorescent (► Fig. 26.3b). It may also be helpful for identifying potential features of other conditions that may mimic dry AMD (e.g., Stargardt disease).

26.2.4 Optical Coherence Tomography Angiography

It is an emerging technology that has shown potential loss of the choriocapillaris in the region of drusen and atrophy. It may also be useful for identification of nonexudative choroidal neovascularization in subclinical wet AMD.

26.3 Critical Work-up

Work-up requires a dilated fundus examination. Ancillary imaging is also often used based on clinical presentation.

26.4 Management

26.4.1 Treatment Options

A multivitamin and mineral supplement, studied by the Age-Related Eye Disease Study (AREDS), comprising vitamins C and E, beta-carotene, zinc, and copper, was found to decrease the progression of AMD in patients with intermediate or advanced AMD. However, there was concern that beta-carotene increased the risk of lung cancer in smokers. AREDS2 supplementation has established equal efficiency with the replacement of beta-carotene with lutein and zeaxanthin. Modification of risk factors, including smoking, is recommended.

Patients should be educated on the chance of progression to advanced AMD. A simplified risk scale from the AREDS study provides guidance on progression risk within 5 years. Risk factors are assigned 1 point each and tallied between both eyes, with the total score ranging from 0 to 4. One point is assigned per eye with at least one large drusen, and 1 point for pigmentary changes. One point is gained if both eyes have intermediate drusen without any large drusen. In patients with advanced AMD in one eye, the eye with advanced disease is given a score of 2, with an additional point given for large drusen and/or pigment changes in the fellow eye. A score of 0 confers a risk of 0.5% progression to advanced AMD in 5 years; score of 1 confers a risk of 3%, 2 a risk of 12%, 3 a risk of 25%, and 4 a risk of 50%.

Extensive research is ongoing for additional therapeutics for dry AMD, including reducing risk of atrophy progression and retinal restoration. At this time, none of these are currently available.

26.4.2 Follow-up

Patients with atrophic or dry AMD are generally followed every 6 to 12 months. Patients with sudden visual decline or change should be seen urgently. This may signify the conversion from dry AMD to neovascular AMD, or the development or foveal involvement of geographic atrophy.

Suggested Reading

[1] Ratnapriya R, Chew EY. Age-related macular degeneration-clinical review and genetics update. Clin Genet. 2013; 84(2):160–166

[2] Bressler SB, Bressler NM. Age-related macular degeneration: non-neovascular early AMD, intermediate AMD, and geographic atrophy A2 - Ryan, Stephen J. In: Sadda SR, Hinton DR, Schachat AP, et al., eds. Retina. 5th ed. London: W.B. Saunders; 2013:1150–1182

[3] Age-Related Eye Disease Study 2 Research Group. Lutein + zeaxanthin and omega-3 fatty acids for age-related macular degeneration: the Age-Related Eye Disease Study 2 (AREDS2) randomized clinical trial. JAMA. 2013; 309 (19):2005–2015

[4] Ferris FL, Davis MD, Clemons TE, et al. A simplified severity scale for age-related macular degeneration: AREDS Report No. 18. Archives of ophthalmology (Chicago, IL: 1960) 2005;123:1570–1574

27 Wet Age-Related Macular Degeneration

Jennifer C.W. Hu and Justis P. Ehlers

Summary

Age-related macular degeneration (AMD) is the leading cause of irreversible visual impairment in older individuals in the United States. There are two different forms of AMD: "dry" nonneovascular and "wet" neovascular. This chapter will focus on the neovascular or "wet" form of AMD where there is neovascularization of the underlying choroidal vessels that can lead to leakage of fluid, retinal pigment epithelial detachment, and hemorrhage in the eye. Symptoms include metamorphopsia, scotomata, and blurry vision; patients may not initially be aware of their vision loss due to compensation by the fellow eye. Various imaging modalities are useful to diagnose neovascular AMD, differentiate it from other pathologies, and evaluate treatment options.

Keywords: choroidal neovascularization, drusen, neovascular age-related macular degeneration

27.1 Features

Neovascular age-related macular degeneration (NVAMD) is a leading cause of irreversible visual impairment in older individuals in the United States. In NVAMD, there is choroidal neovascularization (CNV) which can result in leakage of fluid, retinal pigment epithelial detachment, and hemorrhage. Though the wet form is less common than the dry form, it accounts for 90% of the cases of acute vision loss due to AMD.

27.1.1 Common Symptoms

Symptoms include metamorphopsia, scotomata, and blurry vision. If the fellow eye has good visual acuity, the disease may seem asymptomatic due to compensation from the fellow eye.

27.1.2 Exam Findings

Drusen are an early characteristic finding of both types of AMD. In addition, NVAMD often have findings related to the presence of CNV, including intraretinal fluid, subretinal fluid, intraretinal hemorrhage, subretinal hemorrhage, and pigment epithelial detachments (▶ Fig. 27.1, ▶ Fig. 27.2). The CNV may be visible as a gray/green subretinal lesion. End-stage NVAMD is frequently characterized by subretinal fibrosis and disciform scarring.

27.2 Key Diagnostic Tests and Findings

27.2.1 Optical Coherence Tomography

Optical coherence tomography (OCT) has become the gold standard for the detection of exudative activity due to NVAMD. Intraretinal (i.e., hyporeflective intraretinal cystic changes) and/or subretinal fluid (i.e., hyporeflective subretinal space between retina and retinal pigment epithelium [RPE]) are frequently present (▶ Fig. 27.3, ▶ Fig. 27.4). Additional OCT findings may include outer retinal/ellipsoid zone attenuation, subretinal

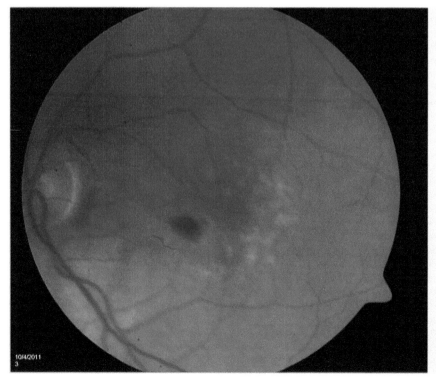

Fig. 27.1 Color fundus photo of new-onset neovascular age-related macular degeneration with retinal hemorrhage and scattered macular drusen.

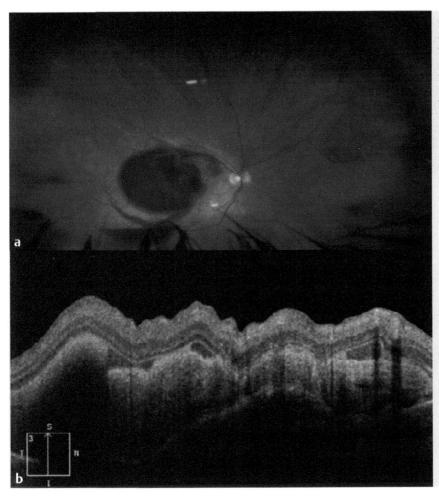

Fig. 27.2 (a) Ultra-widefield fundus photo with extensive subretinal hemorrhage and significant vision loss due to neovascular age-related macular degeneration. (b) Optical coherence tomography demonstrates retinal irregularity and subretinal hyperreflective material consistent with hemorrhage overlying a prominent hemorrhagic pigment epithelial detachment.

hyperreflective material, increased outer retinal reflectivity, and sub-RPE fluid/pigment epithelial detachments (▶ Fig. 27.2). RPE tears may also be visualized on OCT (▶ Fig. 27.5).

CNV classification based on OCT features and CNV location is also utilized to describe the disease. Type 1 CNV are characterized by sub-RPE hyporeflective heterogeneous material (▶ Fig. 27.4). Type 2 CNV are frequently seen as subretinal hyperreflective material located above the RPE. Type 3 CNV or retinal angiomatous proliferation lesion often demonstrate intraretinal cystic changes and possible hyperreflective foci associated with vascular proliferations. Type 3 CNV also has a staging system based on extent/location of lesion (e.g., intraretinal, intraretinal/subretinal, intraretinal/subretinal/sub-RPE).

In addition to its diagnostic role, OCT plays a key role in evaluation of treatment response and determining whether the treatment is needed or not (e.g., PRN dosing) or guiding the length of treatment interval (e.g., treat-and-extend dosing).

27.2.2 Fluorescein Angiography

This historic gold standard for identifying CNV is now less frequently used for NVAMD (▶ Fig. 27.6). Fluorescein angiography (FA) facilitates identification of CNV through visualization of dye leakage (e.g., hyperfluorescence) and helps characterize CNV features (e.g., occult, classic). Blockage due to hemorrhage

and staining related to fibrosis may also be present. FA is now more frequently used when the diagnosis is unclear or treatment response is suboptimal.

27.2.3 Indocyanine Green Angiography

Similar to FA, indocyanine green (ICG) angiography is now used less frequently in NVAMD due to the emergence of OCT. However, in select patient populations ICG angiography has an important role in differentiating polypoidal choroidal vasculopathy (PCV) from more traditional NVAMD. ICG angiography may reveal feeder vessels, CNV vascular plaques, and saccular polyps within the vascular network (▶ Fig. 27.7).

27.2.4 Optical Coherence Tomography Angiography

Optical coherence tomography angiography (OCTA) is emerging as a new diagnostic technique for NVAMD. OCTA will frequently demonstrate abnormal flow signatures consistent with CNV that facilitate diagnosis (▶ Fig. 27.8). In addition, OCTA has demonstrated the presence of CNV in nonexudative (i.e., no fluid on OCT) NVAMD. Identification of these lesions may impact the follow-up interval. The role for OCTA in treatment decision-making remains less clear.

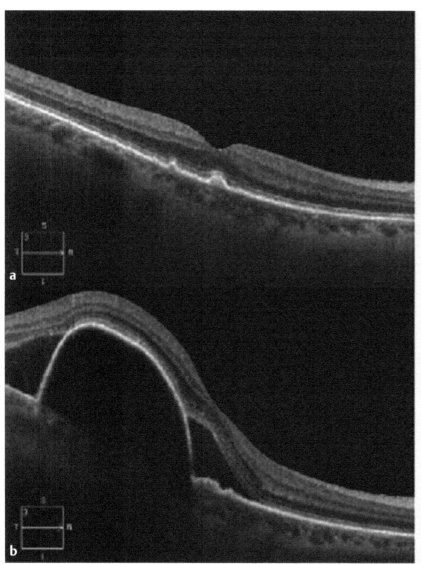

Fig. 27.3 **(a)** Spectral domain optical coherence tomography at initial presentation with nonneovascular age-related macular degeneration with moderate drusen and no evidence of exudation. **(b)** Conversion to neovascular age-related macular degeneration with new-onset vision loss, large pigment epithelial detachment, and subretinal fluid.

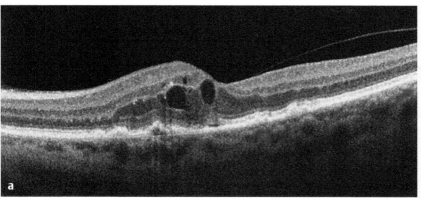

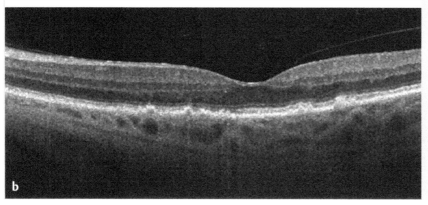

Fig. 27.4 Optical coherence tomography (OCT) with recent conversion to neovascular age-related macular degeneration exhibiting drusen, trace subretinal fluid, and intraretinal fluid. **(a)** Focal subretinal pigment epithelial hyporeflective material is present, likely reflecting type 1 choroidal neovascularization. **(b)** Following anti-vascular endothelial growth factor therapy, OCT demonstrates complete resolution of intraretinal and subretinal fluid.

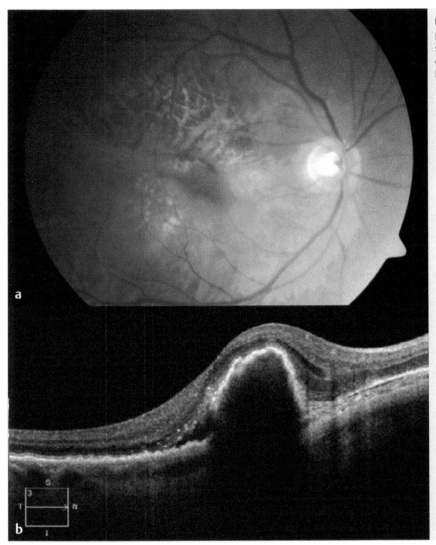

Fig. 27.5 (a) Fundus photograph demonstrating prominent retinal pigment epithelium (RPE) tear scrolling through under the fovea. **(b)** Optical coherence tomography confirming subfoveal large RPE tear and associated subretinal fluid.

27.3 Critical Work-up

The main evaluation needed in NVAMD is to rule out other causes of CNV. Primary ocular pathologies such as myopic CNV, idiopathic, choroidal rupture related, angioid streak related, and others may also be associated with CNV. Inflammatory CNV must also be considered. Subretinal hemorrhage and/or intraretinal hemorrhage may also be seen in conditions other than CNV, including retinal arterial microaneurysm and diabetic retinopathy.

27.4 Management

27.4.1 Treatment Options

Anti-Vascular Endothelial Growth Factor

Anti-vascular endothelial growth factor (VEGF) therapy has become the gold standard therapy for NVAMD. These therapeutics have been transformational for the management of NVAMD

by preserving and potentially improving visual acuity. The intravitreal injections are frequently given either on a treat-and-extend or PRN regimen. Treatment and visit burden are still challenges due to the need for ongoing therapy. Extensive research on longer-duration agents, combination therapy, and extended drug delivery systems is under way. Potential risks of intravitreal injections include endophthalmitis and retinal detachment.

Photodynamic Therapy

With the advent of anti-VEGF therapy, photodynamic therapy (PDT) has become a second-line therapeutic option for NVAMD. It is still occasionally used in eyes with insufficient response to anti-VEGF therapy. In PDT, a photosensitizing agent, verteporfin, is injected systemically and then the photodynamic therapy is applied to the CNV area. Although not often used for traditional NVAMD, PDT still has a significant role in the management of PCV. Potential risks of PDT include central vision loss due to nonperfusion and transient photosensitivity.

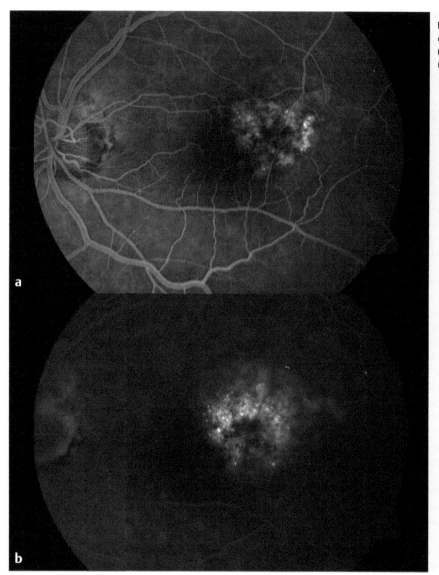

Fig. 27.6 (a) Fluorescein angiogram demonstrating early hyperfluorescence, and (b) late leakage consistent with choroidal neovascularization.

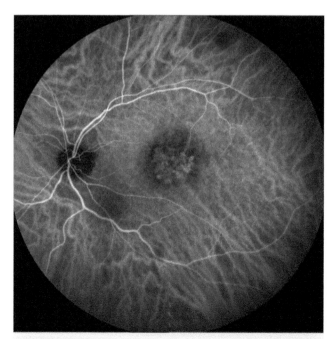

Fig. 27.7 Indocyanine green angiography in neovascular age-related macular degeneration demonstrating vascular plaque.

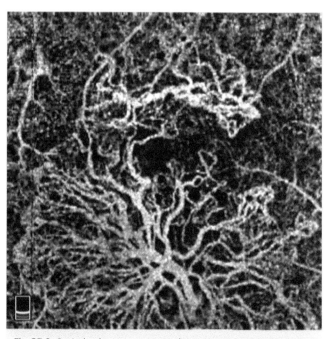

Fig. 27.8 Optical coherence tomography angiography demonstrating choroidal neovascularization.

27.4.2 Follow-up

Patients with NVAMD must be followed up closely for disease activity. Eyes with asymptomatic CNV may sometimes be observed but must be watched carefully for disease progression. Follow-up frequency is most commonly dictated by the treatment regimen utilized. PRN treatment requires frequent (i.e., monthly) follow-up intervals to maximize outcomes. Treat-and-extend regimens use disease activity to dictate follow-up intervals which typically ranges from 6 to 12 weeks, based on response to therapy.

Suggested Reading

[1] Klein R, Klein BEK, Knudtson MD, Meuer SM, Swift M, Gangnon RE, et al. Fifteen-year cumulative incidence of age-related macular degeneration: the Beaver Dam Eye Study. Ophthalmology. 2007; 114(2):253–262

[2] Solomon SD, Lindsley K, Vedula SS, Krzystolik MG, Hawkins BS. Anti-vascular endothelial growth factor for neovascular age-related macular degeneration. In: Cochrane Database of Systematic Reviews. John Wiley & Sons, Ltd; 2014

[3] Nunes RP, Rosenfeld PJ, Filho CA, Yehoshua Z, Martidis A, Tennant MTS. Age-related macular degeneration. In: Ophthalmology. 4th ed. Saunders; 2014:580–599

[4] Photodynamic therapy of subfoveal choroidal neovascularization in age-related macular degeneration with verteporfin: one-year results of 2 randomized clinical trials–TAP report. Treatment of age-related macular degeneration with photodynamic therapy (TAP) Study Group. Arch Ophthalmol. 1999; 117(10):1329–1345

[5] Amoaku WM, Chakravarthy U, Gale R, et al. Defining response to anti-VEGF therapies in neovascular AMD. Eye (Lond). 2015; 29(6):721–731

28 Polypoidal Choroidal Vasculopathy

Keiko Kataoka and Hiroko Terasaki

Summary

Polypoidal choroidal vasculopathy (PCV) is characterized by an abnormal vascular network that originates from choroidal vessels and terminates in polypoidal vessel dilations. Distinguishing between PCV and neovascular age-related macular degeneration (NVAMD) is critical, as PCV has a higher risk of massive hemorrhage compared with that seen in NVAMD due to the rupture of polyps. Eyes with PCV have some typical findings, such as the appearance of orange–red nodule-like lesions and serosanguineous subretinal or subretinal pigment epithelial lesions on fundus examination, the identification of which is the first step in determining the presence of polypoidal lesions. Multiple scans of the entire macular area with optical coherence tomography (OCT) are necessary to find sharp-peaked pigment epithelial detachment (PED) with notch sign or nodule-like moderate hyperreflectivity relating to polyps. To date, indocyanine green angiography (ICG) is the gold standard for diagnosing PCV and identifying polypoidal lesions and branching vascular network expansion. OCT angiography is a new imaging modality and is useful for detecting blood flow signal associated with polyps inside sharp-peaked PED. Thus, a combination of multimodal images can lead to higher accuracy in the diagnosis of PCV. This chapter describes key findings related to polypoidal lesions with multimodal images including OCT, ICG, and OCT angiography. In addition, treatment options including anti-vascular endothelial growth factor therapy and verteporfin photodynamic therapy are also discussed.

Keywords: branching vascular network, indocyanine green angiography, OCT angiography, optical coherence tomography, polypoidal choroidal vasculopathy, polypoidal lesions

28.1 Features

Polypoidal choroidal vasculopathy (PCV) is known to be more common in people of Asian and African ancestry. Clinically, PCV is characterized by polypoidal aneurysmal dilations of network vessels originating in the choroid and is considered by some to be one of the subtypes of neovascular age-related macular degeneration (NVAMD), although the precise pathogenesis of PCV is still controversial.

28.1.1 Common Symptoms

Metamorphopsia, blurred vision, or scotoma in the central or paracentral vision. It may be asymptomatic because the lesions of PCV are located beneath the retinal pigment epithelium (RPE) or they may be located outside the macular area.

28.1.2 Exam Findings

Orange–red nodule-like subretinal lesions can be found on fundus examination or color fundus images (▶ Fig. 28.1). Serosanguineous pigment epithelial detachment (PED), serous retinal detachment, and/or subretinal hemorrhage are found in most active cases (▶ Fig. 28.2). Massive subretinal and sub-RPE hemorrhage can also be seen when polypoidal lesions are ruptured.

28.2 Key Diagnostic Tests and Findings

28.2.1 Optical Coherence Tomography

Anterior sharp protrusion of RPE with relatively moderate internal reflectivity relating to polyps (▶ Fig. 28.3, ▶ Fig. 28.4). Once polyps cause active leakage around them, large serous or hemorrhagic PED can be found. A notch sign in the RPE of a PED or moderate hyperreflective nodule-like lesions along the basal RPE or inside PED are both suggestive of the presence of polypoidal lesions. Round hyporeflective or moderate hyperreflective areas surrounded by hyperreflective rings beneath RPE

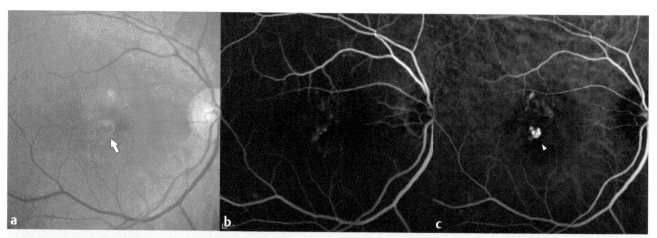

Fig. 28.1 (a) Orange–red nodule-like subretinal lesions (*arrow*) in the color fundus image. (b) Fluorescein angiography shows occult-like hyperfluorescence. (c) Indocyanine green angiography delineates multiple nodule-like lesions (*arrowhead*) with branching vascular network.

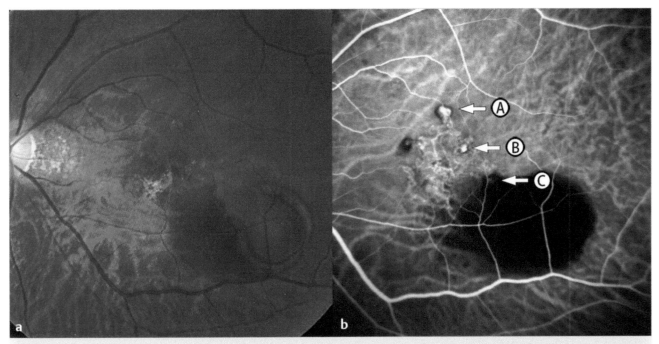

Fig. 28.2 (a) Subretinal hemorrhage and hemorrhagic pigment epithelial detachment in the color fundus image. (b) Indocyanine green angiography demonstrates multiple polypoidal lesions (*arrows A and B*) connected with branching vascular network. Hazed polypoidal lesion in the hemorrhage (*arrow C*).

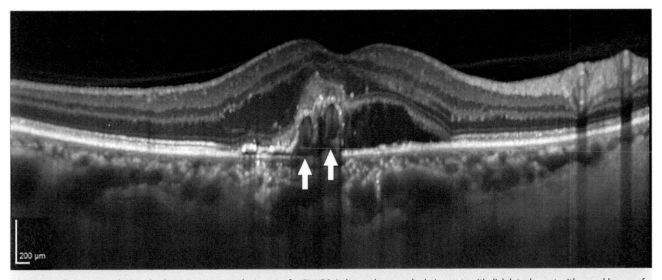

Fig. 28.3 The associated optical coherence tomography image of ▶ Fig. 28.1 shows sharp-peaked pigment epithelial detachment with round lumen of polyps (*arrows*).

suggest lumens of polyps (▶ Fig. 28.3). Branching vascular networks (BVN) can be found adjacent to the sharp or large PED as lower RPE elevation filled with moderate hyperreflectivity (▶ Fig. 28.4). These may be best seen with en face optical coherence tomography (OCT) or C-scan review. At the site of lower RPE elevation, a hyperreflective thin line between the RPE and Bruch's membrane, named the "double-layer sign," may also be noted. However, the double-layer sign can be seen in not only BVN but also type-1 choroidal neovascularization (CNV). Serous

retinal detachment and subretinal hyperreflective material associated with subretinal hemorrhage and/or fibrin are often observed around polypoidal lesions with less intraretinal edema than with NVAMD. Enhanced depth images of spectral-domain OCT or swept-source OCT can be useful in detecting thick choroid called "pachychoroid." It is reported that choroidal thickness in eyes with PCV was greater than that in eyes with NVAMD. Thus, pachychoroid on OCT imaging is helpful in detecting PCV.

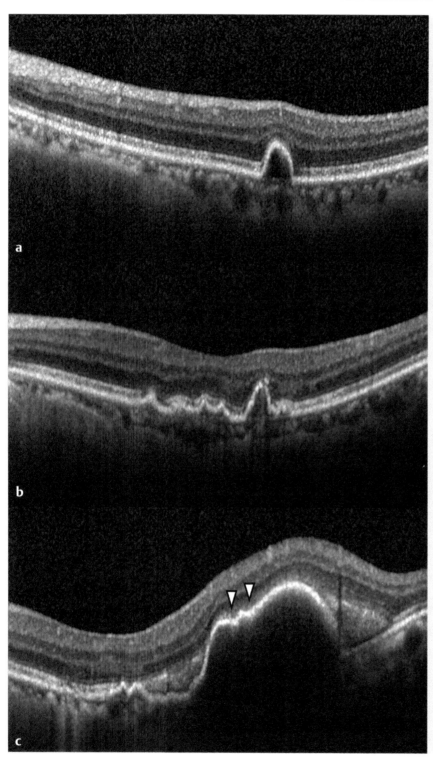

Fig. 28.4 The associated optical coherence tomography (OCT) of the (a–c) lesions in ▶ Fig. 28.3. (a,b) Each OCT demonstrates the B-scan at the polypoidal lesions without exudate and (c) with the large hemorrhagic pigment epithelial detachment (PED). Note the notch signs at the large hemorrhagic PED (*arrowheads*).

28.2.2 Fluorescein Angiography or Ultra-Widefield Fluorescein Angiography

Due to the location of the lesions in PCV, fluorescein angiography (FA) is not as useful in identifying polyps, and it frequently has similar appearance to traditional occult CNV or minimally classic CNV type (▶ Fig. 28.1). FA can be useful for evaluating other conditions that may mimic PCV.

28.2.3 Indocyanine Green Angiography

Indocyanine green angiography (ICGA) is considered the gold standard to detect polypoidal lesions and differentiate PCV from NVAMD and other macular diseases. Polypoidal lesions

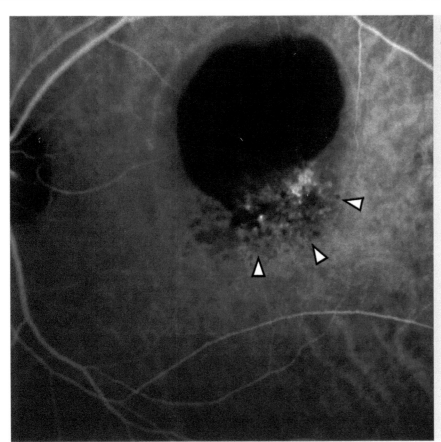

Fig. 28.5 Indocyanine green angiography demonstrates blocking area related to a large pigment epithelial detachment (PED) and branching vascular network adjacent to PED (*arrowheads*). No polypoidal lesion was detected.

delineated as nodular areas or grape-like clusters are seen on ICGA within approximately 6 min following the injection of ICG. It is sometimes difficult to detect polypoidal lesions due to the blocking effect from massive hemorrhage or large PED around polyps. Only the vascular network adjacent to the large blocked hypofluorescent area can be seen as a key sign in suggesting the presence of polyps in the blocked hypofluorescent area (▶ Fig. 28.5). Early-phase dynamic CNV can provide images of a feeder vessel of BVN. Pulsation of polyps may also be detected by dynamic ICG angiography.

28.2.4 Optical Coherence Tomography Angiography

Although still emerging as a diagnostic, flow images of OCT angiography (OCTA) are useful in detecting blood flow in sharp-peaked PED which suggests polypoidal lesions of PCV. Polypoidal lesions are sometimes found more easily on B-scan flow images of OCTA than on ICGA (▶ Fig. 28.6).

28.3 Critical Work-up

No systemic work-up is typically needed with PCV. The primary goal is to rule out other potential diagnoses and make the diagnosis of PCV, which can sometimes be challenging. Multimodal imaging as outlined, including potentially OCT, ICGA, and OCTA (▶ Fig. 28.6).

28.4 Management

28.4.1 Treatment Options

The main goals of PCV treatment are reducing the risk of hemorrhage and managing active disease. It is important to resolve polypoidal lesions, as they have a risk of rupture and subsequent massive hemorrhage.

Anti-Vascular Endothelial Growth Factor

Historically, PCV was considered to be relatively resistant against anti-vascular endothelial growth factor (VEGF) monotherapy compared with NVAMD. However, recent studies with aflibercept have suggested potential good response to anti-VEGF monotherapy. Bimonthly injections of aflibercept for PCV showed 55.4% complete and 32.5% partial resolution of polypoidal lesions.

Photodynamic Therapy and Combination Therapy

Another option for treating PCV is combination therapy with verteporfin photodynamic therapy (PDT) and anti-VEGF therapy. Combination therapy with PDT and ranibizumab has been reported to be superior to ranibizumab monotherapy in the complete regression of polypoidal lesions (69.3 vs 34.7%) and in the number of injections needed (four times vs. seven times for

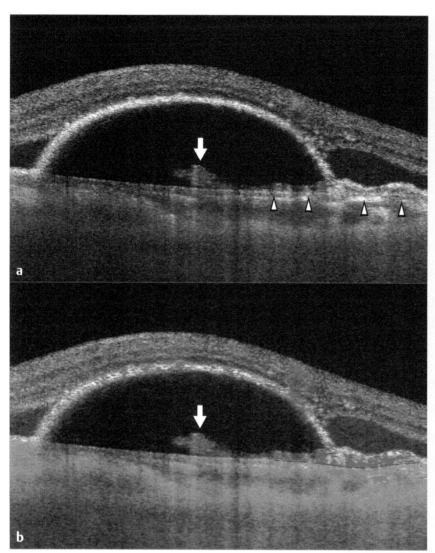

Fig. 28.6 The associated optical coherence tomography (OCT) and flow image by OCT angiography (OCTA) of ▶ Fig. 28.5. **(a)** OCT demonstrates a nodular appearance with moderate hyperreflectivity (*arrow*) and branching vascular network extending into pigment epithelial detachment (*arrowheads*). **(b)** Flow image of OCTA demonstrating the flow signals above and below Bruch's membrane are shown in *red* and *green*, respectively. The flow signals demonstrate the nodular appearance (*arrow*).

12 months). PDT may carry an increased risk of retinal hemorrhage during treatment.

28.4.2 Follow-up

Careful long-term follow-up with fundus examination and OCT scan of the entire macula area is needed. Even after apparent regression of polypoidal lesions, newly formed lesions often occur from residual BVN.

Suggested Reading

[1] Chung SE, Kang SW, Lee JH, Kim YT. Choroidal thickness in polypoidal choroidal vasculopathy and exudative age-related macular degeneration. Ophthalmology. 2011; 118(5):840–845

[2] Koh AH, Chen LJ, Chen SJ, et al. Expert PCV Panel. Polypoidal choroidal vasculopathy: evidence-based guidelines for clinical diagnosis and treatment. Retina. 2013; 33(4):686–716

[3] Yamamoto A, Okada AA, Kano M, et al. One-year results of intravitreal aflibercept for polypoidal choroidal vasculopathy. Ophthalmology. 2015; 122(9): 1866–1872

[4] Koh A, Lai TYY, Takahashi K, et al. EVEREST II study group. Efficacy and safety of ranibizumab with or without verteporfin photodynamic therapy for polypoidal choroidal vasculopathy: a randomized clinical trial. JAMA Ophthalmol. 2017; 135(11):1206–1213

29 Age-Related Choroidal Atrophy

Richard F. Spaide

Summary

Situated between the sclera and Bruch's membrane, the choroid acts as the vascular layer of the eye. Most of the choroid is occupied by blood vessels, with the remaining tissue being melanocytes and stromal tissue. More than 70% of all of the blood flow to the eye goes to the choroid, and it has one of the lowest amounts of oxygen extraction of any tissue. The retinal circulation, which is about 5% of the blood flow to the eye, supplies the inner and middle retina; the choroid supplies the outer retina and is the only source for the avascular fovea. The choroid has additional functions such as acting as a heat sink, absorbing stray light, participating in immune response and host defense, and it is an integral part in the process of emmetropization.

While some diseases are related to the choroid being too thick, other pathological conditions are associated with a thinner choroid. These include some inflammatory diseases after disease resolution, pathologic myopia, and age-related choroidal atrophy (ARCA). One of the more common correlates with a thin choroid in an older patient is pseudodrusen (i.e., subretinal drusenoid deposits), in the context of which geographic atrophy, type 2, and type 3 neovascularization may develop. Optical coherence tomography and fundus photography are helpful imaging modalities.

Keywords: age-related choroidal atrophy, pseudodrusen, subretinal drusenoid deposits

29.1 Features

Choroidal thickness depends on race, age, refractive error, and to a lesser extent on gender; the thickness also shows diurnal variation. A very rough rule of thumb is the subfoveal choroidal thickness in a 50-year-old emmetrope is about 250 to 300 μm and decreases by 2 to 4 μm per year. An average 80-year-old may have an expected choroidal thickness of 200 μm. However, some nonmyopic people may have choroidal thicknesses much less than this and develop what is called age-related choroidal atrophy (ARCA).

29.1.1 Common Symptoms

Difficulty in adapting to dim illumination or bright sunlight. Decreased visual acuity if the choroidal thickness is less than 30 μm.

29.1.2 Exam Findings

The easily recognizable fundus appearance includes a rarefaction of choroidal vessels, yellowish-colored choroidal vessels, the central macular granular pigmentary changes, and subretinal drusenoid deposits (SDD; ▶ Fig. 29.1, ▶ Fig. 29.2). With decreasing choroidal thickness, the pigmentary changes become more prominent. The choroid is typically thinner toward the nerve, and in ARCA patients, the choroidal thinning may progress to where peripapillary atrophy develops because the remaining choroid is unable to provide sufficient support for the surrounding tissue. Eyes with SDD show prolonged dark adaptation. Over time SDD can regress with associated loss of the outer retinal architecture, with thinning of the outer nuclear layer and ellipsoid zone attenuation; this is called outer retinal atrophy. SDD preferentially form in areas with high rod concentration. Type 2 and type 3 choroidal neovascularization may develop in the context of SDD. Because ARCA and the often accompanying SDD affect the perifoveal macula, a small focus of neovascularization or geographic atrophy affecting the fovea can be associated with a greater loss of visual function than the size of the offending lesion would suggest.

29.2 Key Diagnostic Tests and Findings

29.2.1 Optical Coherence Tomography

Optical coherence tomography (OCT) is the key diagnostic for identification of ARCA. In the first description of ARCA, the mean choroidal thickness in evaluated patients was 69.3 μm, although the upper cut-off was 125 μm. Both a thin choroid and a much lower proportion of the choroid being occupied by vessel lumens is frequently present. Some patients have a thickness of 30 μm or less and typically have associated decreased visual acuity.

29.2.2 Fundus Photography

Fundus imaging may be useful to document clinical findings. Sometimes the yellow color changes of the choroidal vessels are more readily apparent in fundus photographs. Autofluorescence imaging does not show loss of the retinal pigment epithelium unless there is concurrent geographic atrophy.

29.3 Critical Work-up

Fundus examination and OCT are the critical evaluation components for making the diagnosis of ARCA.

29.4 Management

29.4.1 Treatment Options

No current treatment for ARCA is available. If choroidal neovascularization develops, intravitreal anti-vascular endothelial growth factor agents should be considered. Patients with marked thinning of the choroid usually need more light and higher contrast material to read easily. Use of electronic means such as a tablet or a computer monitor may make reading easier.

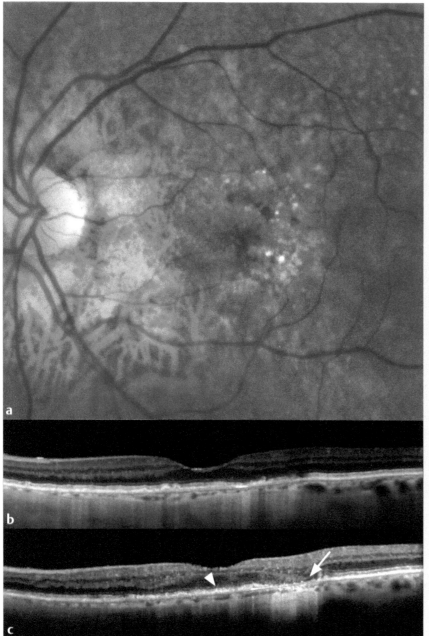

Fig. 29.1 **(a)** Color photograph showing age-related choroidal atrophy with scattered pseudodrusen (also known as subretinal drusenoid deposits) and some drusen. **(b)** The subfoveal choroidal thickness is 58 μm; note the relative avascularity of the choroid. **(c)** One year later, there was loss of the ellipsoid zone in the central fovea (*arrowhead*) and early geographic atrophy with subsidence of the retina, loss of the outer nuclear layer and outer retinal architecture, and hypertransmission.

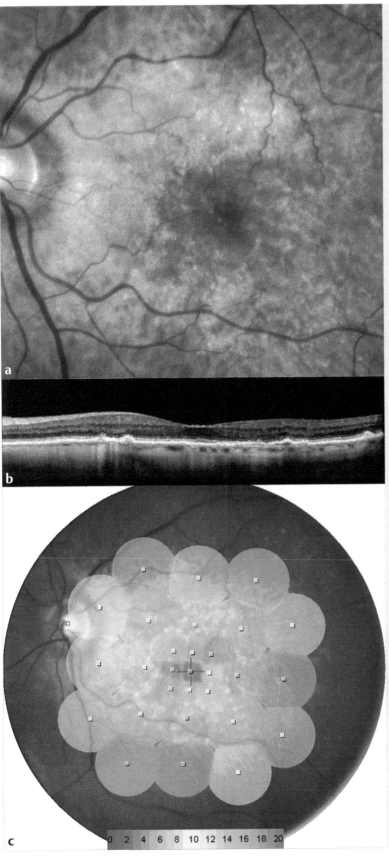

Fig. 29.2 (a) Fundus photo demonstrating drusen and pigmentary changes in the macula and an extensive array of pseudodrusen peripheral to the macula. Note the tessellation of the fundus, a sign of choroidal thinning and the yellowish appearance of the choroidal vessels in the nasal macula. (b) The optical coherence tomography image shows a subfoveal choroidal thickness of 81 μm. (c) Microperimetry shows decreased threshold sensitivity.

29.4.2 Follow-up

Patients should be followed regularly (i.e., every 6–12 months) for the development of complications, such as choroidal neovascularization.

Suggested Reading

[1] Spaide RF. The choroid. In: Spaide RF, Ohno-Matsui K, Yannuzzi LA, eds. Pathologic Myopia. New York: Springer; 2014

[2] Mrejen S, Spaide RF. Optical coherence tomography: imaging of the choroid and beyond. Surv Ophthalmol. 2013; 58(5):387–429

[3] Spaide RF. Age-related choroidal atrophy. Am J Ophthalmol. 2009; 147(5): 801–810

30 Myopic Degeneration and Myopic Foveoschisis

Makoto Inoue and Yuji Itoh

Summary

Pathologic myopia is usually associated with chorioretinal abnormalities such as lacquer cracks, myopic choroidal neovascularization, chorioretinal atrophy, and pigmentary degeneration. These abnormalities are the causes of the visual impairments in eyes with pathologic myopia. As the axial length is elongated and the posterior curvature of the eye is extruded posteriorly in highly myopic eyes, the retina and choroid are abnormally stretched and thin. This leads to the development of the myopic degenerative changes. Imaging, including optical coherence tomography, is important to detect changes associated with myopic traction maculopathy and choroidal neovascularization.

Keywords: choroidal neovascularization, lacquer cracks, macular retinoschisis, myopic degeneration, pathologic myopia

30.1 Features

Pathologic myopia is usually associated with chorioretinal abnormalities such as lacquer cracks, myopic choroidal neovascularization (CNV; ► Fig. 30.1), chorioretinal atrophy, and pigmentary degeneration. These abnormalities are the causes of the visual impairments in eyes with pathologic myopia. As the axial length is elongated and the posterior curvature of the eye is extruded posteriorly in highly myopic eyes, the retina and choroid are abnormally stretched and thin. This leads to the development of the myopic degenerative changes. Myopic traction maculopathy develops in three stages—beginning with a macular retinoschisis and foveoschisis followed by the development of a foveal detachment which subsequently progresses to a macular hole retinal detachment (MHRD) or a macular hole (MH; ► Fig. 30.2, ► Fig. 30.3, ► Fig. 30.4). Vitreous pockets can also be present due to tangential traction by the posterior vitreous cortex, contributing to the development of myopic tractional maculopathy.

30.1.1 Common Symptoms

It is sometimes asymptomatic. The patient may experience decreased visual acuity, metamorphopsia.

30.1.2 Exam Findings

Minimal findings may be present. Areas of retinal pigment epithelium (RPE) hyper- and hypopigmentation are frequently present. Macular and/or peripapillary atrophy may be noted. Posterior staphyloma may be present. A myopic CNV appears as a hypopigmented spot with possible subretinal hemorrhage and hyperpigmentation at the border of the CNV (► Fig. 30.1). Lacquer cracks are typically linear hypopigmented lesions secondary to breaks in Bruch's membrane.

30.2 Key Diagnostics and Tests

30.2.1 Optical Coherence Tomography

Optical coherence tomography (OCT) frequently demonstrates concave curvature of the posterior segment of the eye. Dome-shaped macula may also be present. Myopic CNV appears as subretinal hyperreflective lesions with or without intraretinal fluid, subretinal fluid, subretinal hemorrhage, or RPE detachments. Increased outer retinal reflectivity is often seen in the presence of CNV. Myopic traction maculopathy has multiple OCT features, such as possible intraretinal fluid, subretinal fluid, macular hole, and vitreoretinal interface abnormalities. In MHRD, significant subretinal fluid is noted on OCT.

30.2.2 Fluorescein Angiography or Ultra-Widefield Fluorescein Angiography

Fluorescein angiography (FA) is most frequently utilized to evaluate the presence of CNV. Lacquer cracks, observed as linear transmission defects in the early and transit phases of FA, represent mechanical breaks of the Bruch's membrane, RPE, and choriocapillaris complex. Patchy window defects and RPE atrophy in eyes with myopic degenerative changes can be detected at the macula and around the optic disc.

A myopic CNV appears as a hyperfluorescent spot with a well-demarcated rim of hypofluorescence indicating a type 2 CNV located above the RPE layer. Associated hemorrhages around a myopic CNV are seen in blocked hypofluorescent spots in early images of FA. Leakage from the myopic CNV is seen in the late phase images.

30.2.3 Optical Coherence Tomography Angiography

The role for optical coherence tomography angiography (OCTA) in myopic degeneration is still emerging. It may be particularly useful for identifying CNV in cases where the diagnosis is unclear.

30.3 Management

30.3.1 Treatment Options

CNV Management

Anti-vascular endothelial growth factor (anti-VEGF) therapy is considered the first-line treatment for myopic CNV. Studies suggest that myopic CNV may be more responsive and may have less of a treatment burden than CNV associated with age-related macular degeneration. Photodynamic therapy (PDT) has also been used for myopic CNV but is now second line behind VEGF inhibitors.

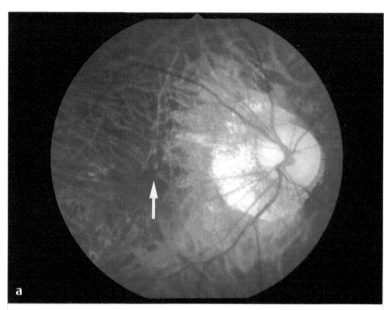

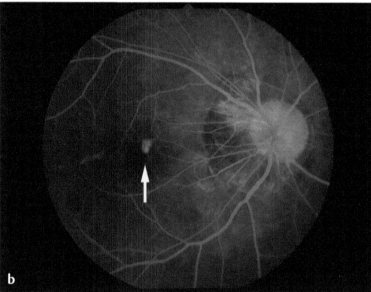

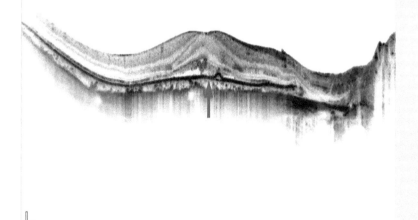

Fig. 30.1 Fundus photograph, fluorescein angiography (FA), and optical coherence tomographic (OCT) images of myopic (−14.0 D) choroidal neovascularization (CNV). **(a)** Fundus photograph showing peripapillary atrophy and myopic CNV (*arrow*) at the fovea. **(b)** FA shows hyperfluorescence at the myopic CNV (arrow) with leakage at the late stage. **(c)** Horizontal OCT image showing a subfoveal CNV (*arrow*) above the retinal pigment epithelium layer with subretinal fluid and hyperreflective material above the CNV.

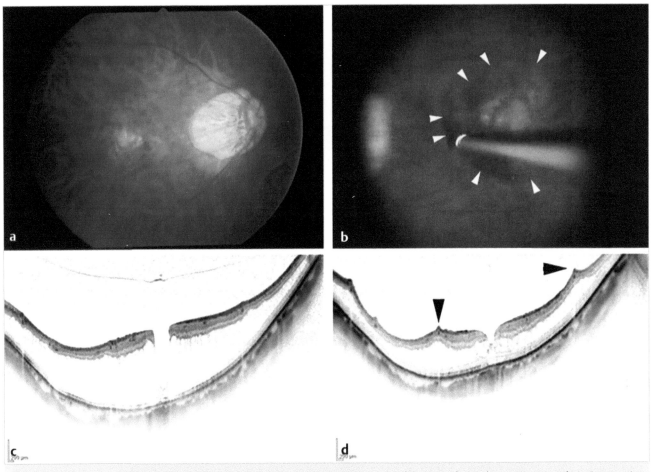

Fig. 30.2 **(a,b)** Fundus photograph and **(c,d)** optical coherence tomographic (OCT) images of the eye with macular myopic retinoschisis. Preoperative photograph and OCT image showing macular retinoschisis. **(c)** Intraoperative photograph of fovea-sparing internal limiting membrane (ILM) peeling showing trimming by a vitreous cutter of an inverted ILM (*arrowheads*) made visible by brilliant blue G staining. **(d)** Postoperative OCT image showing a reduction of retinoschisis, although the arteriolar traction (*arrowheads*) remains.

Tractional Maculopathy Management

Observation should be considered in eyes with minimal visual symptoms. Spontaneous resolution of myopic traction maculopathy is occasionally seen in eyes with a spontaneous relief of the vitreous traction by a posterior vitreous detachment or relief of internal limiting membrane (ILM) traction after spontaneous dehiscence of the ILM.

Surgical intervention with vitrectomy and often ILM peeling procedures are the standard approach to traction maculopathy. Removal of the vitreous cortex that adheres to the retina without removing the ILM has been shown to be effective in treating myopic traction maculopathy. Fovea-sparing ILM peeling in which the ILM is peeled around the fovea with a donut shape has been used to potentially reduce the risk of postoperative MH (▶ Fig. 30.2). Newer techniques, such as an inverted ILM flap technique have been reported to be effective in closing persistent larger-diameter MHs. The ILM is not completely removed from the retina around the MH but is inverted to form a cover over the MH. This is also considered for MHRD to achieve retinal reattachments and MH closure (▶ Fig. 30.4). Gas tamponade is also frequently used at the time of vitrectomy. MH and MHRD development following surgical intervention is a feared complication.

Macular buckling is also utilized as a surgical repair option for myopic MH and MHRD. Utilizing the buckle element, direct support is provided in the area of the staphyloma which reduces the posterior elongation of the eye. Suprachoroidal macular buckling with viscoelastic materials has also been described for traction maculopathy.

30.4 Follow-up

Patients without active CNV are typically followed every 6 to 12 months. If CNV is suspected, follow-up is usually dictated by ongoing management and may be as frequent as monthly.

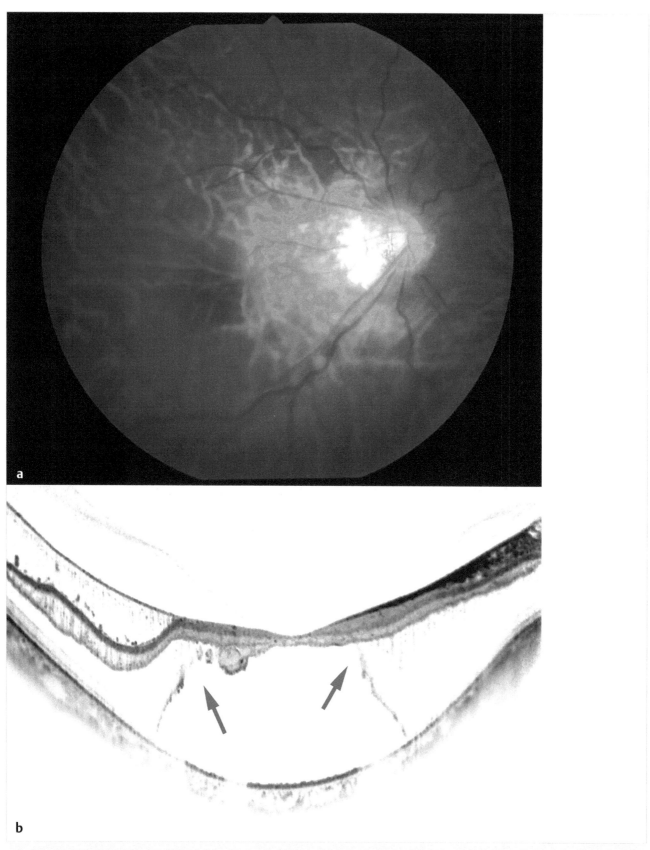

Fig. 30.3 (a) Fundus photograph and (b) optical coherence tomographic (OCT) image demonstrating myopic macular schisis and foveal detachment. OCT image of a vertical scan showing retinoschisis and foveal detachment. The posterior hyaloid is attached to the fovea. Outer retinal holes (*arrows*) can be seen at the edge of the foveal detachment.

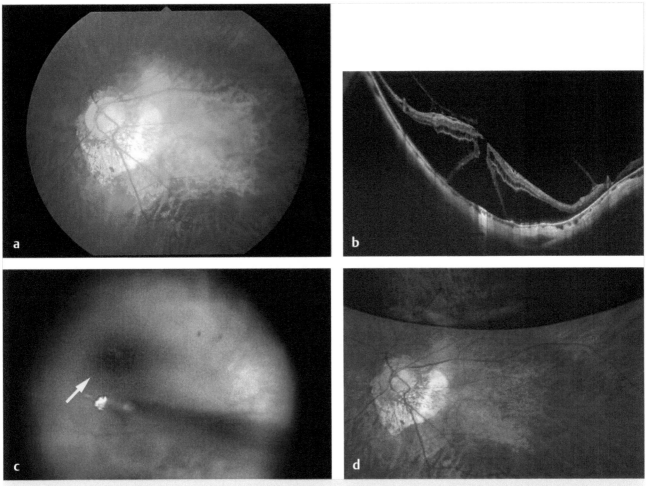

Fig. 30.4 Fundus photograph and optical coherence tomographic (OCT) images of eye with macular retinoschisis and full-thickness macular hole. **(a)** Fundus photograph demonstrating macular hole and schisis. **(b)** OCT image of a vertical scan showing retinoschisis, foveal detachment, and macular hole. **(c)** Intraoperative photograph of the inverted internal limiting membrane (ILM) technique showing ILM was peeled toward the macular hole (*arrow*) after the ILM was made visible by brilliant blue G staining. The ILM was inverted and placed over the macular hole. **(d)** Fundus photograph showing successful repair.

Suggested Reading

[1] Shimada N, Ohno-Matsui K, Yoshida T, Sugamoto Y, Tokoro T, Mochizuki M. Progression from macular retinoschisis to retinal detachment in highly myopic eyes is associated with outer lamellar hole formation. Br J Ophthalmol. 2008; 92(6):762–764

[2] Taniuchi S, Hirakata A, Itoh Y, Hirota K, Inoue M. Vitrectomy with or without internal limiting membrane peeling for each stage of myopic traction maculopathy. Retina. 2013; 33(10):2018–2025

[3] Shimada N, Sugamoto Y, Ogawa M, Takase H, Ohno-Matsui K. Fovea-sparing internal limiting membrane peeling for myopic traction maculopathy. Am J Ophthalmol. 2012; 154(4):693–701

[4] Michalewska Z, Michalewski J, Adelman RA, Nawrocki J. Inverted internal limiting membrane flap technique for large macular holes. Ophthalmology. 2010; 117(10):2018–2025

[5] Takahashi H, Inoue M, Koto T, Itoh Y, Hirota K, Hirakata A. Inverted internal limiting membrane flap technique for treatment of macular hole retinal detachment in highly myopic eyes. Retina. 2018; 38(12):2317–2326

31 Angioid Streaks

Robert J. Courtney

Summary

Angioid streaks are characterized by pale red to deep brown lines of varying width that radiate from the optic nerve, often emulating retinal vessels in their course. While clinical exam is usually sufficient to recognize prototypical cases, multimodal imaging is useful in demonstrating the level of pathology to be breaks within a calcified Bruch's membrane. Roughly half of cases are related to an underlying systemic disorder (e.g., pseudoxanthoma elasticum) and any novel presentation warrants further systemic evaluation. Choroidal neovascularization (CNV) is the most significant ocular complication and accounts for the majority of vision loss. Intravitreal injection of inhibitors of vascular endothelial growth factor is effective in treating CNV, but there is no known treatment or prevention of the causal Bruch's membrane pathology.

Keywords: angioid streaks, Bruch membrane, choroidal neovascularization, fluorescein angiography, fundus autofluorescence, near-infrared imaging, optical coherence tomography, peau d'orange, pseudoxanthoma elasticum

31.1 Features

Angioid streaks are an ocular pathology of striking clinical appearance. The streaks present as reddish breaks in Bruch's membrane that radiate and branch from the nerve, often emulating the course of the major retinal vessels. Angioid streaks are most commonly associated with pseudoxanthoma elasticum (PXE), but have also been described in association with Paget's disease, Ehlers–Danlos syndrome, hemoglobinopathies, and approximately half of cases are idiopathic. The fundamental defect appears to be calcification of Bruch's membrane, which leads to a brittle character that is predisposed to spontaneous breaks and the development of choroidal neovascularization (CNV). Less frequently, traumatic choroidal rupture may occur with minimal force. Although CNV may be treated with anti-vascular endothelial growth factor (VEGF) intravitreal injections, some patients progress to disciform scar formation or macular atrophy.

31.1.1 Common Symptoms

It is typically asymptomatic unless CNV or hemorrhage develops which presents as vision loss and/or metamorphopsia.

31.1.2 Exam Findings

Pale gray, pink, red, or brown radiating cracks in Bruch's membrane emanate from the disc, a zone of peripapillary atrophy, or a peripapillary ring of similar appearance can be seen; often associated with disc drusen, pattern dystrophy of the macula, and a mottled appearance of the temporal macula known as "peau d'orange" (▶ Fig. 31.1). A subtle, diffuse opacification of Bruch's membrane with obscuration of the choroidal vessels, presumably from pathologic calcification, extends from the disc to the area of peau d'orange where the calcification of Bruch's is less confluent; the streaks frequently terminate at this border. In late stages, macular retinal pigment epithelial (RPE) atrophy and/or disciform scarring may be present, obscuring the streaks.

31.2 Key Diagnostic Tests and Findings

31.2.1 Optical Coherence Tomography

Breaks in Bruch's membrane correspond to the streaks. Breaks may be associated with focal detachment or absence of the

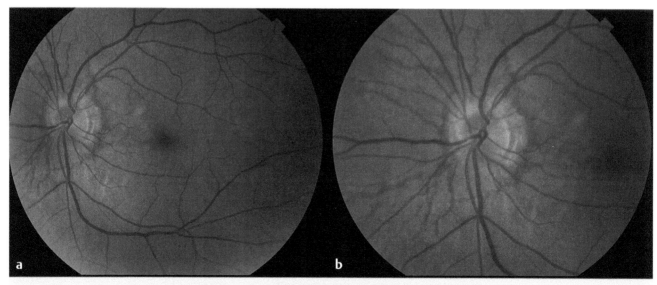

Fig. 31.1 (a,b) Color fundus photo of the left eye demonstrating characteristic appearance of angioid streaks.

overlying RPE; underlying choriocapillaris may also be absent (▶ Fig. 31.2 and ▶ Fig. 31.3). There may be fibrous tissue ingrowth at the breaks. CNV is typically seen in association with these breaks, and may have associated intra- and/or subretinal fluid. Enhanced reflectance is also noted at the most external aspect of the RPE–Bruch's membrane reflectivity band, perhaps secondary to calcification of Bruch's membrane.

31.2.2 Fluorescein Angiography or Ultra-Widefield Fluorescein Angiography

Variable demonstration of streaks is unapparent to stippled RPE staining. If CNV is present, it is typically in the form of classic lesions with significant leakage (▶ Fig. 31.4).

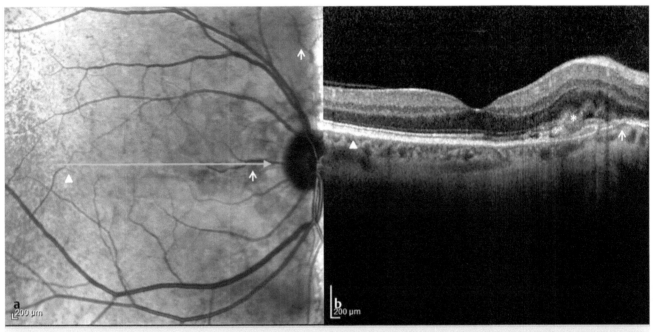

Fig. 31.2 (a) Near-infrared reflectance (NIR) image and (b) optical coherence tomography (OCT) in the right eye of the same patient as ▶ Fig. 31.1 demonstrating angioid streaks and corresponding breaks in Bruch's membrane (*arrows*). The temporal area of peau d'orange apparent as a granular pattern of reflectance on NIR is seen as greater speckling at the basal aspect of the retinal pigment epithelial band on OCT (*arrowheads*). There is an active choroidal neovascularization membrane with subretinal fluid and disruption of retinal architecture (*asterisk*).

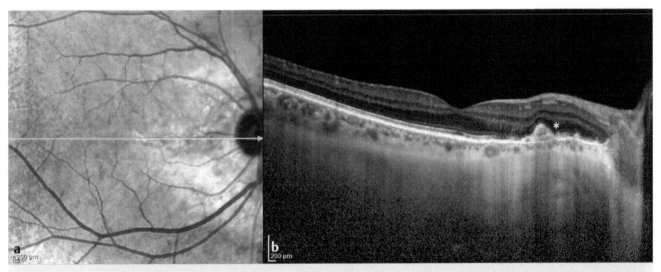

Fig. 31.3 (a,b) Optical coherence tomography and near infrared reflectance image of the same eye 1 month after treatment with bevacizumab showing significant reduction in choroidal neovascularization activity (*asterisk*).

31.2.3 Indocyanine Green Angiography

Streaks may be hypercyanescent, hypocyanescent, or stippled. This technique demonstrates streaks more reliably than fluorescein angiography (FA) and aids in demonstrating CNV. It shows peau d'orange pattern well.

31.2.4 Fundus Autofluorescence

This technique may or may not demonstrate streaks. When present streaks appear as variably banded pattern of hyper- and hypo-autofluorescence (▶ Fig. 31.5). Patients with PXE may show hyper-autofluorescent flecks characteristic of pattern dystrophy.

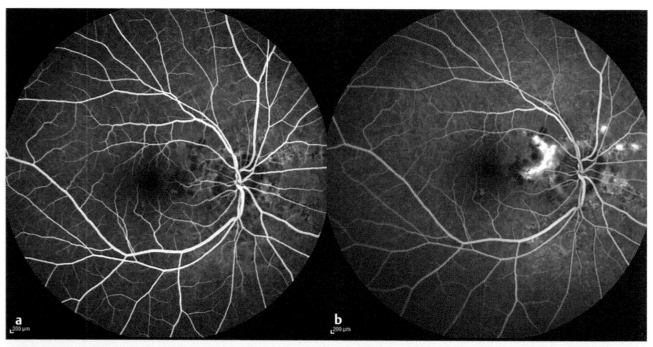

Fig. 31.4 (a) Early and **(b)** mid-late phase fluorescein angiogram of the right eye at presentation of the same eye demonstrating blocked hypofluorescence corresponding to hemorrhage, mottled retinal pigment epithelium staining at the base of the streaks, and leakage from the choroidal neovascularization.

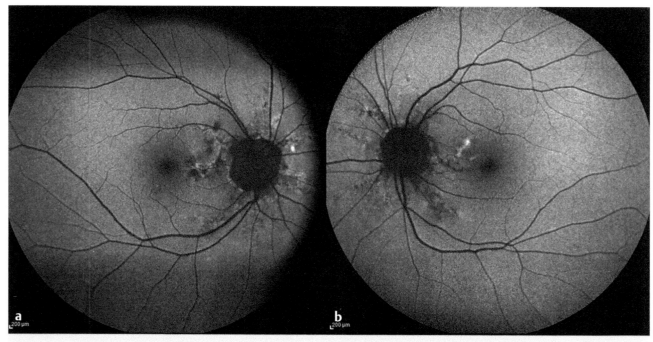

Fig. 31.5 (a,b) Fundus autofluorescence of the same patient showing mottled hypo- and hyper-autofluorescence of the streaks in both eyes.

31.2.5 Optical Coherence Tomography Angiography

This technique may be useful for demonstrating CNV.

31.2.6 Near Infrared Reflectance

Streaks appear dark black against the usual gray background of the fundus (▶ Fig. 31.2, ▶ Fig. 31.3). It is more sensitive than color, autofluorescence, and angiography at detecting the streaks; peau d'orange is also more readily demonstrated as highly reflective flecks within a dull background. Pattern dystrophy typically not well visualized.

31.3 Critical Work-up

Dermatology consult/skin biopsy for PXE, alkaline phosphatase blood test for Paget's disease (if elevated, perform bone scan and X-ray), and hemoglobin electrophoresis if blood dyscrasia suspected. Review of systems to guide additional systemic testing.

31.4 Management

31.4.1 Treatment Options

There is no treatment if the condition is asymptomatic and there is no CNV. Avoid ocular trauma, use protective eyewear when appropriate. Anti-VEGF treatment is currently first-line treatment for CNV. Many CNV lesions are quite responsive to VEGF inhibitors and often require fewer injections than CNV in age-related macular degeneration.

31.4.2 Follow-up

Close follow-up is warranted if CNV is present given the potential lost productivity in this relatively young patient population and high frequency of recurrences.

Suggested Reading

[1] Martinez-Serrano MG, Rodriguez-Reyes A, Guerrero-Naranjo JL, et al. Long-term follow-up of patients with choroidal neovascularization due to angioid streaks. Clin Ophthalmol. 2016; 11(11):23–30

[2] Spaide RF. Peau d'orange and angioid streaks: manifestations of Bruch membrane pathology. Retina. 2015; 35(3):392–397

[3] Charbel Issa P, Finger RP, Holz FG, Scholl HP. Multimodal imaging including spectral domain OCT and confocal near infrared reflectance for characterization of outer retinal pathology in pseudoxanthoma elasticum. Invest Ophthalmol Vis Sci. 2009; 50(12):5913–5918

[4] Zweifel SA, Imamura Y, Freund KB, Spaide RF. Multimodal fundus imaging of pseudoxanthoma elasticum. Retina. 2011; 31(3):482–491

32 Best Disease

Daniel R. Agarwal and Elias I. Traboulsi

Summary

Best disease, also known as Best vitelliform macular dystrophy, is most commonly an autosomal dominant (AD) maculopathy with variable expressivity that can significantly affect vision. First described in 1905, it is most typically characterized by a yolk-like macular lesion generally detected in the 2nd decade of life. In some patients, the lesion collapses and the material in it scrambles, usually with additional vision loss. Best disease is caused by mutations in *BEST1* gene that codes for bestrophin. While most cases are AD, autosomal recessive (AR) inheritance has also been described and the totality of diseases caused by mutations in *BEST1* are referred to as bestrophinopathies. Patients with AR Best disease can present with vision loss, central serous detachments, multiple small vitelliform lesions, and yellowish subretinal deposits. The electrooculogram is characteristically abnormal with a preserved electroretinogram in both AD and some patients with the AR forms. Complications from Best disease include the formation of choroidal neovascular membranes that can further degrade vision. As a pleomorphic genetic disease with two modes of inheritance, genetic testing and counseling are vital parts of the treatment process to help guide family members on the likelihood and implications of having Best disease.

Keywords: autosomal dominant, autosomal recessive, bestrophinopathy, BEST1, Best disease, Electrooculogram, vitelliform

32.1 Features

Autosomal dominant (AD) cases have early age of onset and diagnosis occurs in early childhood to teenage years. In a minority of patients, a choroidal neovascular membrane (CNVM) can form in the setting of surrounding atrophy. Vision may also decline due to fibrosis or geographic atrophy. Autosomal recessive (AR) cases have vision loss in the first or second decades of life and worse vision than those with AD form of disease. Genetic testing for Best disease reveals a mutation in the *BEST1* gene encoding the bestrophin protein that is located in the basolateral membrane of the retinal pigment epithelium (RPE). Over 100 mutations in the *BEST1* gene have been reported.

32.1.1 Common Symptoms

It may be asymptomatic with normal vision in the early stages. Other symptoms include reduction in central visual acuity and/or metamorphopsia.

32.1.2 Exam Findings

Best disease can progress at variable rates not corresponding to the classical staging of the disease. It can also present as a multifocal process, especially in the recessive form, with several vitelliform lesions in the retina.

Autosomal Dominant Best Disease

Traditionally described with a progressive staging system. However, many patients may remain in the same stage that they were in at the time of diagnosis.
- Stage 1: posterior pole will look normal on fundus examination and vision is normal.
- Stage 2: some RPE window and granularity defects may be seen with or without a yellow foveal dot.
- Stage 3: a yellow, well-circumscribed, homogeneous, "yolk-like" appearing (vitelliform) macular lesion is present (▶ Fig. 32.1). Vision may be slightly reduced.

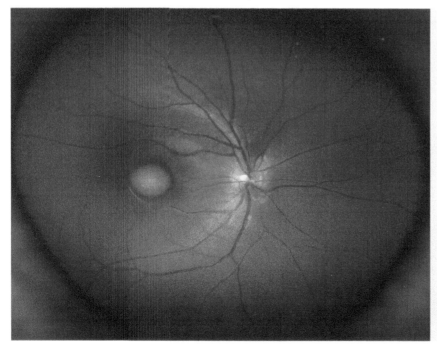

Fig. 32.1 Fundus photograph demonstrating the classic "yolk-like" round vitelliform lesion in the macula.

- Stage 4: characterized by a layering of the vitelliform lesion due to fluid resorption, resulting in a pseudohypopyon appearance as the material moves inferiorly (▶ Fig. 32.2).
- Stage 5: the vitelliruptive stage. The lesion will "scramble" and vision can significantly decrease.
- Stage 6: characterized by RPE atrophy.
- Stage 7: the cicatricial stage. Choroidal neovascularization (CNV) may be present, which often is bilateral and symmetric (▶ Fig. 32.3).

Autosomal Recessive Best Disease

This form often presents with hyperopia. Cystoid macular edema or extensive subretinal fluid are present, sometimes encompassing most of the macula. Single or multiple vitelliform lesions may be visible with flecks inside and outside the macula (▶ Fig. 32.4). Subretinal fibrosis is more common than in the AD form. CNVMs may also occur. Genetic testing reveals mutations in both *BEST1* alleles, with patients being most commonly compound heterozygotes.

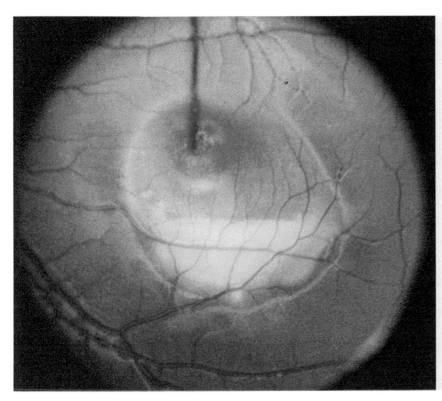

Fig. 32.2 Layering of the vitelliform lesion from fluid resorption resulting in a pseudohypopyon appearance.

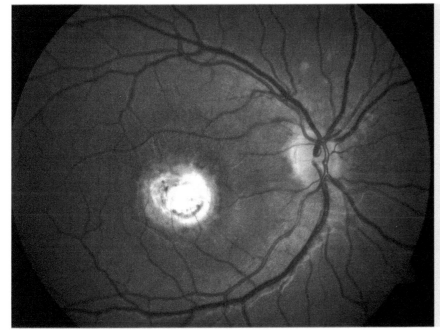

Fig. 32.3 Advanced Best disease with subretinal fibrosis in the center of the macula.

32.2 Key Diagnostic Tests and Findings

32.2.1 Optical Coherence Tomography

Autosomal Dominant Best Disease

Early findings include normal retinal anatomy or subtle changes to the outer retina. As the disease progresses to the intermediate stages, splitting and elevation can occur between the retina and the RPE. Serous retinal detachments may be identified. In the vitelliform stage, the retina is elevated with hyperreflective material visible in the subretinal space corresponding to the vitelliform lesion. Some patients will have a pseudohypopyon with an upper layer of clear fluid and a lower layer of yellow pigment separated by a well-delineated irregular horizontal line that is well visualized on vertically oriented scans. Photoreceptor loss can occur as the hyperreflective material decreases with outer retinal atrophy. A "fibrotic pillar" in the sub-RPE space near the fovea is observed which elevates the retina and is associated with subretinal fluid and a decrease in vision (▶ Fig. 32.5).

Autosomal Recessive Best Disease

Can reveal serous detachments, subretinal fluid, cystoid macular edema, hyperreflective vitelliform lesions, and hyperreflective central scars.

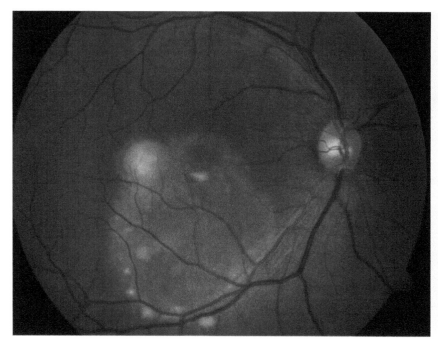

Fig. 32.4 Autosomal recessive bestrophinopathy with multifocal vitelliform lesions visible inside and outside the macula.

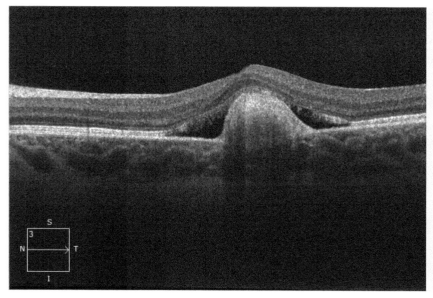

Fig. 32.5 Optical coherence tomographic findings demonstrating a classic "fibrotic pillar" appearance seen in Best disease patients.

32.2.2 Fluorescein Angiography or Ultra-Widefield Fluorescein Angiography

Autosomal Dominant Best Disease

Initially, fluorescein angiography (FA) in this case demonstrates early stage blocked fluorescence from the vitelliform lesion. When the vitelliform lesion "scrambles," underlying atrophy of the RPE and choriocapillaris can lead to window defects.

Autosomal Recessive Best Disease

FA can reveal vitelliform staining or leakage secondary to CNVM.

32.2.3 Fundus Autofluorescence

Autosomal Dominant Best Disease

Abnormally high levels of lipofuscin accumulation can contribute to increased autofluorescence particularly in the stages when vitelliform lesions are present (▶ Fig. 32.6). In later stages, autofluorescence may disappear as the retina becomes atrophic.

Autosomal Recessive Best Disease

Serous detachments can appear autofluorescent. Smaller vitelliform lesions can show significant hyper-autofluorescence.

32.2.4 Electroretinogram

While the full-field electroretinogram (ffERG) will be normal in AD Best disease, the ERG may be abnormal in some patients with severe AR bestrophinopathy. Multifocal ERG (mfERG) reveals deficits consistent with OCT imaging and fundus examination.

32.2.5 Electrooculogram

It shows abnormally low Arden ratio in both AD and AR Best disease (< 1.55 light peak/dark trough; normal > 2.0); one of a few diseases where the electrooculogram (EOG) will provide clinically relevant findings.

32.2.6 Optical Coherence Tomography Angiography

It is an emerging technology for use in Best disease. OCT angiography (OCTA) may be considered to evaluate for the presence of CNV.

32.3 Critical Work-up

Initial examination of all Best disease patients should comprise obtaining a family history, performing a dilated fundus examination, and securing molecular genetic testing. OCT imaging and fundus autofluorescence can be performed as well to help evaluate the lesion. FA and OCTA may be considered if CNV is suspected. EOG testing may also be conducted, if necessary. Immediate family members should undergo examinations looking for evidence of Best disease because of the variable expressivity and the AD and AR modes of inheritance.

32.4 Management

32.4.1 Treatment Options

Currently there are no treatments. Low vision aides can be used to help compensate for deficits in central vision caused by the disease. If CNV occurs, intravitreal anti-VEGF injections may be considered.

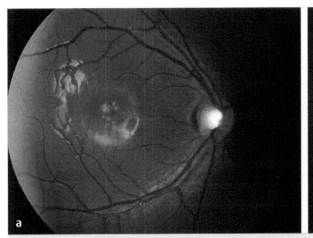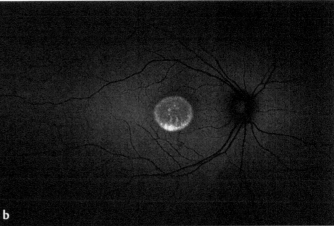

Fig. 32.6 (a) Best disease with scrambling of the vitelliform lesion on fundus photography and (b) fundus autofluorescence with hyper-autofluorescence corresponding to areas of lipofuscin accumulation.

32.4.2 Follow-up

Regular examinations (e.g., every 6–12 months) are advised to monitor disease progression and look for CNV in all patients with Best disease. Family members may benefit from examination and genetic counseling.

Suggested Reading

[1] Johnson AA, Guziewicz KE, Lee CJ, et al. Bestrophin 1 and retinal disease. Prog Retin Eye Res. 2017; 58:45–69

[2] MacDonald IM, Lee T. Best vitelliform macular dystrophy. In: Adam MP, Ardinger HH, Pagon, RA, et al., eds. GeneReviews. Seattle, WA: University of Washington; 2013. Available at: https://www.ncbi.nlm.nih.gov/books/NBK1167/. Accessed September 3, 2017

[3] Sohn EH, Mullins RF, Stone EM. Macular dystrophies. In: Schachat AP, Sadda SR, Hinton DR, et al, eds. Ryan's Retina. 6th ed. Elsevier Inc.; 2018:953–996

[4] Leroy BP. Bestrophinopathies. In: Traboulsi E, ed. Genetic Diseases of the Eye. 2nd ed. Oxford, UK: Oxford University Press; 2012:426–436. Available at: http://oxfordmedicine.com/10.1093/med/9780195326147.001.0001/med-9780195326147-chapter-28

33 Adult Vitelliform Macular Dystrophy

Matthew R. Starr and Sophie J. Bakri

Summary

Adult vitelliform macular dystrophy (AVMD) is a pattern dystrophy typically affecting the fovea bilaterally later in life. Pattern dystrophies are a collection of macular diseases characterized by various patterns of pigment deposition within the retinal pigment epithelium (RPE). The lesions are round or ovoid, symmetric, elevated, subretinal, and may contain a central cluster of dark pigment. Patients are typically discovered to have AVMD during routine ophthalmological exam or may complain of mild decrease in central vision, scotomas, or metamorphopsia. The disease is very similar to milder forms of Best disease, although the lesions associated with AVMD are typically smaller, occur later in life, and patients do not always have abnormalities on electrooculogram. In addition, it can frequently mimic age-related macular degeneration in older patients. The two are best distinguished using genetic testing as AVMD is associated with a mutation of the gene *PRPH2* while Best Disease has a mutation of the *BEST1* gene. AVMD is generally slowly progressive with patients maintaining good reading vision throughout life. The lesions may atrophy over time and rarely, choroidal neovascularization may develop which can be treated with intravitreal anti-vascular endothelial growth factor agents.

Keywords: adult vitelliform macular dystrophy, adult-onset foveomacular vitelliform dystrophy, pattern dystrophy, peculiar foveomacular dystrophy, peripherin

33.1 Features

Adult vitelliform macular dystrophy (AVMD) is generally regarded as a separate entity from juvenile-onset vitelliform macular dystrophy or Best Disease. AVMD has also been known by several other names, including adult-onset foveomacular vitelliform dystrophy (AOFVD), adult vitelliform dystrophy, and pattern dystrophy. Pattern dystrophies are a collection of macular diseases characterized by various patterns of pigment deposition within the retinal pigment epithelium (RPE) of which AVMD is a subset. Compared to Best disease, AVMD typically begins later in life (typically between 40 and 60 years of age), and the lesions are smaller (about 1/2 to 1/3 disc diameters in size; ► Fig. 33.1). AVMD is typically associated with somatic mutations of the gene *PRPH2* on chromosome 6, although there are cases of families where multiple members have AVMD. *PRPH2* is responsible for producing a protein called peripherin 2, a stabilizing glycoprotein found in the outer segments of rods and cones. Loss of peripherin 2 leads to photoreceptor cell loss and accumulation of lipofuscin within the RPE. If older patients are found to have defects in *BEST1* and not *PRPH2* then they are suffering from Best disease and not AVMD. The lesions in Best disease can also display layering of the yellow subretinal pigment in dependent areas of the lesion which is typically not seen in AVMD. This would eliminate any confusion regarding the distinction between AVMD and a milder form of Best disease.

33.1.1 Common Symptoms

Frequently discovered incidentally on routine ophthalmological exams. Symptoms may include scotomata, metamorphopsia, and/or decrease in central vision. If choroidal neovascularization (CNV) develops, visual changes may develop more acutely.

33.1.2 Exam Findings

Bilateral, round, or oval subretinal yellow deposits with a central cluster of dark pigment located in the fovea of each eye are classic findings (► Fig. 33.1a). The lesions are generally symmetric and can also be associated with scattered peripheral drusen (► Fig. 33.1f, g). Later in the course of AVMD, the lesions may atrophy and/or CNV may develop. If several vitelliform lesions are noted on funduscopic exam, entities such as exudative multifocal vitelliform maculopathy or paraneoplastic vitelliform maculopathy must be excluded before making the diagnosis of AVMD.

33.2 Key Diagnostic Tests

33.2.1 Optical Coherence Tomography

Optical coherence tomographic images show discrete, dome-shaped, subfoveal, and homogeneously hyperreflective lesions located between the RPE and the retina (► Fig. 33.1c). These areas can later collapse leading to loss of the ellipsoid zone and RPE. Clefts of hyporeflective areas mimicking subretinal fluid may also be noted.

33.2.2 Fluorescein Angiography or Ultra-Widefield Fluorescein Angiography

Early in AVMD, the subretinal deposits may cause blocking on fluorescein angiography (FA), revealing an area of hypofluorescence surrounded by a small ring of hyperfluorescent staining early in the FA without evidence of leakage late in the FA (► Fig. 33.1d, ► Fig. 33.1e). If CNV is present, evidence of leakage will be present. Later in AVMD, the vitelliform material can atrophy leading to window defects.

33.2.3 Indocyanine Green Angiography

Early in AVMD, vitelliform lesions are hypocyanescent with no hypercyanescent ring; they remain hypocyanescent through the late stages with a hypercyanescent border developing in some patients.

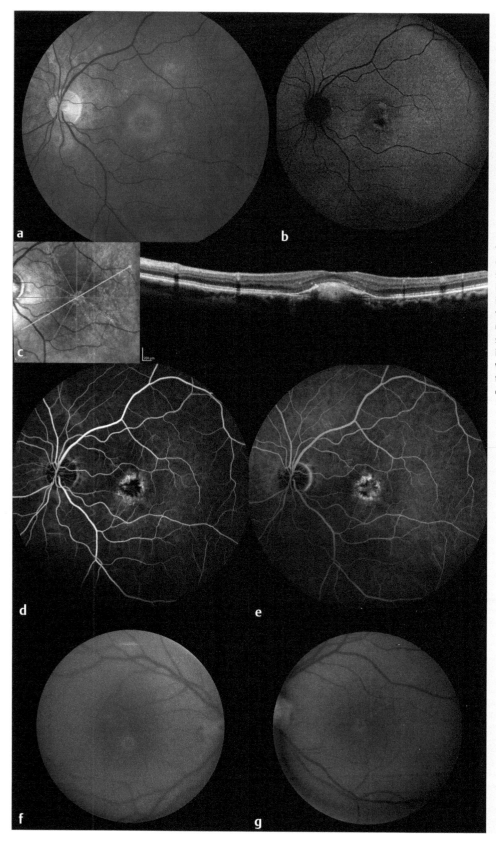

Fig. 33.1 (a) Color photo of the left eye with a round, yellow, subfoveal lesion with a central pigment clump. (b) Fundus autofluorescence with a central hypo-autofluorescent lesion surrounded by an irregular hyper-autofluorescent ring centered at the fovea. (c) Optical coherence tomography of the left eye with an ovoid, subretinal, hyperreflective lesion centered at the fovea with a small amount of overlying subretinal fluid and overlying loss of the ellipsoid zone. Early stage fluorescein angiogram at 44 seconds which shows blocking centrally over the fovea consistent with the yellow subretinal lesion on color photos. (d) There is a surrounding irregular hyperfluorescent ring that does not increase in size or leak on a (e) later fluorescein angiogram at 8 minutes. (f,g) Fundus photo with bilateral, symmetric, about 1/3 disc diameter in size, yellow, subretinal lesions with a central pigment clump. Note the parafoveal yellow, drusen-like deposits in both eyes.

33.2.4 Fundus Autofluorescence

Subretinal lesions may have variable autofluorescence and are typically hypo-autofluorescent due to central blocking but may show hyper-autofluorescence surrounding the hypo-autofluorescent area (▶ Fig. 33.1b). Typically, the vitelliform material exhibits hyper-autofluorescence. The yellow peripheral deposits will resemble hyper-autofluorescent lesions early on in the disease changing to hypo-autofluorescent lesions as the deposits atrophy.

33.2.5 Optical Coherence Tomography Angiography

Possible reduced flow density in the superficial retinal vascular layer, deep retinal vascular layer, and choriocapillary layer. The foveal avascular zone may remain normal. OCT angiography may also be helpful for identifying CNV.

33.2.6 Electrooculogram

May or may not be abnormal as not all patients will have an Arden ratio less than 1.4 (normal being > 1.8). This is in contrast to Best disease in which all patients generally have an abnormal electrooculogram.

33.3 Management
33.3.1 Treatment Options

In the absence of CNV, no specific treatment is available. Intravitreal anti-vascular endothelial growth factors are frequently used for CNV management.

33.3.2 Follow-up

Disease progression is generally slow and patients are often able to maintain fairly good visual acuity. Central vision may slowly decrease and patients can be observed every 6 to 12 months for progression of disease. If CNV is suspected, more frequent follow-up is indicated. Genetic testing is now advocated by some clinicians for better categorization of the disease process and potential hereditary implications.

Suggested Reading

[1] Gass JD. A clinicopathologic study of a peculiar foveomacular dystrophy. Trans Am Ophthalmol Soc. 1974; 72:139–156

[2] Fagerberg L, Hallström BM, Oksvold P, et al. Analysis of the human tissue-specific expression by genome-wide integration of transcriptomics and antibody-based proteomics. Mol Cell Proteomics. 2014; 13(2):397–406

[3] Johnson AA, Guziewicz KE, Lee CJ, et al. Bestrophin 1 and retinal disease. Prog Retin Eye Res. 2017; 58:45–69

[4] Treder M, Lauermann JL, Alnawaiseh M, Heiduschka P, Eter N. Quantitative changes in flow density in patients with adult-onset foveomacular vitelliform dystrophy: an OCT angiography study. Graefes Arch Clin Exp Ophthalmol. 2017

34 Pattern Dystrophy

Amy S. Babiuch and Elias I. Traboulsi

Summary

Pattern dystrophies (PDs) include a group of genetically determined retinal disorders, of which, a major subset have been associated with mutations in the *PRPH2* gene, also known as *peripherin/RDS*. The phenotype of patients with mutations in this gene is extremely heterogeneous and includes macular pattern-like pigmentary changes, atrophic maculopathy, and a clinical picture that resembles classic retinitis pigmentosa.

Gass described pattern dystrophies in five categories based on clinical findings alone. These include adult-onset foveomacular vitelliform dystrophy, butterfly-shaped pattern dystrophy, reticular dystrophy, multifocal pattern dystrophy simulating Stargardt disease/fundus flavimaculatus, and fundus pulverulentus. Typical characteristics of PDs include progressive retinal pigment epithelium alterations often accompanied by yellow-dark subretinal material generally involving the macula and posterior pole. Most patients are asymptomatic until their fourth or fifth decade, following which some may experience progressive vision loss due to ensuing chorioretinal atrophy or development of choroidal neovascularization.

Keywords: adult-onset foveal macular vitelliform dystrophy, butterfly-shaped pattern dystrophy, fundus flavimaculatus, Stargardt disease, reticular dystrophy

34.1 Features

Pattern dystrophies (PDs) include a group of genetically determined retinal disorders, of which, a major subset have been associated with mutations in the *PRPH2* gene, also known as *peripherin/RDS*. The phenotype of patients with mutations in this gene is extremely heterogeneous and includes macular pattern-like pigmentary changes, atrophic maculopathy, and a clinical picture that resembles classic retinitis pigmentosa.

Gass described pattern dystrophies in five categories based on clinical findings alone. These include adult-onset foveomacular vitelliform dystrophy, butterfly-shaped pattern dystrophy, reticular dystrophy, multifocal pattern dystrophy simulating Stargardt disease/fundus flavimaculatus, and fundus pulverulentus. Typical characteristics of PDs include progressive retinal pigment epithelium (RPE) alterations often accompanied by yellow-dark subretinal material generally involving the macula and posterior pole. Most patients are asymptomatic until their fourth or fifth decade, following which some may experience progressive vision loss due to ensuing chorioretinal atrophy or development of choroidal neovascularization.

PDs have been classified into prominent categories. For more details on adult-onset vitelliform dystrophy, see Chapter 33, Adult Vitelliform Macular Dystrophy. In multifocal pattern dystrophy simulating Stargardt disease/fundus flavimaculatus there is autosomal dominant inheritance of mutations in the *peripherin/RDS* gene with variable expressivity and reduced penetrance. Butterfly-shaped pattern dystrophy has autosomal dominant mutations in the *PRPH2 peripherin/RDS* gene. A locus

on 5q21.2-q33.2 is also associated with pattern dystrophy. Finally, reticular dystrophy is uncommon with only a few pedigrees reported with possible autosomal dominant or autosomal recessive transmission.

34.1.1 Common Symptoms

Adult Vitelliform Macular Dystrophy

See Chapter 33, Adult Vitelliform Macular Dystrophy.

Multifocal/Fundus Flavimaculatus-Like Dystrophy

Vision is generally good until about the fifth decade, after which vision may remain stable or begin to decline.

Butterfly-Shaped Pattern Dystrophy

Mostly identified on routine ophthalmologic exam; mostly asymptomatic.

Reticular Dystrophy

Usually asymptomatic, vision may be minimally affected in later stages of disease if atrophic changes occur.

34.1.2 Exam Findings

Adult Vitelliform Macular Dystrophy

See Chapter 33, Adult Vitelliform Macular Dystrophy.

Multifocal/Fundus Flavimaculatus-Like Dystrophy

Bilateral, symmetric yellowish pisciform flecks at the level of the RPE are noted throughout the posterior pole, and beyond the vascular arcades (▶ Fig. 34.1). Macular findings may range from various patterns of yellow or gray deposits to well-demarcated chorioretinal atrophy. Clinical findings can be highly variable ranging from minimal findings to a retinitis pigmentosa-like appearance.

Butterfly-Shaped Pattern Dystrophy

Bilateral central accumulation of material at the level of the RPE that appears pigmented or yellow-white, and in the configuration of "arms" or "wings" extending outward in a spoke-like pattern and surrounded by a zone of depigmentation.

Reticular Dystrophy

A meshwork of pigmented spots/lines at the level of the RPE in the macula, described as having a "knotted fishnet" appearance (▶ Fig. 34.2).

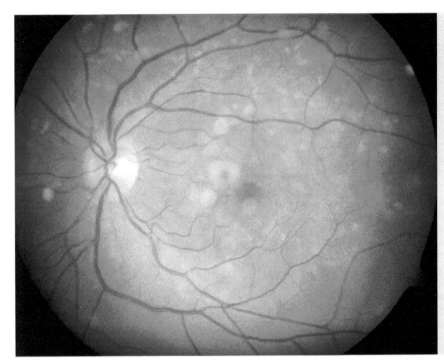

Fig. 34.1 Fundus photograph of multifocal pattern dystrophy simulating Stargardt disease/fundus flavimaculatus revealing yellowish pisciform flecks at the level of the retinal pigment epithelium throughout the posterior pole.

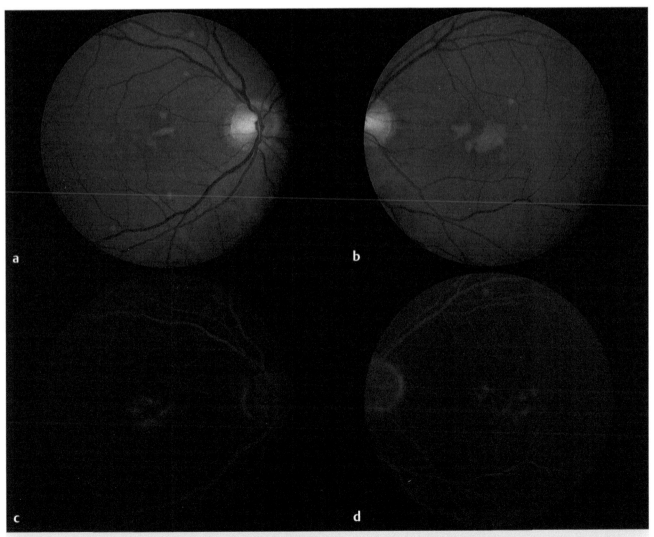

Fig. 34.2 **(a,b)** Butterfly pattern dystrophy demonstrating bilateral central accumulation of material at the level of the retinal pigment epithelium (RPE) that appears pigmented or yellow-white, and in the configuration of "arms" or "wings" extending outward. **(c,d)** The yellowish-white deposits block fluorescence while areas of RPE loss exhibit window defect and hyperfluorescence without leakage on fluorescein angiography. Genetic testing revealed a mutation in the *PRPH2* gene.

34.2 Key Diagnostic Tests and Findings

34.2.1 Optical Coherence Tomography

Adult Vitelliform Macular Dystrophy

See Chapter 33, Adult Vitelliform Macular Dystrophy.

Multifocal/Fundus Flavimaculatus-Like Dystrophy

Focal areas of attenuation of the photoreceptor layer and RPE.

Butterfly-Shaped Pattern Dystrophy

Areas of ellipsoid zone (EZ) disruption with external limiting membrane (ELM) remaining intact; presence of hyperreflective deposits in the subfoveal region at the level of the RPE and extending up to the ELM.

Reticular Dystrophy

Focal thickening of the RPE appearing as bumps with overlying interruption of the EZ. Hyperreflective retinal clumps in the outer retinal layer and elevations in the outer limiting membrane have also been described.

34.2.2 Fluorescein Angiography or Ultra-Widefield Fluorescein Angiography

Adult Vitelliform Macular Dystrophy

See Chapter 33, Adult Vitelliform Macular Dystrophy.

Multifocal/Fundus Flavimaculatus-Like Dystrophy

Areas of hyperfluorescence on early and late phases sometimes with an adjacent or central hypofluorescent spot without leakage. Absence of the "dark choroid" as seen in Stargardt (*STDG1*) disease.

Butterfly Dystrophy

Yellowish-white deposits block fluorescence while areas of RPE loss exhibit window defect and hyperfluorescence without leakage (▶ Fig. 34.3).

Reticular Dystrophy

The deposits are hypofluorescent from early through late stage with hyperfluorescent lesion borders.

34.2.3 Fundus Autofluorescence

Adult Vitelliform Macular Dystrophy

See Chapter 33, Adult Vitelliform Macular Dystrophy.

Multifocal/Fundus Flavimaculatus-Like Dystrophy

Multiple areas of hyperautofluorescence are seen that may or may not correspond with the flecks on fundus examination. Areas of hypoautofluorescence may be present in the areas of RPE atrophy.

Butterfly Dystrophy

Mixed pattern of hyper- and hypoautofluorescence at the macula. The hyperautofluorescence corresponds to areas of the yellowish white deposits (RPE lipofuscin) and the hypoauto-fluorescence corresponds to areas of RPE atrophy.

Reticular Dystrophy

The reticular deposits demonstrate hyperautofluorescence. Areas of hypoautofluorescence may be also present in a reticular pattern.

34.2.4 Electroretinography

Adult Vitelliform Macular Dystrophy

See Chapter 33, Adult Vitelliform Macular Dystrophy.

Multifocal/Fundus Flavimaculatus-Like Dystrophy

Full-field electroretinogram (ERG) is normal in early stage of disease but if disease advances, cone and rod function become compromised at the panretinal level.

Butterfly Dystrophy

Full-field ERG and dark adaptation is generally normal.

Reticular Dystrophy

ERG is usually normal.

34.2.5 Electrooculography

Adult Vitelliform Macular Dystrophy

See Chapter 33, Adult Vitelliform Macular Dystrophy.

Multifocal/Fundus Flavimaculatus-Like Dystrophy

Can be normal or subnormal.

Butterfly Dystrophy

Can be subnormal.

Reticular Dystrophy

Can be normal or subnormal.

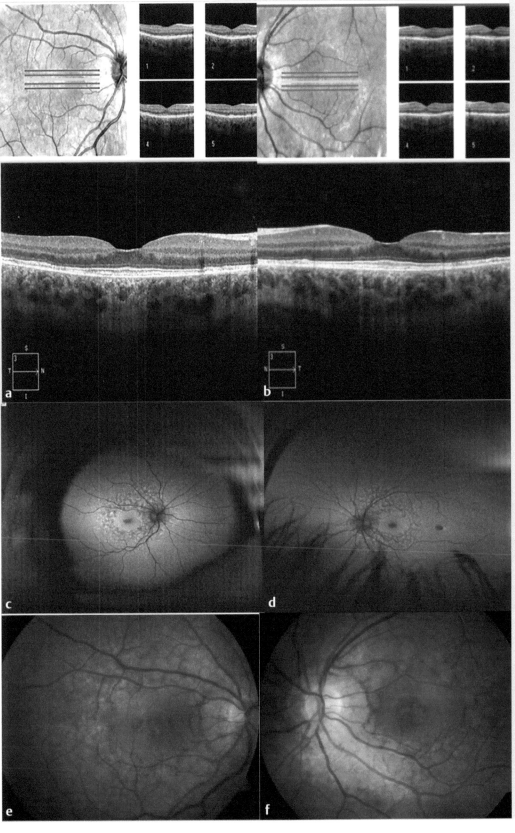

Fig. 34.3 Reticular dystrophy. **(a,b)** Spectral-domain optical coherence tomography of both eyes reveals focal thickening of the retinal pigment epithelium appearing as bumps with some areas of overlying interruption of the ellipsoid zone. **(c,d)** Ultra-widefield fundus autofluorescence of both eyes demonstrates hyperautofluorescence of the reticular deposits intermixed with some areas of hypoautofluorescence. **(e,f)** Fundus photography of both eyes reveals a meshwork of pigmented spots at the level of the retinal pigment epithelium in the macula, the "knotted fishnet" appearance.

34.3 Critical Work-up

In addition to comprehensive ophthalmic exam and appropriate imaging, genetic testing is now advocated by some clinicians for better categorization of the disease process and potential hereditary implications.

34.4 Management

34.4.1 Treatment Options

Observation and patient education, including Amsler grid as choroidal neovascularization can rarely occur, for each of these PD categories. Genetic testing confirms the diagnosis in cases that occur due to mutations in *PRPH2*. Genetic counseling and evaluation of family members should be considered.

Suggested Reading

[1] Agarwal A. Gass' Atlas of Macular Diseases. 5th ed. Elsevier; 2012

[2] Boon CJ, van Schooneveld MJ, den Hollander AI, et al. Mutations in the peripherin/RDS gene are an important cause of multifocal pattern dystrophy simulating STGD1/fundus flavimaculatus. Br J Ophthalmol. 2007; 91(11): 1504–1511

[3] Boon CJ, den Hollander AI, Hoyng CB, Cremers FP, Klevering BJ, Keunen JE. The spectrum of retinal dystrophies caused by mutations in the peripherin/RDS gene. Prog Retin Eye Res. 2008; 27(2):213–235

[4] Kumar V, Kumawat D. Multimodal imaging in a case of butterfly pattern dystrophy of retinal pigment epithelium. Int Ophthalmol. 2017(March)

[5] Zerbib J, Querques G, Massamba N, et al. Reticular pattern dystrophy of the retina: a spectral-domain optical coherence tomography analysis. Am J Ophthalmol. 2013; 156(6):1228–1237

35 Macular Telangiectasia

S. Amal Hussnain and Yasha S. Modi

Summary

Macular telangiectasia type 2 (MacTel 2), the most common macular telangiectatic disorder, is an idiopathic, bilateral condition that manifests in the fifth or sixth decade of life as neurosensory retinal atrophy and ectatic capillaries in the macula. Findings in MacTel 2 encompass an oval area around the fovea, but are more predominant temporally. Fundus features include parafoveal retinal graying, ectatic capillaries, and inner retinal crystalline deposits, with later-stage retinal pigment epithelium (RPE) migration along dilated venules. Unmasking of autofluorescence in the fovea due to loss of photopigments is an early and characteristic feature. Fluorescein angiography shows ectatic capillaries and late hyperfluorescence resulting from leakage of affected vessels as well as staining of the outer retina. Optical coherence tomography (OCT) is perhaps the most useful imaging modality in MacTel 2 diagnosis and displays loss of ellipsoid zone, inner or outer retinal cavitated spaces, RPE migration, and potentially subretinal neovascularization as a later-stage complication. OCT angiography is an emerging technology that can be used to detect vascular changes and a decrease in vessel density at the level of both superficial and deep capillary plexus. Vision loss in MacTel 2 primarily results from neurosensory retinal atrophy and neovascularization. While there is no established treatment for MacTel 2, anti-vascular endothelial growth factor agents have demonstrated efficacy in treating late-stage neovascular complications.

Keywords: ectatic capillaries, idiopathic juxtafoveal telangiectasia, idiopathic perifoveal telangiectasia, MacTel, macular telangiectasia, Müller cells, retinal crystals, retinal graying

35.1 Features

The Macular Telangiectasia Project proposed the classification of several retinal telangiectatic disorders into two distinct groups, now termed macular telangiectasia type 1 and type 2. Macular telangiectasia type 1 is considered a unilateral disorder characterized by aneurysms, lipid exudation, and retinal ischemia, but typically no neovascularization. This chapter will focus on the more commonly encountered macular telangiectasia type 2 (MacTel 2), an idiopathic, bilateral disorder that manifests in the fifth or sixth decade of life as neurosensory retinal atrophy and ectatic capillaries in the macula. Gass and Blodi staging represents chronological changes seen on fundus exam and fluorescein angiography in MacTel 2 (or Idiopathic Juxtafoveolar Retinal Telangiectasis Group 2A, as they termed it; ▶ Table 35.1). In addition, MacTel 2 has also been described based on the presence of neovascularization: a non-proliferative stage characterized by atrophy and a proliferative stage marked by neovascularization. The prevalence of 0.02 to 0.1% for MacTel 2 reported in studies from the United States, Australia, and Africa is based solely on grading of color fundus photographs and likely underestimates the true prevalence. A slight predilection toward women, 64% in the Mac Tel Project, was

shown. Known systemic associations include diabetes and hypertension. A genetic link is suspected, given bilaterality and autosomal dominant pattern of inheritance, but the relationship is likely polygenic as no single causative gene has been identified.

35.1.1 Common Symptoms

Slow loss of vision, distorted vision, trouble reading, and scotomata are some symptoms.

35.1.2 Exam Findings

Parafoveal retinal graying or loss of transparency, ectatic capillaries, and inner retinal crystalline deposits thought to be Müller cell footplates encompass an oval area around the fovea, but are invariably more predominant temporally. Dilated venules with blunt ends dive at right angles (e.g., right angle venules) toward the deeper retina in the fovea and are associated with retinal pigment epithelium (RPE) hypertrophy and pigment migration into the retina (▶ Fig. 35.1).

35.2 Key Diagnostic Tests and Findings

35.2.1 Optical Coherence Tomography

Changes in retinal thickness or reflectivity with thinning is first noted in the outer nuclear layer in the temporal region, but may be masked by thickening from concurrent vascular leakage that manifests as hyperreflectivity of inner retinal layers. Intraretinal and subretinal hyperreflectivity may be present and results from RPE migration and choroidal neovascularization, respectively.

A frequent and significant change is disruption of photoreceptors that results in loss of reflectivity from the ellipsoid zone and can be accompanied by early cavitary changes (▶ Fig. 35.2). These areas correlate with increased fundus autofluorescence (FAF) due to the absence of blue light absorbing photopigment (▶ Fig. 35.3). Hyporeflective cystoid cavities are also seen in

Table 35.1 Gass and Blodi clinical staging of MacTel 2 (Idiopathic Juxtafoveolar Retinal Telangiectasis Group 2A)

Stage 1	No changes on ophthalmoscopy; minimal capillary dilation and mild late staining of the outer retina temporally on fluorescein angiography
Stage 2	Perifoveolar graying and minimal telangiectasia on ophthalmoscopy; evidence of capillary telangiectasia temporal to the fovea on fluorescein angiography
Stage 3	Dilated, blunted venule(s) diving at right angle on ophthalmoscopy; permeability changes underlying right angle venules on fluorescein angiography
Stage 4	Retinal pigment epithelium hyperplasia in proximity to right angle venule(s)
Stage 5	Subretinal neovascularization

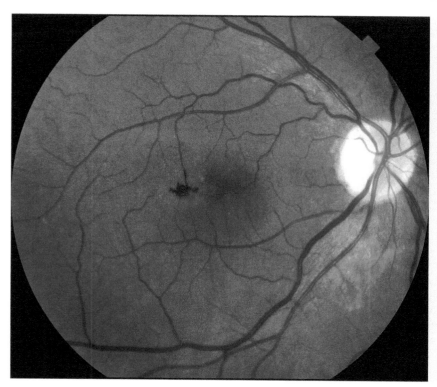

Fig. 35.1 Fundus photograph in MacTel 2 demonstrating parafoveal graying, telangiectatic vessels, and inner retinal crystalline deposits. Retinal pigment epithelium migration is visualized along a right angle dilated venule diving into the deep retina.

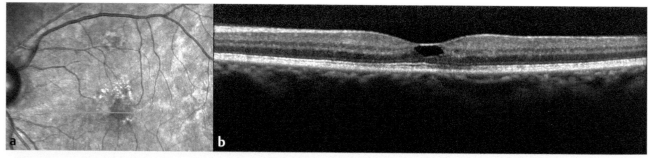

Fig. 35.2 (a,b) Optical coherence tomography in MacTel 2 displaying early cavitary change with internal limiting membrane draping over it. Attenuation of the ellipsoid zone is also evident temporal to the fovea.

both the inner and outer retina and likely result from atrophy of retinal layers (as opposed to exudation which do not show leakage or pooling on fluorescein angiography [FA]). These cavities often have a characteristic appearance of missing retinal tissue rather than the addition of fluid to the retina. The contour of the inner retina may be unchanged even in the presence of fluid. With progressive atrophy over time, these cavities may decrease in size and eventually collapse (► Fig. 35.4).

35.2.2 Fluorescein Angiography or Ultra-Widefield Fluorescein Angiography

Early appearance of telangiectatic vessels and late hyperfluorescence are the two hallmark findings (► Fig. 35.5). It is proposed that late hyperfluorescence results from leakage of affected vessels and staining of the outer retina.

35.2.3 Fundus Autofluorescence

Relative hyper-autofluorescence in the fovea is seen due to unmasking of foveal autofluorescence from loss of both luteal pigment and photopigments in photoreceptors. Hypo-auto-fluorescence is possible due to blockage from RPE plaques (► Fig. 35.3).

35.2.4 Optical Coherence Tomography Angiography

Microvascular alterations are believed to first occur in the deep capillary plexus and then extend to the superficial capillary plexus. Anastomosis with choroidal vasculature can result in subretinal neovascularization. Retinal–retinal anastomosis may also occur where an arteriole is seen feeding a dilated venule at the level of deep capillary plexus (► Fig. 35.6).

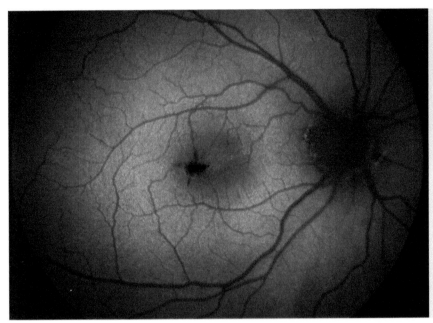

Fig. 35.3 Fundus autofluorescence (FAF) of the same patient with MacTel 2. The fovea is relatively hyper-autofluorescent due to loss of pigments that absorb excitation light and mask the FAF signal in the normal fovea. The retinal pigment epithelium plaque temporal to the fovea results in hypo-autofluorescence by blocking the FAF signal.

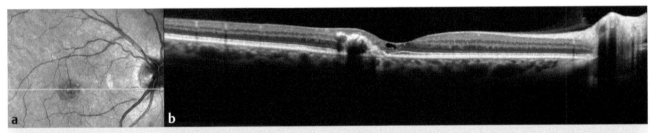

Fig. 35.4 (a,b) Optical coherence tomography in MacTel 2 displaying late findings of retinal atrophy predominantly involving the temporal margin of the fovea, a collapsed cystoid space, focal ellipsoid zone disruption, and increased temporal hyperreflectivity corresponding to retinal pigment epithelium migration.

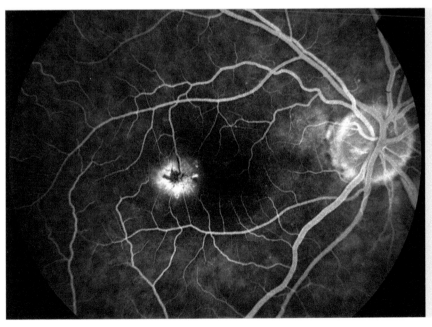

Fig. 35.5 Fluorescein angiogram in the late phase shows diffuse hyperfluorescence more predominant temporally.

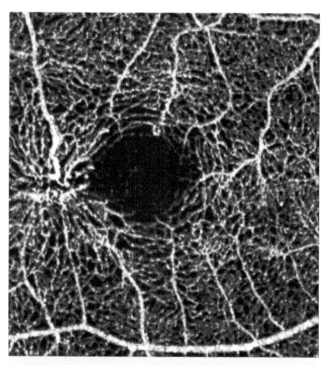

Fig. 35.6 Optical coherence tomography angiography in MacTel 2 depicting retinal–retinal anastomosis. A dilated venule is being fed by an arteriole at the level of deep capillary plexus.

35.3 Critical Work-up

In addition to comprehensive ophthalmic exam and imaging, patients should be evaluated for diabetes given the association between MacTel 2 and diabetes.

35.4 Management

35.4.1 Treatment Options

Central vision loss in MacTel 2 results from non-proliferative causes, such as neurosensory retinal atrophy, retinal cavitation progressing to full-thickness macular hole, or proliferation of neovascular membranes. In the absence of neovascularization, no intervention has been shown to be effective in a large controlled trial. A phase III clinical trial to determine efficacy of ciliary neurotrophic factor against progressive photoreceptor loss in MacTel 2 is currently ongoing. Surgery for macular holes in MacTel 2 has lower success compared to idiopathic macular holes since the underlying pathophysiology in MacTel 2 hole formation is atrophy as opposed to traction. Anti-vascular endothelial growth factor agents have been shown to benefit patients that progress to the proliferative stage of MacTel 2.

Suggested Reading

[1] Gass JD, Blodi BA. Idiopathic juxtafoveolar retinal telangiectasis. Update of classification and follow-up study. Ophthalmology. 1993; 100(10):1536–1546

[2] Yannuzzi LA, Bardal AM, Freund KB, Chen KJ, Eandi CM, Blodi B. Idiopathic macular telangiectasia. Arch Ophthalmol. 2006; 124(4):450–460

[3] Charbel Issa P, Gillies MC, Chew EY, et al. Macular telangiectasia type 2. Prog Retin Eye Res. 2013; 34:49–77

[4] Jindal A, Choudhury H, Pathengay A, Flynn HW, Jr. A novel clinical sign in macular telangiectasia type 2. Ophthalmic Surg Lasers Imaging Retina. 2015; 46(1):134–136

36 Retinitis Pigmentosa

Meghan J. DeBenedictis and Aleksandra Rachitskaya

Summary

Retinitis pigmentosa (RP), a group of hereditary retinal degenerative diseases, is characterized by the degeneration of photoreceptor cells. Night blindness and visual field constriction are common symptoms, with additional color and central vision loss over time. Optical coherence tomography often reveals ellipsoid zone loss and retinal atrophy. Fundus autofluorescence may also be helpful. A perifoveal hyperautofluorescent ring has been proposed as an indicator of potential progression. Patients should be thoroughly worked up to distinguish RP from other hereditary retinal degenerative diseases and other diseases with similar clinical presentations. Various treatments are being tested, such as gene therapies and vitamin A therapy. The Argus II Retinal Prosthesis system is currently the only FDA-approved treatment for patients with advanced RP.

Keywords: Argus, gene therapy, genetics, inherited retinal disease, retinitis pigmentosa, syndrome

36.1 Features

Retinitis pigmentosa (RP) is a group of genetically and phenotypically heterogeneous conditions affecting approximately 1 in 4,000 individuals. RP can be inherited in an autosomal dominant (15–25%), autosomal recessive (5–20%), or X-linked (5–15%) manner. To date, 22 genes have been identified to cause dominant RP, 39 genes identified to cause recessive RP, and 2 genes identified to cause X-linked RP. There are also numerous syndromic forms of RP, such as Usher and Bardet–Biedl syndromes. RP is characterized by degeneration of rod and cone photoreceptor cells. Sector RP is an atypical form of RP which involves only one or two quadrants of the retina showing clinical signs of the disease (pigmentary changes and visual field loss). It is usually characterized by bilateral symmetrical retinal degeneration in the inferior nasal quadrant. The majority of sector RP cases are the result of mutations in the *RHO* gene.

36.1.1 Common Symptoms

Symptoms and age of onset may be highly variable. Nyctalopia and constriction of visual field are usually the initial symptoms, with diminished color vision and central vision loss over time due to affected cone photoreceptor cells. Loss of light perception may be observed in severe cases.

36.1.2 Exam Findings

Optic nerve pallor, attenuated vessels, bone spicules in mid and far peripheral retina, vitreous cells, and posterior subcapsular lens opacities may be present (▶ Fig. 36.2).

36.2 Key Diagnostic Tests and Findings

36.2.1 Optical Coherence Tomography

Progressive reduction in the total thickness of various outer retinal structures is seen on optical coherence tomography (OCT). In fact, ellipsoid zone bandwidth has been proposed as a tool to monitor disease progression. Foveal preservation is often seen, particularly early in the disease, with outer retinal loss in the surrounding retina (▶ Fig. 36.1). Occasionally, cystoid macular edema may be present.

36.2.2 Fundus Autofluorescence

Hypoautofluorescent areas corresponding to the areas of outer retinal atrophy are seen. In the macular region, a perifoveal hyperautofluorescent ring has been proposed to serve as an indicator of prognosis with posterior migration of the ring indicating progression of the disease (▶ Fig. 36.3). The sectoral distribution of sectoral RP may also be demonstrated by fundus autofluorescence (FAF; ▶ Fig. 36.4).

36.2.3 Visual Field Testing

Kinetic and static visual field testing typically shows progressive scotomas in the mid periphery. As disease progresses, the small islands of vision remaining in the far peripheral field and in the visual axis slowly disappear (▶ Fig. 36.5).

36.2.4 Electroretinography

Reduced rod and cone response amplitudes and a prolonged time interval to peak rod or cone responses are seen on full-field electroretinography (ffERG). Amplitudes of the a- and b-waves are either reduced or nondetectable.

36.2.5 Fundus Photography

Optic disc pallor, attenuated retinal arterioles, and peripheral intraretinal pigment deposits known as bone spicules are observed.

36.2.6 Genetic Testing

Multiple clinical laboratories offer testing, though labs may vary in methodology, genes tested, interpretation of results/style of test reports, cost, and turn-around time. Positive genetic test results may allow for recurrence risk counseling, testing of other family members, provision of prognostic information, and ability to participate in potential clinical trials such as gene

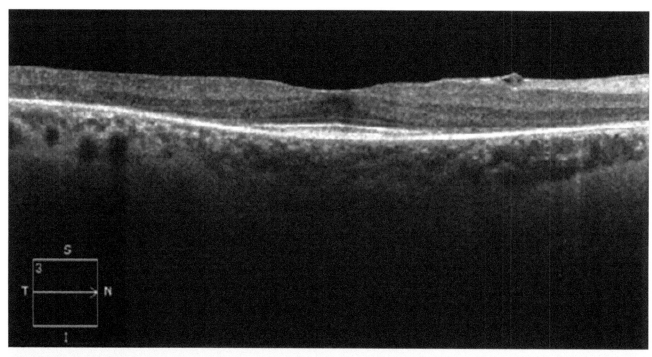

Fig. 36.1 Optical coherence tomography in retinitis pigmentosa demonstrating perifoveal ellipsoid zone and outer nuclear loss. Foveal preservation is seen.

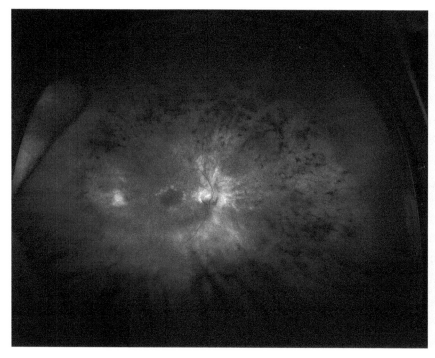

Fig. 36.2 Ultra-widefield photography of retinitis pigmentosa with 360-degree bone spicule pigmentation, optic nerve pallor, and vessel attenuation.

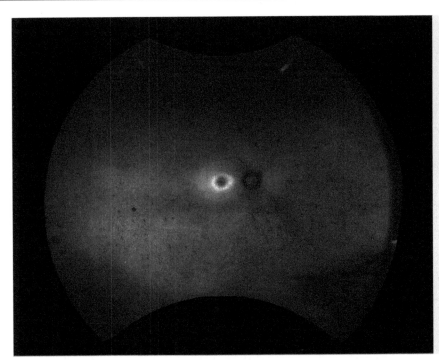

Fig. 36.3 Ultra-widefield fundus autofluorescence image in retinitis pigmentosa exhibiting hyperfluorescent macular ring.

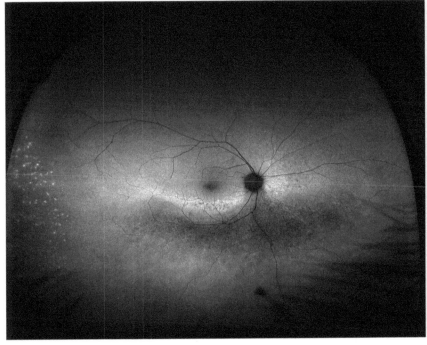

Fig. 36.4 Ultra-widefield fundus autofluorescence image with sector retinitis pigmentosa.

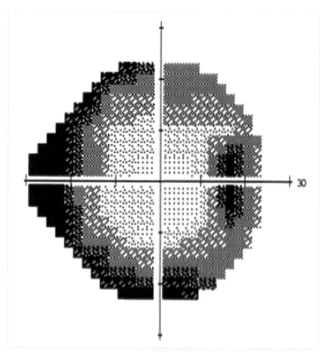

Fig. 36.5 Visual field demonstrated peripheral vision loss in retinitis pigmentosa.

therapy. Genetic testing should be obtained through a certified genetic counselor as comprehensive testing may yield incidental, inconclusive, and unexpected findings. Depending on the laboratory and testing methodology utilized, diagnostic genetic test results can be obtained in over 50% of patients.

36.3 Critical Work-up

RP may be characterized as nonsyndromic or syndromic. In syndromic RP, patients have RP as a feature due to an underlying systemic genetic syndrome (▶ Table 36.1). Thus, careful attention to medical history is crucial for making an accurate clinical diagnosis and ensuring proper medical management and patient referrals. Associated symptoms and conditions in ▶ Table 36.1 should be screened for at time of diagnosis. Much like nonsyndromic RP, the various types of syndromic RP exhibit significant genetic heterogeneity and variable expressivity.

RP should be distinguished from other hereditary retinal degenerative diseases including, but not limited to achromatopsia, choroideremia, cone-rod dystrophies, Leber congenital amaurosis, and Stargardt disease. In addition, similar clinical presentation can be seen in posterior uveitis, ocular syphilis, trauma, old artery occlusion, and retinal toxicity from systemic medications. Age of onset, presenting symptoms, and clinical examination findings are helpful in differentiating these conditions. Thus, a thorough work-up should include ERG, visual field testing, fundus photography, FAF, OCT, systemic review to assess for syndromic RP (refer to ▶ Table 36.1), and genetic testing.

36.4 Management

36.4.1 Treatment Options

Argus II Retinal Prosthesis System

The Argus II Retinal Prosthesis system is currently the only FDA-approved treatment for patients with advanced RP. In order to qualify, patients must be 25 years of age or older, have bare or no light perception in both eyes, and have a history of useful formed vision. The device is designed to provide visual function to patients by providing electrical stimulation to the remaining inner retina, resulting in the generation of phosphenes. It does not treat or reverse the underlying disease pathology.

Gene Therapy

A number of gene therapy trials are currently under way in the United States and Europe for hereditary retinal degenerative diseases, including some of the genes that can cause RP. The first gene therapy, voretigene neparvovec-rzyl, was approved for RP caused by biallelic *RPE65* mutations. This therapeutic is delivered by subretinal injection.

Vitamin A Therapy

Studies have shown some benefit from taking vitamin A and docosahexaenoic acid (DHA). When RP patients were treated with a combination of these two compounds, they had a slower rate of decline of their ERG amplitudes compared to those who did not receive treatment. Combinations of vitamin A supplementation with a diet high in omega-3 fatty acids (≥ 0.20 g/d) have also demonstrated a slower rate of vision decline compared to patients whose diet was low in omega-3 fatty acids.

Low Vision Aids

Referrals to a low vision therapist and orientation and mobility specialist are vital to assist patients with proper cane skills and provide them with technical devices and resources to allow them to use the level of vision they have to the fullest extent.

36.4.2 Follow-up

Yearly examinations should be performed to monitor disease progression and assess for secondary ocular findings such as cataracts and cystoid macula edema. In addition, referral to an ophthalmic genetic counselor should be offered in order to obtain genetic testing and discuss recurrence risks to family members. It is imperative, when obtaining a family history and counseling on recurrence risks, not to discount any inheritance pattern as incomplete penetrance has been observed, de novo mutations in dominant genes can occur, and female carriers of X-linked RP may be symptomatic. Consideration should be given to gender, age of onset of disease, and progression in affected family members.

Table 36.1 Syndromic retinitis pigmentosa diseases with associated systemic findings.

	Retinal dystrophy	Hearing loss	Seizures	MRI abnormalities	Developmental delay/MR	Anosmia	Ataxia	Truncal obesity	Cardiac defects	Cardiomyopathy	Polydactyly	Hypogonadism	Renal anomalies	Respiratory abnormalities	Liver anomalies	Skin findings	Skeletal anomalies
Alstrom syndrome	X	X			X	X		X		X		X	X	X	X	X	X
Bardet Biedl syndrome	X	X			X	X	X	X	X		X	X	X		X		X
Joubert syndrome	X			X	X		X				X		X	X	X		X
Kearns-Sayre syndrome	X	X	X	X			X		X	X			X				
Neuronal ceroid lipofuscinosis (features may vary by type)	X		X	X	X		X							X			
Refsum disease	X	X				X	X		X	X						X	X
Senior Loken syndrome	X												X				
Usher syndrome	X	X															

Note: This table is not comprehensive and does not include every genetic syndrome where retinitis pigmentosa is a feature.

Suggested Reading

[1] Hartong DT, Berson EL, Dryja TP. Retinitis pigmentosa. Lancet. 2006; 368 (9549):1795–1809

[2] Birch DG, Locke KG, Wen Y, Locke KI, Hoffman DR, Hood DC. Spectral-domain optical coherence tomography measures of outer segment layer progression in patients with X-linked retinitis pigmentosa. JAMA Ophthalmol. 2013; 131 (9):1143–1150

[3] Lima LH, Burke T, Greenstein VC, et al. Progressive constriction of the hyper-autofluorescent ring in retinitis pigmentosa. Am J Ophthalmol. 2012; 153(4): 718–727, 727.e1–727.e2

[4] Glöckle N, Kohl S, Mohr J, et al. Panel-based next generation sequencing as a reliable and efficient technique to detect mutations in unselected patients with retinal dystrophies. Eur J Hum Genet. 2014; 22(1):99–104

[5] Berson EL, Rosner B, Sandberg MA, Weigel-DiFranco C, Willett WC. ω-3 intake and visual acuity in patients with retinitis pigmentosa receiving vitamin A. Arch Ophthalmol. 2012; 130(6):707–711

37 Cone Dystrophy

Huber Martins Vasconcelos, Jr. and Paul Yang

Summary

Cone dystrophy is an inherited retinal degeneration characterized by primary degeneration of the cone photoreceptors with or without secondary involvement of the rod photoreceptors. Symptoms are progressive and include loss of visual acuity, central scotoma, dyschromatopsia, hemeralopia, and photoaversion. Rarely, patients may present with syndromic manifestations that include delayed milestones with or without significant intellectual delay, and other neurosensory, metabolic, and multiorgan disease. Cone dystrophy may be inherited in an autosomal dominant, autosomal recessive, or X-linked pattern. Key findings may include macular pigment changes, macular atrophy, and yellow fleck deposits. In severe or advanced disease, these findings may be concentrated in the macula, but widespread throughout the fundus. Important diagnostic work-up include full-field electroretinography, ultra-widefield fundus autofluorescence, optical coherence tomography, and widefield perimetry. Genetic testing is most useful as an adjunctive tool to confirm clinical suspicion, inheritance pattern, and potential for eligibility in clinical trials. There is no approved treatment available at this time; however, there are currently multiple clinical trials investigating the efficacy and safety of small molecule treatment, retinal gene therapy, and stem cell therapy in *ABCA4*-associated Stargardt fundus dystrophy.

Keywords: cone dystrophy, cone-rod dystrophy, inherited retinal degeneration, dyschromatopsia, Stargardt fundus dystrophy

37.1 Features

Cone dystrophy is a category of inherited retinal degenerations that is characterized by primary degeneration of the cone photoreceptors with or without secondary involvement of the rod photoreceptors, which are typically affected in more severe or advanced disease. In these cases, cone-rod dystrophy is a more accurate description; however, for the purposes of this chapter, cone dystrophy will be used as an all-inclusive term. In addition, the progressive nature of cone dystrophy differentiates it from the stationary cone dysfunction syndromes (e.g., achromatopsia, oligocone trichromacy, blue cone monochromatism), which will not be discussed here.

37.1.1 Common Symptoms

Typically presents between childhood and young adulthood. Slowly progressive loss of visual acuity over many years and decades, central scotoma, dyschromatopsia, hemeralopia, and photoaversion are common. Nystagmus is rare given that patients typically have good vision early in life. However, with advanced disease and severe loss of central vision, patients may develop strabismus and even nyctalopia.

37.1.2 Exam Findings

The most notable finding is bilateral decreased visual acuity and color discrimination deficits that accompany a spectrum of macular changes that may include blunted macula with loss of foveal reflex, mild pigment mottling, bull's eye pigment changes, or well-demarcated area of macular atrophy (▶ Fig. 37.1). The presence of yellow subretinal fleck deposits in the macula or posterior pole may be suggestive of Stargardt fundus dystrophy from mutations in *ABCA4* gene. In severe and advanced disease, there may be waxy disc pallor, vascular attenuation, diffuse confluent nummular atrophy, and pigment changes throughout the posterior pole and fundus with residual preservation of the far periphery.

37.2 Key Diagnostic Tests and Findings

37.2.1 Optical Coherence Tomography

Spectral domain optical coherence tomography (SD-OCT) is an increasingly important imaging modality for the diagnosis and monitoring of cone dystrophy. Common findings are outer retina layer attenuation with a pattern of foveal and/or perifoveal loss of the ellipsoid zone (EZ) (i.e., inner segment/outer segment junction; ▶ Fig. 37.1). In more advanced cases, there is atrophy of the retinal pigment epithelium (RPE), wherein the transition zones between preserved and atrophic macular RPE are often marked by a section of hyperreflective choroid due to differences in the OCT signal penetration (▶ Fig. 37.1). When yellow fleck deposits are evident, they are seen as scattered focal spots of subretinal hyperreflective thickening with or without adjacent EZ attenuation. The integrity of the foveolar EZ island is typically correlated with the visual acuity. Thus, the extent of foveolar involvement can be monitored as a marker of disease progression.

37.2.2 Fluorescein Angiography or Ultra-Widefield Fluorescein Angiography

Commonly, a window defect from RPE atrophy and staining of fleck deposits (also easily observable on OCT and fundus autofluorescence [FAF]) may be present. With the advent of OCT, fluorescein angiography (FA) is less commonly used in the diagnosis of cone dystrophy. Historically, a dark choroid was a useful tool in the diagnosis of Stargardt fundus dystrophy; however, modern FA imaging systems often utilize automatic exposure settings that may diminish the prominence of a dark choroid. FA is still used for the evaluation of choroidal neovascularization which can be a rare complication of cone dystrophy.

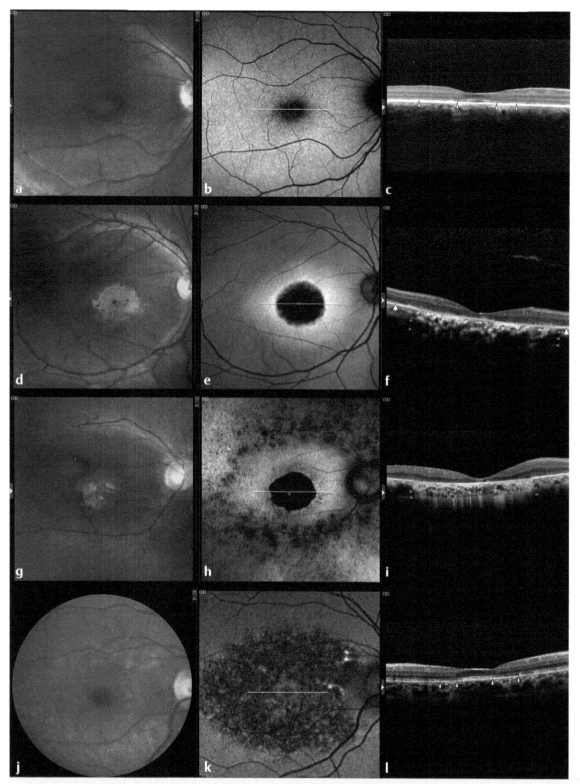

Fig. 37.1 Spectrum of cone dystrophy. **(a–c)** Milder disease with pigment mottling of the macula, which appear as mottled macular hypo-autofluorescence on fundus autofluorescence, and perifoveal attenuation of the ellipsoid zone (EZ or inner segment/outer segment) layer (*white arrowheads* show the transition zones) on OCT. **(d–f)** More advanced disease with macular atrophy, macular hypo-autofluorescence with hyper-autofluorescent ring, and macular attenuation of the ellipsoid zone (*white arrowheads*) and RPE (*red arrowheads* show the resulting hyperreflective appearance of the underlying choroid). **(g–i)** More severe disease with findings similar to B, except with the addition of perimacular ring of atrophy and mottled hypo-autofluorescence, and diffuse attenuation of the ellipsoid zone. **(j–l)** Different phenotype with generalized mottling of pigment and hypo-autofluorescence of the macula with perifoveal attenuation of the ellipsoid zone (*white arrowheads*).

37.2.3 Fundus Autofluorescence

Intense hyper-autofluorescent flecks that correlate with yellow deposits on examination in cases of suspected Stargardt fundus dystrophy. Less specific hyper-autofluorescent findings include a perifoveal ring (▶ Fig. 37.1b), which can also be seen in rod-cone dystrophy or autoimmune retinopathy. The spectrum of macular and fundus hypo-autofluorescence include a mottled (▶ Fig. 37.1a,d), discrete round (▶ Fig. 37.1b), or diffuse nummular pattern, which is generally correlated with RPE atrophy as seen on OCT. Some patients exhibit both a discrete round macular and mottled perimacular hypo-autofluorescence pattern (▶ Fig. 37.1c). The overall hypo-autofluorescent pattern is more specific for cone dystrophy using ultra-widefield FAF, wherein it is readily apparent that the macular or posterior pole is predominantly affected compared to the mid and far peripheral retina. In addition, areas of hypo-autofluorescence on ultra-wide FAF are usually well correlated with scotomas on visual field (▶ Fig. 37.2).

37.2.4 Electroretinography

Amplitude and timing of the cone-dependent waveforms are attenuated and prolonged, respectively, whereas rod-dependent waveforms are normal or attenuated to a lesser degree in

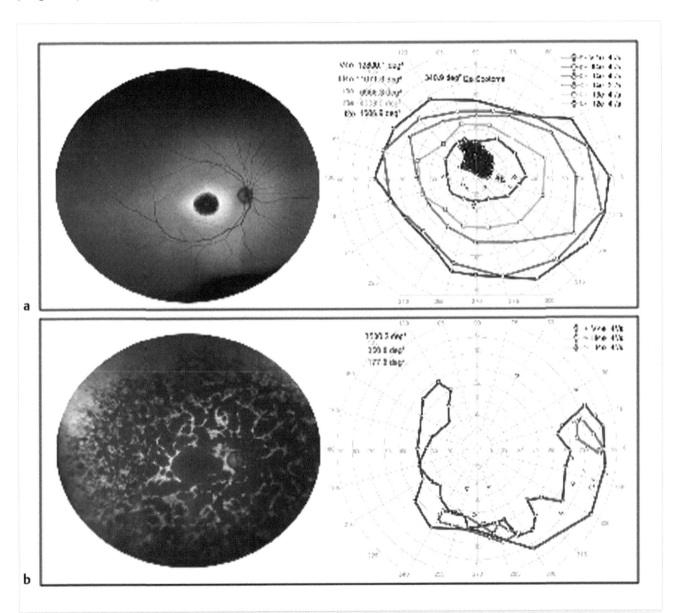

Fig. 37.2 Ultra-widefield fundus autofluorescence and widefield perimetry. **(a)** Mild-moderate disease with macular hypo-autofluorescence and normal autofluorescence of the mid and far peripheral retina on ultra-wide fundus autofluorescence, which correlate with an eccentrically located central scotoma (due to eccentric fixation) and intact peripheral isopters on widefield kinetic perimetry. **(b)** Severe advanced disease with hypo-autofluorescence concentrated in the macula and widespread throughout the fundus with residual normal autofluorescence only in the far peripheral retina. Widefield kinetic perimetry shows large scotoma affecting the central and midperipheral visual fields with residual far peripheral islands of response that correlate with the preserved far peripheral retina.

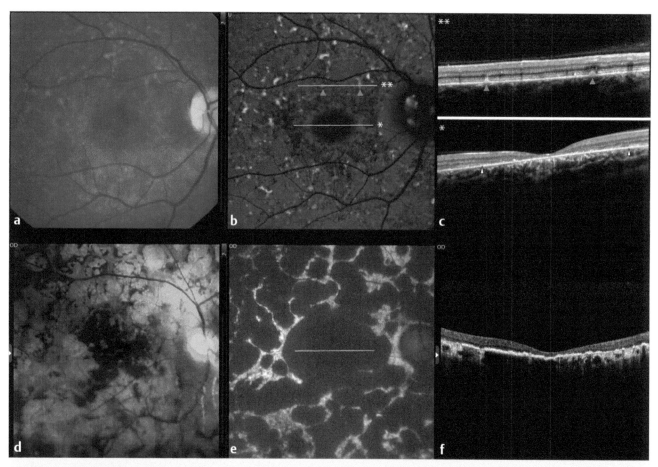

Fig. 37.3 (a–f) Full-field electroretinography in cone dystrophy. Rod-dependent responses to scotopic dim stimulus show waveforms that are only mildly attenuated compared with normal, whereas cone-dependent responses to photopic single and 30 Hz stimuli show waveforms that are more severely attenuated and prolonged compared with normal.

full-field electroretinography (▸ Fig. 37.3). Rarely, the rod-dependent waveforms may exhibit supernormal amplitudes in specific forms of cone dystrophy associated with mutations in *KCNV2* gene. Multifocal ERG (mfERG) is an adjunct modality typically used to characterize or diagnose focal macular cone dysfunction, especially in occult cases. However, mfERG is not specific to or diagnostic of a generalized cone dystrophy, because it can be abnormal in numerous maculopathies and advanced rod-cone dystrophies. mfERG cannot assess the function of rod photoreceptors to determine the proportion of rod versus cone dysfunction.

37.2.5 OCTA

Abnormal vascular features have been observed, but diagnostic value remains to be determined.

37.2.6 Perimetry

Absolute or relative central scotoma with or without involvement of central fixation is common; however, this can also be observed in maculopathies. Widefield perimetry is a more useful diagnostic tool for cone dystrophy, as it can be demonstrated that the central field is much more affected than the mid and far peripheral fields (▸ Fig. 37.2). The most commonly used

widefield manual kinetic perimeter is the Goldmann; however, the Octopus 900 is becoming a more useful widefield perimeter that can perform semiautomated quantitative kinetic perimetry, as well as widefield-automated static perimetry. In advanced cases of cone dystrophy with poor or eccentric fixation, the results of perimetry can be challenging to interpret due to low reliability. Nevertheless, with proper instruction and monitoring of fixation, useful data can be collected. Alternatively, microperimetry can be a more reliable tool for monitoring disease progression when fixation is limited. While microperimetry is limited to the central field, it automatically monitors and quantifies fixation and, on follow-up testing, ensures that the static grid is projected onto the same area of the macula.

37.2.7 Genetic Testing

Genetic testing in cone dystrophy is not yet a sensitive screening tool, and does not replace clinical assessment and work-up. Genetic testing is most useful as an adjunctive tool to confirm clinical suspicion, inheritance pattern, and potential for eligibility in clinical trials. One exception is Stargardt fundus dystrophy, which has a higher rate of positive genetic confirmation due to the specific phenotype of fleck deposits in most cases of *ABCA4*-associated disease. While single gene testing

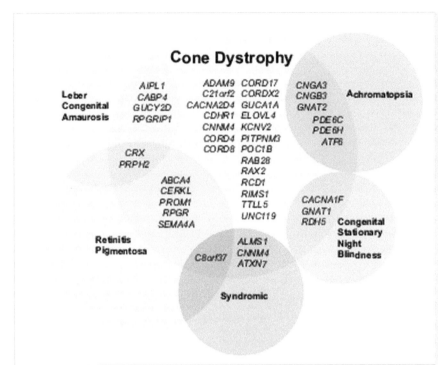

Fig. 37.4 Cone dystrophy genes and possible alternate phenotypes. Syndromic category includes Alstrom syndrome (*ALMS1*), Bardet-Biedl syndrome (*C8orf37*), Jalili (*CNNM4*) syndrome, and spinocerebellar ataxia (*ATXN7*).

may be useful in conditions with highly specific phenotype, next-generation large panel testing is more useful given the prevalence of overlapping phenotype and potential syndromic associations (▶ Fig. 37.4). Certain genes that cause cone dystrophy may also be associated with retinitis pigmentosa, Leber congenital amaurosis, congenital stationary night blindness, or achromatopsia.

37.3 Critical Work-up

Cone dystrophy may be associated with syndromic conditions (e.g., Bardet-Biedl syndrome, Alstrom syndrome, Jalili syndrome, or spinocerebellar ataxia). Patients with syndromic manifestations usually have a history of delayed milestones with or without significant intellectual delay, and other neurosensory, metabolic, and multiorgan disease. Family history is an important part of the initial assessment, which helps in determining the likelihood of a genetic etiology. Cone dystrophy may be inherited in any fashion, so a positive family history is usually indicative of dominant or X-linked disease. However, a negative family history does not rule out genetic disease, as autosomal recessive or de novo dominant cone dystrophy is still possible.

37.4 Management
37.4.1 Treatment Options

There is no approved treatment available at this time; however, there are currently multiple clinical trials investigating the efficacy and safety of small molecule treatment, retinal gene therapy, and stem cell therapy in *ABCA4*-associated Stargardt fundus dystrophy. General guidelines for nutritional supplementation in patients with inherited retinal degeneration include a diet rich in green leafy vegetables (lutein, zeaxanthin) and fish oil (omega-3 fatty acids). High-dose vitamin A is specif-

ically discouraged in *ABCA4*-associated disease, as it has been shown to exacerbate retinal degeneration in animal models. The use of sun glasses with ultraviolet protection, and avoidance or cessation of smoking, is also recommended.

37.4.2 Follow-up

In general, disease progression in inherited retinal degenerations is relatively slow, occurring over the course of years to decades. Annual exam with imaging and perimetry is usually sufficient for monitoring disease progression. The most important considerations during follow-up is the need to refer to low vision services for consultation regarding low vision refraction needs, tools, and adaptive devices such as bioptic telescopes. Patients who are legally blind should be referred for services at the State Commission for the Blind. If genetic testing is being pursued, the patient should be subsequently referred to a genetic counselor for counseling regarding interpretation of the test results and impact on other family members. If the patient develops signs of multisystem disease or delayed development, they must be referred for additional evaluation by a medical geneticist for the possibility of an associated syndrome. Referral to an ophthalmic geneticist for additional evaluation or co-management is always acceptable.

Suggested Reading

[1] Roosing S, Thiadens AA, Hoyng CB, Klaver CC, den Hollander AI, Cremers FP. Causes and consequences of inherited cone disorders. Prog Retin Eye Res. 2014; 42:1–26

[2] Michaelides M, Hardcastle AJ, Hunt DM, Moore AT. Progressive cone and cone-rod dystrophies: phenotypes and underlying molecular genetic basis. Surv Ophthalmol. 2006; 51(3):232–258

[3] Thiadens AA, Phan TM, Zekveld-Vroon RC, et al. Writing Committee for the Cone Disorders Study Group Consortium. Clinical course, genetic etiology, and visual outcome in cone and cone-rod dystrophy. Ophthalmology. 2012; 119(4):819–826

38 Paraneoplastic Retinopathies

Omar S. Punjabi and Dilraj Grewal

Summary

Paraneoplastic and autoimmune retinopathies are a group of immunological disorders that lead to retinal degeneration due to retinal antigens being aberrantly recognized as autoantigens. These include cancer-associated retinopathy, melanoma-associated retinopathy, bilateral diffuse uveal melanocytic proliferation, and presumed non-paraneoplastic autoimmune retinopathy. This group of disorders is associated with presence of antiretinal antibodies and is clinically associated with hetero-geneous and diverse retinal findings associated with bilateral, progressive, and painless visual deterioration associated with electroretinographic findings of abnormal rod, cone, and/or bipolar cell responses.

Various laboratory techniques, including immunohistochem-istry, Western blot, and enzyme-linked immunosorbent assay, have been described for the detection of circulating antiretinal antibodies in patient sera.

Keywords: autoimmune retinopathy, BDUMP, cancer-associated retinopathy, melanoma-associated retinopathy, paraneoplastic retinopathy

38.1 Features

Cancer-associated retinopathy (CAR) is a photoreceptor degen-erative disorder, representing a remote effect of various types of tumors and is associated with presence of various types of antiretinal antibodies in the blood, such as recoverin. This con-dition typically presents with bilateral, often asymmetric, pro-gressive vision loss over days to years. It typically affects both cones and rods. There may be arteriolar attenuation, arteriolar sheathing, and periphlebitis later in some cases. Melanoma-associated retinopathy (MAR) commonly presents after the melanoma has been diagnosed, often at the stage of metastases. It is typically seen in patients with metastatic cutaneous or uveal melanoma and is more common in men than in women. Bilateral diffuse uveal melanocytic proliferation (BDUMP) is a rare paraneoplastic syndrome resulting in bilateral vision loss. This is generally associated with a systemic cancer, which may not be recognized at the time of the ocular signs and symptoms. Non-paraneoplastic autoimmune retinopathy (npAIR) is the most common form of AIR and can be similar in phenotype and electrophysiological findings to CAR. Patients need to be fully investigated for an occult malignancy before a diagnosis of npAIR can be considered. Onset has been reported at a younger age than CAR, and there is often a strong family or medical his-tory of autoimmune disease.

38.1.1 Common Symptoms

CAR

Photoaversion, prolonged glare after light exposure, reduced visual acuity, decreased color perception, and central scotomas are all indicators of cone dysfunction; nyctalopia, prolonged dark adaptation, midperipheral (ring) scotomas, and more extensive peripheral visual field deficits are indicators of rod dysfunction. The visual symptoms are typically worse than the clinical signs.

MAR

Sudden onset of shimmering, flickering, pulsating photopsias, difficulty seeing in the dark, and progressive visual loss over several months. There is peripheral visual field depression or midperipheral visual field loss.

BDUMP

Bilateral vision loss.

npAIR

Progressive, painless visual deterioration, scotomas, and visual field defects. Very similar symptoms to CAR.

38.1.2 Exam Findings

CAR

Fundus initially appears normal. Optic disc pallor is often not seen in early disease and is much more likely in established dis-ease (▶ Fig. 38.1).

MAR

Fundus appearance ranging from normal to optic nerve pallor, vessel attenuation, retinal pigment epithelium (RPE) changes, and the presence of vitreous cells.

BDUMP

Bilateral, multiple, subtle round, or oval subretinal patches in the RPE; multiple elevated pigmented and nonpigmented uveal melanocytic tumors with diffuse uveal tract thickening; exuda-tive retinal detachments; and rapid cataract development.

npAIR

Clinically, very similar to CAR, but the onset has been reported at a younger age, and there is often a strong family or medical history of autoimmune disease.

38.2 Key Diagnostic Tests and Findings

38.2.1 Optical Coherence Tomography

CAR/npAIR

Spectral domain optical coherence tomography (SD-OCT) has shown loss of outer-retinal structures such as the ellipsoid zone

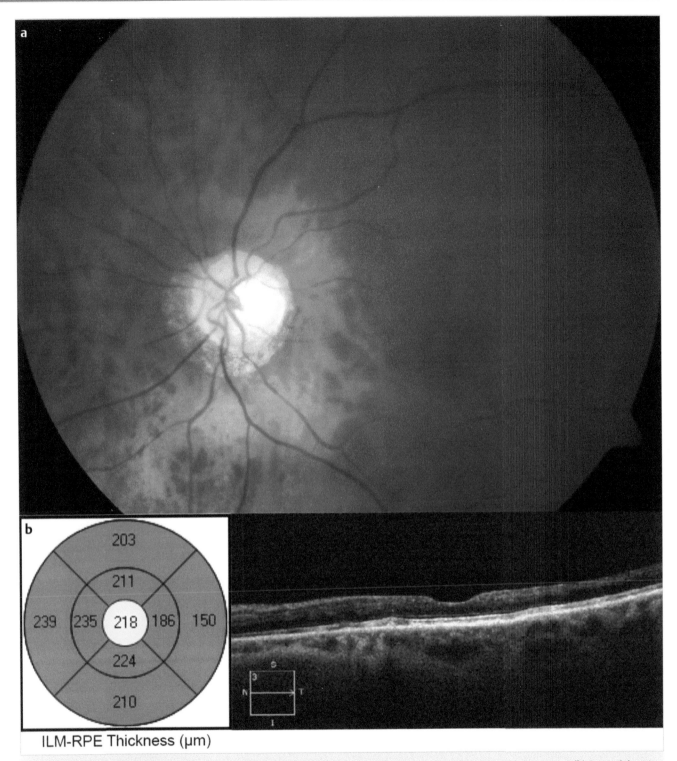

ILM-RPE Thickness (µm)

Fig. 38.1 (a) Fundus photograph in cancer-associated retinopathy (CAR) demonstrating optic nerve pallor and vessel attenuation. (b) Spectral domain optical coherence tomography in CAR with generalized retinal atrophy noted on both retinal thickness map and the B-scan.

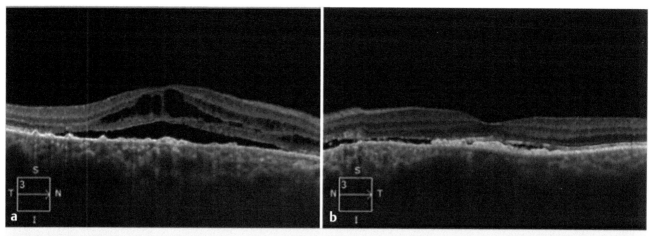

Fig. 38.2 (a,b) Spectral domain optical coherence tomography in bilateral diffuse uveal melanocytic proliferation demonstrating multiple areas of retinal pigment epithelium elevation and choroidal thickening with associated subretinal fluid and macular edema.

(i.e., EZ, previously referred to as the inner segment/outer segment junction), the external limiting membrane, and the outer nuclear layer (▶ Fig. 38.1). Mild cystic spaces and occasionally mild schisis-like changes may be present. Generalized atrophy may also be present. The mild schisis-like changes in the setting of outer retinal atrophy is highly suspicious for pathologic anti-retinal antibodies.

MAR

MAR may be associated with serous or vitelliform detachments of the neurosensory retina and subretinal accumulation of hyperreflective material in the posterior pole.

BDUMP

Choroidal and RPE thickening may be present with variable subretinal fluid and macular edema (▶ Fig. 38.2).

38.2.2 Fundus Autofluorescence

CAR

Areas of hyper-autofluorescence which have been shown to correspond to the loss of outer retina. Some cases show a parafoveal ring of abnormally enhanced autofluorescence with normal autofluorescence inside the ring and a hypo-autofluorescent retina outside the ring.

MAR

Hyper-autofluorescence may be associated with vitelliform-like lesions.

BDUMP

Variable hyper- and hypo-autofluorescence may be present at involved areas (▶ Fig. 38.3).

38.2.3 Electroretinography

CAR/npAIR

There may be abnormalities of both the a- and b-waves, and in some instances, selective involvement of the b-wave. Significant reduction in electrical activity may be present.

MAR

May have a characteristic pattern of a markedly reduced dark-adapted b-wave indicating compromised bipolar cell function, and a normal dark-adapted a-wave (negative appearance) indicating normal photoreceptor cell function, which is seen in approximately half of the patients. The characteristic alteration of the light-adapted a-wave morphology and the b-wave amplitude results from a selective dysfunction of the "ON" bipolar cells. All patients have an abnormal ERG.

38.2.4 Antiretinal Antibodies

The sensitivity and specificity for autoretinal antibodies can vary significantly. It is important to interpret the results of the test in the context of the clinical picture. The presence of autoretinal antibodies may not be pathologic.

CAR

The presence of antiretinal antibodies (such as anti-recoverin and alpha-enolase, Tubby-like protein 1, heat shock cognate protein 70, glyceraldehyde 3-phosphate dehydrogenase, and anti-carbonic anhydrase II antibody) may precede the detection of tumor.

MAR

Retinal antibodies may be present, particularly of bipolar cell, also including antibodies against transducin, rhodopsin, arrestin, CAII, interphotoreceptor retinoid-binding protein, bestrophin, a-enolase, myelin basic protein, and rod outer segment proteins.

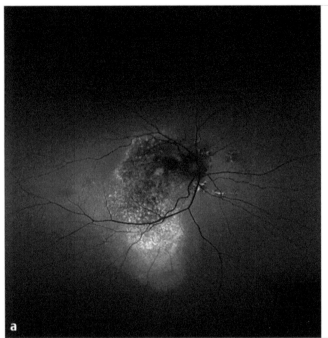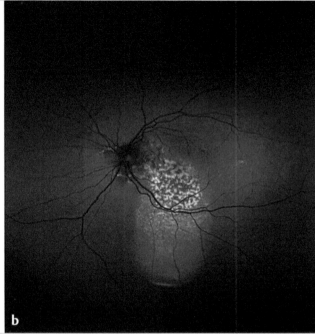

Fig. 38.3 (a,b) Fundus autofluorescence in bilateral diffuse uveal melanocytic proliferation related to metastatic bladder cancer showing multiple areas of retinal pigment epithelium hypofluorescence and hyperfluorescence in the macula of both eyes.

npAIR

Antiretinal antibodies against recoverin, the IPL, the inner retinal layer (35-kDa antibody against retinal Müller cell–associated antigen), a-enolase, CAII, and rod transducin-a have been described.

38.3 Management

38.3.1 Treatment Options

CAR

There is no established treatment protocol, and the evidence for therapeutic intervention is relatively limited. Long-term immunosuppression with cyclosporine, azathioprine, oral prednisone, and intravenous immunoglobulin (IVIg) are probably the most widely studied treatment options.

MAR

Although several treatment modalities including oral, sub-Tenon, or intravenous corticosteroids; plasmapheresis; IVIg; azathioprine; gabapentin; and X-irradiation of metastases or cytoreductive surgery have been described, overall the treatment of the visual loss associated with MAR has been disappointing.

BDUMP

Approximately 30 cases of BDUMP have been reported in the literature. The average survival from initial presentation has been approximately 17 months. Retention of visual acuity is poor, but intervention with corticosteroids, plasmapheresis, chemotherapy, and radiotherapy may be considered.

npAIR

Triple-therapy regimen consisting of cyclosporine (100 mg/day), azathioprine (100 mg/day), and prednisone (20–40 mg/day) has been utilized. In addition, IVIg, infliximab, and intravitreal triamcinolone acetate have been attempted.

Suggested Reading

[1] Weleber RG, Watzke RC, Shults WT, et al. Clinical and electrophysiologic characterization of paraneoplastic and autoimmune retinopathies associated with antienolase antibodies. Am J Ophthalmol. 2005; 139(5):780–794

[2] Spaide RF, Curcio CA. Anatomical correlates to the bands seen in the outer retina by optical coherence tomography: literature review and model. Retina. 2011; 31(8):1609–1619

[3] Arai Y, Kajihara S, Masuda J, et al. Position-independent, high-level, and correct regional expression of the rat aldolase C gene in the central nervous system of transgenic mice. Eur J Biochem. 1994; 221(1):253–260

[4] Adamus G, Ren G, Weleber RG. Autoantibodies against retinal proteins in paraneoplastic and autoimmune retinopathy. BMC Ophthalmol. 2004; 4:5

[5] Ohta K, Kikuchi T, Yoshida N. Slowly progressive non-neoplastic autoimmune-like retinopathy. Graefes Arch Clin Exp Ophthalmol. 2011; 249(1):155–158

39 Congenital Stationary Night Blindness

Laryssa A. Huryn, Brett G. Jeffrey, and Catherine A. Cukras

Summary

Congenital stationary night blindness encompasses a group of disorders that have a spectrum of clinical and electrophysiologic findings as well as molecular causes. The primary symptom is night blindness and dark adaptation deficiencies; however, not every patient is symptomatic. Full-field electroretinography is critical in the evaluation of these patients, as it reflects the underlying protein dysfunction and helps differentiate them from progressive retinal degenerations.

Keywords: albipunctatus, congenital stationary night blindness, electronegative ERG, nyctalopia, Oguchi disease

39.1 Features

Congenital stationary night blindness (CSNB) encompasses many disorders that have a spectrum of clinical and electrophysiologic findings as well as molecular causes. The gene associations are as follows:

- CSNB1 (complete):
  - X-linked (*NYX*) (▶ Fig. 39.1).
  - Autosomal recessive (*GRM6, TRPM1, GPR179, LRIT3*).
- CSNB2 (incomplete):
  - X-linked (*CACNA1F*) (▶ Fig. 39.2).
  - Autosomal recessive (*CABP4, CACNA2D4*).

- Riggs:
  - Autosomal dominant (*RHO, GNAT1, PDE6B*).
  - Autosomal recessive (*SLC24A1, GNAT1*).
- CSNB fundus with abnormalities:
  - Autosomal recessive (Oguchi [▶ Fig. 39.3]: *SAG, GRK1*; fundus albipunctatus [▶ Fig. 39.4]: *RLBP1, RPE65, RDH5*).

39.1.1 Common Symptoms

Difficulty seeing under dim light conditions that not all patients are aware of, but final dark-adapted thresholds are elevated by approximately 2 to 3 $\log_{10}$ units. Color discrimination is unaffected and visual acuity is usually mildly affected (median = 20/40). Amblyopia may be observed secondary to strabismus.

39.1.2 Exam Findings

Refractive changes vary, but high myopia is often seen in CSNB1 and CSNB2. Nystagmus may be present in young individuals. Patients with CSNB most often have a normal fundus; however, other less common forms have distinctive fundus findings. A fundus of abnormal appearance in association with CSNB includes Oguchi disease (golden-yellow fundus reflex which disappears with long dark adaptation [Mizuo-Nakamura phenomenon]) and fundus albipunctatus (numerous small, white-yellow lesions scattered across the retina from the posterior pole to midperiphery, sparing the macula).

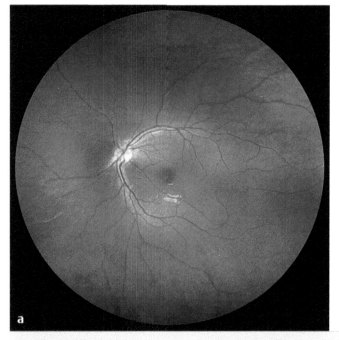

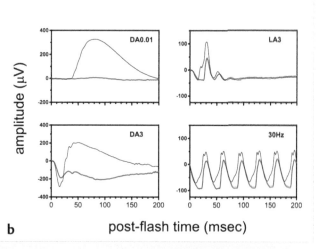

Fig. 39.1 CSNB1 (complete)—*NYX*. A 10-year-old boy with a history of nystagmus, strabismus, and nyctalopia. His best corrected visual acuity is 20/50 in the right eye and 20/63 in the left with myopic correction of −9.00 + 1.75 × 045 OD and −5.00 + 1.75 × 160 OS. **(a)** His visual field is full on Goldmann testing and fundus examination is normal. Full-field ERG demonstrates the electronegative waveform in response to bright flash (DA3) and no measurable response to a dim stimulus (DA0.01). **(b)** Under photopic conditions, the LA3 response has a distinct flattened trough followed by a sharp rising late response that produces a characteristic sawtooth appearance to 30-Hz flicker. Genetic testing revealed a mutation in *NYX*.

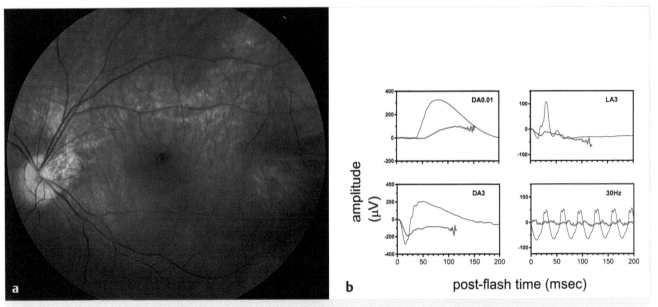

Fig. 39.2 CSNB2 (incomplete)—*CACNA1F.* A 16-year-old boy with no history of nyctalopia or nystagmus. His best corrected visual acuity is 20/80 in the right eye and 20/40 in the left with myopic correction of −17.25 + 4.00 × 089 OD and −15.50 + 1.75 × 119 OS. His visual field was full on Goldmann testing and color vision normal. **(a)** Fundus exam demonstrates myopic changes. Full-field ERG: Under scotopic conditions, the dim flash response (DA0.01) is reduced but clearly present, and the bright flash response (DA3) demonstrates the electronegative waveform. **(b)** The photopic ERG (LA3) is barely detectable and there is no measurable 30-Hz flicker ERG. Patient ERG responses are truncated at 10 to 150 ms due to blinks following the flash. Genetic testing revealed a mutation in *CACNA1F.* (Courtesy of Brian Brooks, NIH).

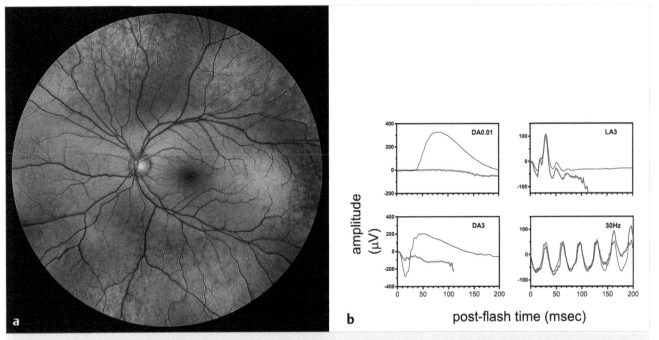

Fig. 39.3 Oguchi disease—*SAG.* **(a)** A 13-year-old boy with nyctalopia and a golden sheen to the fundus with confirmed *SAG* mutation. Full-field ERG: Under scotopic conditions, the DA0.01 and DA3 ERGs resemble those observed for CSNB1. **(b)** However, under photopic conditions (LA3 and 30 Hz), the ERGs have normal amplitudes and implicit times.

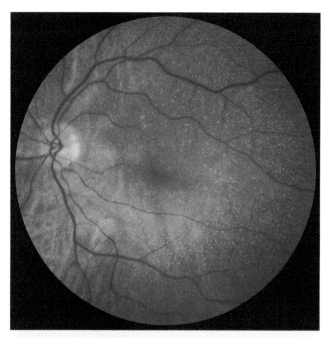

Fig. 39.4 Fundus albipunctatus. A 61-year-old female with a family history of fundus albipunctatus presenting with a lifelong history of nyctalopia and numerous small white-yellow lesions within the retina.

39.2 Key Diagnostic Tests and Findings

39.2.1 Electroretinography

Full-field electroretinography is critical in the evaluation of patients with possible CSNB to differentiate them from progressive conditions such as X-linked retinitis pigmentosa or cone dystrophy. Responses reflect underlying protein dysfunction (▶ Fig. 39.1, ▶ Fig. 39.2, ▶ Fig. 39.3).

Normal/Myopic Fundus

For the dark-adapted response to a bright flash (ISCEV DA3 or DA10), both CSNB1 and CSNB2 have an electronegative ERG, characterized by significantly reduced b-wave amplitude in the setting of a normal/near-normal a-wave amplitude. CSNB1 under scotopic conditions has no measurable response to a dim stimulus (DA 0.01). Under photopic conditions, the LA3 response has a distinct flattened trough followed by a sharp rising late response that produces a characteristic sawtooth response to 30-Hz flicker. CSNB2 under scotopic conditions has a reduced but still clearly present dim flash stimulus (DA 0.01). Photopic ERGs (LA3 and 30-Hz flicker) are markedly reduced in amplitude. Riggs CSNB has no measurable response to a dim stimulus (DA 0.01) under scotopic conditions. The scotopic bright flash response (DA3 or DA10) resembles the photopic ERG recorded

to a bright flash (LA10). Photopic ERGs are normal/near normal in amplitude and timing.

Abnormal Fundus

In fundus albipunctatus after 30 minutes of dark adaptation, DA0.01 response is undetectable, and there is an electronegative waveform with bright flash. Cone flicker responses are delayed and only mildly decreased. Although this ERG may resemble the Riggs type of CSNB, unlike the Riggs type, prolonged dark adaptation (3–12 hours) results in nearly complete recovery of rod-mediated ERG. In Oguchi disease, changes after 30-minute dark adaptation are similar to that of fundus albipunctatus. Scotopic responses will also increase in amplitude after prolonged dark adaptation. However, the scotopic bright flash ERG will only be normal to a single flash. The ERG response will revert to an electronegative ERG for subsequent flashes.

39.3 Critical Work-up

As electronegative ERG is a hallmark of this diagnosis, it should be noted that this ERG can also be observed in other monogenic retinal diseases (for which there are usually additional retinal findings) and in adults with cancer- and melanoma-associated retinopathy (for which there are often no notable retinal findings) but warrants additional medical work-up.

39.4 Management

39.4.1 Treatment Options

Currently, there is no treatment available for patients with CSNB. Patients should be reassured with the knowledge that this is generally a stationary disease. They should be offered genetic testing and counseled on inheritance patterns and risk to future offspring.

39.4.2 Follow-up

Routine screening with cycloplegic refraction in the pediatric population to ensure proper spectacle correction and amblyopia treatment.

Suggested Reading

[1] Boycott KM, Sauvé Y, MacDonald IM. X-Linked Congenital Stationary Night Blindness. January 16, 2008 [Updated April 26, 2012]. In: Adam MP, Ardinger HH, Pagon RA, et al., eds. GeneReviews® [Internet]. Seattle, WA: University of Washington; 1993–2018. Available at: https://www.ncbi.nlm.nih.gov/books/NBK1245/. Accessed April 12, 2019

[2] Zeitz C, Robson AG, Audo I. Congenital stationary night blindness: an analysis and update of genotype-phenotype correlations and pathogenic mechanisms. Prog Retin Eye Res. 2015; 45:58–110

[3] McCulloch DL, Marmor MF, Brigell MG, et al. ISCEV standard for full-field clinical electroretinography (2015 update). Doc Ophthalmol. 2015; 130(1):1–12

40 Albinism

Atalie C. Thompson and Lejla Vajzovic

Summary

Albinism is a rare inherited disorder of melanin biosynthesis that can be broadly classified into oculocutaneous albinism and ocular albinism. Ocular signs and symptoms include photophobia, pendular nystagmus, strabismus, refractive errors, poor visual acuity, iris transillumination defects, hypopigmentation of the retinal pigment epithelium, and foveal hypoplasia. Those with oculocutaneous albinism also have depigmented hair and skin. Magnetic resonance imaging demonstrates asymmetric hyper-decussation at the chiasm and fundus autofluorescence patterns reveal decreased macular pigment. Optical coherence tomography has helped provide insight into the structural and developmental differences of the optic nerve and retina in patients with albinism, and shows foveal hypoplasia, a thicker central macular thickness, and decreased perifoveal thickness of the inner and outer retinal layers. Patients with life-threatening systemic syndromes such as Chédiak-Higashi and Hermansky-Pudlak should be co-managed with a hematologist. Patients with albinism should undergo genetic testing and counseling and have an annual ophthalmic examination. Eye muscle surgery may be pursued as part of the management of strabismus and nystagmus in some patients.

Keywords: foveal hypoplasia, ocular albinism, oculocutaneous albinism

40.1 Features

Albinism is a rare genetically heterogeneous inherited disorder of impaired melanin biosynthesis that is characterized by specific changes in the eye and visual pathway with or without reduced pigmentation of the skin and hair. There are two main forms: oculocutaneous albinism (OCA) and ocular albinism (OA). Patients with OA have only the ocular and optic changes that result from reduced melanin pigment during development, while those with OCA also have depigmentation of the skin, hair, and eyelashes.

OA can arise from either autosomal recessive or X-linked recessive mutations, while all subtypes of OCA have an autosomal recessive inheritance pattern. Autosomal recessive ocular albinism (AROA) results from mutations in *TYR* and *TYRP1*, while X-linked mutations in the *GPR143* gene at Xp22.2 lead to OA1, the Nettleship-Falls variant of OA (MIM #300500). Different genetic mutations can lead to variable phenotypic expression. Patients with mutations in the tyrosinase (*TYR*) gene on chromosome 11q14-q21 develop OCA type 1 (OCA1), which is characterized by white hair and fair skin. However, those with OCA1B (MIM #606952) can develop some melanin pigment in their eyes, hair, and skin, while those with OCA1A (MIM #2031100) do not develop any melanin pigment. Patients with OCA2 have mutations in the OCA2 gene (chromosome 15q12-q13, MIM #203200). Less commonly, patients can develop OCA3 from mutations on the tyrosinase-related protein 1 (*TYRP1*) gene. Patients with OCA3 tend to develop a milder phenotype. Those with *SLC45A2* mutations develop OCA4 (MIM #606574), which is characterized by a wide array of phenotypic expression. A new gene *OCA5* (MIM #615312) has been identified on chromosome 4q24, and *OCA6* (MIM#203100) is due to mutations on *SLC24A5* on chromosome 1q21.1. In rare circumstances, OCA is associated with potentially fatal systemic syndromes such as Chédiak-Higashi (CHS) and Hermansky-Pudlak (HPS).

40.1.1 Common Symptoms

Extreme photophobia and glare symptoms result from light easily entering and scattering inside the eyes. Systemic syndromes can have life-threatening and debilitating comorbidities (e.g., frequent pyogenic sinopulmonary or skin infections and peripheral neuropathy in CHS; blood clotting disorders, and ceroid accumulations in the lungs and kidneys in HPS).

40.1.2 Exam Findings

A pendular sensory nystagmus develops due to poor development of the optic system. During infancy, the patient's eye movements may have a low frequency and large amplitude that later evolve into the more distinct fast and slow phases in adulthood. Because they have a positive angle kappa, they often have the external appearance of pseudoexotropia. Concomitant strabismus and loss of stereopsis are possible and may lead to a head tilt. Patients with albinism who have less pigment have worse visual acuity, though visual acuity tends to be better at near than distance because convergence helps dampen the nystagmus at near.

On slit lamp exam, albinos demonstrate speckled or diffuse transillumination defects and variable depigmentation of the iris (▶ Fig. 40.1). Patients with more severe OCA1A can have light blue to pink irides, while those with less severe forms, like OCA1B, may have green or brown irides. Patients with OCA2, -3, and -4 may have better visual acuity than patients with OCA1 and can demonstrate increases in pigmentation over time in the iris, skin, choroid, and retinal pigment epithelium (RPE). Hypopigmentation of the RPE may reveal visible choroidal macular vessels on dilated fundus exam, and foveal hypoplasia leads to absence of the foveal pit and the foveal light reflex (▶ Fig. 40.2). Patients with OA and AROA demonstrate similar ocular findings to OCA but have normal pigmentation of the skin and hair.

40.2 Key Diagnostic Tests and Findings

40.2.1 Optical Coherence Tomography

Absence of the foveal pit, or foveal hypoplasia, is classically seen (▶ Fig. 40.3). Thicker central macular thickness may be present (possibly from delayed and arrested migration of the inner retinal layer from the fovea during development), but the perifoveal retinal thickness is reduced in both the outer and inner retinal layers. Incomplete maturation of the optic nerve

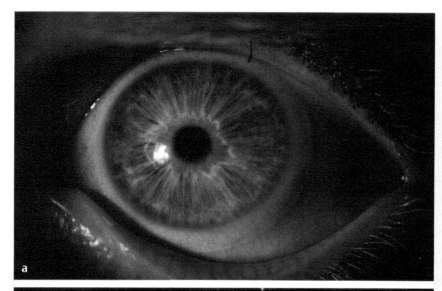

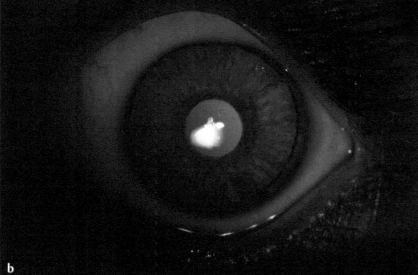

Fig. 40.1 (a) Slit-lamp photograph of the left eye with (b) transillumination defects of the iris due to oculocutaneous albinism. (Photographer, Michael P. Kelly.)

head is possible as evidenced by a significantly smaller median cup area and cup-to-disc ratio. The retinal nerve fiber layer is significantly thinner in albinism and correlates with ganglion cell layer thickness at the central fovea.

40.2.2 Fundus Autofluorescence

Lack of hypo-autofluorescence in the macula due to absent macular pigment (▶ Fig. 40.4).

40.2.3 Magnetic Resonance Imaging

Excessive over-decussation of the fibers in the chiasm.

40.2.4 Visual Evoked Potential

Three-lead visual evoked potential will be asymmetric due to the asymmetric decussation at the chiasm.

40.3 Critical Work-up

All patients with albinism should undergo a full ophthalmic exam during early childhood to aid in the detection and management of amblyopia, strabismus, nystagmus, and refractive errors. Patients/families should also meet with a genetics specialist both for genetic testing and genetic counseling. Referral to support groups may be beneficial to the patient and family. Due to their increased risk for squamous and basal cell carcinomas of the skin, patients should periodically be evaluated by a dermatologist. Specialists in hematology can further assist in the diagnosis and management of patients with CHS and HPS. Due to the high risk of hemorrhaging, hematology should be consulted prior to elective ocular surgeries and perioperative plasmapheresis may be required for patients with HPS. Demonstration of giant granules and inclusion bodies in leukocyte precursor cells on bone marrow biopsy is pathognomonic for CHS.

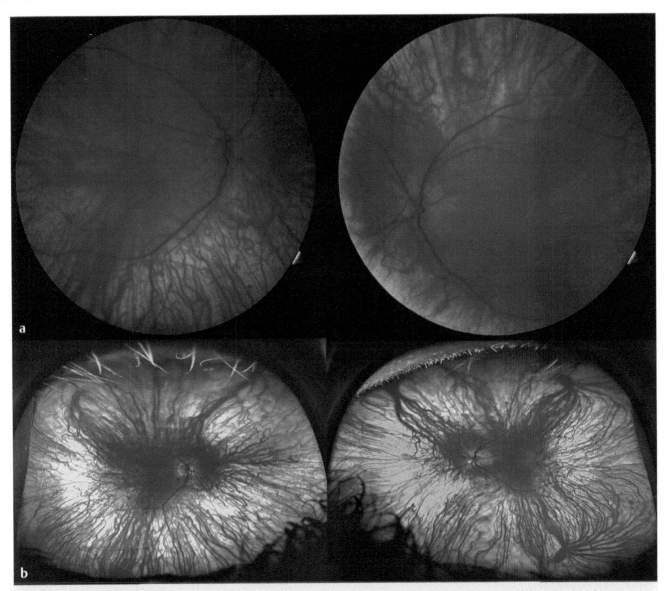

Fig. 40.2 (a) Fundus photographs of hypoplastic foveas of the right and left eye. (b) Ultra-widefield fundus photos of the right and left eye demonstrate visible choroidal vessels due to retinal pigment epithelium hypopigmentation. (Photographer, Michael P. Kelly.)

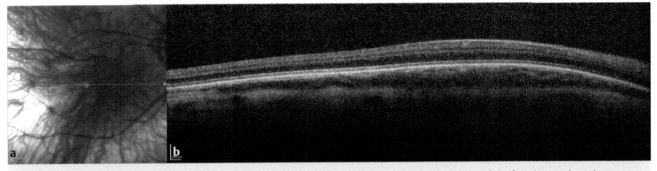

Fig. 40.3 (a,b) Spectral domain-optical coherence tomography demonstrates foveal hypoplasia with absence of the foveal pit in the right eye. (Photographer, Michael P. Kelly.)

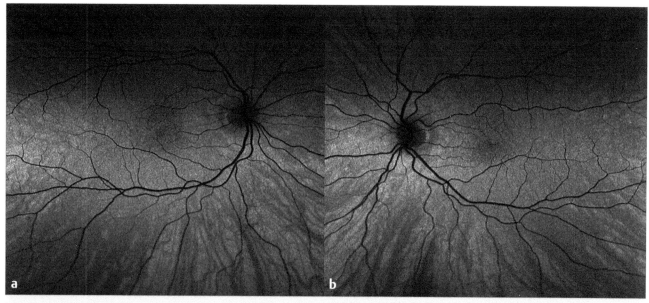

Fig. 40.4 (a,b) Fundus autofluorescence demonstrates absent macular pigment in the right and left eye. (Photographer, Michael P. Kelly.)

40.4 Management

40.4.1 Treatment Options

There are currently no cures for albinism or its associated systemic syndromes. For symptomatic management, patients should wear sunglasses to reduce their sensitivity to light and wear long sleeves, hats, and sunscreen for protection from ultraviolet rays. Corrective lenses for refractive errors may help improve visual function, especially in patients with strabismus where vision may range from hypermetropia to myopia with or without astigmatism. Patients may elect to undergo eye muscle surgery for management of nystagmus and strabismus.

40.4.2 Follow-up

Patients with OCA and OA should undergo a full ophthalmic examination by an ophthalmologist every year. Although visual outcomes are dependent on the severity of the disease, they have a normal expected lifespan and intellectual development.

Suggested Reading

[1] Gargiulo A, Testa F, Rossi S, et al. Molecular and clinical characterization of albinism in a large cohort of Italian patients. Invest Ophthalmol Vis Sci. 2011; 52(3):1281–1289

[2] Kim J, Elshatory YM, Pathak AK, Adamopoulou C. Albinism—EyeWiki. Available at: http://eyewiki.aao.org/Albinism. Accessed September 30, 2017

[3] McCafferty BK, Wilk MA, McAllister JT, et al. Clinical insights into foveal morphology in albinism. J Pediatr Ophthalmol Strabismus. 2015; 52(3):167–172

[4] Lee H, Purohit R, Sheth V, et al. Retinal development in albinism: a prospective study using optical coherence tomography in infants and young children. Lancet. 2015; 385 Suppl 1:S14

[5] Mohammad S, Gottlob I, Sheth V, et al. Characterization of abnormal optic nerve head morphology in albinism using optical coherence tomography. Invest Ophthalmol Vis Sci. 2015; 56(8):4611–4618

41 Gyrate Atrophy

Matteo Scaramuzzi and Elias I. Traboulsi

Summary

Gyrate atrophy of the choroid and retina is a rare, genetically determined, autosomal recessive, slowly progressive chorioretinal dystrophy featuring hyperornithinemia to levels 10 to 15 times above normal, caused by a deficiency of the mitochondrial matrix enzyme ornithine aminotransferase (OAT). Ornithine accumulation leads to a retinal degeneration characterized by scalloped areas of atrophy in the midperipheral retina that coalescence centrally and peripherally with the advancing disease. Symptoms include nyctalopia and decreased visual acuity due in some cases to cystoid macular edema, posterior subcapsular cataract, or rarely from choroidal neovascularization (CNV). Diagnosis is primarily clinical, supported by plasma high ornithine levels. Molecular genetic testing for mutations in *OAT* gene confirms the clinical diagnosis. Fluorescein angiography and optical coherence tomography are helpful in detecting macular complications.

A better understanding of the pathogenetic mechanisms will lead to more effective treatment strategies in the future. Current treatments include dietary restriction of arginine, vitamin B_6 supplementation, topical or oral carbonic anhydrase inhibitors, and treatments for rare cases of associated CNV.

Keywords: choroidal neovascularization, gyrate atrophy, macular edema, ornithine

41.1 Features

Gyrate atrophy (GA) of the choroid and retina is a rare, genetically determined, autosomal recessive, slowly progressive chorioretinal dystrophy characterized by sharply demarcated areas of chorioretinal atrophy in the midperipheral retina. This dystrophy was first reported in 1973, and more than 200 cases have since been described with about one-third from Finland. The main feature of this disease is the hyperornithinemia with levels 10 to 15 times above normal due to a deficiency of the mitochondrial matrix enzyme ornithine aminotransferase (OAT). Ornithine is a nonessential amino acid majorly converted to glutamate by OAT and subsequently to proline in the urea cycle. The *OAT* gene is located on 10q26 and found is expressed highly in the retina, liver, and kidney. Over 50 mutations have been described to date. OAT mutations lead to ornithine accumulation, which is toxic for ocular structures such as corneal endothelium, iris smooth muscle, ciliary body, photoreceptors, and especially the retinal pigment epithelium (RPE). The atrophic areas in the midperipheral retina show a marked loss of the choroidal vessels, including the choriocapillaris, RPE, and photoreceptors. The normally appearing areas in the posterior pole show focal areas of photoreceptor cell loss, shortening of outer segments in the transitional area, and absence in the atrophic areas.

41.1.1 Common Symptoms

Nyctalopia begins in the first and second decades of age (usually of mild and slowly progressive nature) and possible restriction of peripheral field vision. Visual acuity is usually preserved in the early stages but may decrease primarily from foveal involvement or secondarily from cystoid macular edema or cataracts. Blindness usually occurs in most untreated patients in the fifth decade of life.

41.1.2 Exam Findings

The fundus shows peripheral small, geographic, sharply demarcated enlarging and merging scalloped areas of atrophy of the RPE and choriocapillaris during the earlier and intermediate stages and a tendency for pigment clumping to occur at the margins of such lesions. Occasional patients have peripapillary atrophic lesions that progress in size in a similar way that progressive lesions do. Atrophy begins in midperipheral and peripheral areas, in a garland-shaped fashion, and then coalesces and progresses centrally and peripherally. In advanced stages, the disease involves the entire fundus, with relative sparing of the macula. The optic disc and retinal arterioles usually are normal until the late stages of the disease (▶ Fig. 41.1). Posterior vitreous detachment, epiretinal membranes, macular hole, choroidal neovascularization (CNV), and cystoid macular edema have been observed. Moderate to severe myopia is found in most patients. Posterior subcapsular cataracts generally appear in the second decade of life. Extraocular manifestations have rarely been associated with GA. The most common are electromyographic abnormalities, although very few patients complain of slight muscle weakness. Electroencephalograms or electrocardiograms also may be abnormal in some patients.

41.2 Key Diagnostic Tests and Findings

41.2.1 Optical Coherence Tomography

A fundamental tool to detect macular defects that are difficult to define with ophthalmoscopy. Hyporeflective cystic spaces secondary to macular edema (▶ Fig. 41.2), macular hole, epiretinal membrane, or vitreomacular traction have been described. Hyperreflective deposits could be seen in inner retinal layers, suggesting the gliotic response to ongoing cell death. Interestingly, in older GA patients, outer retinal tubulation corresponding to the arrangement of degenerating photoreceptor cells may be present.

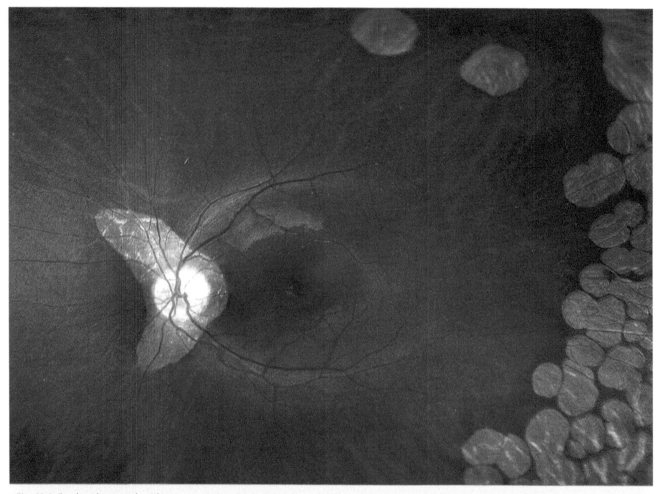

Fig. 41.1 Fundus photograph with gyrate atrophy, showing the classical midperipheral and peripheral confluent areas of chorioretinal atrophy. Note boomerang-shaped atrophic lesion at the optic nerve head.

41.2.2 Fluorescein Angiography or Ultra-Widefield Fluorescein Angiography

Hyperfluorescence in the areas of chorioretinal atrophy, often larger than clinically visible atrophic areas corresponding to window defects.

41.2.3 Electroretinography

Subnormal in the early stages of the disease, with marked reduction or nondetectable a- and b-wave responses in later stages. The rod responses are affected more severely in the early stages. A delayed cone implicit time response could be seen with 30-Hz flicker stimulus.

41.2.4 Electrooculography

Usually not reduced until later stages of the disease.

41.2.5 Visual Field

Defects correspond to the atrophic areas. Field loss begins in the midperipheral area as regionally dense scotomas eventually coalescing to form a ring scotoma. Progressive field loss ultimately leaves the patient with only small residual central fields.

41.2.6 Ornithine Measurements

High ornithine levels are found in urine, plasma, aqueous humor, and cerebrospinal fluid, often 10 to 20 times higher than normal. There is no evidence of correlation of age or severity with the concentration of ornithine in plasma. Ornithine levels decrease significantly with dietary restriction and vitamin B_6 supplementation.

41.2.7 Genetic Testing

A definitive diagnosis can be obtained by identifying the underlying mutations in the *OAT* gene on chromosome 10.

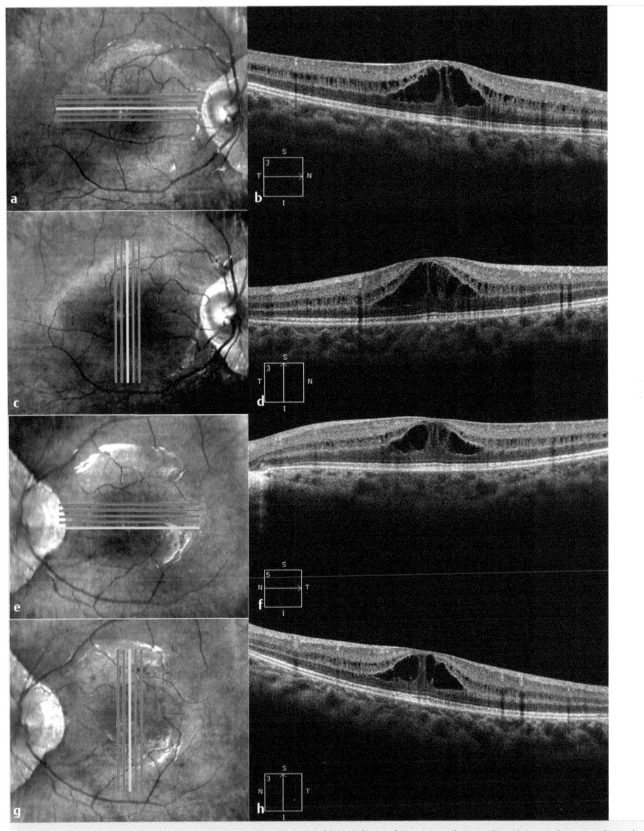

Fig. 41.2 (a–d) Optical coherence tomography of the right eye and **(e–h)** the left eye of the patient shown in **Fig. 41.1**, revealing cystoid macular edema.

41.3 Critical Work-up

While GA has typical fundus features, a GA-like fundus phenotype with a possible autosomal dominant inheritance pattern and normal plasma ornithine levels has also been described. GA also has some phenotypic similarities to myopic degeneration and hereditary choroidal atrophy. In the later stage, it may clinically resemble choroideremia. Some cases of retinitis pigmentosa sometimes may resemble GA. In GA, however, the pigment clumps usually are denser and associated with the atrophic lesions. The history of night blindness and fundus appearance of scalloped areas of atrophy of the RPE and choroid are suggestive of the diagnosis (▶ Fig. 41.1).

41.4 Management

41.4.1 Treatment Options

As with other inherited retinal degenerative disorders, a better understanding of the pathogenetic mechanisms will lead to more effective treatment strategies in the future.

Diet

As the function of OAT enzyme is dependent on pyridoxine (vitamin B_6) as a cofactor, supplementation treatment with oral vitamin B6 has been tried. Vitamin B_6-responsive patients with the following mutations: V332 M, A226V, T181 M, E318K, and G237D constitute less than 5% of cases and appear to have a milder disease and a better visual function.

As ornithine is derived mainly from arginine, a low-protein diet with near-total elimination of arginine has been studied. Results are controversial. No improvement or arrest of the chorioretinal degeneration is shown with short-term use of the diet. However, long-term studies are encouraging, showing a reduction of ornithine levels, a slower progression of chorioretinal lesions, and a reduction in loss of retinal function if the diet is started early, continued for several years, and plasma ornithine levels are maintained below six times the normal range. With the widespread use of optical coherence tomography, macular edema has been discovered to be a more common finding than previously recognized, even in the early stages of the disease. The management of the macular edema remains includes diet modification, carbonic anhydrase drops, and vitamin B_6 supplementation.

Steroids

The pathogenesis of macular edema in GA is not yet known. A likely hypothesis is a disruption of blood–retinal barrier. Intravitreal triamcinolone injection has been demonstrated to temporarily reduce macular edema in a case report.

Carbonic Anhydrase Inhibitor

Assuming an imbalance of the distribution of RPE membrane-bound carbonic anhydrase isozyme in the pathogenesis of the edema, oral carbonic anhydrase inhibitors such as acetazolamide were used as a treatment with good response, indicating that these factors play a role in the genesis of the edema. One case example with macular edema secondary to GA treated with topical dorzolamide drops three times a day (baseline, ▶ Fig. 41.2) resulted in a significant reduction over a 4-month period and almost complete resolution after 10 months (▶ Fig. 41.3).

Choroidal Neovascularization

CNV is infrequent in GA but can accelerate visual loss. Antivascular endothelial growth factor therapy is typically utilized for CNV management.

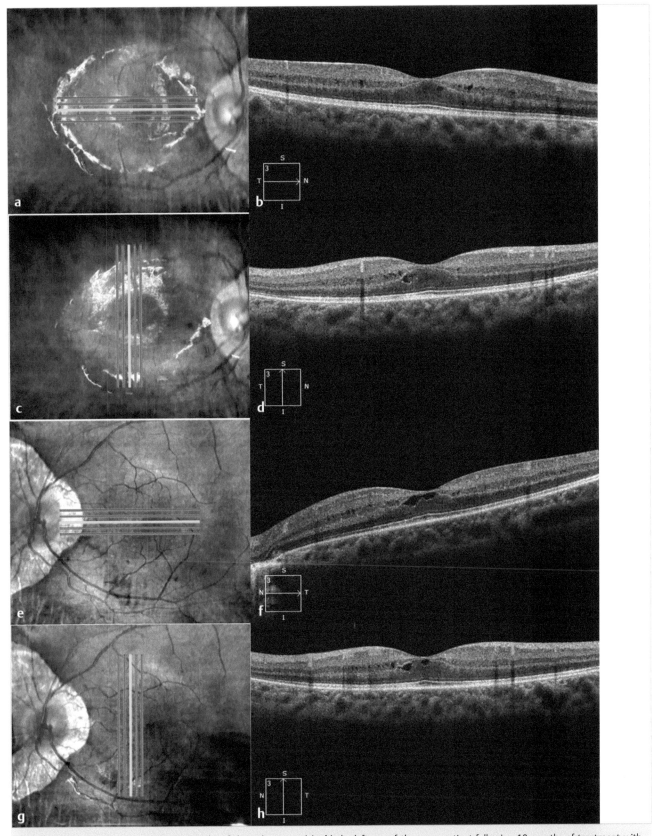

Fig. 41.3 (a–d) Optical coherence tomography of the right eye and (e–h) the left eye of the same patient following 10 months of treatment with dorzolamide, a low-protein diet, and vitamin B$_6$ supplementation, demonstrating significant improvement in the amount of cystoid macular edema.

41.4.2 Follow-up

Patients with GA should be followed every 6 to 12 months and more frequently if complications such as CNV or macular edema are present.

Suggested Reading

[1] Traboulsi EI. Genetic Diseases of the Eye. New York, NY: Oxford University Press; 2012

[2] Sergouniotis PI, Davidson AE, Lenassi E, Devery SR, Moore AT, Webster AR. Retinal structure, function, and molecular pathologic features in gyrate atrophy. Ophthalmology. 2012; 119(3):596–605

[3] Oliveira TL, Andrade RE, Muccioli C, Sallum J, Belfort R, Jr. Cystoid macular edema in gyrate atrophy of the choroid and retina: a fluorescein angiography and optical coherence tomography evaluation. Am J Ophthalmol. 2005; 140 (1):147–149

[4] Kaiser-Kupfer MI, Caruso RC, Valle D, Reed GF. Use of an arginine-restricted diet to slow progression of visual loss in patients with gyrate atrophy. Arch Ophthalmol. 2004; 122(7):982–984

[5] Piozzi E, Alessi S, Santambrogio S, et al. Carbonic Anhydrase Inhibitor with Topical NSAID Therapy to Manage Cystoid Macular Edema in a Case of Gyrate Atrophy. Eur J Ophthalmol. 2017; 27(6):e179–e183

42 Choroideremia

Ruben Jauregui and Stephen H. Tsang

Summary

Choroideremia is chorioretinal dystrophy that presents with symptoms of nyctalopia and constricting visual fields. The disorder is inherited in an X-linked manner and thus is mostly seen in males, although female carriers can also present with characteristic findings on examination but are rarely symptomatic. In addition to fundus examination, a variety of imaging modalities can aid in the correct diagnosis of choroideremia. Recent developments in gene therapy and its application on clinical trials offer a potential treatment for this disease.

Keywords: Choroideremia, chorioretinal dystrophy, female carriers, gene therapy, nyctalopia, peripheral vision loss, X-linked

42.1 Features

Choroideremia is X-linked chorioretinal dystrophy characterized by progressive degeneration and atrophy of the retinal pigment epithelium (RPE), choriocapillaris, and retina. First described by Mauthnuer in 1872, its prevalence is estimated to be between 1 in 50,000 and 1 in 100,000. Choroideremia is caused by mutations in the *CHM* gene, localized to the long arm of the X chromosome at Xq21.2, which encodes for Rab escort protein 1. This protein is involved in intracellular trafficking in both RPE cells and photoreceptors and is considered to play an important role in the removal of outer segment discs by the RPE. As intracellular trafficking is affected, the RPE and photoreceptor cells die prematurely. Given the X-linked nature of the disease, it is mostly seen in males.

42.1.1 Common Symptoms

Nyctalopia in the first or second decades of life; peripheral vision loss over the next three to five decades; central visual acuity is often maintained until the fifth decade of life. Once degeneration affects the macula, rapid deterioration of central vision occurs.

42.1.2 Fundus Findings

Findings on dilated fundus examination parallel the progression of symptoms (▶ Fig. 42.1). Early in the disease, the midperiphery photoreceptors, primarily the rods, are affected. This is followed by progressive atrophy with loss of peripheral field and night vision. Patchy areas of depigmentation are seen peripherally and spread centripetally. Well-defined regions of atrophy with scalloped borders develop where the underlying large choroidal vessels and sclera are visible. An island of preserved RPE around the macula is preserved until the late stages in the disease course.

42.2 Key Diagnostic Tests and Findings

42.2.1 Optical Coherence Tomography

Increased central retinal thickness early in the disease when visual acuity is unaffected. As the disease progresses and visual acuity declines, slow thinning of the central retina is observed. Cystoid macular edema is a common observable complication. Outer retinal tubulation signifies end-stage photoreceptor degeneration.

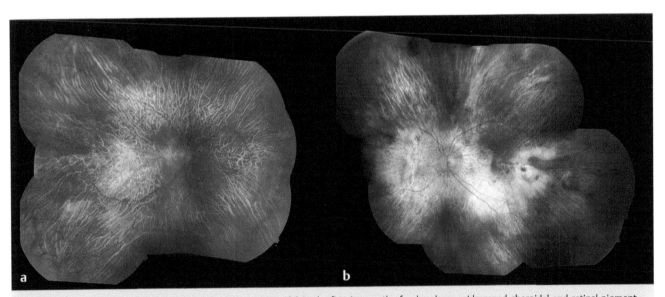

Fig. 42.1 Fundus photographs of two choroideremia patients. **(a)** In the first image, the fundus shows widespread choroidal and retinal pigment epithelium (RPE) atrophy, with the underlying larger choroidal vessels visible. Characteristic pigment clumping at the level of RPE is also seen peripherally. **(b)** The fundus of this patient shows an advanced stage of the disease. An island of spared RPE is seen around the macula, but there is widespread choroidal and RPE atrophy on the periphery. On the center of the posterior pole, the atrophy has advanced to the stage where the underlying white sclera is visible.

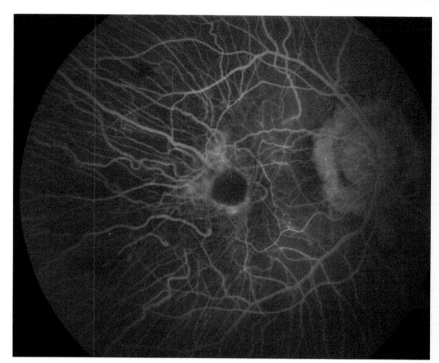

Fig. 42.2 Late-phase fluorescein angiogram in choroideremia. The areas of atrophic retinal pigment epithelium (RPE) and choriocapillaris appear as hypofluorescent with prominent visualization of the choroidal vessels. In contrast, the island of spared RPE around the macula and optic nerve appears as hyperfluorescent as the dye is able to penetrate through the choriocapillaris.

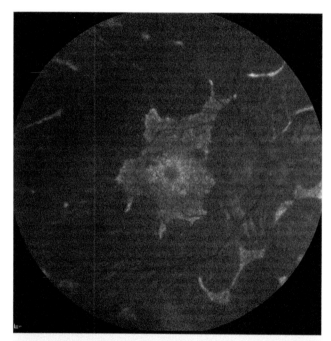

Fig. 42.3 Fundus autofluorescence of a patient with choroideremia demonstrating widespread chorioretinal atrophy as areas of hypoautofluorescence. An area of spared retinal pigment epithelium (RPE) on the macular area is observed. The borders between spared and atrophic RPE are sharp and well-demarcated.

42.2.2 Fluorescein Angiography or Ultra-Widefield Fluorescein Angiography

Areas of atrophic RPE and choriocapillaris appear hypofluorescent, in contrast to the islands of preserved RPE and chorioca-

pillaris, which appear hyperfluorescent as the dye is able to perfuse the choriocapillaris (▶ Fig. 42.2).

42.2.3 Fundus Autofluorescence

Early loss of peripheral autofluorescence with subsequent centripetal loss is seen. The patchy hypofluorescent areas of atrophy generally present with sharp edges and can help in identifying atrophic areas not apparent on fundus examination (▶ Fig. 42.3).

42.2.4 Electroretinography

Abnormalities are detected early in the disease, with reduced scotopic responses seen before photopic responses are affected. As the disease progresses, both responses become gradually extinguished.

42.2.5 Visual Fields

Reduced retinal sensitivity in the equatorial retina, developing of a ring scotoma, and loss of peripheral visual fields.

42.2.6 Genetic Testing

Female carriers are generally asymptomatic, and even in the rare cases where they are symptomatic, their disease is less severe than that of male patients. Carriers may have mild RPE mottling in the periphery, classically described as "motheaten," and a pattern of hypofluorescent speckles can be observed in fundus autofluorescence imaging (▶ Fig. 42.4, ▶ Fig. 42.5). The macula is otherwise unaffected. The phenotypic variability seen in carriers is due to lyonization, in which one copy of the X chromosome is randomly silenced in embryogenesis.

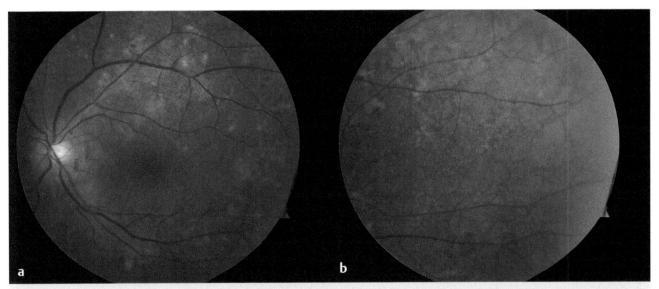

Fig. 42.4 (a) Fundus photographs of a female carrier of choroideremia demonstrating characteristic retinal pigment epithelium mottling in the periphery (b) with reticular degeneration also visualized at high magnification.

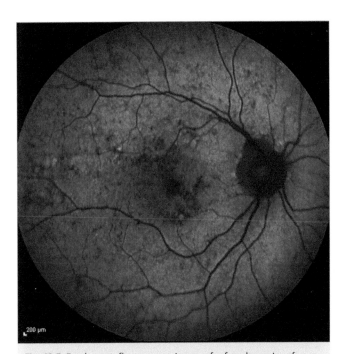

Fig. 42.5 Fundus autofluorescence image of a female carrier of choroideremia demonstrating speckles of hypofluorescence throughout the posterior pole. This reticular pattern is characteristically observed in choroideremia carriers.

42.3 Critical Work-up

In the diagnosis of choroideremia, other retinal pathologies that present with nyctalopia and visual field loss should be ruled out. Differential diagnoses include retinitis pigmentosa, gyrate atrophy, Bietti crystalline dystrophy, and thioridazine toxicity.

42.4 Management

Genetic counseling is recommended for the patient and the family. Although there is no treatment available, recent investigational therapies have focused on retinal gene therapy as a way to replace the defective gene via viral vectors. Studies show promise in the treatment of choroideremia via gene therapy as they show tolerability of humans to the viral vector and signs of visual improvement in these patients. In addition, the Choroideremia Natural History Study is a multicenter US-based study that is under way to evaluate disease progression. This study would help in understanding clinical endpoints of disease progression and subsequently establish endpoints for the deployment of gene therapy.

Suggested Reading

[1] Khan KN, Islam F, Moore AT, Michaelides M. Clinical and genetic features of choroideremia in childhood. Ophthalmology. 2016; 123(10):2158–2165

[2] Heon E, Alabduljalil T, McGuigan DB, III, et al. Visual function and central retinal structure in choroideremia. Invest Ophthalmol Vis Sci. 2016; 57(9): OCT377–OCT387

[3] MacLaren RE, Groppe M, Barnard AR, et al. Retinal gene therapy in patients with choroideremia: initial findings from a phase 1/2 clinical trial. Lancet. 2014; 383(9923):1129–1137

[4] Edwards TL, Jolly JK, Groppe M, et al. Visual acuity after retinal gene therapy for choroideremia. N Engl J Med. 2016; 374(20):1996–1998

43 Stargardt Disease

Sruthi Arepalli and Justis P. Ehlers

Summary

Stargardt disease is the most commonly inherited macular dystrophy in children and adults. It can present with a wide variety of symptoms and fundus findings. Vision loss can be mild or severe on initial presentation. Most commonly, fundus findings include bull's-eye maculopathy, foveal pigmentary changes, atrophy, and/or pisciform flecks in the retinal pigment epithelium. Optical coherence tomography reveals loss of foveal architecture and photoreceptors with disease progression. There is no cure for Stargardt disease and patients should be counseled on genetic transmission.

Keywords: ABCA4, ellipsoid zone, fundus, macular dystrophy, retinal pigment epithelium

43.1 Features

Stargardt disease is the most commonly inherited macular dystrophy, with prevalence ranging from 1 in 8,000 to 1 in 10,000. Diagnosis can be difficult as the disease has an incredibly heterogeneous presentation, with varied age of onset and clinical findings. Patients usually present in childhood to early adulthood, but there have been cases described in patients up to the age of 50. Autosomal recessive mutations in the gene *ABCA4* are the leading cause, with as many as 1 in 20 people carrying a mutation. Mutations in this gene are also linked to various other retinal dystrophies, including cone, "cone–rod," "rod–cone," and retinitis pigmentosa. In a small percentage of the population, other genes, including *ELOVL4, PRPH2,* or *BEST1* are linked to Stargardt development.

The *ABCA4* gene encodes for a retinal adenosine triphosphate-binding transporter, ABCR, which is located on the outer segments of cones and rods. ABCR transports the end products of the visual cycle from the photoreceptors to the retinal pigment epithelium (RPE). Without ABCR, biretinoid products accumulate in the outer segments of photoreceptors, which are ultimately digested by the RPE. In the RPE, the biretinoids react with other compounds to form a toxic by-product, N-retinylidene-N-retinylethanolamine (A2E), which leads to the accelerated formation of lipofuscin and death of the RPE with the subsequent decline of the overlying photoreceptors. Several hundred disease-causing mutations have been found in the *ABCA4* gene, creating a myriad of phenotypes. More drastic variants of the genotype, including nonsense mutations, are linked to earlier and more severe expression, while missense mutations are often linked to milder phenotypes.

43.1.1 Common Symptoms

Central vision loss or paracentral scotomas are characteristic, with preservation of the full visual field. Presenting visual acuity ranges from 20/20 to light perception. Patients may have no visual symptoms and are diagnosed when incidental findings are found on routine examination.

43.1.2 Exam Findings

Variable findings such as subtle fundus manifestations (e.g., blunted foveal reflex, mild RPE changes, fine granular yellow-white accumulations in the macula) can precede perceived vision loss. The most common findings are a result of the accumulated A2E and lipofuscin, creating white, yellow, or orange flecks in the RPE. Flecks are typically oblong and often connect at oblique angles, which resemble a fishtail ("pisciform"). The distribution of flecks differs, localized to the macula in some, extending to the equator in others (▶ Fig. 43.1). The number, color, and borders of these flecks vary between patients, creating an even more complex clinical picture. In addition to flecks, pigmentary changes and bull's-eye maculopathy (e.g., atrophy) may develop (▶ Fig. 43.2, ▶ Fig. 43.3). Subretinal fibrosis can accompany the flecks in select patients with severe disease. In some patients, the accumulation of material of A2E and lipofuscin in the RPE results in brown discoloration in the macula and choroidal vessels loss on ophthalmoscopy (▶ Fig. 43.4). The peripapillary RPE is typically spared, even with extensive disease.

43.2 Key Diagnostic Tests and Findings

43.2.1 Optical Coherence Tomography

Demonstrates loss of foveal architecture, including the degeneration of photoreceptors and RPE atrophy. Consecutive scans can monitor disease progression, especially the ellipsoid zone (EZ) loss, as this has been linked to visual acuity in patients (▶ Fig. 43.3c). En face EZ integrity thickness maps can quantify the percentage of foveal EZ atrophy or attenuation, which was shown to be significantly higher than normal controls and significantly correlated to decreased visual acuity.

43.2.2 Fluorescein Angiography or Ultra-Widefield Fluorescein Angiography

Areas of atrophy and pisciform flecks appear hyperfluorescent. Possible accumulation of A2E in the RPE blocks the transmission of light to the choroidal circulation (i.e., "the silent choroid").

43.2.3 Fundus Autofluorescence

Can detect and monitor areas of atrophy and lipofuscin flecks in the RPE. Atrophy is hypofluorescent, while flecks appear either hyper- or hypofluorescent (▶ Fig. 43.1b, ▶ Fig. 43.2b, ▶ Fig. 43.3b). Fundus autofluorescence (FAF) patterns may be linked to visual prognosis and risk of atrophy progression.

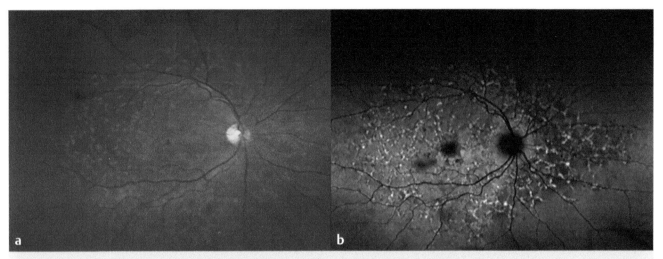

Fig. 43.1 **(a)** Fundus photograph of the right eye with Stargardt disease with widespread pisciform flecks up to the arcades and foveal pigmentary changes. **(b)** Fundus autofluorescence shows the same flecks as hyperfluorescent and atrophy at the fovea.

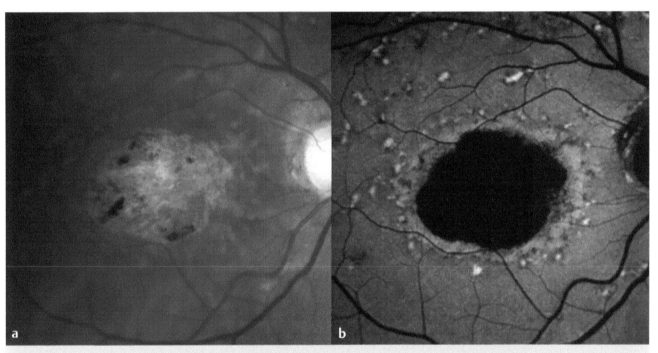

Fig. 43.2 **(a)** Fundus photograph showing advanced disease with foveal atrophy and surrounding retinal pigment epithelium (RPE) flecks. **(b)** Fundus autofluorescence shows the same area of atrophy as hypofluorescent with surrounding flecks in the RPE as hyperfluorescent.

43.2.4 Electroretinography

Usually unremarkable due to photoreceptor loss typically limited to the fovea. However, in patients with severe disease and widespread cone and photoreceptor loss, the widefield electroretinography may be impacted.

43.3 Critical Work-up

As Stargardt disease is most commonly inherited in an autosomal recessive fashion, genetic testing is frequently imple-

mented to provide genetic counseling for family members. Imaging can support the diagnosis, especially in subtle cases.

43.4 Management

43.4.1 Treatment Options

There is no cure for Stargardt disease. Research investigating gene therapy are underway. Vitamin A supplementation is discouraged as this may accelerate the formation of toxins through the visual cycle.

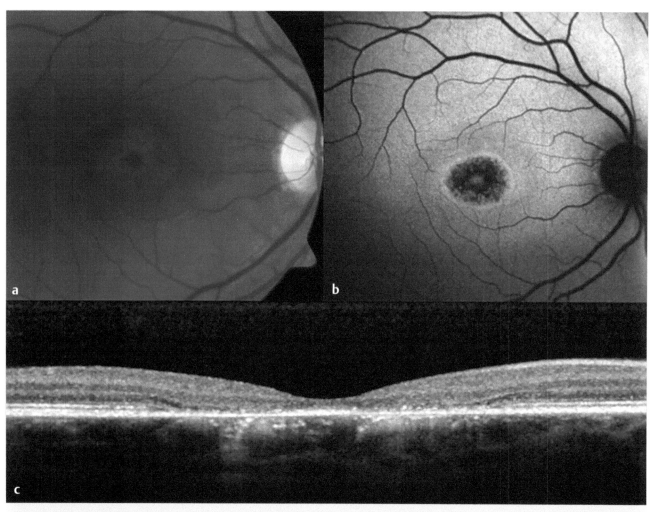

Fig. 43.3 **(a)** Fundus photograph with bull's-eye maculopathy. **(b)** Fundus autofluorescence with correlating hypofluorescence surrounding the maculopathy. **(c)** Optical coherence tomography through the area of atrophy showing outer retinal atrophy, including ellipsoid zone loss.

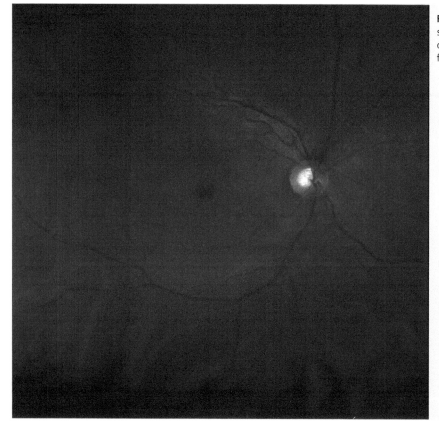

Fig. 43.4 Fundus photograph of the right eye, showing loss of choroidal vasculature from the opaque retinal pigment epithelium in the macula from lipofuscin accumulation.

43.4.2 Follow-up

Patients should be followed on an annual basis to monitor visual acuity and possible progression of atrophy. Serial optical coherence tomography and FAF can help monitor the progression of the disease as well.

Suggested Reading

[1] Sohn EH, Mullins RF, Stone EM. Chapter 42 – Macular Dystrophies A2 – Ryan, Stephen J. In: Sadda SR, Hinton DR, Schachat AP et al., eds. Retina. 5th ed. London: W.B. Saunders; 2013:852–890

[2] Arepalli S, Traboulsi EI, Ehlers JP. Ellipsoid zone mapping and outer retinal assesment in Stargardt disease. Retina. 2018; 38(7):1427–1431

[3] Tanna P, Strauss RW, Fujinami K, Michaelides M. Stargardt disease: clinical features, molecular genetics, animal models and therapeutic options. Br J Ophthalmol. 2017; 101(1):25–30

[4] Fujinami K, Lois N, Mukherjee R, et al. A longitudinal study of Stargardt disease: quantitative assessment of fundus autofluorescence, progression, and genotype correlations. Invest Ophthalmol Vis Sci. 2013; 54(13):8181–8190

44 Cobblestone Degeneration

Kevin Wang and Justis P. Ehlers

Summary

Pavingstone (cobblestone) degeneration is a peripheral retinal condition characterized by multiple rounded, punched-out areas of chorioretinal atrophy with prominent underlying choroidal vessels and pigmented borders. Lesions are yellow–white regions of depigmentation caused by areas of atrophy, which can occur singly or coalesce into bands. It is observed in 27% of patients over 20 years of age with incidence increasing with age. There is no association with retinal tears or detachment, and prophylaxis treatment is not recommended.

Keywords: cobblestone degeneration, pavingstone degeneration

44.1 Features

Pavingstone (cobblestone) degeneration is a peripheral retinal degeneration characterized by multiple rounded, punched-out areas of chorioretinal atrophy with prominent underlying choroidal vessels and pigmented borders (▶ Fig. 44.1). Lesions are yellow–white regions of depigmentation caused by chorioretinal atrophy, which can occur singly or coalesce into bands. It is observed in 27% of patients over 20 years of age with incidence increasing with age.

44.1.1 Common Symptoms

Asymptomatic.

44.1.2 Exam Findings

Peripheral retinal multiple rounded, punched-out areas of chorioretinal atrophy with prominent underlying choroidal vessels and pigmented borders.

44.2 Key Diagnostic Tests and Findings

None required.

44.3 Critical Work-up

None required.

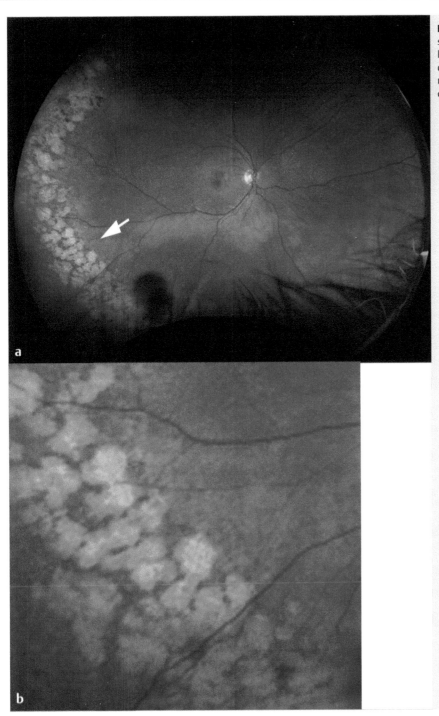

Fig. 44.1 (a) Ultra-widefield fundus photograph showing peripheral scalloped atrophic white lesions with pigmented borders pavingstone/cobblestone degeneration (*arrow*). **(b)** High magnification view of pavingstone/cobblestone degeneration.

44.4 Management

44.4.1 Treatment Options

No treatment is required. There is no association with retinal tears or detachment, and prophylaxis treatment is not recommended.

44.4.2 Follow-up

No specific follow-up is required for pavingstone degeneration.

Suggested Reading

[1] O'Malley P, Allen RA, Straatsma BR, O'Malley CC. Paving-stone degeneration of the retina. Arch Ophthalmol. 1965; 73:169–182

Part V

Other Macular Disorders

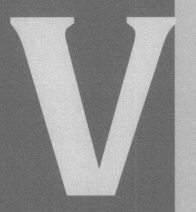

45 Central Serous Chorioretinopathy and Pachychoroid Disease

Belinda C.S. Leong and K. Bailey Freund

Summary

Central serous chorioretinopathy (CSCR) remains a poorly understood condition for which optimal management continues to challenge ophthalmologists and retinal specialists. In 2013, the term pachychoroid (Greek: παχύς, thick) was introduced, which led to the inclusion of CSCR into a broader range of conditions, all manifesting varying degrees of inner choroidal thinning, dilated choroidal veins termed "pachyvessels," and choroidal vascular hyperpermeability on indocyanine green angiography (ICGA). These entities, referred to as the pachychoroid disease spectrum, include CSCR, pachychoroid pigment epitheliopathy, pachychoroid neovasculopathy with the potential to progress to aneurysmal type 1 neovascularization (polypoidal choroidal vasculopathy), focal choroidal excavation, and peripapillary pachychoroid syndrome.

Imaging modalities important for diagnosis and guiding treatment include optical coherence tomography (OCT), fluorescein angiography, ICGA, fundus autofluorescence, and OCT angiography. Treatment options for some of these conditions include thermal laser, photodynamic therapy, intravitreal antivascular endothelial growth factor therapy, and mineralocorticoid receptor antagonists.

Keywords: central serous chorioretinopathy, corticosteroids, pachychoroid, photodynamic therapy

45.1 Features

Central serous chorioretinopathy (CSCR) was first described by von Graefe in 1866 as "relapsing central luetic retinitis" and by Bennett in 1955 as "central serous retinopathy" associated with a primary choroidal pathology. A history is often elicited in these patients of a psychological stressor occurring at peak symptom onset, sleep deprivation, and/or a history of exogenous corticosteroid exposure. In 2013, the term pachychoroid was introduced as a descriptive term for choroidal morphologic and pachymetric features of CSCR, which were recognized as residing within a broader range of conditions referred to as the pachychoroid disease spectrum. These include the following:

- Acute CSCR (▶ Fig. 45.1, ▶ Fig. 45.2).
- Chronic CSCR (▶ Fig. 45.3, ▶ Fig. 45.4).
- Pachychoroid pigment epitheliopathy (PPE) or *form fruste* CSCR.

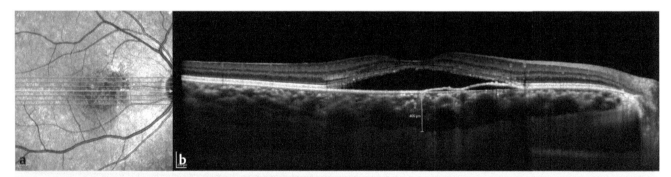

Fig. 45.1 Acute central serous chorioretinopathy. (a) Spectral domain optical coherence tomography (b) with enhanced depth imaging demonstrates serous macular detachment associated with a nasal serous pigment epithelial detachment. Prominent Haller's layer vessels (pachyvessels) within a thickened choroid are evident. The inner choroidal layers are attenuated beneath the area of detachment.

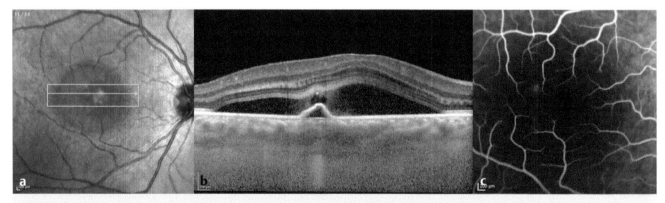

Fig. 45.2 (a,b) Acute central serous chorioretinopathy demonstrating acute focal leakage point emanating from the pigment epithelial detachment peak as a central lucency among the fibrinous subretinal fluid. (c) This was confirmed on fluorescein angiography. A pachyvessel underlies this area.

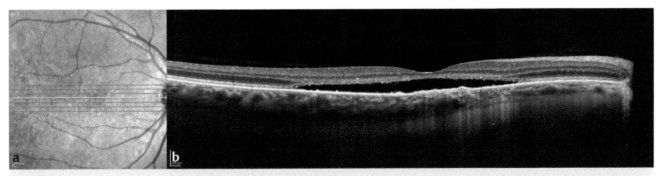

Fig. 45.3 (a,b) Chronic central serous chorioretinopathy. Enhanced depth imaging optical coherence tomography demonstrates neurosensory detachment and a shallow irregular pigment epithelial detachment over a thickened choroid with attenuated inner choroidal layers and pachyvessels. The overlying foveal macular thickness is reduced due to loss of outer retinal tissue.

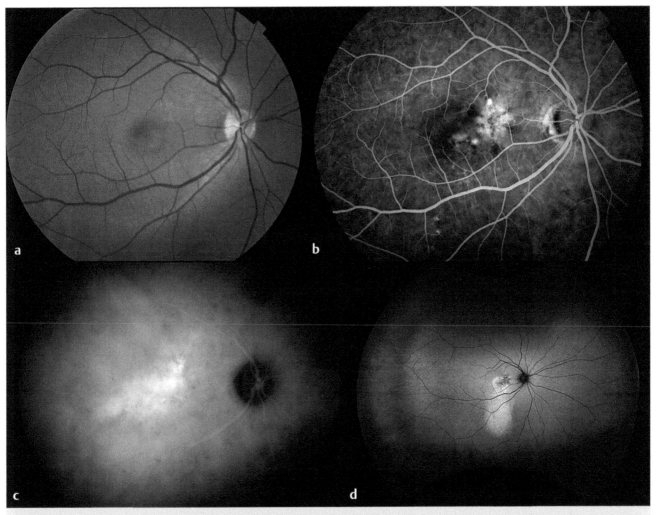

Fig. 45.4 Chronic central serous chorioretinopathy with recurrent serous detachment. **(a)** Color fundus photograph demonstrates reduced choroidal tessellation at the posterior pole. **(b)** Arteriovenous-phase fluorescein angiography shows two focal leakage points overlying a staining pigment epithelial detachment. **(c)** Midphase indocyanine green angiography shows central choroidal vascular hyperpermeability. **(d)** Fundus autofluorescence demonstrates mottled hypoautofluorescence centrally and inferior hyperfluorescence due to the chronic descending subretinal fluid.

- Pachychoroid neovasculopathy (a late complication of PPE) (▶ Fig. 45.5).
- Focal choroidal excavation.
- Other complications:
  - Bullous exudative retinal detachment: a rare manifestation due to the breakdown of physiological mechanisms governing outer retinal hydration resulting in neurosensory detachment of over 10 disc diameters.
  - Aneurysmal type 1 neovascularization (NV; previously known as polypoidal choroidal vasculopathy).
  - Peripapillary pachychoroid syndrome: a newly defined condition with pachychoroid features located around the optic nerve.

45.1.1 Common Symptoms

Common symptoms and examination findings are outlined in ▶ Table 45.1.

45.2 Key Diagnostic Tests and Findings

Relevant investigations and associated findings are summarized in ▶ Table 45.2. Optical coherence tomography (OCT), fluorescein angiography (FA), fundus autofluorescence (FAF), indocyanine green angiography (ICGA), and OCT angiography (OCTA) all have potentially important roles in diagnosis.

45.3 Critical Work-up

Systemic work-up is usually unnecessary. However, medications and supplements should be reviewed to identify any potential triggers for disease activity. Imaging is typically guided based on presentation. When available, enhanced depth imaging OCT and/or swept-source OCT may help identify relevant choroidal findings. FAF and FA may also be considered to

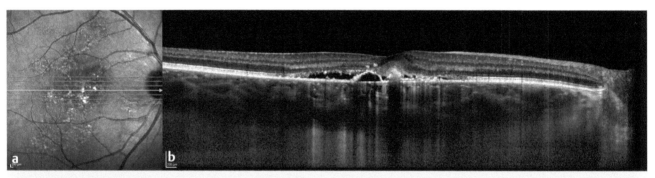

Fig. 45.5 (a,b) Treatment-naive pachychoroid neovasculopathy. A thickened choroid is present with attenuated inner choroidal layers and pachyvessels. There is an irregular pigment epithelial detachment with hyperreflective sub-retinal pigment epithelium contents. A shallow serous detachment with an area of subretinal hyperreflective material overlies the type 1 neovascular lesion.

Table 45.1 Common symptoms and clinical findings in CSCR and the pachychoroid disease spectrum

Condition	Common symptoms	Examination findings
Acute CSCR	Painless acute/subacute decrease in central vision with metamorphopsia, micropsia, and a hypermetropic shift. Spontaneous resolution	Serous RD with or without serous PED. Reduced fundus tessellation
Chronic CSCR	Prolonged and/or relapsing and remitting decrease in central vision with metamorphopsia, micropsia, and a hypermetropic shift for 6 mo or longer	Subfoveal/parafoveal subretinal fluid that appears more fibrinous in nature. RPE and outer retinal disruption, including both atrophy and pigment aggregation. Reduced fundus tessellation
PPE	Often asymptomatic	RPE changes reminiscent of CSCR occurring without evidence of subretinal fluid. Changes may be central or peripapillary. Reduced fundus tessellation
Pachychoroid NV	Central or paracentral decrease in vision and/or distortion when exudation occurs centrally. May be asymptomatic when fluid is eccentric to the fovea	RPE changes reminiscent of CSCR. Subretinal, intraretinal, and/or sub-RPE fluid in the absence of soft drusen. Hemorrhage is rare unless aneurysms occur. Reduced fundus tessellation
Aneurysmal type 1 NV 2° to pachychoroid disease	As per pachychoroid NV, but symptomatic exudation is more common	As per pachychoroid NV, but lipid and hemorrhage are more common
Bullous exudative RD	Similar to chronic CSCR with visual symptoms over a greater proportion of the visual field	Gravitating bullous RD with turbid subretinal fluid. Multiple PEDs of varying size. Polygonal or crescent-shaped RPE tears may be present
PPS	Similar to chronic CSCR with symptoms preferentially prevalent adjacent to the blind spot (optic nerve) extending to fixation	Single or multiple PEDs. Reduced fundus tessellation. Peripapillary RPE changes. Choroidal folds may be present

Abbreviations: CSCR, central serous chorioretinopathy; NV, neovasculopathy; PED, pigment epithelial detachment; PPE, pachychoroid pigment epitheliopathy; PPS, peripapillary pachychoroid syndrome; RD, retinal detachment; RPE, retinal pigment epithelium.

Table 45.2 Key diagnostic tests and findings in CSCR and the pachychoroid disease spectrum

Modality	Acute CSCR	Chronic CSCR	PPE	Pachychoroid NV	Aneurysmal type 1 NV 2° to chronic CSCR	Bullous exudative RD	PPS
OCT (EDI mode ideal)	Serous RD. Discrete single or multiple serous PEDs may be present. Subretinal fibrinous material with a central lucency may be seen at the sites of active leakage. Diffuse or focal increase in choroidal thickness. Pachyvessels beneath sites of leakage	Subretinal fluid with subretinal hyperreflective material. Outer retinal atrophy and intraretinal fluid may be present. Diffuse or focal increase in choroidal thickness, often with hyporeflective cavities. Attenuated inner choroidal layers over pachyvessels beneath areas of fluid and RPE alteration	Overall thickened choroid on EDI-OCT, especially at sites of pigmentary epitheliopathy. Diffuse or focal increase in choroidal thickness. Attenuated inner choroidal layers over pachyvessels beneath sites of RPE alteration	Shallow irregular RPE detachment corresponding to type 1 NV. Attenuated inner choroidal layers over pachyvessels. May show subretinal, intraretinal, and/or sub-RPE fluid. May show subretinal hyperreflective material (fibrin). Absence of soft drusen	Peaked PEDs at the site of aneurysms with shallow irregular PED corresponding to the BVN of type 1 NV. Attenuated inner choroidal layers and pachyvessels beneath BVN. Possible overlying subretinal fluid, hemorrhage, and/or fibrin. Absence of soft drusen	Multiple PEDs of varying size, especially in the posterior pole. Subretinal hyperreflective material (fibrin) is common. Gravitating bullous serous RD with turbid fluid. RPE tears may be present and/or RPE "blowouts" at PED edge. Attenuated inner choroidal layers and pachyvessels. Hyperreflective lesions at choriocapillaris level and hyperreflective choroidal vessel walls	Peripapillary choroidal thickening with attenuated inner choroidal layers and pachyvessels. Intraretinal and/or subretinal fluid extending from the temporal margin of the optic disc without evidence of cavitary optic disc anomalies or advanced glaucomatous cupping. Associated atrophy of the RPE and outer retinal bands at the temporal optic disc margin producing choroidal hypertransmission
FA	Focal leakage at the level of the RPE typically in a smokestack or inkblot pattern. May be multiple focal leaks	Early phase hyperfluorescence in areas of retinal atrophy. Diffuse leakage at RPE level in midphase	Areas of RPE hypo- and hyperfluorescence at sites of RPE changes corresponding to relative RPE window defects and focal RPE thickening	Patterns of poorly defined (occult) choroidal NV	Patterns of poorly defined (occult) choroidal NV with late-phase hyperfluorescent staining of and/or leakage from aneurysms (polyps)	Multifocal intense leakage at PED sites. May show RPE blowouts at PED edge. Some leaks may track inferiorly (unlike the typical smokestack). May show nonperfusion and terminal capillary telangiectasias with chronic exudative RD. Ultra-widefield is preferred	Granular transmission hyperfluorescence without focal areas of leakage. Late hyperfluorescent staining in ring-like configuration immediately surrounding optic disc associated with potential mild leak. Gravitational tracks may be present

Table 45.2 (continued)

Modality	Acute CSCR	Chronic CSCR	PPE	Pachychoroid NV	Aneurysmal type 1 NV 2° to chronic CSCR	Bullous exudative RD	PPS
ICGA	Midphase CVH, which may be multifocal or localized to areas of leakage present on FA. Dilated choroidal veins. Areas of choroidal vascular hypoperfusion. Similar ICGA abnormalities are often seen in unaffected fellow eyes	Dilated choroidal veins. Multifocal midphase CVH. Areas of choroidal vascular hypoperfusion	Dilated choroidal veins and midphase CVH corresponding to areas of RPE abnormalities	Dilated choroidal veins. Multifocal midphase CVH. Late-staining plaque corresponding to type 1 NV	Dilated choroidal veins. Multifocal midphase CVH. Late-staining plaque corresponding to (BVN) type 1 NV. Hypercyanescent aneurysms, which may show "washout" (inactive) or late hypercyanescent leakage (active)	Ultra-widefield imaging shows dilated choroidal veins and extensive multifocal regional CVH partially obscured by bullous RD	Peripapillary dilated choroidal veins and multifocal midphase CVH
FAF	Often subtle changes, including focal areas of hyper- and hypoautofluorescence and/or mild granularity. Mild hyperautofluorescence corresponding to the area of serous RD	Nonspecific mottling corresponding to known RPE changes. Gravitating tracks of hypo- and hyperautofluorescence. Annular pigment epitheliopathy and/or spoke-like hyperautofluorescence may be present. Zonal areas of hyper- and hypoautofluorescence in areas of prior or persistent serous detachment	Focal areas of hypo- and/or hyperautofluorescence in areas of RPE change. Absence of FA patterns related to serous RD	Nonspecific focal areas of hyper- and hypoautofluorescence	Nonspecific focal areas of hyper- and hypoautofluorescence	Confluent or granular hypo- and/or hyperfluorescence. RPE tears and "blowouts" are hypofluorescent	Granular or mottled peripapillary changes. May show gravitational tracks of RPE abnormalities
OCTA	Nonspecific alterations of inner choroidal flow signal	Areas of reduced inner choroidal flow signal	Nonspecific alterations of inner choroidal flow signal	Tangled network of neovascular flow signal	Branching or tangled network of neovascular flow signal with aneurysms typically located at the margin of the lesion	Areas of reduced inner choroidal flow signal	Nonspecific alterations of inner choroidal flow signal

Abbreviations: BVN, branching vascular network; CSCR, central serous chorioretinopathy; CVH, choroidal vascular hyperpermeability; EDI, enhanced depth imaging; FA, fluorescein angiography; FAF, fundus autofluorescence; ICG, indocyanine green; ICGA, indocyanine green angiography; NV, neovasculopathy; OCT, optical coherence tomography; OCTA, OCT angiography; PED, pigment epithelial detachment; PPE, pachychoroid pigment epitheliopathy; PPS, peripapillary pachychoroid syndrome; RD, retinal detachment; RPE, retinal pigment epithelium.

evaluate for typical features of CSCR. In cases of suspected NV, ICGA and OCTA can also be particularly helpful.

45.4 Management

45.4.1 Treatment Options

The majority of acute CSCR cases resolve over weeks to months without intervention or with education on the reduction of stressors and the elimination of exogenous corticosteroids. Observation is typically the first choice of management in these cases.

Thermal Laser

An option in persistent acute or chronic CSCR if the site of leakage at the retinal pigment epithelium (RPE) level is small, singular, and extrafoveal. The application of thermal laser to the leakage site aims to close it. However, the underlying choroidal pathology remains untreated.

Photodynamic Therapy

Photodynamic therapy (PDT) with verteporfin is used to treat anomalous choroidal vasculature in persistent acute CSCR or chronic CSCR and to target NV in pachychoroid neovasculopathy and aneurysmal type 1 NV. Intravenous verteporfin followed by nonthermal laser reacts with oxygen in the target tissue to release free radicals, which damage vascular endothelium. Treatment parameters commonly used with PDT for CSCR include half-dose, half-fluence, full-dose, and full-fluence.

Antivascular Endothelial Growth Factor Intravitreal Therapy

Targeting vascular endothelial growth factor (VEGF) with intravitreal anti-VEGF therapy is a well-established treatment for neovascular age-related macular degeneration and other retinal disease driven by angiogenesis and vascular permeability. The role in reducing permeability at the level of the choriocapillaris and RPE has not been established in CSCR; however, intravitreal anti-VEGF therapy has been used to treat exudation from type 1 NV secondary to chronic CSCR and pachychoroid neovasculopathy.

Mineralocorticoid Receptor Antagonists

Both endogenous and exogenous corticosteroids (of which mineralocorticoids are a subset) are risk factors for CSCR manifestation. Mineralocorticoid receptors are present in the retina and choroid and hence may be a target to address an underlying mechanism in this disease process. Eplerenone and spironolactone are readily available competitive inhibitors of mineralocorticoid receptors used in the treatment of hypertension and cardiac failure. As potassium-sparing diuretics, serum potassium levels require close monitoring. Some studies have reported improvements in visual acuity and subretinal fluid with variable associated anatomic improvement in central macular and choroidal thickness.

45.4.2 Follow-up

Acute CSCR patients may be followed every 4 to 12 weeks, based on symptoms and severity of exacerbation. If clinically inactive, the follow-up interval can be extended to every 6 to 12 months. The follow-up frequency of patients with other pachychoroid diseases is dependent on clinical severity. When active treatment is considered, the frequency of treatment, monitoring for treatment response, and consideration of additional treatment can all vary considerably at the discretion of the treating ophthalmologist.

Suggested Reading

[1] Balaratnasingam C, Lee WK, Koizumi H, Dansingani K, Inoue M, Freund KB. Polypoidal choroidal vasculopathy—a distinct disease or manifestation of many? Retina. 2016; 36(1):1–8

[2] Chung H, Byeon SH, Freund KB. Focal choroidal excavation and its association with pachychoroid spectrum disorders—a review of the literature and multimodal imaging findings. Retina. 2017; 37(2):199–221

[3] Dansingani KK, Gal-Or O, Sadda SR, Yannuzzi LA, Freund KB. Understanding aneurysmal type 1 neovascularization (polypoidal choroidal vasculopathy): a lesson in the taxonomy of 'expanded spectra'—a review. Clin Exp Ophthalmol. 2018; 46(2):189–200

[4] Pang CE, Freund KB. Pachychoroid neovasculopathy. Retina. 2015; 35(1):1–9

[5] Warrow DJ, Hoang QV, Freund KB. Pachychoroid pigment epitheliopathy. Retina. 2013; 33(8):1659–1672

46 Hypotony Maculopathy

Nathan E. Cutler and Justis P. Ehlers

Summary

Hypotony maculopathy is a condition characterized by low intraocular pressure (IOP) and fundus abnormalities, including choroidal folds, chorioretinal folds, macular edema, optic nerve edema, and/or vascular tortuosity. Risk factors include young age, myopia, and glaucoma filtering procedures. Visual symptoms can range from asymptomatic to metamorphopsia and central vision loss. Diagnostic testing with optical coherence tomography and fluorescein angiography demonstrates distinctive chorioretinal folds. Prompt normalization of IOP often results in excellent visual recovery.

Keywords: chorioretinal folds, hypotony maculopathy, intraocular pressure

46.1 Features

Dellaporta first clinically described hypotony and reduced vision following glaucoma procedures or perforating eye injuries in 1954. Years later, Gass used the term "hypotony maculopathy" to highlight the macular changes and visual dysfunction sometimes present in eyes with hypotony. Reduced intraocular pressure (IOP) can cause decreased central vision as a result of folding in the choroid, neurosensory retina, and the retinal pigment epithelium (RPE). As hypotony develops, the outer sclera becomes edematous, resulting in a corresponding reduction to the inner surface area of the eye wall. That compression or reduction of inner scleral size causes the inner choroid and retinal layers to undulate and leads to vision loss (▶ Fig. 46.1). Causes of hypotony can be from decreased aqueous production such as in severe inflammatory conditions or from increased aqueous outflow due to a number of conditions such as wound leak, overfiltration after glaucoma surgery, or cyclodialysis clefts. Hypotony maculopathy is reported in 10 to 20% of cases of glaucoma filtering surgery with an increased incidence seen after the introduction of antimetabolites, particularly mitomycin C. In addition to delayed wound healing and greater risk of wound leak, mitomycin C has been found to be toxic to the ciliary body, causing decreased aqueous production. Risk factors also include younger age, myopia, and male gender. It is believed that the reduced scleral rigidity found in young and myopic eyes facilitates the inward collapse of the scleral wall during hypotony. Choroidal effusion and diabetes have been found to be associated with decreased risk of developing hypotony maculopathy.

46.1.1 Common Symptoms

Decreased central vision and metamorphopsia are common. Choroidal thickening and retinal folds can cause relative hyperopia due to axial shortening of the eye. Mild anatomical changes can be asymptomatic.

46.1.2 Exam Findings

Hypotony or recent hypotony is a requisite finding for diagnosis. There is no consensus definition, and upper limits of 5 to 9 mm of Hg have been used in clinical studies. The true definition of hypotony should be any value that causes characteristic functional and structural changes. In rare cases, hypotony maculopathy features may be seen with a "relative hypotony" after a sudden reduction of the IOP to low normal levels from significantly higher levels.

Choroidal/chorioretinal folds in the posterior pole are the characteristic examination finding. The folds are usually broad, have yellow crests with dark narrow troughs, and most often radiate outward from the optic disc and usually appear in a stellate pattern around the fovea, though sometimes their orientation can be random. In long-standing cases of low IOP, the pigmented lines from RPE migration and hyperplasia may persist even after the resolution of the hypotony. Optic nerve edema is sometimes present due to anterior bowing of the lamina cribrosa and subsequent reduction of axoplasmic transport. Vascular tortuosity with or without vascular engorgement can be seen. Cystoid macular edema is a rare finding.

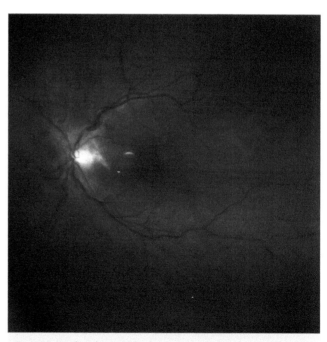

Fig. 46.1 Fundus photograph of an eye with hypotony maculopathy, showing radial chorioretinal folds, mild optic nerve edema, and tortuous vessels in the posterior pole.

46.2 Key Diagnostic Tests and Findings

46.2.1 Optical Coherence Tomography

Demonstrates choroidal/chorioretinal folds, including subtle alterations demonstrated as undulating Bruch's membrane/RPE. In addition, intraretinal fluid and/or subretinal fluid may also be occasionally identified. Review all radial or cube line scans as the orientation of chorioretinal folds can be found in any axis (▶ Fig. 46.2).

46.2.2 Fluorescein Angiography or Ultra-Widefield Fluorescein Angiography

Choroidal folds and striking bands of alternating hyper- and hypofluorescence. Hyperfluorescent streaks correspond to the crests of choroidal folds where the RPE is relatively thin. Leakage may be seen at the optic nerve.

46.2.3 Indocyanine Green Angiography

Can demonstrate alternating hyper- and hypofluorescent bands similar to fluorescein angiography. Hyperfluorescent bands are often thicker in indocyanine green angiography due to underlying choroidal congestion. Dilation and tortuosity of the choroidal vessels can also be seen.

46.2.4 Ultrasonography

B-scan can show flattening and thickening of the sclera and choroid in the posterior pole (▶ Fig. 46.3). Ultrasound biomicroscopy can be helpful for determining the cause of hypotony in the case of a cyclodialysis cleft or ciliary body detachment.

46.3 Critical Work-up

Chorioretinal folds can be found in several conditions without associated hypotony. Any condition that leads to a reduction in the inner surface area of the sclera can result in folds. The simple mnemonic "THIN RPE" can be used to remember a number of conditions that can lead to chorioretinal folds (i.e., Tumors, Hypotony, Inflammation and idiopathic, choroidal Neovascular membranes, Retrobulbar mass, Papilledema, and Extraocular hardware). In cases of chorioretinal folds and normal IOP, pursue additional testing to rule out the conditions listed above.

46.4 Management

46.4.1 Treatment Options

Treatment depends on the correction of the underlying cause for the hypotony and restoration of normal IOP. Prompt IOP correction can prevent permanent vision loss.

In the cases of postoperative hypotony, wound leaks need to be closed with either a bandage contact lens if small or definitive suture closure for larger and more posterior leaks.

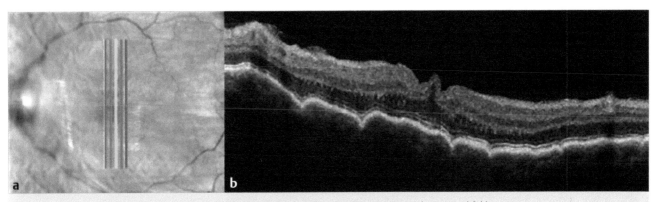

Fig. 46.2 (a,b) Optical coherence tomography of hypotony maculopathy, showing prominent chorioretinal folds.

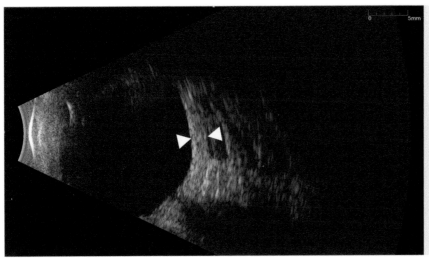

Fig. 46.3 B-scan ultrasound of hypotony maculopathy, showing flattening of the posterior pole and thickening of the choroid (*white arrowheads* indicate the thickened choroid).

Overfiltration after glaucoma surgery might require autologous blood injection in or around the bleb, suturing the scleral flap closed, or the use of a patch graft. Cyclodialysis cleft closure can be achieved through a variety of methods, including topical mydriatics, laser therapy, or surgery. In cases of inflammatory conditions, topical or more often systemic corticosteroids are indicated. In cases of persistent retinal folds despite normalization of IOP, a few reports have shown success with pars plana vitrectomy with or without internal limiting membrane peeling and gas tamponade. Perfluorocarbon has also been used to help flatten the posterior retina intraoperatively.

46.4.2 Follow-up

Prompt detection and subsequent correction of hypotony have a good prognosis for recovery of vision. Prolonged chorioretinal folds may lead to irreversible structural changes in the macula and a poor visual outcome despite the resolution of the hypotony. However, with the resolution of hypotony, the improvement in visual acuity can be obtained even several years after the initial instance of hypotony.

Suggested Reading

[1] Gass JDM. Hypotony maculopathy, Chapter 34. In: Bellows JG, ed. Contemporary Ophthalmology. Honoring Sir Stewart Duke-Elder. Baltimore, MD: Williams & Wilkins, 1972:343–366

[2] Bindlish R, Condon GP, Schlosser JD, D'Antonio J, Lauer KB, Lehrer R. Efficacy and safety of mitomycin-C in primary trabeculectomy: five-year follow-up. Ophthalmology. 2002; 109(7):1336–1341, discussion 1341–1342

[3] Fannin LA, Schiffman JC, Budenz DL. Risk factors for hypotony maculopathy. Ophthalmology. 2003; 110(6):1185–1191

[4] Pederson JE. Ocular hypotony. Trans Ophthalmol Soc U K. 1986; 105(Pt 2): 220–226

[5] Duker JS, Schuman JS. Successful surgical treatment of hypotony maculopathy following trabeculectomy with topical mitomycin C. Ophthalmic Surg. 1994; 25(7):463–465

47 Cystoid Macular Edema

Nandini Venkateswaran and Jayanth Sridhar

Summary

Cystoid macular edema is a thickening of the macula with multiple cyst-like areas of fluid and retinal swelling. Causes vary and can include vascular diseases such as diabetes mellitus and vein occlusions, inflammatory conditions, inherited conditions, and medication use. One of the most common etiologies is in the postoperative period and particularly after cataract surgery. Symptoms include compromised vision, loss of color vision, contrast sensitivity, metamorphopsia, central scotomas, and micropsia. Multiple imaging modalities can assist with diagnosis and various treatment options that can be employed to achieve visual improvement.

Keywords: cystoid macular edema, pathogenesis, diagnostic imaging modalities

47.1 Clinical Features

Cystoid macular edema (CME) is a retinal condition in which there is thickening of the macula with cystic fluid spaces within the macula. In many cases, abnormal vascular permeability leads to the breakdown of the blood–retina barrier and subsequent intracellular and extracellular fluid accumulation. This process is thought to be driven primarily by retinal ischemia and/or increase in inflammatory mediators; direct macular traction after shifts in the vitreous has also been shown to play a role. Causes vary and can include vascular disease such as diabetes mellitus and vein occlusions, inflammatory conditions such as uveitis, inherited conditions such as retinitis pigmentosa (RP), and medication use including prostaglandins and epinephrine. One of the most common etiologies occurs following intraocular surgery, particularly after cataract surgery (referred to as Irvine–Gass syndrome) with an incidence ranging from 0.2 to 20%. CME can also occur after other types of intraocular surgical procedures, including penetrating keratoplasty, glaucoma drainage implant surgery, intraocular lens fixation procedures, pars plana vitrectomy with or without epiretinal membrane peeling, and scleral buckling. Nonleaking CME may also occur due to specific etiologies (e.g., juvenile retinoschisis, Goldmann-Favre disease, nicotinic acid maculopathy, certain subtypes of RP, and the use of antimicrotubule agents) that are not due to increased vascular permeability.

47.1.1 Common Symptoms

Decreased vision, blurred vision, loss of color vision or contrast sensitivity, metamorphopsia, central scotomas, and micropsia.

47.1.2 Exam Findings

Clinical signs include loss of the normal foveal reflex, retinal thickening, and cystic spaces in the foveal region on funduscopy. In some cases, vitritis and optic nerve swelling can be observed as well. Underlying vascular disease can be ascertained with clinical findings such as retinal exudates, cotton wool spots, retinal hemorrhages, and retinal vascular tortuosity.

47.2 Key Diagnostic Tests and Findings

47.2.1 Optical Coherence Tomography

Possible retinal thickening with the formation of intraretinal cystic fluid pockets within the outer plexiform layer and vitreomacular interface abnormalities such as vitreomacular traction or epiretinal membranes that can contribute to CME formation (▶ Fig. 47.1, ▶ Fig. 47.2).

47.2.2 Fluorescein Angiography or Ultra-Widefield Fluorescein Angiography

Dilation of the foveal capillaries in early phases and leakage into the cystoid spaces possibly forming classic petaloid leakage pattern in the foveal region in late phases. Late phases may also show leakage of the optic disc (▶ Fig. 47.3). Fluorescein angiography (FA) may also help assess macular ischemia and other potential underlying etiologies (e.g., diabetic retinopathy). Ultra-widefield fluorescein angiography can exhibit leakage in the peripheral retina that can have a honeycomb-like

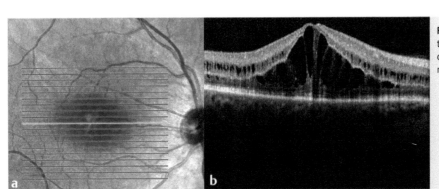

Fig. 47.1 (a,b) Macular optical coherence tomography showing intraretinal cysts in the outer plexiform layer consistent with cystoid macular edema.

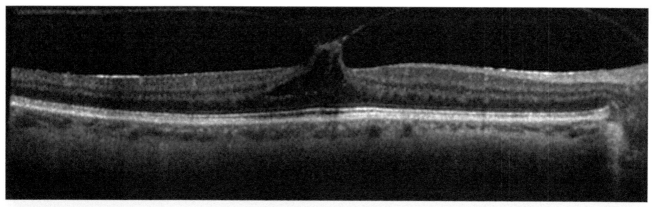

Fig. 47.2 Macular optical coherence tomography demonstrating vitreomacular traction with resultant cystoid macular edema.

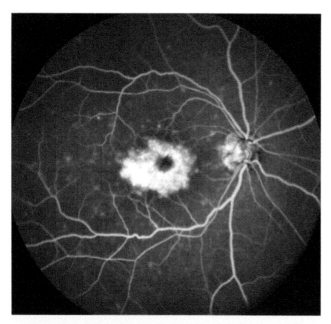

Fig. 47.3 Late-phase fluorescein angiography images show leakage into the cystoid spaces forming the classic petaloid leakage pattern in the foveal region along with staining of the optic disc.

appearance. Lack of leakage on FA changes the differential diagnosis for the etiology.

47.2.3 Fundus Autofluorescence

Intraretinal cysts appear as hyperautofluorescent areas in the macular region.

47.2.4 Fundus Photography

Color fundus photography can show loss of the normal foveal reflex along with radially oriented cystic spaces in the foveal region (▶ Fig. 47.4).

47.3 Critical Work-up

Work-up should be tailored toward determining the underlying etiologies. Thorough patient history and physical examination are crucial. A medical history of diabetes mellitus, hypertension, hyperlipidemia, or obesity or an ocular history of glaucoma can predispose patients to CME secondary to diabetic or hypertensive retinopathy or retinal vein occlusions. Ocular inflammatory conditions such as anterior uveitis, posterior scleritis, sarcoidosis, toxoplasmosis, birdshot chorioretinopathy, Behcet syndrome, Eales disease, and Vogt–Koyanagi–Harada syndrome as well as retinal degenerations such as RP can be associated with CME. A review of medication use can reveal the use of agents such as topical epinephrine or oral nicotinic acid or niacin that can cause CME formation. Prior ocular surgeries, such as penetrating keratoplasties, intraocular lens fixation procedures, glaucoma drainage implants, scleral buckles, and pars plana vitrectomies can lead to CME. In particular, complex cataract surgery with posterior capsular rupture and resultant aphakia, severe iris trauma, vitreous traction at the wound, and vitreous loss are associated with a high incidence that typically manifests 3 to 12 weeks postoperatively. Cataract surgery in diabetic patients with or without comorbid diabetic macular edema can often accelerate CME, often leading to a worse visual outcome. Consider conditions that cause CME but do not demonstrate leakage on FA in the differential diagnosis (e.g., juvenile retinoschisis, Goldmann-Favre disease, nicotinic acid maculopathy, certain subtypes of RP, and the use of antimicrotubule agents). In conjunction with a comprehensive history and ocular examination, optical coherence tomography and FA are the primary imaging modalities used to arrive at the final diagnosis.

47.4 Management

47.4.1 Treatment Options

Treatment options include medical and surgical modalities and depend ultimately on the underlying etiology. Options include topical nonsteroidal anti-inflammatory drugs (NSAIDs), corticosteroids, antivascular endothelial growth factor (anti-VEGF) agents, carbonic anhydrase inhibitors (CAIs), and surgical intervention for significant vitreoretinal interface abnormalities.

Nonsteroidal Anti-Inflammatory Drugs

Topical NSAIDs inhibit cyclooxygenase enzymes and thereby reduce the production of proinflammatory prostaglandins. They are typically employed in the postoperative period.

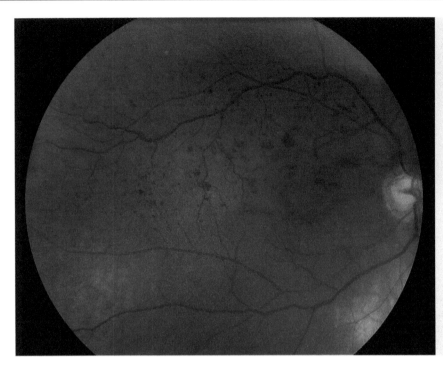

Fig. 47.4 Color fundus photograph showing loss of the normal foveal reflex associated with superotemporal intraretinal hemorrhages, indicating a branch retinal vein with associated cystoid macular edema.

Corticosteroids

Steroids inhibit inflammatory mediators and leukostasis, reduce fibrin deposition, and enhance the barrier function of vascular endothelial tight junctions. They can be administered topically, periocularly in the sub-Tenon's space, intravitreally, and orally. Corticosteroids have shown most utility in postoperative CME and CME occurring due to underlying ocular inflammatory conditions.

Antivascular Endothelial Growth Factor

The primary role for anti-VEGF agents in the management of CME is in the eyes with the underlying diabetic component to the CME or other ischemic retinopathies (such as retinal vein occlusion).

Carbonic Anhydrase Inhibitors

These medications change the polarity of the ionic transport systems in the retinal pigment epithelium (RPE), allowing increased fluid transport across RPE from the subretinal space with subsequent reduction in edema. CAIs are often used in nonleaking CME, such as in cases of CME due to antimicrotubule agents or CME associated with RP. Topical or systemic therapy may be used.

Surgical Intervention

In cases of vitreoretinal interface abnormalities, surgical intervention may resolve CME that is refractory to medical therapy. Vitrectomy can be performed to release the posterior hyaloid, eliminate vitreomacular traction, and remove epiretinal membranes.

47.4.2 Follow-up

CME may be self-limiting and observation may be considered based on symptoms and severity. Evaluation is typically performed every 1 to 3 months during the early treatment period to assess response to therapeutics and evaluate any adverse effects from the chosen treatment (e.g., elevated intraocular pressure with steroids). Treatment is frequently approached in a stepwise fashion from least invasive to more invasive. Final visual acuity after CME development may eventually be limited by permanent retinal structural change alterations, including photoreceptor atrophy, lamellar hole formation, and reactive pigment epithelium changes, particularly in chronic cases.

Suggested Reading

[1] Rotsos TG, Moschos MM. Cystoid macular edema. Clin Ophthalmol. 2008; 2 (4):919–930

[2] Scholl S, Kirchhof J, Augustin AJ. Pathophysiology of macular edema. Ophthalmologica. 2010; 224 Suppl 1:8–15

[3] Chu CJ, Johnston RL, Buscombe C, Sallam AB, Mohamed Q, Yang YC, United Kingdom Pseudophakic Macular Edema Study Group. Risk factors and incidence of macular edema after cataract surgery: a database study of 81984 eyes. Ophthalmology. 2016; 123(2):316–323

[4] Staurenghi G, Invernizzi A, de Polo L, Pellegrini M. Macular edema. Diagnosis and detection. Dev Ophthalmol. 2010; 47:27–48

48 Choroidal Folds

Jaya B. Kumar and Justis P. Ehlers

Summary

Although uncommon, choroidal (i.e., chorioretinal) folds represent an important and distinct clinical exam finding that warrants a thorough work-up to evaluate for ocular, orbital, and potential systemic conditions. Optical coherence tomography, fluorescein angiography, indocyanine green angiography, and ultrasonography are important diagnostics. Treatment options vary depending on underlying etiology.

Keywords: choroidal folds, hypotony, hyperopia, retrobulbar mass, uveal effusion syndrome

48.1 Features

Chorioretinal folds (CRFs) are anatomically characterized by undulations of the inner choroid, Bruch's membrane, and overlying retinal pigment epithelium. This clinical appearance results from underlying choroidal alterations that push the overlying Bruch's membrane into folds.

48.1.1 Common Symptoms

Usually, asymptomatic; metamorphopsia or blurry vision possible, depending on the underlying etiology.

48.1.2 Exam Findings

CRFs typically present as alternating yellow and dark bands, usually horizontally oriented and radiating from the optic nerve. The following exam findings can help determine etiology of the folds, including presence of a relative afferent pupillary defect (e.g., optic nerve head disorders, retrobulbar mass), abnormalities on external exam (e.g., proptosis for thyroid eye disease and orbital mass), anterior segment exam for wound leak (e.g., hypotony), and posterior segment exam for optic nerve edema, drusen, choroidal detachment, choroidal mass, and scleral buckle.

48.2 Key Diagnostic Ophthalmic Tests and Findings

48.2.1 Optical Coherence Tomography

May reveal subtle to significant CRFs. Rarely, intraretinal fluid may be present.

48.2.2 Fluorescein Angiography or Ultra-Widefield Fluorescein Angiography

Can be particularly helpful in cases where folds are suspected but exam findings are mild or difficult to discern. Typical findings include the early increase in background choroidal fluorescence and alternating bands of hyper- and hypofluorescence corresponding to crests and valleys of CRF. In uveal effusion syndrome, fluorescein angiography can demonstrate leopard spots of hyper- and hypofluorescence.

48.2.3 Indocyanine Green Angiography

Possible granular choroidal hyperfluorescence in uveal effusion syndrome.

48.2.4 Ultrasonography

Thickening and occasional flattening of the sclera on B-scan. May facilitate identification of a retrobulbar mass.

48.3 Critical Work-up

Patient history should investigate any recent trauma, surgery, headaches, blurry vision, metamorphopsia, and medications. In addition to clinical exam and key diagnostics, consider magnetic resonance imaging brain and orbits to evaluate retrobulbar or intracranial process and systemic imaging (CT chest/abdomen/pelvis) for suspected metastasis. There are many differential diagnoses to consider: hypotony following glaucoma surgery, wound leaks, and cyclodialysis cleft (▶ Fig. 48.1); uveal effusion syndrome (idiopathic exudative detachment of choroid, ciliary body, and retina usually associated with scleral thickening and hyperopia); retrobulbar/orbital mass lesions (benign or malignant tumors and orbital abscess) (▶ Fig. 48.2); idiopathic folds (diagnosis of exclusion, usually seen in young hyperopic patients) (▶ Fig. 48.3); inflammatory from thickening and inflammation of the sclera (e.g., posterior scleritis); Vogt–Koyanagi–Harada syndrome; thyroid eye disease, autoimmune etiologies; scleral buckle; intraocular neoplastic conditions (e.g., choroidal metastasis); choroidal neovascularization (CNV) with fibrotic contraction; optic nerve head disorders (e.g., papilledema); medications associated with choroidal folds, including topiramate and bimatoprost; and space flight-associated neuro-ocular syndrome (i.e., reported during and after long-duration space flights, which includes optic disc edema, choroidal and retinal folds, hyperopia, and retinal nerve fiber infarcts).

48.4 Management

48.4.1 Treatment Options

Manage underlying etiology. Options include repair of the surgical wound, excision for retrobulbar mass, oral prednisone or other anti-inflammatory agents for scleritis, oral prednisone or scleral thinning procedure/scleral windows for uveal effusion syndrome, antivascular endothelial growth factor for CNV, discontinuation of offending medication (topiramate or bimatoprost), and observation for idiopathic folds.

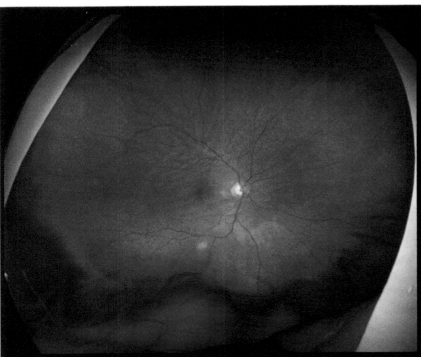

Fig. 48.1 Widefield image demonstrates choroidal folds 2 weeks after trabeculectomy.

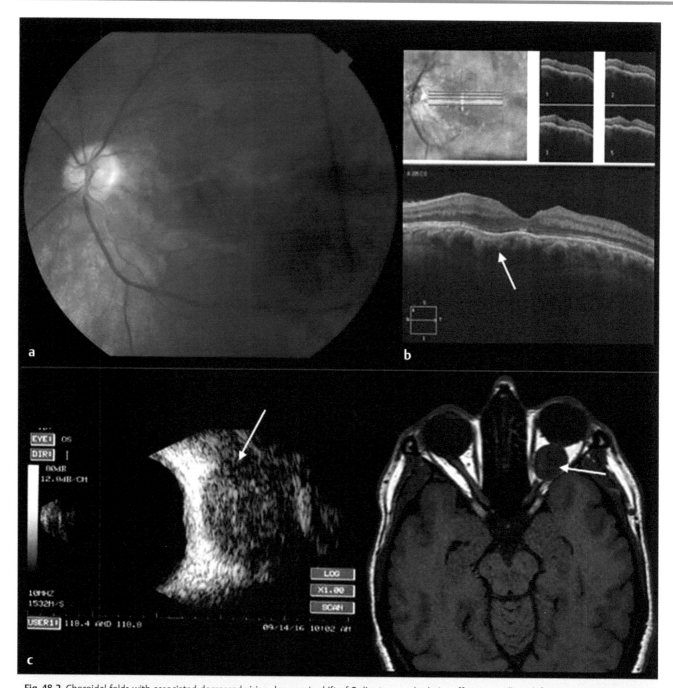

Fig. 48.2 Choroidal folds with associated decreased vision, hyperopic shift of 5 diopters, and relative afferent pupillary defect were present. Fundus photography demonstrating optic nerve pallor, (a) retinal pigment epithelium clumping and hypopigmentation in macula, and (b) choroidal folds demonstrated on optical coherence tomography. (c) Further imaging revealed a large hypoechogenic mass on ultrasonography, and MRI T1 axial scan showed a well-circumscribed left intraconal heterogeneous mass compressing lateral and medial rectus muscles and displacement of left optic nerve.

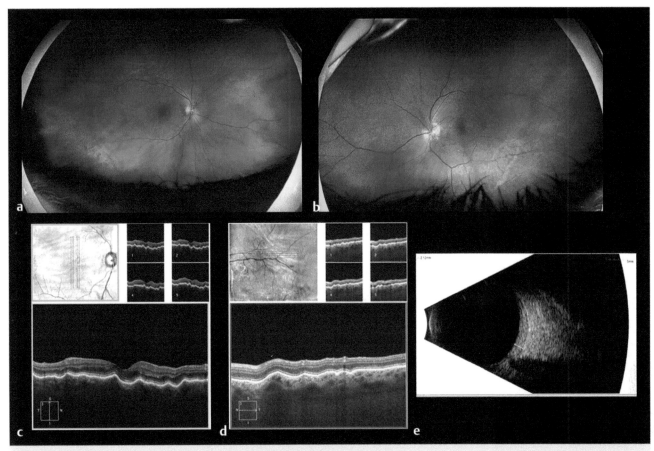

Fig. 48.3 Bilateral idiopathic choroidal folds and retinoschisis demonstrated in **(a,b)** widefield images and **(c,d)** optical coherence tomography. **(e)** Ultrasonography showed symmetric choroidal thickening 2.12 mm and no orbital mass.

48.4.2 Follow-up

Follow-up is dictated by underlying etiology and specific management strategy for that etiology.

Suggested Reading

[1] Olsen TW, Palejwala NV, Lee LB, Bergstrom CS, Yeh S. Chorioretinal folds: associated disorders and a related maculopathy. Am J Ophthalmol. 2014; 157 (5):1038–1047

[2] MW BCaJ. Uveal Effusion Syndrome and Hypotony Maculopathy. In: Schachat AP WC, Hinton DR, Sadda SR, Wiedemann P, ed. Ryan's Retina. Vol. 1. New York: Elsevier; 2018:1484–2495

[3] Freund KB SD, Mieler WF, Yannuzzi LA. Inflammation. In: Freund KB SD, Mieler WF, Yannuzzi LA, ed. The Retina Atlas. 2nd ed. China: Elsevier Health Sciences; 2016:279–398

[4] Kupersmith MJ, Sibony PA, Feldon SE, Wang JK, Garvin M, Kardon R, OCT Sub-Study Group for the NORDIC Idiopathic Intracranial Hypertension Treatment Trial. The effect of treatment of idiopathic intracranial hypertension on prevalence of retinal and choroidal folds. Am J Ophthalmol. 2017; 176:77–86

[5] Gualtieri W, Janula J. Topiramate maculopathy. Int Ophthalmol. 2013; 33(1): 103–106

49 Optic Pit-Related Maculopathy

Shangjun (Collier) Jiang and Netan Choudhry

Summary

Optic pit-related maculopathy is caused by intraretinal and/or subretinal fluid accumulation from congenital structural defects in the optic nerve head. Optic disc pits are detected as hypo- or hyperpigmented, oval-shaped excavations on fundus exam. Optical coherence tomography and fluorescein angiography can be used as diagnostic imaging and to track treatment response. Nonsurgical management with laser photocoagulation may temporarily alleviate fluid accumulation but does not provide long-term benefit. Surgical methods such as vitrectomy can successfully resolve fluid accumulation and improve visual acuity for the long term.

Keywords: optic nerve, optic pit, optical coherence tomography, vitrectomy

49.1 Features

Optic disc pits (ODPs) are a congenital deformity of the optic pit that affects men and women equally, with a prevalence of 1 in 11,000 people. Structural defects in the optic nerve head cause a disruption of the physiologic opening where the vitreous cavity and subarachnoid space meet each other. Thus, vitreous and/or cerebrospinal fluid can migrate into the subretinal space or within the retina and cause optic pit-related maculopathy.

49.1.1 Common Symptoms

Often asymptomatic and detected incidentally. When ODPs are complicated by macular changes such as intraretinal fluid accumulation, serous retinal detachment, and/or retinal pigment changes, they may be accompanied with more significant vision loss: metamorphopsia, micropsia, blurred vision, and/or central scotoma. Peripheral visual field loss may also be present.

49.1.2 Exam Findings

ODPs may resemble hypo- or hyperpigmented, oval-shaped excavations in the optic nerve during routine fundus examinations (▶ Fig. 49.1). Typically, these pits are solitary and gray, although multiple ODPs may also be detected in the optic nerve as yellow or black.

49.2 Key Diagnostic Tests and Findings

49.2.1 Optical Coherence Tomography

A schisis-like separation between the inner and outer retina due to fluid accumulation from the ODP. Fluid accumulation may also result in a serous retinal detachment characterized by hyporeflective subretinal fluid (▶ Fig. 49.2).

49.2.2 Fluorescein Angiography or Ultra-Widefield Fluorescein Angiography

Typically, early hypofluorescence and late hyperfluorescence of the ODP (▶ Fig. 49.3) with often minimal leakage in the area of retinal edema/detachment.

49.2.3 Fundus Autofluorescence

Not a primary modality for evaluation, however, the ODP can appear slightly hypoautofluorescent compared to the surrounding disc, which is devoid of retinal pigment epithelium cells. In the presence of a serous detachment secondary to ODP, the macula can appear hyperautofluorescent (▶ Fig. 49.4).

49.2.4 Optical Coherence Tomography Angiography

May reveal vascular perfusion anomalies related to the ODP.

49.2.5 Perimetry Testing

May reveal visual field defects such as an enlarged blind spot and a paracentral arcuate scotoma.

49.3 Critical Work-up

Differential diagnoses to consider include optic nerve coloboma, choroidal and scleral crescent, tilted disc syndrome,

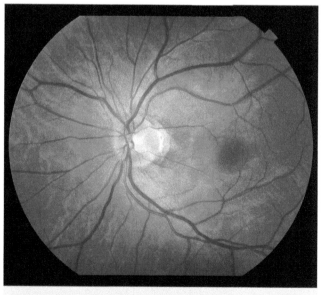

Fig. 49.1 Color fundus photograph of an optic disc pit in the left eye, showing a hypopigmented, oval-shaped excavation in the optic nerve.

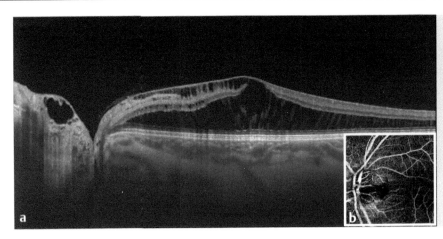

Fig. 49.2 (a) Swept-source optical coherence tomography (OCT) of a left eye with an optic disc pit (ODP) maculopathy, showing a schisis-like separation between the inner and outer retinal layers. (b) Swept-source OCT angiography of the left eye, indicating decreased vascular perfusion to the area of the ODP.

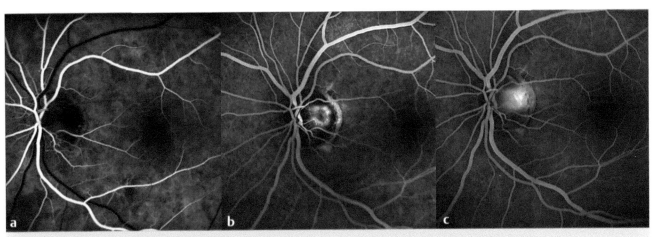

Fig. 49.3 (a–c) Fluorescein angiography of a patient with an optic disc pit demonstrating progressive staining of the pit as the study progresses but no leakage or hyperfluorescence within the retina.

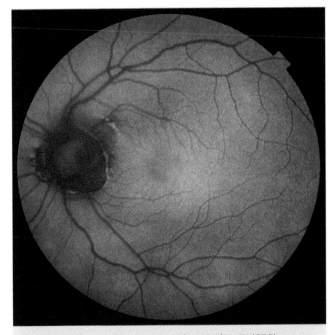

Fig. 49.4 Fundus autofluorescence with optic disc pit (ODP) maculopathy. The ODP appears hypoautofluorescent compared to the surrounding disc, which is devoid of retinal pigment epithelium cells, and the macula appears hyperautofluorescent due to the presence of subretinal and intraretinal fluid.

circumpapillary staphyloma, hypoplastic disc, morning glory disc anomaly, and glaucomatous optic neuropathy.

49.4 Management

49.4.1 Treatment Options

Nonsurgical Management

A variety of therapies have been trialed in the treatment of serous detachments secondary to ODP. Oral corticosteroids have not been found to be effective. Macular fluid accumulation may initially decrease, but the response is only temporary as the reaccumulation of fluid results in further maculopathy. Laser photocoagulation alone has not been proven to be effective. When laser is used as an adjunct to vitrectomy and intravitreal gas injection, it may enhance effectiveness by creating a barrier against intraretinal and subretinal fluid migration.

Surgical Management

Pars plana vitrectomy with laser photocoagulation and gas tamponade has been the mainstay of therapy for ODPs since the late 1980s (▶ Fig. 49.5). A combination of vitrectomy alone or in combination with internal limiting membrane peeling with gas

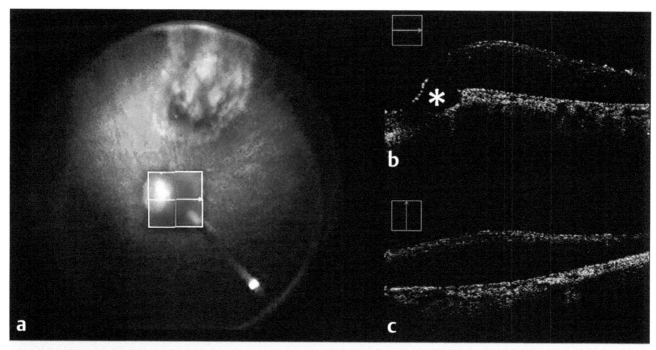

Fig. 49.5 (**a**) Intraoperative fundus image of an optic disc pit (ODP) with peripheral retinochoroidal coloboma. Horizontal (**b**) and vertical (**c**) intraoperative optical coherence tomography of an ODP, demonstrating macular edema from the ODP. Courtesy of Rishi Gupta.

has been reported with variable success rates. Laser photocoagulation in conjunction with pars plana vitrectomy is also considered as an option to produce a juxtapapillary scar that creates a barrier against fluid accumulation. Fluid resolution is often slow following surgical procedures. Macular buckling has also been reported for ODP. In this procedure, an L-shaped silicone buckle is implanted to the posterior globe to cause a buckling effect under the macula, creating a barrier to fluid flow between the optic nerve anomaly and the macula.

49.4.2 Follow-up

Follow-up frequency is based on active symptoms and the presence of macular fluid. Optical coherence tomography is used for surveillance of macular complications and to follow for the resolution after surgical intervention. In asymptomatic ODPs without macular complications, annual follow-up is typically sufficient.

Suggested Reading

[1] Moisseiev E, Moisseiev J, Loewenstein A. Optic disc pit maculopathy: when and how to treat? A review of the pathogenesis and treatment options. Int J Retina Vitreous. 2015; 1(1):13

[2] Jain N, Johnson MW. Pathogenesis and treatment of maculopathy associated with cavitary optic disc anomalies. Am J Ophthalmol. 2014; 158(3): 423–435

[3] Bjornsson HD, Nezgoda JT, Leng T. Optic Pits – EyeWiki. Available at: http://eyewiki.aao.org/Optic_Pits. Published 2014. Accessed September 16, 2017

[4] Shah SD, Yee KK, Fortun JA, Albini T. Optic disc pit maculopathy: a review and update on imaging and treatment. Int Ophthalmol Clin. 2014; 54(2):61–78

VI

50 Bacterial Endophthalmitis

Edmund Tsui, Nitish Mehta, and Yasha S. Modi

Summary

Endophthalmitis is a rare but vision-threatening condition resulting from exogenous or endogenous inoculation of intraocular tissues by microorganisms with a subsequent severe inflammatory reaction. Endophthalmitis can be further subdivided into endogenous, postprocedural/surgical (e.g., postintravitreal injection, postcataract, bleb-related), and post-traumatic endophthalmitis. Depending on the causative organism and mechanism of inoculation, endophthalmitis may present with varying degrees of decreased vision, eye pain, and redness and a varying combination of signs of ocular inflammation, including anterior chamber cell, hypopyon, vitritis, choroiditis, subretinal abscess, and retinitis. Prompt diagnosis with vitreous aspiration or pars plana vitrectomy and initiation of intravitreal and/or systemic antibiotics is critical in preserving visual acuity in this ocular emergency.

Keywords: abscess, blebitis, endogenous endophthalmitis, endophthalmitis, hypopyon, postoperative, retinitis, trauma, vitritis

50.1 Features

50.1.1 Endogenous Endophthalmitis

Endogenous endophthalmitis results from the hematogenous spread of microorganisms (bacteria, fungi, or mycobacteria) from distant foci to intraocular structures and accounts for 2 to 8% of all cases of endophthalmitis.

- Risk factors:
  - Recent hospitalization.
  - Diabetes mellitus.
  - Immunosuppression.
  - Intravenous drug use.
  - Others: Indwelling catheters, urinary tract infection, organ abscesses, and endocarditis.
- Causative organisms:
  - Several series have identified fungal organisms as the culprit in the majority of cases (in developed countries). The most commonly isolated fungal species is *Candida*, followed by *Aspergillus*.
  - In bacterial endogenous endophthalmitis, gram-positive species (*Staphylococci* and *Streptococci)* predominate in isolates from Western countries, whereas gram-negative strains (especially *Klebsiella)* are the main culprit in East Asian countries. Bacterial endogenous endophthalmitis is more common than fungal causes in East Asian countries. *Klebsiella* infections are associated with rapid progression of the disease and poor visual outcome.

Endophthalmitis following intravitreal injection of anti-vascular endothelial growth factor (anti-VEGF) agent or steroid is rare (i.e., < 1 per 1,000 injections) and typically occurs acutely following the procedure.

- Risk factors:
  - Talking, coughing, and sneezing should be avoided during the injection procedure. Studies have suggested that potential ocular surface contamination with oral flora may be a risk factor.
  - The use of povidone-iodine to sterilize the ocular surface is recommended as a preinjection sterilizing agent.
  - The use of bladed lid speculums, the hemisphere of injection, conjunctival displacement, and type of anti-VEGF agent have not been definitively shown to alter risk.
  - The use of postoperative antibiotics has not been shown to decrease the risk of postinjection endophthalmitis and was shown to increase the rate of antibiotic resistance.
- Causative organisms:
  - Coagulase-negative *Staphylococcus* and *Streptococcus* species are the most common isolates in postinjection endophthalmitis.

50.1.2 Sterile Endophthalmitis

Noninfectious endophthalmitis, also referred to as sterile endophthalmitis or postinjection vitritis, is believed to be an inflammatory reaction to a drug or drug delivery vehicle. Although hypopyon, fibrin in the anterior chamber, and pain are less common, all vitreous inflammation postintravitreal injections must be suspected as infectious endophthalmitis.

Toxic anterior segment syndrome following intraocular surgery has a similar presentation to sterile postoperative inflammation (limbus to limbus corneal edema, frequently presents without pain, less vitritis compared to infectious endophthalmitis); however, this inflammation is usually greatest on postoperative day 1, whereas an infectious endophthalmitis typically presents after 2 or more days. The etiology is unknown but is believed to be a severe inflammatory immune response to various factors introduced during the procedure (e.g., detergents, residual viscoelastic, and preservatives).

50.1.3 Postcataract Surgery Endophthalmitis

Endophthalmitis following cataract surgery is a rare but feared complication.

- Incidence:
  - Reported worldwide to be 0.03 to 0.2%.
- Risk factors:
  - Posterior capsular rupture.
  - Manual intracapsular and extracapsular cataract extraction.
  - Clear corneal incisions, silicone intraocular lenses, male gender, and age greater than 85 years have also been identified as risk factors.
- Causative organisms:
  - The source likely originates from ocular surface and/or skin flora.

- Coagulase-negative *Staphylococcus* is the most commonly isolated organism, followed by *Staphylococcus aureus* and *Streptococcus* species.
- Chronic postoperative endophthalmitis is rare and occurs more than 6 weeks after surgery. These infections are typically due to indolent bacteria such as *Propionibacterium acnes*, *Staphylococcus epidermidis*, or fungi, such as *Candida* or *Aspergillus*. Patients are generally misdiagnosed as having chronic or recurrent uveitis postcataract surgery due to their indolent course.

50.1.4 Bleb-Related Endophthalmitis

During a filtering glaucoma surgery, a bleb is created and as a result, the aqueous humor is only separated from the external environment by a thin conjunctival barrier. When this barrier is disrupted, this allows for the introduction of bacteria into the bleb (i.e., blebitis) and ultimately into the eyes (bleb-related endophthalmitis [BRE]). The onset of BRE may be early (< 1 month postoperatively) or delayed (> 1 month).
- Incidence: Approximately 1%.
- Risk factors: Nasally or inferiorly located bleb due to increased exposure to the tear film, bleb leakage, use of antimetabolites, blepharitis, and bleb revisions.
- Causative organisms:
  - One-third of cases are attributed to *Streptococcus* species, followed by *Staphylococcus* and gram-negative species.
  - Early BRE is most commonly from coagulase-negative *Staphylococcus* and *S. aureus*.
  - Delayed-onset BRE is attributed to more virulent microorganisms, such as *Streptococcus* and *Haemophilus* species.

Glaucoma drainage implants, such as Ahmed glaucoma valve or Baerveldt glaucoma implant, have also been associated with endophthalmitis; the major risk factor is conjunctival erosion over the tube.
- Commonly isolated organisms include *Staphylococcus* species, *Streptococcus pneumoniae*, and *Pseudomonas aeruginosa*.

50.1.5 Post-Trauma Endophthalmitis

After penetrating injury or globe rupture, inoculation of the intraocular tissue with foreign material may result in a particularly fulminant manifestation of endophthalmitis.
- Incidence:
  - Incidence of trauma-related endophthalmitis ranges from 0 to 16.5%.
- Risk factors:
  - Presence of intraocular foreign body (IOFB), injury occurring in a rural setting, ruptured lens capsule, contaminated injury with organic matter, delayed repair of globe, and vitreous prolapse through wound.
- Causative organisms:
  - Coagulase-negative *Staphylococci* and *Streptococci* species.
  - *Bacillus*, *Pseudomonas*, *Klebsiella*, and *Clostridium* species are seen and are associated with a fulminant and rapid progression.
  - Soil contamination and IOFB are associated with a higher incidence of *Bacillus* infections.

- Polymicrobial infections are also more common with penetrating globe injuries compared to other causes of endophthalmitis.
- *Aspergillus* species are the most prevalent fungal cause of post-traumatic endophthalmitis.

50.2 Symptoms

Eye redness, pain, photophobia, floaters, and decreased vision in the setting of ocular trauma, ocular surgery, intravitreal injection, or systemic illness (e.g., fever, chills, nausea, vomiting, and other signs associated with the underlying systemic etiology) may be present in endophthalmitis.

50.2.1 Exam Findings

Signs of various types of endophthalmitis include vitreous haze/cell, anterior chamber inflammation, vitreous exudates, visible arteriolar septic emboli, uveal tissue abscesses (▶ Fig. 50.1), hypopyon (▶ Fig. 50.2), whitened bleb with surrounding conjunctival injection (▶ Fig. 50.3), and necrotizing retinitis.

50.3 Key Diagnostic Tests and Findings

50.3.1 Optical Coherence Tomography

If there is a view of the posterior segment, vitreous inflammation on optical coherence tomography can present as multiple discrete hyper-reflective foci in the vitreous cavity and posterior hyaloid thickening. Hyper-reflective foci can be seen to aggregate on the posterior hyaloid or retinal surface. Retinal and/or choroidal abscesses appear as discrete hyper-reflective masses confined to the retina in the former, and discrete hyper-reflective masses that elevate the retinal pigment epithelium in the latter (▶ Fig. 50.4). Varying degrees of retinal hyper-reflectivity and layer obscuration may be present, depending on the location and severity of the retinitis.

50.3.2 Fluorescein Angiography or Ultra-Widefield Fluorescein Angiography

Fluorescein angiography may demonstrate vascular leakage from vasculitis if media permits proper imaging.

50.3.3 Ultrasonography

Ultrasound is an important modality in endophthalmitis to identify the extent of vitritis and membrane formation in the setting of a media opacity and no posterior segment view. Vitreous inflammation and exudate will appear as diffuse or compartmentalized hyperechogenicity of the vitreous cavity (▶ Fig. 50.5). Choroidal or retinal abscesses, if present, will appear as dome-shaped elevations. Chorioretinal thickening may also be present.

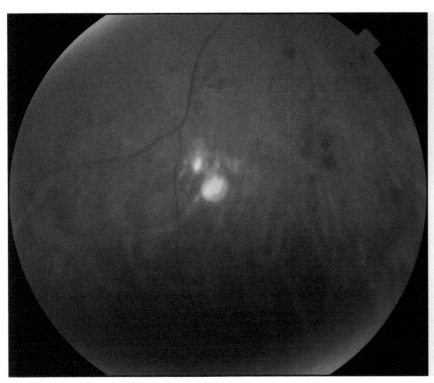

Fig. 50.1 Color fundus photograph following partial treatment of methicillin-sensitive *Staphylococcus aureus* endophthalmitis with resolving vitritis and a persistent yellow–white choroidal abscesses.

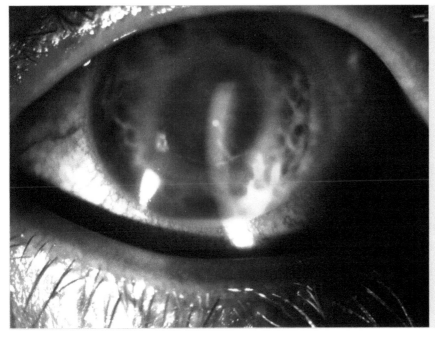

Fig. 50.2 Anterior segment photograph of an eye with a hypopyon with suspected bacterial endophthalmitis following cataract surgery.

Ultrasound is also a useful adjunct to detect retained IOFBs in trauma cases.

50.4 Critical Work-up

Ocular fluid testing of vitreous specimen obtained by vitreous tap or pars plana vitrectomy is preferred. Aqueous tap may also be considered. Consider aerobic/anaerobic stains/culture, fungal stains/culture, and additional specialized stains/culture as appropriate. Real-time polymerase chain reaction when available may be used to obtain more rapid diagnosis but does not offer antibiotic susceptibility. Systemic investigation and examination are critical for suspected endogenous endophthalmitis. Perform thorough systemic evaluation, including complete physical examination (including a full skin check), blood and urine cultures, and imaging as appropriate. Consider inpatient admission to expeditiously complete this work-up and begin systemic treatment.

50.5 Management

50.5.1 Treatment Options

Prompt collection of vitreous cultures followed by intravitreal antimicrobials is the general paradigm in the treatment of endophthalmitis. Commonly employed broad-spectrum intravitreal antibiotics include vancomycin (1 mg/0.1 mL) combined with ceftazidime (2.25 mg/0.1 mL) and moxifloxacin (400 µg/0.1 mL) monotherapy. Commonly employed broad-spectrum intravitreal antifungals include intravitreal amphotericin (5 µg/0.1 mL) and voriconazole (50 µg/0.1 mL). A repeat injection of intravitreal antibiotics may also be considered 36 to 60 hours after initial treatment if there is no stabilization and improvement.

Consider pars plana vitrectomy based on visual acuity, clinical severity, and response to intravitreal therapeutics. Postcataract surgery endophthalmitis with visual acuity of light perception was demonstrated to benefit from immediate vitrectomy compared to eyes with better visual acuity. Anti-inflammatory measures such as topical steroids, intravitreal short-acting steroids, and/or systemic steroids are often considered to help reduce the inflammatory severity. Concurrent retinal detachments in the setting of endophthalmitis portend a poor outcome and should be managed with pars plana vitrectomy and/or scleral buckle with long-acting gas or silicone oil tamponade.

Left untreated, endophthalmitis carries a poor prognosis with severe to complete vision loss. Early diagnosis and treatment before the destruction of delicate intraocular tissue is the single greatest factor to preserve functional vision. Initial visual acuity

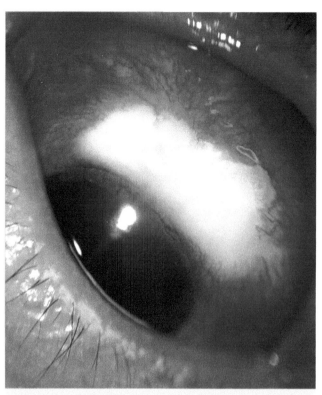

Fig. 50.3 External photograph of bleb-related endophthalmitis with diffuse conjunctival injection and a whitened bleb.

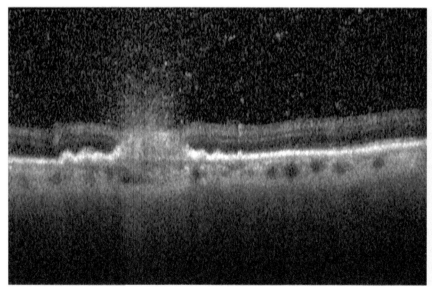

Fig. 50.4 Spectral domain optical coherence tomography B-scan of choroidal abscesses manifesting as a dense chorioretinal hyper-reflective lesion with overlying hyper-reflective vitreous foci.

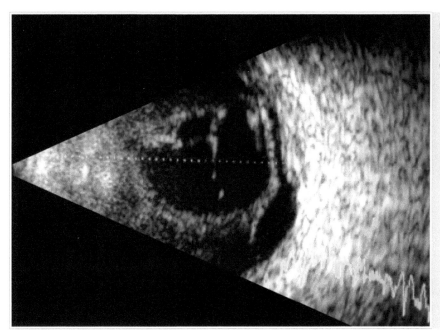

Fig. 50.5 B-scan ultrasonography demonstrating loculated hyperechoic areas within the vitreous consistent with vitreous inflammation in endogenous endophthalmitis.

has a significant correlation with final visual acuity in all types of endophthalmitis. Proper identification of the culprit microbe is paramount, as patients with methicillin-resistant *S. aureus*, *Klebsiella*, or *Aspergillus* endogenous endophthalmitis carry higher rates of poor final visual outcome and enucleation.

Suggested Reading

[1] Bhavsar AR, Glassman AR, Stockdale CR, Jampol LM, Diabetic Retinopathy Clinical Research Network. Elimination of topical antibiotics for intravitreous injections and the importance of using povidone-iodine: update from the diabetic retinopathy clinical research network. JAMA Ophthalmol. 2016; 134 (10):1181–1183

[2] Cao H, Zhang L, Li L, Lo S. Risk factors for acute endophthalmitis following cataract surgery: a systematic review and meta-analysis. PLoS One. 2013; 8(8): e71731

[3] Zahid S, Musch DC, Niziol LM, Lichter PR, Collaborative Initial Glaucoma Treatment Study Group. Risk of endophthalmitis and other long-term complications of trabeculectomy in the Collaborative Initial Glaucoma Treatment Study (CIGTS). Am J Ophthalmol. 2013; 155(4):674–680, 680.e1

[4] Ahmed Y, Schimel AM, Pathengay A, Colyer MH, Flynn HW, Jr. Endophthalmitis following open-globe injuries. Eye (Lond). 2012; 26(2):212–217

[5] Endophthalmitis Vitrectomy Study Group. Results of the Endophthalmitis Vitrectomy Study. A randomized trial of immediate vitrectomy and of intravenous antibiotics for the treatment of postoperative bacterial endophthalmitis. Arch Ophthalmol. 1995; 113(12):1479–1496

51 Fungal Endophthalmitis

Durga S. Borkar and Sunir J. Garg

Summary

Fungal endophthalmitis is characterized by intraocular inflammation involving the vitreous and anterior chamber of the eye due to endogenous or exogenous fungal infection. Clinical presentation of fungal endophthalmitis can vary depending on the source, particularly between endogenous and exogenous causes, as well as the causative organism. In contrast to bacterial endophthalmitis, fungal endophthalmitis can have a more indolent course presenting both diagnostic and therapeutic challenges. Treatments include intravitreal and/or systemic antifungal agents, as well as surgical intervention with pars plana vitrectomy. Regardless of treatment modality, visual acuity outcomes tend to be poor.

Keywords: Candida, endophthalmitis, fungal infection, PCR testing, voriconazole

51.1 Features

Fungal endophthalmitis refers to intraocular inflammation involving the vitreous and anterior chamber of the eye due to endogenous or exogenous fungal infection. Clinical presentation of fungal endophthalmitis can vary depending on the source, particularly between endogenous and exogenous causes, as well as the causative organism. Endogenous fungal endophthalmitis occurs through hematogenous spread. Risk factors include a history of intravenous drug use, immunocompromised status, recent hospitalization, diabetes, malignancy, central lines, recent systemic surgery, organ transplantation, liver or renal disease, and ongoing parenteral nutrition. Exogenous fungal endophthalmitis typically occurs in immunocompetent patients after a history of ocular trauma, cataract surgery, or glaucoma filtering surgery. In some cases, fungal endophthalmitis can occur as a sequela of external ocular infection, such as fungal keratitis. Fungal endophthalmitis is uncommon after intravitreal injection or pars plana vitrectomy.

51.1.1 Common Symptoms

Commonly, redness of the eye, decreased vision, pain, photophobia, and floaters; often has a subacute presentation with symptoms worsening over days to weeks.

51.1.2 Exam Findings

Anterior segment exam can initially reveal minimal pathology. Eventually, patients can develop conjunctival injection, scleritis, keratic precipitates, and a hypopyon. Patients with endogenous fungal endophthalmitis often present with single or multiple chorioretinal lesions with overlying focal vitritis ("string of pearls") unlike the commonly diffuse intraocular inflammation seen with bacterial endophthalmitis (▶ Fig. 51.1, ▶ Fig. 51.2). This likely occurs from the fungus spreading from the choroidal and/or retinal circulation into the vitreous. Patients with exogenous fungal endophthalmitis can have a similar presentation; however, findings are also often specific to the cause of the infection (e.g., a patient with fungal endophthalmitis related to fungal keratitis can have a dense anterior chamber reaction, while a patient with fungal endophthalmitis related to trauma may have more diffuse vitritis). Similarly, postcataract fungal endophthalmitis cases can occasionally present with an inflammatory plaque on the back of the intraocular lens implant.

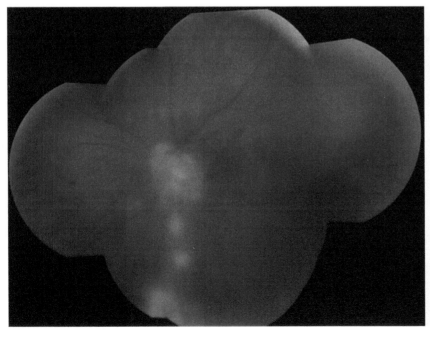

Fig. 51.1 Montage fundus photograph of the left eye revealing peripapillary chorioretinal lesions with overlying focal areas of vitritis in the classic "string of pearls" configuration typical of endogenous fungal endophthalmitis.

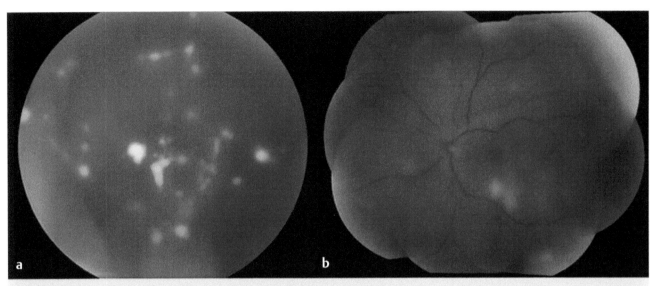

Fig. 51.2 **(a)** Fundus photograph of the left eye with endogenous *Candida* endophthalmitis due to a colonoscopy, treated with oral voriconazole and a single intravitreal voriconazole injection (100 μg). A diffuse vitritis with more focal condensations of vitreous inflammation is seen. **(b)** Montage fundus photograph of the left eye 2 months after treatment shows significantly improved vitritis.

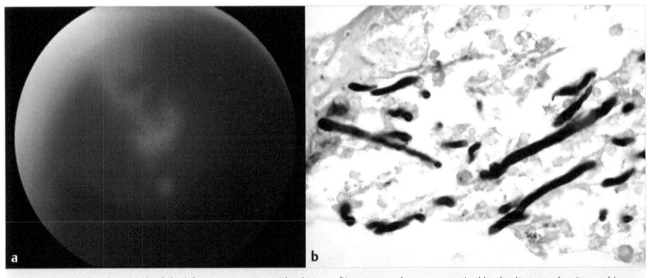

Fig. 51.3 **(a)** Fundus photograph of the left eye in a patient with a history of intravenous drug use, negative blood cultures, and a vitreous biopsy positive for *Aspergillus flavus*. **(b)** Pathology showed numerous, branching septate hyphae.

51.2 Key Diagnostic Tests and Findings

51.2.1 Ultrasonography

B-scan ultrasonography can rule out a retinal detachment in patients with dense vitritis.

51.2.2 Intraocular Fluid Cultures

While cultures and calcofluor white staining are often initially obtained via a vitreous or aqueous fluid aspirate, this can be low yield, particularly in cases of endogenous fungal endophthalmitis that primarily have posterior segment involvement. In these cases, vitreous samples obtained via pars plana vitrectomy can provide a higher yield in obtaining a diagnostic sample. However, fungal species can be difficult to culture even with an appropriate sample, sometimes taking weeks to incubate. The most common causative organisms for fungal endophthalmitis are *Candida* species, followed by *Aspergillus* species (▶ Fig. 51.3). Yeasts, such as *Candida*, more commonly result from an endogenous source, while molds, such as *Aspergillus* and *Cryptococcus* (▶ Fig. 51.4), are more likely to be associated with an exogenous etiology.

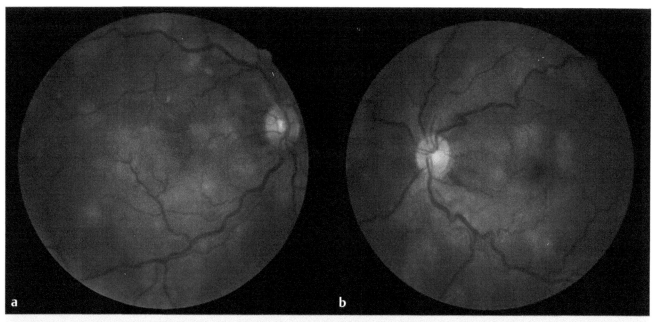

Fig. 51.4 Fundus photographs of the **(a)** right and **(b)** left eyes demonstrate bilateral disseminated cryptococcal endophthalmitis with associated cryptococcal meningitis. Although there is minimal vitritis, diffuse chorioretinal lesions in the macula and periphery are present.

51.2.3 Polymerase Chain Reaction

Because of the difficulty in culturing fungal species, various methods have been proposed to more accurately identify fungal endophthalmitis. One of the most promising methods currently is polymerase chain reaction (PCR) testing of vitreous samples. PCR testing can detect intraocular infection with very small amounts of vitreous fluid and appears to be more sensitive. However, testing can be time-consuming and expensive and is not available in many centers.

51.3 Critical Work-up

In addition to cultures of intraocular fluid, blood and urine cultures should be obtained in cases of suspected endogenous fungal endophthalmitis. Additional testing for fungal endophthalmitis is focused primarily on identifying the organism. Because of the often indolent course and nonspecific findings, fungal endophthalmitis can be a diagnostic challenge, particularly early in the clinical course. It can be misdiagnosed as a myriad of other entities, including conjunctivitis, anterior uveitis, neuroretinitis, panuveitis, and acute retinal necrosis.

51.4 Management

51.4.1 Treatment Options

Treatments include intravitreal and/or systemic antifungal agents, as well as surgical intervention with pars plana vitrectomy with vitreous sampling and intravitreal antifungal medications. Systemically, intravenous amphotericin B has been the traditional treatment. While systemic treatment is necessary for cases of endogenous fungal endophthalmitis in order to treat the causative infection, intravenous amphotericin B can

have significant systemic side effects. Voriconazole is a newer agent that has been shown to be effective and reach therapeutic levels intraocularly after only two oral doses, and oral fluconazole is useful for *Candida*, the most common cause of endogenous fungal endophthalmitis. In cases of exogenous fungal endophthalmitis, intravitreal injection with amphotericin B or voriconazole should be considered. While some cases are managed with medical treatment alone, pars plana vitrectomy along with antifungal medicines may be useful to help remove the infectious burden from the eye, decrease inflammation, and decrease vitreoretinal traction.

51.4.2 Follow-up

Patients need to be followed closely when they have an active infection. Recurrence may occur even after the infection appears quiescent; thus, ongoing surveillance for recurrence remains important. Repeat intravitreal injections of antifungal agents may be necessary. Concomitant steroids should be given cautiously and only once the appropriate antifungal medication has been started. Regardless of treatment modality, visual acuity outcomes tend to be poor with over half of patients having final visual acuities of less than 20/400.

Suggested Reading

[1] Chakrabarti A, Shivaprakash MR, Singh R, et al. Fungal endophthalmitis: fourteen years' experience from a center in India. Retina. 2008; 28(10):1400–1407

[2] Lingappan A, Wykoff CC, Albini TA, et al. Endogenous fungal endophthalmitis: causative organisms, management strategies, and visual acuity outcomes. Am J Ophthalmol. 2012; 153(1):162–16–6.e1

[3] Chee YE, Eliott D. The Role of Vitrectomy in the Management of Fungal Endophthalmitis. Semin Ophthalmol. 2017; 32(1):29–35

[4] Durand ML. Bacterial and Fungal Endophthalmitis. Clin Microbiol Rev. 2017; 30(3):597–613

52 Toxoplasmosis

Akshay S. Thomas and Dilraj Grewal

Summary

Toxoplasma retinochoroiditis is a result of infection with the intracellular protozoan parasite *Toxoplasma gondii*. Ocular toxoplasmosis can be congenital or acquired, and worldwide is the most common cause of inflammation in the back of the eye. Optical coherence tomography, fluorescein angiography, fundus autofluorescence, and ultrasonography are useful diagnostic tests. Mild cases, which do not threaten the macula, are often observed and may resolve without treatment. In more severe cases, treatment options include antiparasitic regimens, steroids, and new therapies currently in development.

Keywords: chorioretinitis, cysts, lesions, retinochoroiditis, Toxoplasma gondii, Toxoplasmosis, vitritis

52.1 Features

Toxoplasma retinochoroiditis is the most common cause of infectious posterior uveitis in immunocompetent individuals and is a result of congenital or acquired infection with the ubiquitous intracellular protozoan parasite *Toxoplasma gondii*. *T. gondii* is a widespread parasite that approximately 25 to 30% of the human population is infected with. Humans can get infected by the consumption of undercooked cyst-contaminated meat products or by sporulated oocysts, which can be found in water, soil, or vegetables. The parasite exists in different morphologic and metabolic stages, which are products of the parasite's sexual cycle in the intestine of cats. After ingestion, the cysts (or oocysts) are disrupted and the bradyzoites are released into the intestinal lumen where they rapidly enter cells and multiply as tachyzoites. Ocular toxoplasmosis can result in a granulomatous panuveitis.

52.1.1 Common Symptoms

Symptoms include eye redness, pain, photophobia, floaters, and blurry vision. In some cases, toxoplasma retinochoroiditis may only have focal overlying vitritis, and hence, some patients with peripheral lesions may be largely asymptomatic.

52.1.2 Exam Findings

Variable based on the extent of involvement but may include keratic precipitates (▶ Fig. 52.1a), anterior chamber cell, scleritis, posterior synechiae, cataract, vitreous cell, vitreous haze, chorioretinal lesions, epiretinal membrane, intraretinal hemorrhages, neuroretinitis (▶ Fig. 52.1b), retinal vasculitis, choroidal neovascularization (CNV), and retinal detachment. Strabismus (often due to poor vision secondary to a macular lesion), nystagmus, and microphthalmia may be present in congenital toxoplasmosis.

The classic description of an active chorioretinal lesion is that of a "headlight in the fog," which refers to the whitish focal area of necrotizing retinochoroiditis that is somewhat visible through the vitreous haze (▶ Fig. 52.1c). Inactive chorioretinal lesions appear as variable pigmented patches of chorioretinal atrophy (▶ Fig. 52.2). It is not uncommon to have reactivation of toxoplasma retinochoroiditis adjacent to a previous lesion in which case lesions in various degrees of evolution are noted. Immunocompromised individuals may have a more atypical presentation with large confluent areas of retinochoroiditis and simultaneous bilateral active disease. Lesions may also present as punctate outer retinal toxoplasmosis (characterized by multifocal, small lesions, which are located in the deep layers of the retina and retinal pigment epithelium. Patients with congenital toxoplasma retinochoroiditis are more likely to have bilateral and macula-involving lesions.

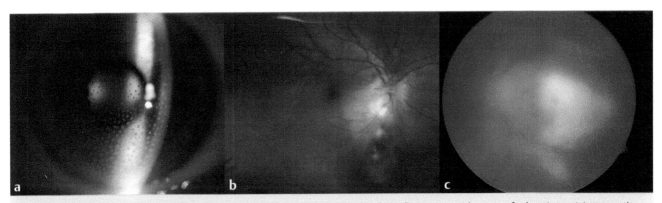

Fig. 52.1 Clinical findings in ocular toxoplasmosis. **(a)** Granulomatous anterior chamber inflammation with mutton-fat keratic precipitates on the corneal endothelium. **(b)** Retinochoroiditis adjacent to the optic nerve with resulting disc edema with the evidence of a previous toxoplasma chorioretinal lesion with hyperpigmentation with the development of a new lesion adjacent to its border. **(c)** "Headlight in the fog" appearance resulting from a whitish area of retinitis seen through the vitreous haze.

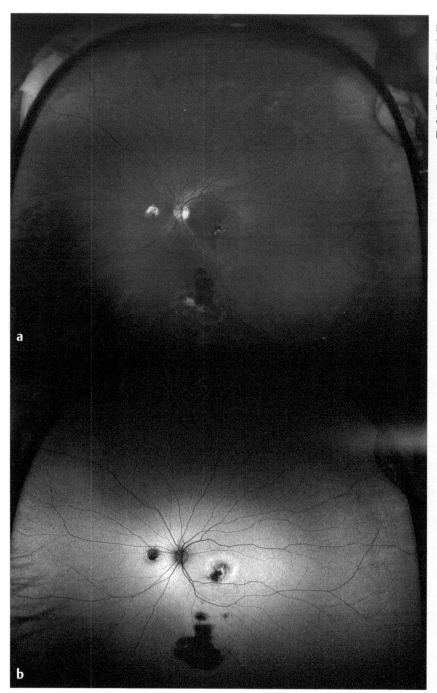

Fig. 52.2 Ultra-widefield imaging in inactive toxoplasma retinochoroiditis. **(a)** Multiple healed pigmented chorioretinal lesions are seen without overlying vitritis. **(b)** Autofluorescence reveals hypoautofluorescence of the lesions due to retinal pigment epithelium (RPE) loss. There is a rim of hyperautofluorescence around the nasal and macular lesions, which may be secondary to photoreceptor loss overlying intact RPE.

52.2 Key Diagnostic Tests and Findings

52.2.1 Optical Coherence Tomography

Active lesions may show disorganization of retinal layers (both inner and outer) in the region of retinitis and vitreous cells adjacent to the area of retinitis (▶ Fig. 52.3a,b). Inactive lesions typically show chorioretinal atrophy. Optical coherence tomography is also useful in detecting intraretinal and subretinal fluid that may be associated with CNV at the site of the chorioretinal

lesion and may reveal epiretinal membrane formation with or without associated distortion of the retina.

52.2.2 Fluorescein Angiography or Ultra-Widefield Fluorescein Angiography

May show diffuse or focal retinal vasculitis. The retinal vasculitis is more often a periphlebitis, though arteriolar inflammation is also possible (▶ Fig. 52.3c). There may be a blockage from

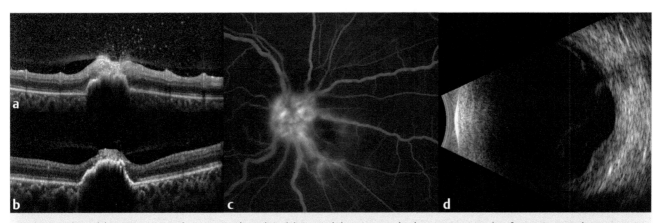

Fig. 52.3 Multimodal imaging in toxoplasma retinochoroiditis. **(a)** Spectral domain optical coherence tomography of an active toxoplasma chorioretinal lesion shows disorganization of the retinal layers, retinal thickening, retinal pigment epithelium (RPE) thickening/elevation, and overlying vitreous hyper-reflective dots consistent with overlying vitritis. **(b)** The same lesion 6 years later showing retinal atrophy, persistent RPE elevation, and resolution of the overlying vitritis. **(c)** Fluorescein angiogram demonstrates blockage from a small juxtapapillary focus of retinitis with perivascular leakage from the adjacent retinal blood vessels and disc. **(d)** B-scan ultrasound shows vitreous hyperechogenicity from vitritis and a focal area of chorioretinal elevation corresponding to a toxoplasma chorioretinal lesion.

pigment deposition in the chorioretinal scar and/or a window defect in areas of atrophy. Fluorescein angiography may additionally help in diagnosing CNV associated with the chorioretinal lesion.

52.2.3 Fundus Autofluorescence

Most often notable for hypoautofluorescence in regions of atrophic scarring (▶ Fig. 52.2b).

52.2.4 Ultrasonography

In cases where significant vitritis prohibits adequate examination of the fundus, B-scan ultrasonography may reveal a focal elevation with overlying vitreous hyperechogenicity (▶ Fig. 52.3d) and traction on the retina, which, if severe, may also present as a tractional retinal detachment.

52.3 Critical Work-up

Acquisition of aqueous samples should be considered for toxoplasma polymerase chain reaction (PCR) testing along with serum samples for toxoplasma immunoglobulin G (IgG) and IgM levels for Goldmann–Witmer coefficient analysis, particularly if the diagnosis is unclear. The Sabin–Feldman dye test is used to measure primarily IgG antibodies and titer is considered positive. IgM antibodies, on the other hand, may persist for 1 year or longer, following acute infection. A negative IgM enzyme-linked immunosorbent assay (ELISA) result in an immunologically normal adult almost always excludes recent infection. For congenital toxoplasmosis, IgA ELISA is a more sensitive test for the detection of infection in the fetus and newborn than IgM. Other causes of uveitis such as sarcoidosis, tuberculosis, and syphilis should be ruled out with antitreponemal antibodies, QuantiFERON Gold testing, angiotensin-converting enzyme levels, and a chest X-ray. In cases with chorioretinal lesions, other causes of necrotizing retinitis such as viral retinitis need to be ruled out as well, typically by

sending aqueous samples for herpes simplex virus, varicella zoster virus, and cytomegalovirus PCR. In patients with atypical findings such as multiple/bilateral lesions, human immunodeficiency virus testing should be performed.

52.4 Management

52.4.1 Treatment Options

Observation

Small extramacular lesions, which do not threaten vision, may be observed without treatment in immunocompetent patients as the disease is often self-limited.

Concurrent Antivirals

In equivocal cases for toxoplasmosis diagnosis, coverage for potential viral retinitis with oral antivirals (e.g., valacyclovir) is appropriate until aqueous PCR results return.

Antiparasitic Regimen

Lesions within the vascular arcades, those in close proximity to the optic disc, or large lesions > 1 disc diameter in size and retinochoroiditis in immunosuppressed patients warrant treatment. There is no clear consensus on the best antiparasitic treatment regimen, but each of the following has been used to treat ocular toxoplasmosis in the United States (▶ Table 52.1).
- Pyrimethamine, sulfadiazine, and folinic acid ("triple therapy").
- Trimethoprim/sulfamethoxazole.
- Azithromycin.
- Atovaquone.
- Oral or intravitreal clindamycin.

Each of the above antiparasitic regimens is typically continued for 5 to 6 weeks until the lesions are consolidated.

Table 52.1 Common treatment regimens for ocular toxoplasmosis

Antiparasitic therapy	Typical dose	Advantages	Disadvantages
Triple therapy: • Pyrimethamine • Sulfadiazine • Folinic acid	• 100-mg loading dose followed by 25–50 mg daily in one to two divided doses • 1 g four times a day • 5 mg once every other day	• Documented safety and efficacy in pregnancy	• Weekly laboratory monitoring required to check for bone marrow suppression
Trimethoprim/sulfamethoxazole	160 mg/800 mg two times a day	• Relatively affordable • Generally well tolerated	• May not be as effective as triple therapy • Not safe for the use in pregnancy
Azithromycin	250 mg one to two times a day	• Relatively affordable • Generally well tolerated • Safe for use in pregnancy	• May not be as effective as triple therapy • Unclear if it provides protection to the fetus in pregnant patients
Atovaquone	750 mg three to four times a day	Effective against both toxoplasma tachyzoite and cyst, thus potentially reducing recurrences	• Expensive • Has not been studied extensively
Clindamycin	• 300 mg four times a day (oral) • 2 mg/0.1 mL (intravitreal)	• Relatively affordable • Generally well tolerated • Safe for use in pregnancy	• May not be as effective as triple therapy

Steroids

Topical and oral steroids may be used in combination with antiparasitic agents, depending on the degree of anterior chamber inflammation and vitritis, respectively. Initiation of oral steroids is typically delayed until antiparasitic agents have been on board for a few days. Intraocular/periocular steroid in patients with ocular toxoplasmosis must be used with extreme caution.

Maintenance Therapy

Maintenance therapy with a reduced dosing schedule of the clinicians' antiparasitic regimen of choice is recommended for the following:
• Immunocompromised patients.
• Patients with multiple episodes of reactivation of retinochoroiditis.
• In a patient undergoing ocular surgery in an eye with inactive toxoplasma retinochoroiditis.

Cysts

Management is often challenging due to the ability of the parasite to form cysts for its survival, effectively avoiding immunosurveillance by the host. Cysts are often impenetrable to host enzymes and it is very difficult to eliminate latent cysts from retinal tissue.

New Therapies

There are several therapeutic agents in the development, including small molecule inhibitors such as artemisinin and enzyme targets such as blocking calcium-dependent protein kinases.

52.4.2 Follow-up

Patients with active inflammation are followed every few days to every 1 to 2 weeks until a response to therapy is noted with the consolidation of the lesions and improvement in inflammation, following which clinic visits are further spaced out based on clinical activity.

Suggested Reading

[1] Holland GN, Lewis KG. An update on current practices in the management of ocular toxoplasmosis. Am J Ophthalmol. 2002; 134(1):102–114

[2] Kim SJ, Scott IU, Brown GC, et al. Interventions for toxoplasma retinochoroiditis: a report by the American Academy of Ophthalmology. Ophthalmology. 2013; 120(2):371–378

[3] Fernandes Felix JP, Cavalcanti Lira RP, Cosimo AB, Cardeal da Costa RL, Nascimento MA, Leite Arieta CE. Trimethoprim-Sulfamethoxazole Versus Placebo in Reducing the Risk of Toxoplasmic Retinochoroiditis Recurrences: A Three-Year Follow-up. Am J Ophthalmol. 2016; 170:176–182

[4] Maenz M, Schlüter D, Liesenfeld O, Schares G, Gross U, Pleyer U. Ocular toxoplasmosis past, present and new aspects of an old disease. Prog Retin Eye Res. 2014; 39:77–106

53 Toxocariasis

Thuy K. Le and Justis P. Ehlers

Summary

Ocular toxocariasis (OT) is a helminthic disease that may cause a large spectrum of ocular complications. It is one of the most common parasitic causes of visual loss in the world, particularly in children. Infection usually results from accidental ingestion of dirt that has been contaminated with dog or cat feces that contain infectious *Toxocara* eggs. Rarely, people can also become infected from eating undercooked meat containing *Toxocara* larvae. OT occurs when the *Toxocara* larvae migrate to the eye with symptoms, including vision loss, eye inflammation, and damage to the retina. Serum and vitreous testing for specific *Toxocara* immunoglobulin G aids in diagnosis and ultrasonography is vital for evaluating leukocoria to help distinguish between other possible diagnoses.

Keywords: granuloma, retinal fold, Toxocara

53.1 Features

Ocular toxocariasis (OT) is a helminthic disease that may cause a large spectrum of ocular complications. It is one of the most common parasitic causes of visual loss in the world, particularly in children. Infection usually results from accidental ingestion of dirt that has been contaminated with dog or cat feces that contain infectious *Toxocara* eggs. Rarely, people can also become infected from eating undercooked meat containing *Toxocara* larvae. OT occurs when the *Toxocara* larvae migrate to the eye with symptoms, including vision loss, eye inflammation, and damage to the retina. Serum and vitreous testing for specific *Toxocara* immunoglobulin G aids in diagnosis and ultrasonography is vital for evaluating leukocoria to help distinguish between other possible diagnoses.

53.1.1 Common Symptoms

Often asymptomatic. Ocular symptoms are usually unilateral and include blurry vision, floaters, and other potential signs of inflammation.

53.1.2 Exam Findings

In its most common form of endophthalmitis, it presents in the retina and vitreous, possibly as a yellow-white lesion and often with vitritis. Retinal detachment and leukocoria may be present, and hypopyon may develop in severe cases. A peripheral granuloma, noted as a white elevated mass, may be present in the peripheral retina and/or ciliary body region with possible falciform folds with associated retinal dragging in late stages. Alternatively, it may present as a posterior granuloma that may have indistinct borders with overlying vitritis in the acute stage (► Fig. 53.1). As the acute inflammation subsides, the granuloma typically becomes more defined and consolidated. In optic papillitis, the optic disc will be elevated with telangiectatic vessels and possible subretinal exudate. Other ophthalmic findings include amblyopia and strabismus.

53.2 Key Diagnostic Tests and Findings

53.2.1 Optical Coherence Tomography

Optical coherence tomography may demonstrate the localization of the granuloma with choroidal involvement and rupture through Bruch's membrane and the retinal pigment epithelium. Outer retinal involvement with possible associated subretinal and intraretinal fluid is seen during the acute inflammatory phase (► Fig. 53.2).

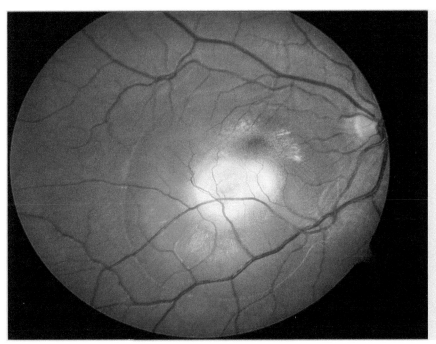

Fig. 53.1 Fundus photograph of a posterior granuloma with whitish subretinal lesion in the macula.

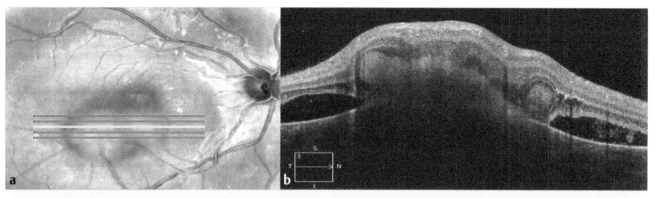

Fig. 53.2 (a,b) Optical coherence tomography over granuloma demonstrating outer retinal involvement from the lesion emerging from the choroid. Associated subretinal fluid is present.

53.2.2 Blood Testing

The current standard testing is an indirect enzyme-linked immunosorbent assay (ELISA) based on the excretory–secretory antigens of *Toxocara canis* and *Toxocara cati*. However, the absence of specific antibodies does not exclude diagnosis as antibodies may be undetectable possibly due to the relatively low parasite numbers. In such cases, the presence of specific antibodies in the aqueous humor can confirm the diagnosis.

53.2.3 Ultrasonography

Ultrasonography is an important ancillary test when fundus examination is not possible due to vitreous opacity and for distinguishing between differential diagnoses, which also present with leukocoria (e.g., calcifications for retinoblastoma and hyaloid remnants for persistent hyperplastic primary vitreous [PHPV]). In cases of severe endophthalmitis, it may demonstrate the inflammatory mass and retinal detachment.

53.3 Critical Work-up

Clinical appearance through slit lamp and indirect ophthalmoscopic examinations are critical to diagnosis as ELISA sensitivity and specificity vary according to the cutoff titer chosen to define a positive test. Differential diagnoses include Coats' disease, retinoblastoma, familial exudative vitreoretinopathy, optic neuritis, persistent fetal vasculature, PHPV, and toxoplasmosis.

53.4 Management

53.4.1 Treatment Options

Medication

For active ocular inflammation, consider topical steroids or periocular injections, and for severe cases, consider oral steroids. Topical cycloplegics may be helpful for severe anterior

segment inflammation and to prevent synechiae formation. The role of anthelmintic therapy is unproven.

Surgery

Pars plana vitrectomy can be performed to obtain vitreous fluid for analysis in cases of unclear etiology, to remove inflammatory tissue, and to treat OT sequelae (e.g., cataracts, epiretinal membranes, retinal detachments, and severe vitreoretinal traction). Surgical removal of subretinal larvae has been reported.

Laser

Laser photocoagulation of mobile subretinal *Toxocara* larvae and to treat choroidal neovascular membrane has been reported.

53.4.2 Follow-up

Consultation with a vitreoretinal specialist and/or pediatric ophthalmologist may be helpful, depending on the need for amblyopia treatment and disease severity. Future prevention should include good hygiene and reduced exposure to contaminated environments.

Suggested Reading

[1] Ehlers JP. Toxocariasis. In JI Maguire et al. Wills Eye Institute Five Minute Opthalmology Consult. Lippincott. 2011.

[2] Hashida N, Nakai K, Nishida K. Diagnostic evaluation of ocular toxocariasis using high-penetration optical coherence tomography. Case Rep Ophthalmol. 2014; 5(1):16–21

[3] Sabrosa NA, Zajdenweber M. Nematode infections of the eye: toxocariasis, onchocerciasis, diffuse unilateral subacute neuroretinitis, and cysticercosis. Ophthalmol Clin North Am. 2002; 15(3):351–356

[4] Shields JA. Ocular toxocariasis. A review. Surv Ophthalmol. 1984; 28(5):361–381

[5] Suzuki T, Joko T, Akao N, Ohashi Y. Following the migration of a Toxocara larva in the retina by optical coherence tomography and fluorescein angiography. Jpn J Ophthalmol. 2005; 49(2):159–161

54 Acute Retinal Necrosis

Jawad I. Arshad and Sunil K. Srivastava

Summary

Acute retinal necrosis (ARN) is occlusive retinitis caused by a viral infection with an associated high risk of vision loss due to macular involvement, retinal detachment, and optic neuropathy. The most common causes of ARN are varicella zoster and herpes simplex viruses. The diagnosis of ARN is based on the presentation of anterior uveitis, vitritis, and the appearance of white- or cream-colored areas of necrotizing retinitis.

Keywords: acute retinal necrosis, herpes zoster, retinal vasculitis, varicella zoster

54.1 Features

Acute retinal necrosis (ARN) is retinitis with occlusive vasculitis caused by a viral infection with an associated high risk of vision loss due to macular involvement, retinal detachment, and optic neuropathy. The most common causes of ARN are varicella zoster and herpes simplex viruses. The American Uveitis Society proposed criteria to establish the clinical diagnosis of ARN. The diagnosis of ARN is based on the presentation of anterior uveitis, vitritis, and the appearance of white- or cream-colored areas of necrotizing retinitis. These areas will often be patchy, can be confluent, and will extend rapidly circumferentially and posteriorly. Retinal detachment is a relatively common side effect of ARN due to diffuse retinal thinning and atrophy and can be seen in up to two-thirds of all patients.

54.1.1 Common Symptoms

May be associated with decreased vision, redness, photophobia, pain, floaters, and flashes. Occasionally, nonocular symptoms of herpetic infection may be present, such as shingles manifesting in the V1 dermatome.

54.1.2 Exam Findings

Anterior chamber findings often reveal cell and keratic precipitates. The vitreous cell is commonly present. Fundus examination will show multiple white- or cream-colored patches of retinitis. Often, intraretinal hemorrhages will be interspersed with retinitis. Vitreous haze is often present, especially in those with a normal immune system (▶ Fig. 54.1). Occlusion of retinal arteries is commonly seen. Atrophic areas of the retina can be seen in those who present with several weeks of symptoms. Retinal detachments can be also seen and are particularly high risk when extensive areas of atrophy are present. Bilateral involvement is common.

54.2 Key Diagnostic Tests and Findings

54.2.1 Optical Coherence Tomography

Optical coherence tomography may demonstrate areas of increased reflectivity in areas of retinal necrosis as well as possible focal hyper-reflective foci in the posterior vitreous, representing areas of vitritis.

54.2.2 Fluorescein Angiography or Ultra-Widefield Fluorescein Angiography

Fluorescein angiography/ultra-widefield fluorescein angiography provides feedback related to overall vascular leakage and extent of nonperfusion. This imaging tool may also be helpful for evaluating treatment response or clinical worsening. Extensive vascular leakage may be present along with nonperfusion in the areas of affected retina.

54.2.3 Fundus Photography

Monitoring early treatment response or clinical worsening can be challenging. Fundus photography, particularly ultra-

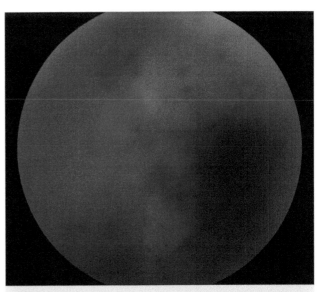

Fig. 54.1 Fundus photograph of the patient with acute retinal necrosis. Vitreous haze prevents a clear view of the retina. Confluent whitening of the retina is present with intraretinal hemorrhage.

widefield imaging, can facilitate disease response to therapeutic intervention and to follow for clinical worsening as well (▶ Fig. 54.2, ▶ Fig. 54.3).

54.3 Critical Work-up

The establishment of the diagnosis in a rapid fashion is critical as the disease can be quickly progressive. Often presumptive treatment may be initiated prior to obtaining positive laboratory findings. Polymerase chain reaction of anterior chamber fluid or vitreous fluid is used to identify the causative virus. The review of systems and targeted laboratory work-up is critical to rule out other infectious causes and to identify potential causes of systemic immune suppression, including human immunodeficiency virus, chemotherapy, or systemic immunosuppressive agents.

54.4 Management

54.4.1 Treatment Options

Pharmacotherapy

Treatment is often initiated with systemic antivirals (IV acyclovir or oral valacyclovir) combined with local intravitreal injections of antivirals (foscarnet or ganciclovir). Following the initiation of antiviral therapy, systemic corticosteroids are often used as adjunctive therapy for the severe inflammation associated with this disease in those who are immunocompetent.

Surgery

Early pars plana vitrectomy is controversial but has been advocated to potentially reduce the risk of retinal detachment, but its effectiveness remains unclear. Surgical repair for retinal detachments in complex usually requires vitrectomy with/ without scleral buckle and endolaser photocoagulation. An extended tamponade with silicone oil is usually needed.

Laser

The role of prophylactic laser is also controversial.

54.4.2 Follow-up

Close follow-up after the presentation is needed to carefully observe the treatment effect and monitor for early retinal detachment. Intravitreal therapy when used is given as often as twice a week. Once inactive, the long-term prognosis is unknown. Cases of contralateral eye involvement occurring years after initial diagnosis have been reported. The use of long-term antiviral prophylaxis is still unclear, though the

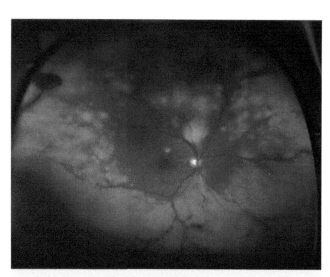

Fig. 54.2 Ultra-widefield fundus photography of immune-compromised patient with varicella zoster virus acute retinal necrosis. Diffuse confluent retinitis is present 360 degrees. A clear view usually indicates an immune-compromised host.

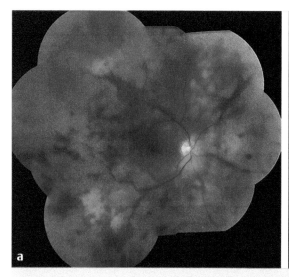
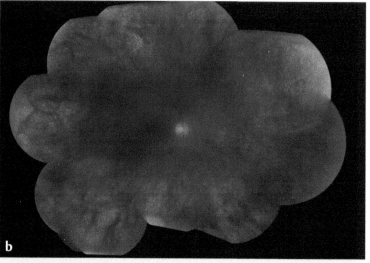

Fig. 54.3 (a) Montage fundus photograph demonstrating extensive retinitis in the patient with varicella zoster virus-associated acute retinal necrosis. (b) Montage fundus photograph following several months of systemic and intravitreal antiviral therapy. Note the pigmentation and thinned peripheral retina.

benefit of protecting the contralateral eye for those who have lost vision in one eye can outweigh the long-term risks associated with antiviral therapy. Lifelong prophylaxis is suggested in patients with comorbid conditions that can cause recurrence as well as those with recurrent infections.

Suggested Reading

[1] Holland GN. Standard diagnostic criteria for the acute retinal necrosis syndrome. Executive Committee of the American Uveitis Society. Am J Ophthalmol. 1994 May; 117(5):663–667

[2] Donovan CP, Levison AL, Lowder CY, Martin DF, Srivastava SK. Delayed recurrence of acute retinal necrosis (ARN): A case series. J Clin Virol. 2016; 80:68–71

[3] Luu KK, Scott IU, Chaudhry NA, Verm A, Davis JL. Intravitreal antiviral injections as adjunctive therapy in the management of immunocompetent patients with necrotizing herpetic retinopathy. Am J Ophthalmol. 2000; 129 (6):811–813

[4] Aizman A, Johnson MW, Elner SG. Treatment of acute retinal necrosis syndrome with oral antiviral medications. Ophthalmology. 2007; 114(2):307–312

[5] Schoenberger SD, Kim SJ, Thorne JE, et al. Diagnosis and treatment of acute retinal necrosis: a report by the American Academy of Ophthalmology. Ophthalmology. 2017; 124(3):382–392

55 Syphilitic Uveitis

Angela J. Verkade and Christina Y. Weng

Summary

Syphilis is often regarded as one of the great masqueraders, as its manifestations in the eye can be easily misinterpreted for those of other more common ocular disorders. However, syphilis remains an important diagnosis on the differential of intraocular inflammation, particularly given that syphilitic infection is on the rise after reaching a nadir in the United States in 2000. In 2013, the rate of primary and secondary syphilis was 5.3 cases per 100,000 Americans and continues to rise, especially in young men who have sex with men. Syphilitic uveitis can occur as little as 6 weeks after initial infection or years later in latent infection. Numerous laboratory studies can aid in the diagnosis of syphilis, but when ocular syphilis is the first presenting sign of disease, a high clinical suspicion combined with a thorough review of systems is required. Ancillary imaging can be helpful, although the diagnosis is made primarily on a clinical and serological basis. While curable if recognized promptly, this condition can lead to permanent loss of vision and systemic complications if treatment is delayed.

Keywords: chorioretinitis, neurosyphilis, penicillin, retinitis, syphilis, Treponema pallidum, uveitis

55.1 Features

Syphilitic uveitis is frequently the presenting manifestation of systemic syphilis caused by the spirochete bacterium *Treponema pallidum*. Primary syphilis is the first stage where patients develop a painless chancre, most commonly located on the genitalia, representing an accumulation of spirochetes that arises 10 to 90 days after inoculation and typically resolves 1 month later. The secondary stage arises 1 to 2 months following the primary stage. Multiple organ systems are involved, and patients can experience fever, headache, malaise, lymphadenopathy, joint pain, mouth ulcers, and characteristic maculopapular rash on the palms and soles. These manifestations typically resolve without intervention. The third stage is the latent phase, an asymptomatic period of indefinite duration. The final phase is the tertiary stage where nearly every organ system is affected. Patients may have gummas or gummata, namely a granulomatous reaction that can occur in skin, liver, bones, heart, brain, or many other tissues. Tertiary syphilis can induce widespread inflammation causing neurologic (e.g., Argyll Robertson pupil and tabes dorsalis) and cardiovascular (e.g., aortic aneurysms and mitral valve insufficiency) complications. Neurosyphilis can occur at any phase of syphilitic infection; any form of ocular involvement should be considered neurosyphilis and treated as such. Syphilitic uveitis can present in many ways, including anterior uveitis, posterior uveitis, panuveitis, vasculitis, and placoid chorioretinitis.

55.1.1 Common Symptoms

Anterior Uveitis

Blurry vision, photophobia, conjunctival injection, headache, epiphora, and pain.

Intermediate Uveitis

Symptoms are similar to those of posterior syphilitic uveitis discussed below.

Posterior Uveitis

Blurry vision, floaters, photopsias, and eye pain.

55.1.2 Exam Findings

Anterior Uveitis

Anterior segment involvement is the most common with granulomatous iridocyclitis, occurring in nearly half of those with ocular syphilis. Syphilitic iridocyclitis may present either as granulomatous inflammation with large keratic precipitates, anterior chamber cell and flare, and iris nodules or as nongranulomatous anterior chamber inflammation. Synechiae, iris atrophy, elevated intraocular pressure, and the rare hypopyon may also be observed. Dilated iris vessels (iris roseolae) occur rarely but are relatively specific for this condition.

Other anterior segment findings include episcleritis, scleritis, or papillary conjunctivitis. Immune-mediated, noninfectious, nonsuppurative interstitial keratitis is considered an immune reaction and can present similarly to anterior uveitis.

Intermediate Uveitis

While syphilitic uveitis can manifest as isolated intermediate uveitis with snowbanks and snowballs in the pars plana, it is much more common to see vitreous inflammation associated with retinal or choroidal inflammation, representing true posterior uveitis.

Posterior Uveitis

T. pallidum is unique in that it can affect all layers of the retina and choroid. As with anterior involvement, posterior uveitis can be focal or diffuse, unilateral, or bilateral. Posterior syphilitic uveitis can manifest as chorioretinitis, vitritis, retinal vasculitis, exudative retinal detachment, panuveitis, and rarely as necrotizing retinitis. Any combination of findings can be seen on examination, including vitreous cell and haze vascular sheathing, retinal whitening, preretinal precipitates, retinal necrosis, chorioretinitis, retinal elevation, hemorrhage, and chorioretinal infiltrate (▶ Fig. 55.1).

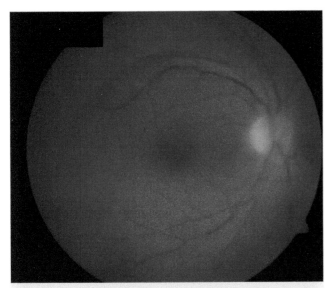

Fig. 55.1 Fundus photograph demonstrating diffuse vitritis with preretinal precipitates and optic nerve head edema.

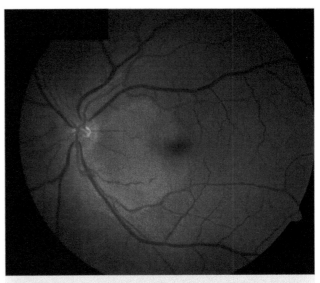

Fig. 55.2 Fundus photograph highlighting a large confluent peripapillary chorioretinal plaque-like infiltrate secondary to syphilis (i.e., posterior placoid chorioretinitis). (Photo courtesy of Petros E. Carvounis, MD.)

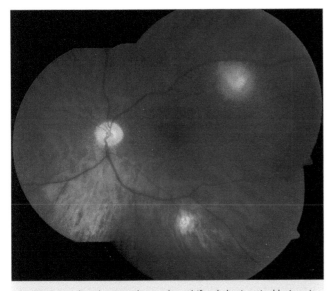

Fig. 55.3 Fundus photograph reveals multifocal chorioretinal lesions in the posterior pole of a patient with syphilitic chorioretinitis. Note the difference in the appearance of the well-circumscribed inactive inferotemporal lesion compared to the creamy active superotemporal lesion with indistinct borders.

Chorioretinitis is a frequent manifestation of posterior syphilitic uveitis. In its confluent form, there are large, multifocal swaths of creamy white retinal infiltrates tending to be similar in size to those seen in viral retinitis, but their cream color differs from the stark white infiltrates classic of viral infections. In the placoid form, more commonly referred to as acute syphilitic posterior placoid chorioretinitis, there is equal involvement of the outer retina and inner choroid. Large, circular, yellowish-gray areas of inflammation present are located in the deep retinal and retinal pigment epithelium (RPE) layers of the posterior

pole and can be singular (▶ Fig. 55.2) or multifocal (▶ Fig. 55.3); they may have overlying vitreous inflammation or even be found adjacent to an area of exudative retinal detachment.

Syphilitic retinitis often presents with a patchy "ground glass" appearance with yellow–white lesions that have indistinct margins and are often associated with retinal vasculitis and vitritis. These lesions can be difficult to differentiate from those of acute retinal necrosis, although they are more likely to affect the posterior pole and tend to have a grayish opacified appearance that differs from the white necrosis seen in herpetic retinitis. Superficial preretinal precipitates are a distinctive clinical pattern of this entity; they are small, creamy white, and may follow the vascular distribution (▶ Fig. 55.4). Areas of the affected retina in syphilitic retinitis tend to heal with minimal disruption of the RPE, but untreated, occlusive vasculitis with resulting complex retinal detachments can occur. Syphilitic occlusive vasculitis can affect arteries, arterioles, capillaries, veins, and venules and may initially present as a nonspecific retinal vein occlusion before eventually progressing to necrotizing retinitis.

In panuveitis and other posterior syphilitic uveitis, the optic disc is commonly affected; the patient may have a relative afferent pupillary defect, and the optic nerve may be swollen with blurred disc margins.

55.2 Key Diagnostic Tests and Findings

55.2.1 Optical Coherence Tomography

Common findings: Preretinal precipitates in syphilitic retinitis, cystoid macular edema, and outer retinal and RPE abnormalities in posterior placoid chorioretinitis (▶ Fig. 55.5); subretinal fluid in exudative retinal detachments. Once the uveitis has resolved, areas of ellipsoid loss may be identified, which may persist in severe disease.

55.2.2 Fluorescein Angiography or Ultra-Widefield Fluorescein Angiography

Posterior involvement may reveal optic disc hyperfluorescence with late leakage or central leakage if macular edema is present. Vasculitis manifests with sheathing and diffuse vascular leakage. In posterior placoid chorioretinitis, plaques may initially appear dark or slightly hyperfluorescent but become progressively more hyperfluorescent as they stain and leak in late frames (▶ Fig. 55.6a). Lesions and late RPE staining resemble leopard spots (also seen once the uveitis resolves due to resultant RPE mottling).

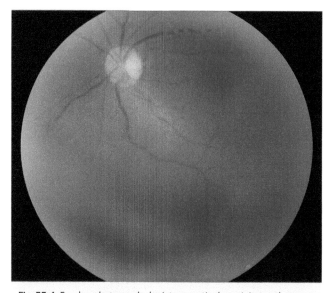

Fig. 55.4 Fundus photograph depicts preretinal precipitates that can be seen in syphilitic retinitis, particularly visible overlying the retinal vessels. Note the vitreous haze from overlying vitritis that is concurrently present. (Photo courtesy of Thomas A. Albini, MD.)

55.2.3 Indocyanine Green Angiography

Both early and late confluent hypocyanescence of placoid lesions are thought to signify profound choroidal inflammation that presumably extinguishes normal choroidal fluorescence due to congestion in areas of vasculitis and can help distinguish this entity from other types of infectious retinitis (▶ Fig. 55.6b). Midperipheral hypercyanescent hotspots and persistent leakage from damaged choroidal vessels may also signify disease chronicity.

55.2.4 Serology

Direct organism detection by polymerase chain reaction of aqueous or vitreous has not been well-studied as a reliable diagnostic method. At present, diagnosis depends on serologic testing for syphilis. The recommended screening algorithm from the Centers for Disease Control and Prevention (CDC) begins with enzyme immunoassays and chemiluminescent immunoassays to detect antibodies to treponemal antigens, followed by reflex testing of positive specimens with a nontreponemal test such as the rapid plasma reagin (RPR). All patients who test positive for syphilis should also be tested for human immunodeficiency virus, given the high prevalence of coinfection.

Nontreponemal Tests

Include RPR and the venereal disease research laboratory tests; if positive, this is considered diagnostic of past or present syphilis.

Treponemal Tests

Include the microhemagglutination assay for *T. pallidum*, fluorescent treponemal antibody absorption, and the *T. pallidum* particle agglutination test, which has largely replaced the former two due to its superior sensitivity and specificity; these tests remain positive for life in infected individuals, but do not necessarily indicate an active infection.

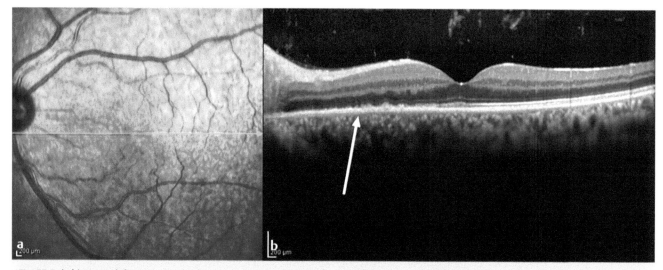

Fig. 55.5 (a,b) Spectral domain optical coherence tomography reveals the area of focal outer retinal, ellipsoid zone, and retinal pigment epithelial atrophy (*arrow*) corresponding to the chorioretinal infiltrate in the patient from ▶ Fig. 55.2. (Courtesy of Petros E. Carvounis, MD.)

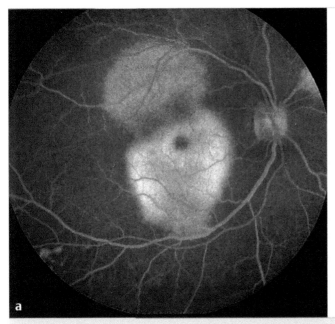
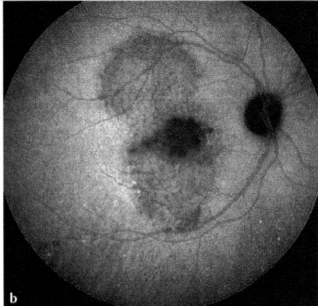

Fig. 55.6 (a) Plaques in posterior placoid chorioretinitis become progressively hyperfluorescent in fluorescein angiography while (b) remaining hypocyanescent even in late indocyanine green angiography. (This image was originally published in the Retina Image Bank website. Author: Annal D. Meleth, MD, MS. Photographer: Kenneth Thompson Title: Syphilis CR/Syphilis Late FA/Syphilis Late ICG. Retina Image Bank. Year: 2017. © the American Society of Retina Specialists.)

55.2.5 Cerebrospinal Fluid Testing

As syphilitic uveitis is considered an extension of neurosyphilis, all affected persons should receive cerebrospinal fluid (CSF) testing. Repeat lumbar punctures should be performed every 6 months until normalized.

55.3 Management

55.3.1 Treatment Options

Penicillin

The favored treatment for all stages. Ocular syphilis with active clinical manifestations should be treated as neurosyphilis and managed with an infectious disease specialist. Adults typically receive aqueous crystalline penicillin G 18 to 24 million units per day administered as 3 to 4 million units intravenously every 4 hours or by continuous infusion for 10 to 14 days. Procaine penicillin 2.4 million units intramuscularly once daily with probenecid 500 mg orally four times per day, both for 10 to 14 days, is an acceptable alternative. Benzathine penicillin 2.4 million units intramuscularly once a week for up to 3 weeks can also be considered. Because penicillin is so effective for syphilis treatment, if a patient is allergic to penicillin, the CDC recommends penicillin desensitization. If the penicillin allergy is life-threatening, doxycycline or tetracycline can be used to treat primary or secondary syphilis. A frequent complication of treatment is the Jarisch–Herxheimer reaction, which is considered to be a type 3 hypersensitivity where an immune complex reaction to treponemal antigens can occur after treatment initiation in approximately one-third of patients. Symptoms consist of a flu-like episode, including fever, chills, headache, malaise, flushing,

and tachycardia. This generally can be treated with supportive care and continuation of penicillin therapy.

Steroids

Benefit is unclear. Topical steroids with cycloplegic drops may assist in controlling anterior inflammation. Intravitreal steroids are rarely used. While there may be a role for oral and periocular steroids (e.g., treatment of associated macular edema), they should only be used once the underlying infection has been treated.

55.3.2 Follow-up

Patients should be followed closely and treated until there is a fourfold decrease in titer of the same nontreponemal test that was used for diagnosis. Additionally, if CSF was initially positive, this should be repeated until a negative result indicates an adequate treatment response. Unfortunately, patients with advanced forms of syphilitic uveitis will often suffer ophthalmic comorbidities such as optic neuropathy, retinal ischemia, cystoid macular edema, or retinal detachment that may preclude visual rehabilitation.

Suggested Reading

[1] Patton ME, Su JR, Nelson R, Weinstock H, Centers for Disease Control and Prevention (CDC). Primary and secondary syphilis—United States, 2005–2013. MMWR Morb Mortal Wkly Rep. 2014; 63(18):402–406

[2] Centers for Disease Control and Prevention. Reverse Sequence Syphilis Screening Webinar. https://www.cdc.gov/STD/Syphilis/RSSS-webinar/Reverse-Sequence-Syphilis-Screening-Webinar.mp4. Accessed October 5, 2017

[3] Davis JL. Ocular syphilis. Curr Opin Ophthalmol. 2014; 25(6):513–518

[4] Workowski KA, Bolan GA, Centers for Disease Control and Prevention. Sexually transmitted diseases treatment guidelines, 2015. MMWR Recomm Rep. 2015; 64 RR-03:1–137

56 Ocular Tuberculosis

Andrea Elizabeth Arriola-López and Thomas A. Albini

Summary

Tuberculosis (TB) infects one-third of the world population, and more than 80% of patients with active tuberculosis are HIV positive and at high risk of developing active disease. Intraocular TB constitutes a very small percentage of uveitis cases in North America and Europe (about 0.5%) but represents a much larger proportion in the developing world (over 30% in some studies in India). In the eye, TB may involve the choroid, retinal vessels, retinal pigment epithelium, outer retina, and vitreous and often two or more structures simultaneously. Clinical presentation includes granulomatous anterior uveitis, intermediate uveitis, and posterior or panuveitis. Routine testing for prior TB exposure includes tuberculous skin testing, an interferon-γ release assay (such as QuantiFERON-TB Gold), or chest X-ray or CT. Multimodal imaging, including optical coherence tomography, fluorescein angiography, fundus autofluorescence, indocyanine green angiography, and ultrasound, is useful as diagnostic tools and for long-term follow-up of the disease. The Center for Disease Control and Prevention recommends a four-drug anti-TB treatment regimen of isoniazid, rifampicin, ethambutol, and pyrazinamide for patients with active tuberculosis.

Keywords: granuloma, intraocular, mycobacteria, QuantiFERON, Tuberculoma, Tuberculosis, Uveitis, serpiginous-like

56.1 Features

Mycobacterium tuberculosis (MTB) infects one-third of the world's population. In the United States, the overall case rate of active TB is rare. Foreign-born persons constitute approximately two-thirds of those cases and as a group had 13 times higher incidence rate than those born in the United States (15.6 vs. 1.2 per 100,000 persons). Human immunodeficiency virus (HIV) positive patients are also at high risk of developing active disease.

The reported prevalence of intraocular tuberculosis (IOTB) varies from 1% in patients with pulmonary TB to over 20% in those with extrapulmonary infection. IOTB accounts for 0.5% of uveitis cases without a known active systemic disease. There are two possible pathophysiological mechanisms: active mycobacterial infection (hematogenous spread of TB into local ocular tissues [choroidal granuloma] or direct exogenous infection of TB into local ocular tissues [conjunctivitis/scleritis/keratitis]) and immunological response without local replication of the infectious agent causing delayed hypersensitivity reaction to TB situated elsewhere in the body (e.g., conjunctival phlyctenule/Eales disease).

56.1.1 Common Symptoms

Systemic

Mostly asymptomatic; cough (sometimes blood-tinged), weight loss, night sweats, and fever when symptoms present.

Ocular

Most commonly blurred vision and light sensitivity.

56.1.2 Exam Findings

Anterior Segment Findings

Broad posterior synechiae, necrotizing and non-necrotizing diffuse or nodular scleritis, episcleritis, and peripheral ulcerative keratitis. Other rare forms can include interstitial keratitis, phlyctenulosis, iris or ciliary body granulomas, and dacryoadenitis.

Posterior Segment Findings

Posterior uveitis is the most common presentation; may manifest as choroidal tubercles, occlusive retinal vasculitis (affecting venous structures, includes chorioretinal inflammation adjacent to the involved vessels), serpiginous-like choroiditis or multifocal serpiginoid choroiditis (MSC), choroidal or optic disc granuloma(s), and optic neuropathy (papillitis, neuroretinitis, and retrobulbar optic neuropathy) (▶ Fig. 56.1).

Retinal Perivasculitis and Multifocal Serpiginoid Choroiditis

Strongly suggestive of ocular tuberculosis.

Choroidal Tuberculomas

Identified in the context of systemic TB (pulmonary/extrapulmonary). Choroidal granulomas may be unifocal or multifocal; typically, white-, cream-, or yellow-colored and may be associated with an exudative retinal detachment.

56.2 Key Diagnostic Tests and Findings

56.2.1 Optical Coherence Tomography

TB choroidal granulomas present as a localized area of adhesion between the retinal pigment epithelium (RPE)–choriocapillaris layer and the overlying neurosensory retina ("contact sign"), surrounded by an area of exudative retinal detachment. Anterior segment optical coherence tomography of anterior lesions reveals a poorly demarcated amorphous lesion in the iridocorneal angle, corneal edema, narrowing and synechiae of the iridocorneal angle, anterior chamber exudates, and cells in presumed ocular TB. Active areas reveal irregular disruption of the outer retinal hyper-reflective bands associated with both the photoreceptors and RPE, as well as pronounced thickening of the underlying choroid. Granularity of the outer photoreceptor layer and proliferating RPE cells indicate the chronicity of the underlying choroidal pathology in cases of TB choroidal

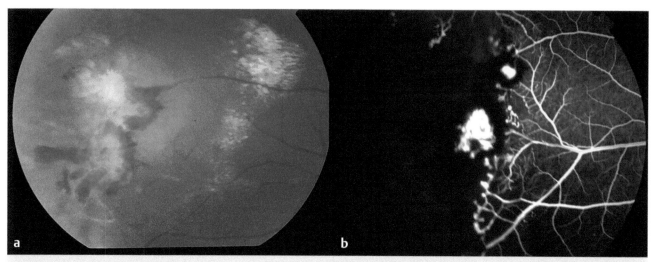

Fig. 56.1 (a) Fundus photograph demonstrating a temporal midperipheral fibrovascular proliferation along with sclerosed blood vessels. (b) Fluorescein angiography shows the area of capillary nonperfusion and hyperfluorescence from the leaking neovascularization. (Courtesy of J. Fernando Arevalo, MD.)

granulomas. Inactive areas show atrophy of the outer retina and underlying choroid.

56.2.2 Fluorescein Angiography or Ultra-Widefield Fluorescein Angiography

Active choroidal granulomas exhibit early hypofluorescence and late hyperfluorescence (▶ Fig. 56.2a,c). Inactive healed tubercles show transmission hyperfluorescence (▶ Fig. 56.2b, d). Large choroidal granulomas may show early hyperfluorescence with a dilated capillary bed, progressive increase in hyperfluorescence, and late pooling of dye in the subretinal space. Serpiginous-like choroiditis shows an initial hypofluorescent active edge with late hyperfluorescence and diffuse staining of the active advancing edge. Active retinal vasculitis shows focal or diffuse staining and leakage from the retinal vasculature, mainly from the veins, and optic disc hyperfluorescence (associated with focal or diffuse capillary leakage), and also identifies the extent of areas of capillary nonperfusion, as well as retinal (border of inactive lesion) and/or optic disc neovascularization. Papillitis and neuroretinitis show early optic disc hyperfluorescence with leakage in the late frames. Fluorescein angiography is also useful in identifying cystoid macular edema characterized by progressive leakage and accumulation of dye in cystic spaces surrounding the fovea with a characteristic "petaloid pattern." Ultra-widefield fluorescein angiography identifies the entire extent of choroidal lesions, areas of retinal capillary nonperfusion, peripheral neovascularization, and detection of disease activity (▶ Fig. 56.1a,b).

56.2.3 Indocyanine Green Angiography

Choroidal granulomas are oval or round hypocyanescent lesions during the dye transit and become isocyanent during the late phases. If the granuloma is occupying full thickness of choroidal stroma, it remains hypocyanescent throughout the study (> 90% granulomas are full thickness). Lesions of tuberculous serpiginous-like choroiditis or MSC lesions manifest as irregular-shaped hypocyanescent lesions during the early and late phases. In the healed stage, indocyanine green angiography shows better delineation of the atrophic choroid.

56.2.4 Fundus Autofluorescence

Four stages in the evolution of tuberculous serpiginoid-like choroiditis have been described. Stage I has acute lesions characterized by a diffuse amorphous halo of hyper-autofluorescence that last for 2 to 4 weeks. Stage II has lesions with well-demarcated hypo-autofluorescent border. During stage III as lesions heal, they acquire predominantly mottled hypo-autofluorescence with some granular hyper-autofluorescence. In stage IV, completely healed lesions/atrophic areas become uniformly hypo-autofluorescent.

56.2.5 Optical Coherence Tomography Angiography

Active tubercular serpiginous-like choroiditis shows choriocapillaris flow void areas (suggestive of hypoperfusion or sluggish flow) appearing as well-delineated hyporeflective zones with few preserved islands of choriocapillaris in the center of the lesion. As the lesions heal, medium-to-large choroidal vessels in the choriocapillaris zone on en face optical coherence tomography angiography can be visualized.

56.2.6 Fundus Photography

Color photographs show choroidal tubercles, solitary choroidal tuberculoma, serpiginous-like choroiditis or MSC, retinal vasculitis, and optic neuropathy. Serial fundus photography (from acute stage to the stage of healing) is useful in the assessment of morphologic evolution of the lesions and detection of vitreous haze.

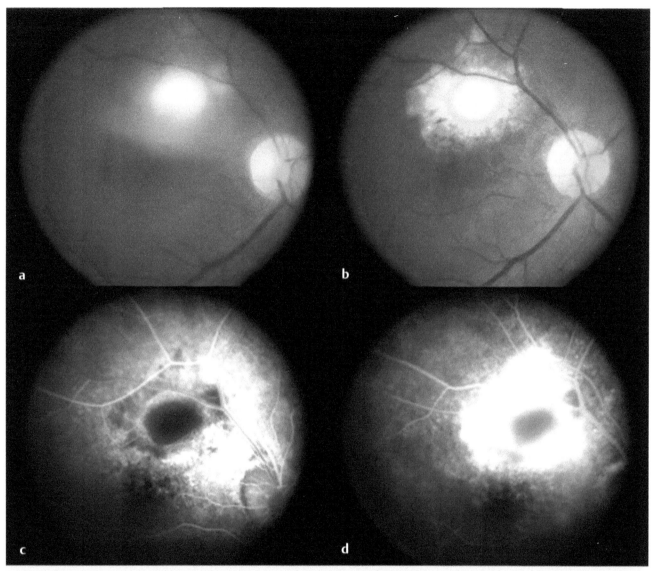

Fig. 56.2 Ocular tuberculosis. **(a)** Fundus color photograph demonstrating active white/yellowish lesion underneath temporal vessels. **(b)** Same eye with healed lesion, pigmentary changes around and radial folds involving the fovea. **(c)** Fluorescein angiography (FA) shows hypofluorescence corresponding to the active lesion. **(d)** FA demonstrates hyperfluorescence around the healed lesion.

56.2.7 Slit Lamp Photography

Documents features such as granulomatous anterior uveitis, mutton-fat keratic precipitates, broad-based posterior synechiae, Koeppe and/or Busacca nodules with mild-to-moderate inflammation, hypopyon, and endophthalmitis-like pictures.

56.2.8 Ultrasonography

Ocular ultrasound B-scan and ultrasound biomicroscopy may present iris or ciliary body masses. Ultrasonographic appearance of choroidal granuloma may show low-to-moderate internal reflectivity.

56.3 Critical Work-up

Routine testing for prior TB exposure includes tuberculous skin testing, interferon-γ release assay, and/or chest X-ray or CT (positive predictive value in excess of 90%, exposure is by no means equivalent to active infection). Microbiological confirmation of MTB might include a positive culture, histological identification of acid-fast bacilli, or polymerase chain reaction (PCR)-based amplification of MTB deoxyribonucleic acid. PCR-based testing might be more likely to be positive in eyes with highly suggestive clinical findings, including retinal vasculitis with vitreous hemorrhage and choroiditis. The gold standard to establish the diagnosis of ocular TB remains a positive culture from the eye.

Diagnosis of presumed ocular TB is made when ocular PCR and/or cultures are negative or lacking in the presence of active uveitis and positive QuantiFERON test (or purified protein derivative [PPD]) and no other kind of uveitis is likely. Supportive criteria include fundus findings consistent with TB (e.g., granuloma, serpiginous-like, retinal vasculitis with areas of multiple, pigmented chorioretinal atrophy along blood vessels), suggestive systemic investigation (e.g., chest imaging and evidence of extrapulmonary TB), known lifetime exposure, endemic origin, and magnitude of PPD or QuantiFERON. Differential diagnosis to consider includes sarcoidosis, syphilis, Lyme disease, HIV, Vogt–Koyanagi–Harada syndrome, amelanotic malignant melanomas (by ultrasound), and serpiginous choroiditis.

56.4 Management

56.4.1 Treatment Options

Systemic management should be coordinated with an infectious disease specialist. The gold standard for dosage of anti-TB treatment (ATT) treatment of pulmonary and extrapulmonary TB is rifampin (450 mg/d if body weight [BW] 50 kg or 600 mg/d if BW > 50 kg), isoniazid (5 mg/kg/d), ethambutol (15 mg/kg/d), and pyrazinamide (25–30 mg/kg/d). Rifampicin alone can lead to MTB resistance. Topical fluoroquinolones (moxifloxacin/ofloxacin) are well-tolerated and well-established ocular therapeutics for ocular surface infection. The Center for Disease Control and Prevention recommends a four-drug ATT regimen for a minimum of 2 months (up to 3–4 months), with subsequent administration of two-drug therapy (isoniazid and rifampicin), for a minimum of 4 months (up to 15 months). Some of the side effects of ATT include liver damage, rash, reduced libido, and general malaise. Corticosteroids are often used along with ATT.

56.4.2 Follow-up

Dependent on specific ocular manifestations, the severity of disease, and risk of vision loss. In general, frequent follow-up with serial multimodal imaging to document progression or regression is essential.

Suggested Reading

[1] Cunningham ET, Jr, Rathinam SR, Albini TA, Chee S-P, Zierhut M. Tuberculous uveitis. Ocul Immunol Inflamm. 2015; 23(1)–2–6

[2] Kee AR, Gonzalez-Lopez JJ, Al-Hity A, et al. Anti-tubercular therapy for intraocular tuberculosis: A systematic review and meta-analysis. Surv Ophthalmol. 2016; 61(5):628–653

[3] Yeh S, Sen HN, Colyer M, Zapor M, Wroblewski K. Update on ocular tuberculosis. Curr Opin Ophthalmol. 2012; 23(6):551–556

[4] Agarwal A, Mahajan S, Khairallah M, Mahendradas P, Gupta A, Gupta V. Multimodal Imaging in Ocular Tuberculosis. Ocul Immunol Inflamm. 2017; 25(1): 134–145

57 Cytomegalovirus Retinitis

Heather M. Tamez and Stephen J. Kim

Summary

Cytomegalovirus (CMV) retinitis remains the most common ocular opportunistic infection in patients with human immunodeficiency virus (HIV) and acquired immunodeficiency syndrome (AIDS), and it can also occur in patients with other causes of immune system compromise. Up to 50% of patients are asymptomatic upon diagnosis while others typically note blurred vision, scotomata, ocular discomfort, and floaters. CMV retinitis is diagnosed clinically based on the relevant patient history of HIV/AIDS or immunosuppression and findings on ophthalmic exam. Three classic patterns of retinitis are recognized: fulminant/edematous, indolent/granular, and frosted branch angiitis. Testing of intraocular fluid for CMV DNA by polymerase chain reaction can aid in establishing the diagnosis in uncertain cases and can be useful when monitoring for disease recurrence. The mainstays of the treatment of CMV retinitis are immune reconstitution, particularly with highly active antiretroviral therapy (HAART) in HIV/AIDS patients, and treatment with systemic antiviral medications. Systemic treatment is not only adequate for treating ocular disease but it also reduces the risk of overall mortality, second eye involvement, and visceral CMV disease. Despite adequate treatment, all patients require regular ophthalmic follow-up after diagnosis of CMV retinitis as patients remain at risk for vision loss related to retinitis progression, retinal detachments, or immune reconstitution uveitis (IRU) even years after initial diagnosis.

Keywords: antiviral therapy, cytomegalovirus, HAART, HIV/AIDS, immunosuppression, immune reconstitution uveitis, posterior uveitis, retinitis

57.1 Features

Cytomegalovirus (CMV) retinitis occurs most frequently in patients with severe immunocompromise as a consequence of acquired immunodeficiency syndrome (AIDS) and is the most common ocular opportunistic infection among these patients. It can also occur in patients with other forms of immunosuppression such as iatrogenic immunosuppression following organ transplantation, hematologic malignancies, and diabetes mellitus. It rarely reported to occur in apparently healthy individuals.

57.1.1 Common Symptoms

CMV retinitis may be asymptomatic in up to 50% of cases. Blurred vision, ocular discomfort, scotomata, and floaters may occur. Complaints characteristic of acute uveitis including pain, photophobia, and redness are typically absent in CMV retinitis.

57.1.2 Exam Findings

CMV retinitis typically presents along with mild anterior chamber inflammation that can include keratic precipitates as well as very mild if any vitritis. Three patterns of classic active retinal lesions have been described. Atypical findings such as severe intraocular inflammation, elevated intraocular pressure, retinal arteritis, and acute retinal necrosis-like retinitis may be more common in patients with CMV retinitis without human immunodeficiency virus (HIV).

Necrotizing

Fulminant hemorrhagic retinitis in the background of retinal necrosis (▶ Fig. 57.1).

Nonnecrotizing

More indolent, granular satellite lesions with little or no hemorrhage. This presentation, in particular, is nearly pathognomonic for CMV retinitis (▶ Fig. 57.2).

Exudative/Frosted Branch Angiitis

Extensive vascular (primarily venous) sheathing (▶ Fig. 57.3).

57.2 Key Diagnostic Tests and Findings

57.2.1 Fundus Photography

CMV retinitis is primarily diagnosed clinically based on relevant patient history (HIV/AIDS status or other immunosuppression) and standard ophthalmic exam. Fundus photography, particularly ultra-widefield imaging, allows for careful documentation to aid in monitoring for treatment response and reactivation or extension as may be evidenced by the extension of active lesions or the appearance of new lesions.

57.2.2 Viral Testing

Detection of CMV DNA by polymerase chain reaction (PCR) in intraocular fluid helps to confirm the diagnosis of CMV retinitis in atypical cases. PCR analysis of intraocular fluid can also aid in the monitoring of treatment response in cases initially diagnosed on clinical grounds.

57.3 Management

57.3.1 Treatment Options

The foundation of treatment for CMV retinitis is addressing the underlying immunodeficiency, if possible. For patients with HIV/AIDS, this means initiating highly active antiretroviral therapy (HAART) in HAART-naive patients and looking for antiviral resistance in patients with low CD4 counts despite appropriate HAART treatment. In patients with iatrogenic immunosuppression, this means reducing these treatments as much as is clinically feasible.

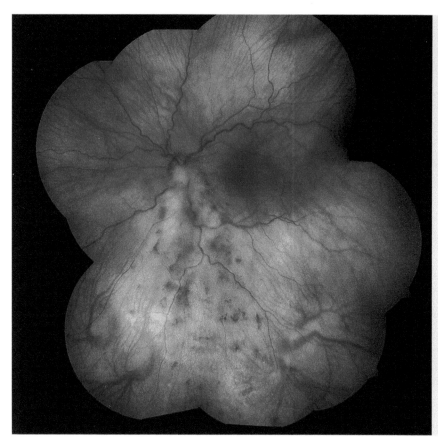

Fig. 57.1 Fundus photograph of hemorrhagic retinitis involving the optic nerve in a patient with cytomegalovirus retinitis in the setting of human immunodeficiency virus.

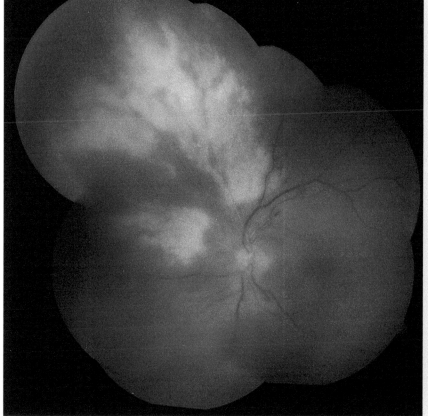

Fig. 57.2 Fundus photograph of classic granular, nonhemorrhagic retinitis of the left eye with satellite lesions in a patient with cytomegalovirus retinitis in the setting of immunosuppression.

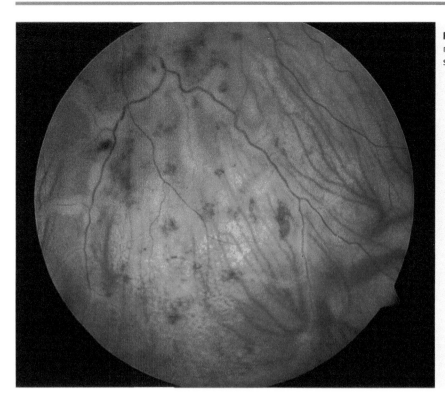

Fig. 57.3 Fundus photograph of hemorrhagic retinitis with extensive primarily venous sheathing.

The treatment of CMV retinitis with antiviral therapy should be systemic (with or without concomitant intraocular therapy). Compared with patients receiving only intraocular therapy for CMV retinitis, those treated with systemic therapy benefited from a 50% reduction in mortality, an 80% reduction in the rate of second eye disease, and a 90% reduction in the incidence of visceral CMV disease. Options for systemic therapy include ganciclovir, valganciclovir, foscarnet, and cidofovir. Systemic therapy may be discontinued when appropriate immune reconstitution has taken place; in patients with HIV/AIDS, this is typically defined as CD4+T-cell count of greater than 100 cells/μL for greater than 6 months. The treatment with intravitreal antivirals is often considered at the discretion of the treating physician, especially in cases of immediately vision-threatening retinitis; however, intraocular treatment does not preclude the necessity of systemic antiviral medications.

57.3.2 Follow-up

Visual and overall prognosis vary significantly, depending upon whether or not a patient is able to achieve immune reconstitution. The regular ophthalmic follow-up to monitor retinitis progression and other complications, including involvement of the contralateral eye, epiretinal membrane formation, retinal neovascularization, cataract formation, optic atrophy, retinal detachments, and immune reconstitution uveitis (IRU) is important. No level of immune reconstitution appears to be fully protective—in a recent study, retinitis progression and complications leading to vision loss all occurred in some patients with CD4 counts of greater than 200 cells/μL. Even

when managed promptly and appropriately, CMV retinitis can lead to rhegmatogenous retinal detachments in up to 30% of patients. Retinal breaks occur in areas of thinned, necrotic retina and can occur when the disease is no longer active. Retinal detachments related to CMV retinitis are often challenging to repair due to the thinned, necrotic tissue and multiple breaks that are characteristic; the use of scleral buckling and silicone oil are often necessary and visual outcomes may be poor. IRU may occur in cases of CMV retinitis following the recovery of immune system function. Risks for the development of IRU include severity of CMV retinitis and treatment with cidofovir. Sequelae of IRU include epiretinal membrane formation, development of cystoid macular edema, retinal neovascularization, cataract formation, and proliferative vitreoretinopathy, all of which can lead to secondary vision loss.

Suggested Reading

[1] Jabs DA, Ahuja A, Van Natta M, Lyon A, Srivastava S, Gangaputra S, Studies of the Ocular Complications of AIDS Research Group. Course of cytomegalovirus retinitis in the era of highly active antiretroviral therapy: five-year outcomes. Ophthalmology. 2010; 117(11):2152–61.e1, 2

[2] Jabs DA, Ahuja A, Van Natta M, Dunn JP, Yeh S, Studies of the Ocular Complications of AIDS Research Group. Comparison of treatment regimens for cytomegalovirus retinitis in patients with AIDS in the era of highly active antiretroviral therapy. Ophthalmology. 2013; 120(6):1262–1270

[3] Lee JH, Agarwal A, Mahendradas P, et al. Viral posterior uveitis. Surv Ophthalmol. 2017; 62(4):404–445

[4] Pathanapitoon K, Tesavibul N, Choopong P, et al. Clinical manifestations of cytomegalovirus-associated posterior uveitis and panuveitis in patients without human immunodeficiency virus infection. JAMA Ophthalmol. 2013; 131 (5):638–645

58 Human Immunodeficiency Virus Retinopathy

Waseem H. Ansari and Justis P. Ehlers

Summary

Ocular features of human immunodeficiency virus (HIV) were first identified in the 1980s. The most common ocular manifestation of HIV is noninfectious occlusive microangiopathy, more commonly known as HIV retinopathy. This pathology is the result of ischemic changes in the retinal nerve fiber layer, resulting in intraretinal hemorrhages and cotton wool spots. HIV retinopathy has been shown to affect almost 50% of patients with acquired immunodeficiency syndrome and 3% of patients with asymptomatic HIV infection. It is difficult to know the true incidence of HIV retinopathy as it is likely underreported due to its asymptomatic presentation. The cause of HIV retinopathy is unknown; various theories have proposed a primary cause involving direction infection of vascular endothelial cells versus a secondary cause involving immune complex deposition or an increased hypercoagulable state.

Keywords: cotton wool spots, HIV retinopathy, telangiectasias

58.1 Features

Ocular features of human immunodeficiency virus (HIV) were first identified in the 1980s. The most common ocular manifestation of HIV is noninfectious occlusive microangiopathy, more commonly known as HIV retinopathy. This pathology is the result of ischemic changes in the retinal nerve fiber layer, resulting in intraretinal hemorrhages and cotton wool spots. HIV retinopathy has been shown to affect almost 58% of patients with acquired immunodeficiency syndrome and 3% of patients with asymptomatic HIV infection. It is difficult to know the true incidence of HIV retinopathy as it is likely underreported due to its asymptomatic presentation. The cause of HIV retinopathy is unknown; various theories have proposed a primary cause involving direction infection of vascular endothelial cells versus a secondary cause involving immune complex deposition or an increased hypercoagulable state.

58.1.1 Common Symptoms

Most remain asymptomatic; potential symptoms include subtle loss of color vision and/or contrast sensitivity, visual field deficits, and subnormal electrophysiological responses thought to occur due to the microischemic infarcts in the retinal nerve fiber layer, which can cause subjective visual changes.

58.1.2 Exam Findings

The most common exam findings are those similar to any occlusive vasculitic disease and can include cotton wool spots, microaneurysms, telangiectatic vascular changes, or intraretinal hemorrhages. Cotton wool spots, seen as fluffy white lesions, are the most characteristic and involve ischemic changes of the nerve fiber layer thought to be caused by retinal vascular disease (▶ Fig. 58.1). They are the earliest sign of HIV retinopathy and seen in approximately half of the patients who have advanced HIV disease. Some studies have also demonstrated increased tortuosity of retinal arterioles and decreased retinal arteriolar caliber compared to normal healthy subjects. Rarely, retinal vascular occlusions have been observed in patients with HIV without any other risk factors.

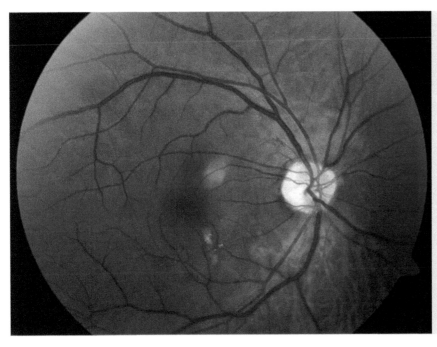

Fig. 58.1 Fundus photograph of human immunodeficiency virus retinopathy, demonstrating retinal whitening and vascular telangiectatic changes.

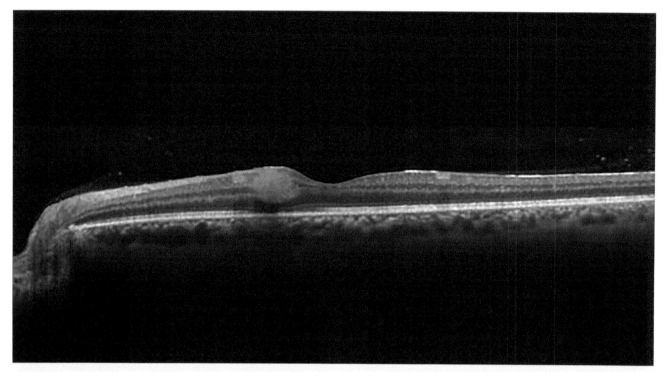

Fig. 58.2 Optical coherence tomography of the retina, demonstrating localized thickening of the inner retina with hyper-reflectivity with shadowing of the outer retina correlating to the area of ischemic changes from human immunodeficiency virus retinopathy.

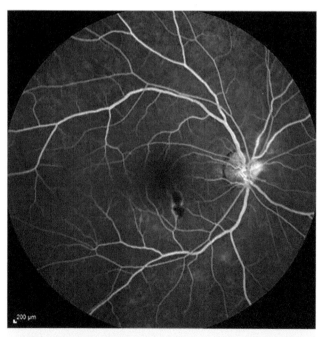

Fig. 58.3 Fluorescein angiogram of the right eye of a patient with human immunodeficiency virus retinopathy. The hypofluorescent area inferior to the fovea is being blocked due to whitening from the cotton wool spot and nonperfusion.

58.2 Key Diagnostic Tests and Findings

58.2.1 Optical Coherence Tomography

Demonstrates similar findings to those in other arterial occlusive diseases. Inner retina is hyper-reflective, causing shadowing of the outer retina with loss of detail in affected areas (▶ Fig. 58.2). These hyper-reflective areas generally correlate to the cotton wool spots seen on retinal examination. Over time, the inner retina can become atrophic and thin due to the chronic retinovascular disease. Cone photoreceptor density is rarely reduced with ellipsoid zone disruption.

58.2.2 Fluorescein Angiography or Ultra-Widefield Fluorescein Angiography

Demonstrate microvascular changes with widespread microaneurysms being the most common, followed by telangiectatic vessels (▶ Fig. 58.3). Both retinal arterial and vein occlusions have been noted in rare cases. Any signs of retinal leakage or vasculitis should draw concern for infectious etiologies.

58.2.3 Optical Coherence Tomography Angiography

Recent studies demonstrate retinal vascular telangiectasias, capillary loops, decreased retinal vascular flow density, and an enlarged foveal avascular zone in patients with clinical evidence of HIV retinopathy. Choroidal vasculature appears unaffected.

58.3 Critical Work-up

HIV retinopathy is generally benign; however, infectious causes of retinopathy must be ruled out. On exam, the cotton wool spots can be differentiated from the infectious retinal whitening from causes such as cytomegalovirus or toxoplasmosis by their appearance. Infectious causes of retinitis can progress rapidly and lead to vision loss through retinal necrosis or devastating complications such as retinal detachments. The cotton wool spots in noninfectious retinopathy tend to be more superficial, have sharp margins, are nonprogressive, and tend to resolve in weeks to months without any treatment. Lesions in infectious retinopathy tend to be larger in size and can be accompanied by inflammatory signs such as vitreous cell and vascular sheathing. If there is suspicion for an infectious etiology, the diagnostic tap should be performed with injection of anti-ineffective agents as needed. Additionally, patients should be referred to appropriate services for the management of HIV, as needed.

58.4 Management

58.4.1 Treatment Options

No treatments are indicated for the diagnosis of HIV retinopathy. Close monitoring for resolution of lesions is indicated.

Additionally, the presence of HIV microangiopathy has been associated with increased mortality. CD4 count is an important predictor of HIV disease; thus, highly active antiretroviral therapy has shown to decrease the incidence of HIV-related ocular complications.

58.4.2 Follow-up

Patients with cotton wool spots should have close follow-up initially to confirm resolution. Cotton wool spots and intraretinal hemorrhages generally resolve without any severe complications. Any patients with signs of progression or the development of newer or aggressive lesions should be worked up to rule out vision-threatening infectious retinitis. Some evidence has shown that progressive visual changes can develop related to changes in the retinal pigment epithelium due to chronic retinal microvascular changes, but these are uncommon. Most patients recover without any permanent visual changes.

Suggested Reading

[1] Lai TY, Wong RL, Luk FO, Chow VW, Chan CK, Lam DS. Ophthalmic manifestations and risk factors for mortality of HIV patients in the post-highly active anti-retroviral therapy era. Clin Exp Ophthalmol. 2011; 39(2):99–104

[2] Mowatt L. Ophthalmic manifestations of HIV in the highly active anti-retroviral therapy era. West Indian Med J. 2013; 62(4):305–312

[3] Plummer DJ, Sample PA, Arévalo JF, et al. Visual field loss in HIV-positive patients without infectious retinopathy. Am J Ophthalmol. 1996; 122(4): 542–549

[4] Arcinue CA, Bartsch DU, El-Emam SY, et al. Retinal Thickening and Photoreceptor Loss in HIV Eyes without Retinitis. PLoS One. 2015; 10(8):e0132996

[5] Riva AAIA, Agrawal R, Jain S, et al. Analysis of Retinochoroidal Vasculature in Human Immunodeficiency Virus Infection Using Spectral-Domain OCT Angiography. Ophthalmol Retina. 2017; 1(6):545–554

59 West Nile Retinopathy

Ijeoma S. Chinwuba and Yasha S. Modi

Summary

West Nile retinopathy is a relatively new disease entity with distinctive ophthalmic manifestations. Newer imaging modalities such as spectral domain optical coherence tomography and ultra-widefield angiography have enabled more detailed study of patterns of West Nile-associated chorioretinitis to study its mechanism of disease. While some transient manifestations can be addressed with symptomatic management, there are other complications such as ischemic retinopathy and optic neuropathy that do not have a specific treatment and may limit visual prognosis.

Keywords: chorioretinitis, occlusive vasculitis, posterior uveitis, West Nile virus

59.1 Features

West Nile virus (WNV) is a zoonotic disease due to a single-stranded RNA flavivirus of the same family as Japanese encephalitis, St. Louis encephalitis, and yellow fever. WNV was first described in Uganda in 1937 and the first case in the Western Hemisphere was reported in 1999 in New York City. Demonstration of ophthalmic involvement was first reported in 2003. One study found 24% of patients with WNV had WNV retinopathy.

59.1.1 Common Symptoms

Ocular

Blurred vision, photophobia, floaters, and diplopia. Vision ranges from normal to moderate–severe impairment and often returns to near baseline. Optic neuropathy, choroidal neovascularization, and vision loss from the occlusive retinal vascular disease have been reported.

Systemic

Most are asymptomatic (i.e., 80%), while approximately 20% develop WN fever and experience high-grade fever, lymphadenopathy, headache, malaise, myalgia, nausea and vomiting, and/or gastrointestinal disorders. WN meningoencephalitis may cause altered mental status and signs of aseptic meningitis. Meningoencephalitis is associated with higher risk of WNV retinopathy. Risk of developing WNV meningoencephalitis is associated with advanced age or the presence of diabetes and mortality is 5 to 10% of patients with the neuroinvasive disease. In addition, the severity of ophthalmic manifestations has also been linked to diabetes.

59.1.2 Exam Findings

Bilateral retinopathy is more common than unilateral lesions and is typically self-limited. Diabetes is a potential risk factor for multifocal chorioretinitis and advanced age is associated with prolonged recovery. Reported ocular presentations of WNV include chorioretinitis, anterior uveitis without focal lesions, occlusive retinal vasculitis and retinal hemorrhages (which may lead to permanent field defects and vision loss), congenital chorioretinal scarring in children born to previously infected mothers, disc edema or optic atrophy (possibly due to mononuclear perivascular inflammation and subsequent occlusion of the posterior ciliary vessels), and sixth nerve palsy.

Chorioretinitis staging is as follows:

- Acute stage: Deep, creamy yellow multifocal nummular chorioretinal lesions with a scattered or circumlinear distribution and an average diameter of 250 μm (range 100–1,500 μm); typically in the midperiphery and may be associated with vitritis.

Chorioretinal streaks in a circumlinear distribution have been variably described but are also seen in multifocal choroiditis and ocular histoplasmosis syndrome. Anterior segment findings may include self-limited uveitis.

- Subacute stage: Pigmentation begins and a cream halo may remain.
- Convalescent stage: Atrophic lesions with sharp margins (▶ Fig. 59.1, ▶ Fig. 59.2).

59.2 Key Diagnostic Tests and Findings

59.2.1 Optical Coherence Tomography

Optical coherence tomography demonstrates deep hyper-reflective lesions extending from the outer nuclear layer to the level of the retinal pigment epithelium (RPE) with associated disruption of the ellipsoid zone in areas of active lesions. Granular hyper-reflective specks at the level of the inner and outer nuclear layers that resolve over the first few weeks after infection are possible. Macular edema is variably present. Areas of outer retinal atrophy and RPE atrophy may be present in areas of previous lesions (▶ Fig. 59.3).

59.2.2 Fluorescein Angiography or Ultra-Widefield Fluorescein Angiography

Findings depend on the age of lesion: early hypofluorescence with late staining in the acute stage, "target lesions" (central hypofluorescence with peripheral hyperfluorescence) in the subacute stage, and uniform window defects with staining in the convalescent stage. Lesions may be more prominent on angiography than on exam and frequently demonstrate a radial or linear arrangement, even appearing "laser like" on diagnostic testing (▶ Fig. 59.2, ▶ Fig. 59.4, ▶ Fig. 59.5).

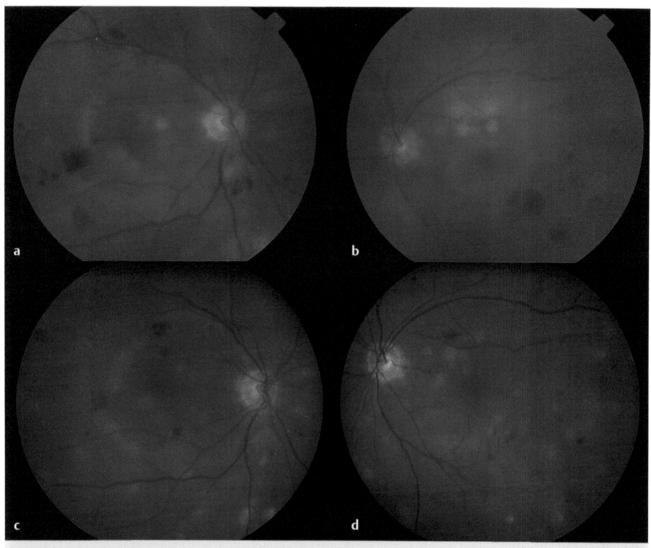

Fig. 59.1 (a,b) Color fundus photograph of acute West Nile chorioretinitis in the right and left eyes, demonstrating yellow chorioretinal lesions, retinal hemorrhages, and vitritis. **(c,d)** Following the resolution of disease activity, chorioretinal lesions are more distinct with some more pigmented and others more depigmented. Vitritis has improved.

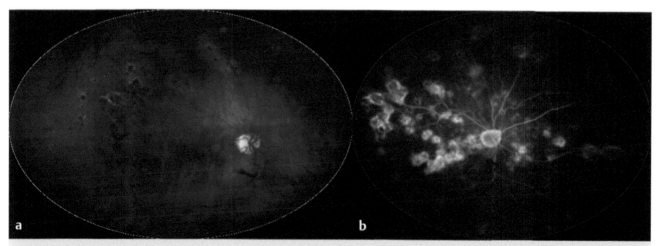

Fig. 59.2 (a) Ultra-widefield fundus photograph of convalescent stage of West Nile retinopathy. **(b)** Ultra-widefield fluorescein angiography of convalescent stage of West Nile retinopathy with staining and window defects related to the chorioretinal lesions.

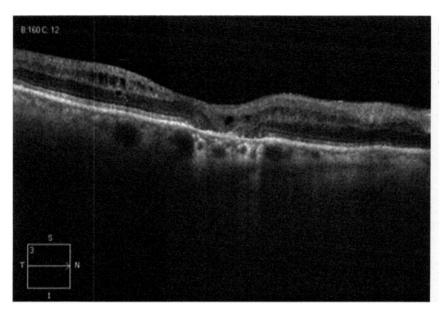

Fig. 59.3 Spectral domain OCT B-scan in convalescent stage of West Nile retinopathy with associated mild macular edema. Outer retinal and retinal pigment epithelium atrophy is present overlying a previous active lesion.

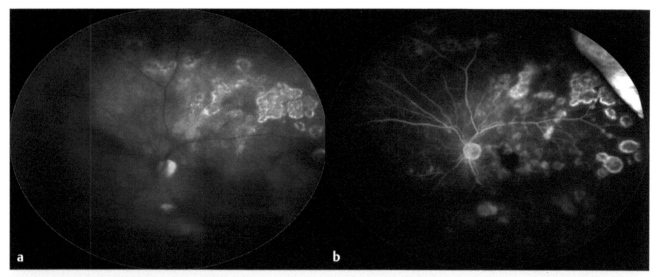

Fig. 59.4 **(a)** Ultra-widefield fundus photograph of convalescent stage of West Nile retinopathy with hyperpigmented discrete "laser-like" lesions. **(b)** Ultra-widefield fluorescein angiography of convalescent stage of West Nile retinopathy with staining and window defects related to the chorioretinal lesions.

59.2.3 Indocyanine Green Angiography

Acute lesions are distinctly hypocyanescent both early and late in the transit window, suggesting possible blocking of the cyanescence from the RPE/outer retinal lesions rather than the initially posited theory of choroidal hypoperfusion. Indocyanine green angiography may identify numerous RPE/choroidal areas of hypoperfusion that may not otherwise correspond to apparent creamy white spots on funduscopic exam or intravenous fluorescein angiography.

59.3 Critical Work-up

Differential diagnoses include multifocal choroiditis, ocular histoplasmosis, sarcoidosis, tuberculosis, and syphilitic chorioretinitis. History and laboratory evaluation can narrow this differential. Infection should be confirmed by WNV-specific immunoglobulin M (IgM) and IgG serologies and confirmatory lumbar puncture for WNV IgM in cerebrospinal fluid with opening pressure for cases of meningoencephalitis. There may be antibody cross-reactivity in individuals vaccinated against yellow fever or Japanese encephalitis or who have been infected by other flaviviruses. Equivocal cases may be confirmed with plaque reduction neutralization assay, particularly when false positives due to cross-reactivity with other flaviviruses are suspected.t

59.4 Management

Management is directed at prevention through mitigation of exposure risk (e.g., mosquito control and the use of insect repellant) and symptomatic care.

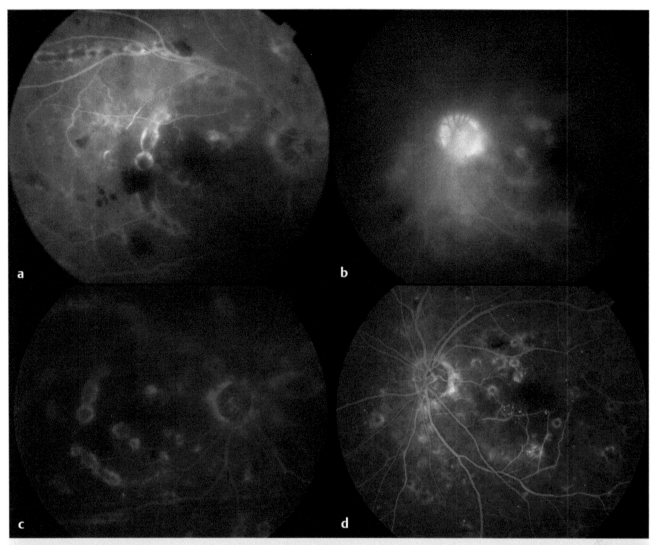

Fig. 59.5 Fluorescein angiography in acute West Nile chorioretinitis in the right and left eyes, demonstrating leakage/staining from laser-like lesions, areas of vascular occlusion, and vascular leakage. **(a,b)** Extensive optic nerve hyperfluorescence is present in the left eye. **(c,d)** Following the resolution of disease activity, chorioretinal lesions demonstrate window defects and staining with the resolution of the vascular leakage and optic nerve hyperfluorescence.

59.4.1 Treatment Options

Supportive care is the mainstay treatment for WNV and WNV retinopathy. Prior experimental treatments described in case reports with variable treatment response include ribavirin, interferon-α-2b, and intravenous immunoglobulin. Topical steroids may be used to treat the anterior uveitis component that occurs acutely. Late-onset complications may rarely include choroidal neovascularization occurring adjacent to the sites of prior chorioretinal scarring, which may be treated with intravitreal antivascular endothelial growth factor therapy.

59.4.2 Follow-up

There are no established follow-up guidelines and interval examination is thus established by the treating physician based on the degree of activity and interventions employed (e.g., treatment of the acute phase with topical corticosteroids).

Suggested Reading

[1] Garg S, Jampol LM. Systemic and intraocular manifestations of West Nile virus infection. Surv Ophthalmol. 2005; 50(1):3–13

[2] Chan CK, Limstrom SA, Tarasewicz DG, Lin SG. Ocular features of west nile virus infection in North America: a study of 14 eyes. Ophthalmology. 2006; 113(9):1539–1546

[3] Wang R, Wykoff CC, Brown DM. Granular Hyperreflective Specks by Spectral Domain Optical Coherence Tomography as Signs of West Nile Virus Infection: The Stardust Sign. Retin Cases Brief Rep. 2016; 10(4):349–353

[4] Learned D, Nudleman E, Robinson J, et al. Multimodal imaging of west nile virus chorioretinitis. Retina. 2014; 34(11):2269–2274

[5] Seth RK, Stoessel KM, Adelman RA. Choroidal neovascularization associated with West Nile virus chorioretinitis. Semin Ophthalmol. 2007; 22(2):81–84

60 Ebola Virus

Jessica G. Shantha and Steven Yeh

Summary

The World Health Organization has identified diseases such as Ebola virus (EBOV) as high priority and is soliciting both national and international partners to develop research strategies, global awareness, and preventive health policies for these pathogens. The first EBOV outbreak was in 1976, and over the last 42 years, there have been over 30 outbreaks with the most recent outbreak in August 2018 in the Democratic Republic of Congo. Moreover, the largest outbreak occurred in West Africa with over 28,000 people infected and 11,000 deaths from 2013 to 2016 with the highest rate of transmission in Sierra Leone, Liberia, and Guinea. This chapter will outline the systemic and ophthalmic manifestations of EBOV as well as discuss potential treatments and vaccines for prevention.

Keywords: Ebola, Ebola virus disease, panuveitis, uveitis, viral persistence

60.1 Features

Ebola is an enveloped, single-strand, negative polarity RNA virus transmitted through direct contact with bodily fluids/tissues from humans (e.g., blood, secretions, semen, saliva, urine, and breast milk) or animal vectors (e.g., bats, chimpanzees, gorillas, and duikers). Infection of macrophages leads to activation and release of cytokines, while dendritic cell activation causes a decrease in cytokine release and T-cell activation with downregulation of key components of the innate immune viral response. These responses cause an increase in vascular permeability, hypovolemic shock, multisystem failure, disseminated intravascular coagulation, hemorrhage, rash, and a high case fatality rate. Given the number of Ebola survivors in the latest outbreak, new observations are being made of the enduring consequences following survival from this hemorrhagic fever. Acute clinical symptoms are summarized and an array of lingering symptoms and signs having affected survivors (as documented from prior outbreaks from the Democratic Republic of Congo and Uganda, as well as more recent evidence from the most recent West African outbreak) follows. Ophthalmic sequelae may include various inflammatory features.

60.1.1 Common Symptoms

Acute Ocular Symptoms

Subconjunctival hemorrhage and vision loss (of unclear etiology due to inability to perform ophthalmic examination acutely) and conjunctival injection have been reported in 48 to 58% of patients during active infection.

Acute Systemic Symptoms

Initially, a flu-like presentation with fever, headache, malaise, and diarrhea. Ebola virus (EBOV) is known to cause a "viral hemorrhagic fever."

Long-Term Sequelae

Arthralgias (may include joint pain or ache without swelling); tenosynovitis (rare), fatigue, headache, abdominal pain, audiologic symptoms (tinnitus, aural fullness, and subjective hearing loss), anxiety, depression, insomnia, alopecia, Ebola virus persistence in immune privileged sites (i.e., reproductive organs, central nervous system, and eye fluid), and tenosynovitis (rare).

60.1.2 Exam Findings

Findings include anterior uveitis, intermediate uveitis, posterior uveitis with chorioretinal scar, panuveitis, and posterior synechiae. Cataract as a secondary complication may present as a uveitic white cataract, posterior subcapsular cataract, and anterior capsular fibrotic plaque (► Fig. 60.1, ► Fig. 60.2, ► Fig. 60.3).

60.2 Key Diagnostic Tests and Findings

60.2.1 Polymerase Chain Reaction

Detection of viral antigens or viral RNA by real-time reverse transcription polymerase chain reaction (RT-PCR). These tests can be positive within 3 days after symptoms develop.

60.2.2 GeneXpert Ebola Virus Assay

Used for rapid testing via an automated cartridge-based system for both RNA extraction and RT-PCR detection of EBOV, nucleoprotein, and glycoprotein (GP) targets.

Advantages include decreased training and technical expertise, faster results, and minimal biosafety requirements.

60.2.3 Serology

Serologic testing for EBOV immunoglobulin M and G.

60.2.4 Fluid Analysis

Ocular fluid analysis has been performed on one survivor with positive EBOV RT-PCR and EBOV culture in a biosafety level 4 (BSL-4) laboratory. Note that eye fluid testing of EBOV RNA by RT-PCR has not been systematically validated to date.

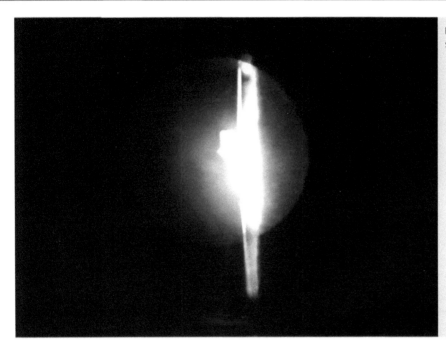

Fig. 60.1 Uveitic white cataract is a known sequela of Ebola virus disease.

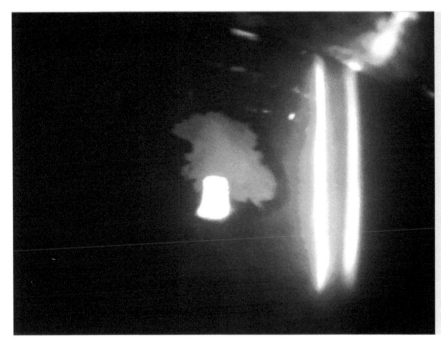

Fig. 60.2 Slit lamp photograph shows uveitic cataract with posterior synechiae in an Ebola virus disease survivor.

60.3 Critical Work-up

Specimens require biosafety level 4 laboratory for testing specimens suspected to be EBOV positive.

60.4 Management

60.4.1 Treatment Options

Therapies

Drug development for EBOV was largely fueled by the concern of the use of the virus as a bioweapon. Several medical countermeasures were studied for the treatment and prevention of acute EVD. Therapeutic strategies included direct virus targeting, modulation of host factors, modulation of the immune response, and clinical management of patient disease, largely through supportive care. Classes of anti-EBOV medications include the following: small molecules (e.g., nucleoside analogs BCX4430, GS-5734, and favipiravir [T-705]) antisense therapies (e.g., small-interfering RNAs [siRNAs]) and immunotherapeutics (e.g., ZMapp cocktail, composed of three monoclonal chimeric antibodies with neutralizing activity targeting EBOV GP).

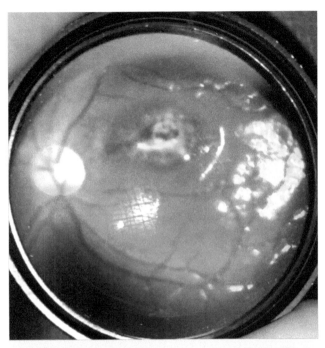

Fig. 60.3 Chorioretinal scars have been observed in Ebola virus disease survivors with posterior uveitis. Further studies are needed to determine if these scarring patterns are due to Ebola versus other infections endemic to West Africa (e.g., toxoplasmosis).

Vaccines

Several vaccine-based strategies have been developed and include conventional vaccines (i.e., heat- or formalin-inactivated EBOV), subunit vaccines (nonviral), virus-like particles, and vector-based vaccines. Within vector-based vaccines, the types of vaccines include vaccinia virus-based, adenovirus-based, and vesiculovirus (vesicular stomatitis virus [VSV])-based candidate vaccines, all of which have been studied in rodent models and nonhuman primates. An open-label, cluster randomized trial showed that recombinant VSV–Zaire EBOV offered significant protection against EVD, with no cases among vaccinated individuals from day 10 after vaccination. A ring vaccination strategy was effective in contributing to disease control in regions of Sierra Leone and Guinea in this vaccine trial and may have future applications.

Suggested Reading

[1] Vine V, Scott DP, Feldmann H. Ebolavirus: An Overview of Molecular and Clinical Pathogenesis. Methods Mol Biol. 2017; 1628:39–50

[2] Mattia JG, Vandy MJ, Chang JC, et al. Early clinical sequelae of Ebola virus disease in Sierra Leone: a cross-sectional study. Lancet Infect Dis. 2016; 16(3): 331–338

[3] Shantha JG, Crozier I, Hayek BR, et al. Ophthalmic manifestations and causes of vision impairment in Ebola virus disease survivors in Monrovia, Liberia. Ophthalmology. 2017; 124(2):170–177

[4] Tiffany A, Vetter P, Mattia J, et al. Ebola virus disease complications as experienced by survivors in Sierra Leone. Clin Infect Dis. 2016; 62(11):1360–1366

[5] Henao-Restrepo AM, Camacho A, Longini IM, et al. Efficacy and effectiveness of an rVSV-vectored vaccine in preventing Ebola virus disease: final results from the Guinea ring vaccination, open-label, cluster-randomised trial (Ebola Ça Suffit!). Lancet. 2017; 389(10068):505–518

61 Zika Virus and the Retina

Peter H. Tang and Darius M. Moshfeghi

Summary

Previously considered an isolated threat to remote regions of Africa and Asia, the Zika virus was transmitted to South America in 2015 and subsequently spread throughout the globe. Researchers first discovered the virus in 1947 from a rhesus monkey in the Zika Forest of Uganda. Less than 10 years later, the first reported cases of human infection occurred in Nigeria. The first Zika virus outbreak occurred in 2007 in the Yap Islands of the Federated States of Micronesia, followed by another in 2013 in French Polynesia. It was confirmed to have spread to Brazil in 2015 and subsequently became a global health emergency. While Zika infection produces a mild flu prodrome in adults, the most dramatic effects have been observed in congenital Zika virus infections (CZI) with the development of microcephaly. Ocular findings associated with CZI were first reported in 2016 and subsequently expanded to include pigment mottling, chorioretinal atrophy, optic nerve abnormalities, iris coloboma, and lens subluxation. With new infections still being reported and the lack of an effective treatment, the Zika virus remains a global epidemiologic and medical challenge.

Keywords: chorioretinopathy, maculopathy, retinopathy, virus, Zika

61.1 Features

The Zika virus belongs to the genus of viruses in the family Flaviviridae, which also includes West Nile, dengue, and yellow fever. These viruses are composed of positive-sense single-stranded RNA enveloped in an icosahedral nucleocapsid. The most common mode of transmission is from the bite of an infected arthropod (e.g., *Aedes aegypti* and *Aedes albopictus* mosquito species) that is endemic to tropical and temperate climate regions. There have also been documented cases of transmission sexually, congenitally, and through blood transfusion and organ transplantation. Furthermore, the virus has recently been detected in other bodily fluids, raising the possibility of potential transmission through nonsexual contact.

Studies have found that infection during the first trimester is linked to the development of microcephaly. While the understanding of the pathophysiology of microcephaly associated with congenital Zika virus infections (CZI) has made tremendous progress, the association of CZI with chorioretinal maculopathy is less well understood. While some believe Zika virus to be the direct cause, these findings may be sequelae of Zika-induced microcephaly. Microcephaly itself has been shown to be associated with chorioretinal degeneration, pigmentary changes, and vascular abnormalities. Thus, it is important to investigate the mechanisms for these findings so as to properly attribute the pathophysiology.

61.1.1 Common Symptoms

Ocular

Vision-threatening fundus abnormalities in infants with CZI. Eye redness in adults.

Systemic

Varies from asymptomatic to mild symptoms, including fever, rash, and joint pain.

61.1.2 Exam Findings

Chorioretinal atrophy and pigment mottling may be present.

61.2 Key Diagnostic Tests and Findings

61.2.1 Serology

The recent development of a serologic test for an immunoglobulin M (IgM) antibody to the virus has improved the screening process. The IgM antibody develops within 1 week after infection and can stay positive for up to 12 weeks afterward. This method has been recommended as a screening method for neonates suspected of having CZI; however, its low specificity and high cross-reactivity to other flaviviruses pose significant challenges. A positive result requires a confirmatory plaque reduction neutralization test performed at the Centers for Disease Control and Prevention (CDC). Furthermore, microcephaly is no longer a required criterion for screening neonates.

61.2.2 Fundus Photography

Possible focal pigment mottling and chorioretinal atrophy (▶ Fig. 61.1). To date, limited diagnostic evaluation of retinal findings has been described such as optical coherence tomography and angiography due to the challenging issues related to examination, including the frequent necessity of performing the exam under anesthesia.

61.3 Critical Work-up

Diagnosis is arduous as the manifestation of clinical symptoms is nonspecific and highly variable. Recently, knowledge of focal pigment mottling and chorioretinal atrophy has been expanded to include hemorrhagic retinopathy in conjunction with vascular abnormalities and torpedo maculopathy. Other flaviviruses such as dengue can produce similar retinal findings; thus, proper serologic confirmation of the Zika virus is crucial.

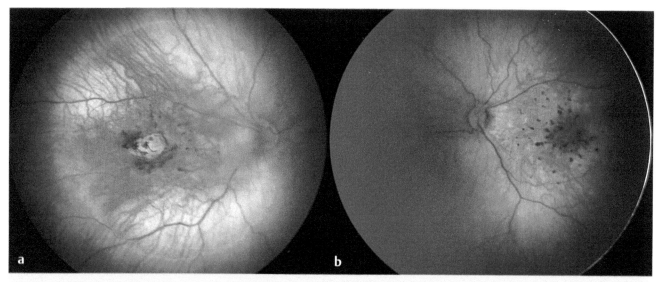

Fig. 61.1 (a,b) Fundus photographs of the child with congenital Zika infection show chorioretinal atrophy of the **(a)** right eye as well as pigmentary changes within the macula of both eyes.

61.4 Management

61.4.1 Treatment Options

Prevention

Currently, the major focus is through epidemiological efforts to educate the population to minimize person-to-person transmission of the Zika virus and increase prophylaxis against mosquito bites in endemic areas, especially for women of childbearing age. There are major government-led projects to decrease the *Aedes* mosquito population through insecticide spraying and other measures. Ongoing efforts to develop a vaccine for the Zika virus are well under way.

Management

Symptomatic management (e.g., bed rest and oral hydration) remains the only intervention. It is estimated that only a small fraction of infected individuals presents with symptoms. Niclosamide has been identified as a possible treatment for males and nonpregnant females as it may reduce the transmission of Zika virus and other Zika-related complications. For infants with CZI, early diagnosis and monitoring are important. While no effective treatments or vaccines currently exist for the retinal and neurological manifestations of CZI, it is important that neonates exposed to the virus in utero receive comprehensive and routine eye examinations and systemic evaluations.

61.4.2 Follow-up

To evaluate for retinal involvement in neonates suspected of CZI, these children should ideally be assessed within 1 month after birth, and the CDC recommends a follow-up eye examination at an age of 3 months regardless of normal findings at the initial examination.

Suggested Reading

[1] Ventura CV, Maia M, Bravo-Filho V, Góis AL, Belfort R, Jr. Zika virus in Brazil and macular atrophy in a child with microcephaly. Lancet. 2016; 387(10015): 228

[2] de Paula Freitas B, de Oliveira Dias JR, Prazeres J, et al. Ocular findings in infants with microcephaly associated with presumed Zika virus congenital infection in Salvador, Brazil. JAMA Ophthalmol. 2016; 134(5):529–535

[3] Williamson PC, Linnen JM, Kessler DA, et al. First cases of Zika virus-infected US blood donors outside states with areas of active transmission. Transfusion. 2017; 57 3pt2:770–778

[4] Swaminathan S, Schlaberg R, Lewis J, Hanson KE, Couturier MR. Fatal Zika virus infection with secondary nonsexual transmission. N Engl J Med. 2016; 375(19):1907–1909

62 Presumed Ocular Histoplasmosis Syndrome

Joseph Daniel Boss and Justis P. Ehlers

Summary

Presumed ocular histoplasmosis syndrome (POHS) is a multifocal chorioretinitis with a theorized infectious etiology from *Histoplasma capsulatum*. POHS is traditionally a clinical diagnosis based on the absence of inflammation and having two or more findings of the triad of small atrophic, "punched-out" chorioretinal lesions, peripapillary atrophy, and macular choroidal neovascularization (CNV) or associated sequelae. POHS is often asymptomatic; however, when the macula is involved, it may cause symptoms ranging from metamorphopsia to profound central vision loss. Treatment is primarily limited to active CNV management with intravitreal anti-vascular endothelial growth factor therapy.

Keywords: chorioretinitis, choroidal neovascularization, histo spots, histoplasmosis, ocular histoplasmosis syndrome, presumed ocular histoplasmosis syndrome

62.1 Features

First described in 1941, presumed ocular histoplasmosis syndrome (POHS), also known as ocular histoplasmosis or ocular histoplasmosis syndrome, has been debated as a separate condition from multifocal chorioretinitis and punctate inner choroidopathy due to a presumed precursor fungal infection. The dimorphic fungus *Histoplasma capsulatum* is the strongly theorized infectious agent based on skin testing for histoplasmin in affected individuals, increased reports of POHS in endemic areas of the protozoan, and reports of histoplasmosis deoxyribonucleic acid found in affected enucleated eyes. Ocular disease is believed to arise after inhalation of spores into the lungs, ultimately resulting in hematogenous dissemination. POHS is controversially linked to endemic areas of the Unites States, including Ohio and Mississippi (the "histo belt") but has been reported throughout the United States and Europe. Numerous theories exist on POHS pathogenesis. One theory includes the choroid being involved via hematogenous transmission at the time of the initial systemic infection. As the focal chorioretinitis resolves, atrophic chorioretinal scars develop. The loss of retinal pigment epithelium (RPE) and Bruch's membrane may result in choroidal neovascularization (CNV). Fragile choroidal neovascular vessels lack proper functioning tight junctions, resulting in leakage of fluid, lipid exudate, and hemorrhages. Chronic remodeling with fibrovascular scarring can subsequently occur, resulting in profound central vision loss when the fovea is affected. The cause of patient-to-patient variation in the initiation of CNV is unknown, with possible underlying genetic predisposition implications based on human leukocyte antigen (HLA)-DRw2 typing. Additional theories for CNV predisposition include hypersensitivity reaction, reinfection, or a larger initial fungal inoculation.

62.1.1 Common Symptoms

Ocular

Often asymptomatic; may be diagnosed incidentally during routine eye examinations. Manifestations can be wide-ranging, depending on the severity and location of chorioretinal lesions. Fovea-involving maculopathy may cause metamorphopsia and central vision loss.

Systemic

Depends on the severity of the exposure and immune status of the host. Most commonly, mild flu-like respiratory symptoms may occur in immunocompetent patients that are not typically diagnosed.

62.1.2 Exam Findings

Clinical diagnosis is based on having two or more findings of the triad of small atrophic, "punched-out" chorioretinal lesions (histo spots), peripapillary atrophy or pigment changes, and maculopathy due to CNV (▶ Fig. 62.1, ▶ Fig. 62.2). Vitreous inflammation, or vitreous cell, is absent. Atrophic lesions tend to be smaller than the optic disc, located in the macula or periphery, asymmetric, and often asymptomatic. CNV sequelae include subretinal and intraretinal hemorrhages, subretinal fluid, and late fibrovascular disciform scarring.

62.2 Key Diagnostic Tests and Findings

62.2.1 Optical Coherence Tomography

Macula-involving lesions help assess atrophic lesions for atrophy, CNV, and fibrous scarring over time. Outer retinal atrophy is present over atrophic lesions. Inactive CNV may be present as a subretinal or sub-RPE consolidated hyperreflective lesion. Active CNV may be associated with increased ellipsoid zone disruption and increased outer retinal reflectivity, in addition to possible intraretinal or subretinal fluid (▶ Fig. 62.3).

62.2.2 Fluorescein Angiography or Ultra-Widefield Fluorescein Angiography

Can aid in assessing for CNV activity (▶ Fig. 62.1).

62.2.3 Fundus Photography

Follow lesions throughout time in patients with asymptomatic peripheral chorioretinal lesions. Widefield fundus photography is preferred when lesions occur peripherally (▶ Fig. 62.2).

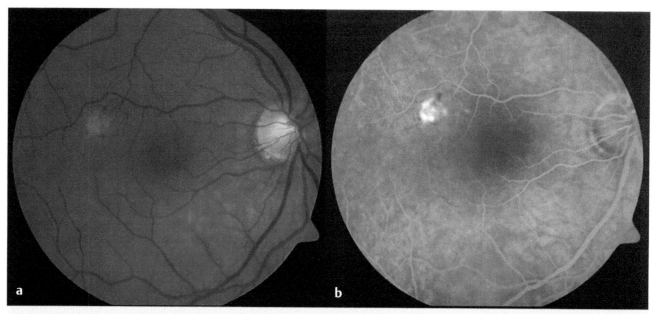

Fig. 62.1 Presumed ocular histoplasmosis. **(a)** Mild peripapillary atrophy temporal to the optic nerve with macular active choroidal neovascularization (yellow lesion). **(b)** Fluorescein angiography in late venous phase of the macular lesion.

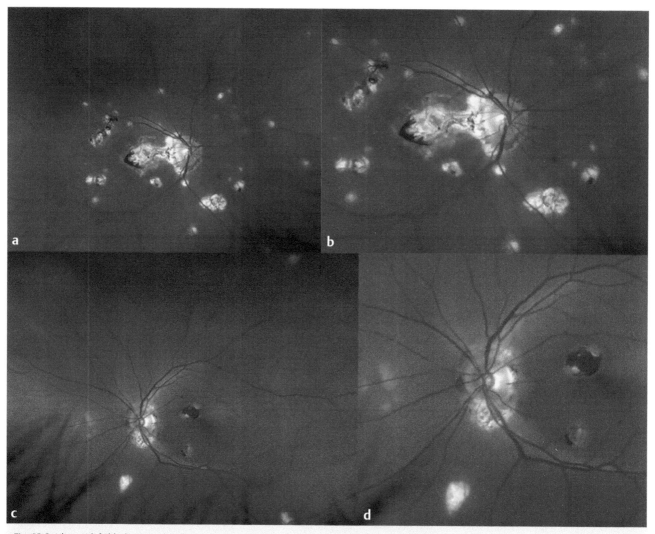

Fig. 62.2 Ultra-widefield photographs of presumed ocular histoplasmosis of a right eye **(a,b)** and left eye **(c,d)** with posterior pole views, demonstrating peripapillary atrophy, scattered peripheral chorioretinal scars, and macular involvement.

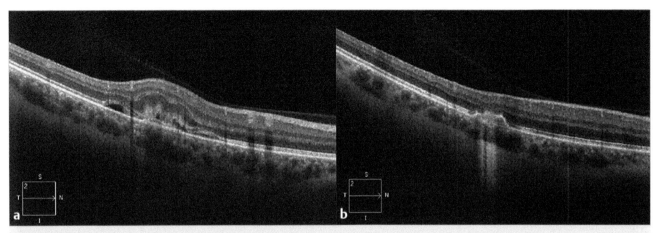

Fig. 62.3 Presumed ocular histoplasmosis. **(a)** Macular OCT showing active subretinal choroidal neovascularization before treatment compared to after treatment with a vascular endothelial growth factor inhibitor **(b)**.

62.2.4 Optical Coherence Tomography Angiography

Similar to fluorescein angiography, optical coherence tomography angiography may provide additional information regarding the presence of CNV throughout the identification of abnormal flow networks consistent with CNV.

62.3 Critical Work-up

POHS remains a clinical diagnosis. Due to lack of significant negative and positive predictive values, routine HLA typing and histoplasmosis skin or serum testing are not typically recommended.

62.4 Management

62.4.1 Treatment Options

The primary focus of treatment in POHS is the management of CNV. There is no established treatment for the prevention of CNV development.

For the management of active CNV, anti-vascular endothelial growth factor (VEGF) therapies have become common. CNV may be particularly responsive to anti-VEGF treatment, requiring fewer treatments than typically seen in neovascular age-related macular degeneration. Historically, CNV was managed with both laser photocoagulation and photodynamic therapy (PDT). Laser may still be considered for lesions that are at least 200 μm from the foveal center. PDT may also be used for CNV, including subfoveal lesions. Intravitreal triamcinolone, targeting a possible underlying inflammatory pathogenesis, has also been described.

62.4.2 Follow-up

Inactive POHS may be followed every 6 to 12 months. Patients with active CNV or history of active CNV should be followed closely and treated if indicated due to the potential serious visual complications if untreated or undertreated.

Suggested Reading

[1] Krause AC, Hopkins WG. Ocular manifestation of histoplasmosis. Am J Ophthalmol. 1951; 34(4):564–566

[2] Spencer WH, Chan C-C, Shen DF, Rao NA. Detection of Histoplasma capsulatum DNA in lesions of chronic ocular histoplasmosis syndrome. Arch Ophthalmol. 2003; 121(11):1551–1555

[3] Meredith TA, Smith RE, Duquesnoy RJ. Association of HLA-DRw2 antigen with presumed ocular histoplasmosis. Am J Ophthalmol. 1980; 89(1):70–76

[4] Macular Photocoagulation Study Group. Krypton laser photocoagulation for neovascular lesions of ocular histoplasmosis. Results of a randomized clinical trial. Arch Ophthalmol. 1987; 105(11):1499–1507

63 Diffuse Unilateral Subacute Neuroretinitis

Sruthi Arepalli, Arthi Venkat, and Sunil K. Srivastava

Summary

Diffuse unilateral subacute neuroretinitis occurs secondary to a subretinal nematode with resultant toxicity to the overlying retina and optic nerve. Due to the mild symptoms that characterize the early phases of the disease, patients usually do not present until the later stages. The fundus examination is typically comprised of crops of rotating evanescent fundus lesions, with late-stage changes including retinal pigment epithelium scarring and optic nerve atrophy. Treatment consists of photocoagulation of the nematode or oral antihelminthic therapy. Despite these measures, the visual return is usually limited.

Keywords: cystoid macular edema, diffuse unilateral subacute neuroretinitis, electroretinogram, fluorescein angiography, nematode, optical coherence tomography, optic nerve atrophy, uveitis

63.1 Features

Diffuse unilateral subacute neuroretinitis (DUSN) is a typically monocular inflammatory condition caused by various subretinal nematodes. DUSN tends to affect younger individuals and is classified into early and late stages, with characteristic findings associated with each. Early disease usually does not result in dramatic vision loss and consists of recurrent, evanescent gray-white or yellow-white clusters of fundus lesions that disappear and reappear in different locations. Later disease, which is linked to more drastic visual decline, is associated with retinal arteriolar narrowing, optic disc atrophy, and degeneration of the retinal pigment epithelium (RPE).

In the United States, the disease burden is highest in the southeast, as well as the northern and Midwestern portions. In the southeast, the majority of cases are linked to a smaller nematode, whereas the larger nematode is usually identified in cases occurring in the northern and Midwestern United States.

The exact pathogenesis of the disease is unknown. The current assumption is that the ocular pathology results from a noxious reaction of the retina and optic nerve to the subretinal organism. In particular, a smaller nematode, *Ancylostoma caninum* (400–1,000 μm in length), and a larger nematode, *Baylisas-*

caris procyonis (1,500–2,000 μm in length), are hypothesized to lead to the disease and are thought to survive in the eye for multiple years. *A. caninum* is also associated with cutaneous larva migrans, which has preceded DUSN in a subset of patients. *B. procyonis* is a parasite found in raccoons and squirrels that causes central nervous system disease. In addition, there have been reports of neural larva migrans in association with DUSN, and serological studies have confirmed the presence of this organism in some patients. Exposure through animal contact is thought to be the mechanism of infection.

63.1.1 Common Symptoms

In early stages, patients may be asymptomatic or experience mild visual decline, scotomas, or floaters. In later stages, the visual decline is greater, including possible worsening of scotomas and floaters.

63.1.2 Exam Findings

In early disease, exam findings mainly consist of rotating crops of gray–white or yellow–white retinal lesions parallel to the path of the nematode. These lesions typically last up to 2 weeks before disappearing and can lead to scarring in late disease stages. Patients may present with optic nerve damage, resulting in an afferent pupillary defect and optic nerve swelling, vitritis, and retinal arteriolar narrowing (▶ Fig. 63.1). Less commonly reported findings include exudative changes, choroidal neovascular membranes, and intra- and subretinal hemorrhage. Rarely, a macular star may develop.

In late stages, exam findings include more profound damage in the same areas above, with RPE degeneration and scarring that may be confused for unilateral retinitis pigmentosa, ocular histoplasmosis, or long-standing atrophy secondary to retinal vascular occlusion (▶ Fig. 63.1). The most common clinical signs, regardless of time of presentation, included subretinal tracks and focal alterations of the RPE (90% each), and small white spots and optic nerve atrophy (80% each).

At either stage of the disease, a motile subretinal nematode may be found with careful fundus examination.

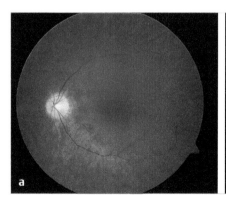
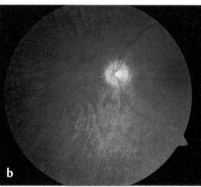

Fig. 63.1 (a) Fundus photograph of diffuse unilateral subacute neuroretinitis, demonstrating vessel attenuation and optic nerve pallor. **(b)** Retinal periphery demonstrates extensive pigmentary changes and vessel attenuation. Possible nematode is noted in the inferonasal area.

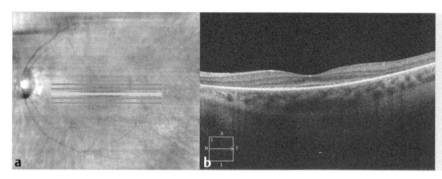

Fig. 63.2 (a,b) Spectral domain optical coherence tomography in diffuse unilateral subacute neuroretinitis, demonstrating extensive outer retinal atrophy with minimal foveal sparing.

63.2 Key Diagnostic Tests and Findings

63.2.1 Optical Coherence Tomography

Generalized retinal atrophy in the areas of involvement, with a significant decrease in inner retinal thickness after disease resolution (▶ Fig. 63.2). Interestingly, even when eyes show no signs of retinal atrophy on examination, the inner nuclear layer is still thinner than the normal contralateral eye on optical coherence tomography.

63.2.2 Fluorescein Angiography or Ultra-Widefield Fluorescein Angiography

In early stages, DUSN lesions exhibit early hypofluorescence and late staining, and retinal vascular leakage and disc hyperfluorescence may also be seen. The similarity of these findings to other inflammatory or "white dot" syndromes contributes to the difficulty of an early accurate diagnosis. Late stages mainly demonstrate window defects due to diffuse RPE wipeout.

63.2.3 Indocyanine Green Angiography

Multiple hypocyanescent spots throughout the fundus, similar to many inflammatory disorders.

63.2.4 Electroretinography

The deviation in electroretinogram (ERG) from normal varies, but in most patients, the b-wave is decreased more than the a-wave, indicating inner retinal loss. In select cases, the death of the nematode resulted in some improvement in ERG. Multifocal ERG shows that the areas of decreased response are specific to the areas of retinal and RPE lesions.

63.3 Critical Work-up

In cases of suspected DUSN, it is important to attempt to locate the nematode through careful examination and treat with photocoagulation if possible. Of note, the lights involved in ophthalmoscopy may cause the nematode to move. In select cases, it can be located with high-magnification fundus photography. Even with careful examination, the nematode may not be found. Although a few reports have shown positive serology in DUSN patients, most agree that there is limited utility in obtaining blood smears or stool studies.

63.4 Management

63.4.1 Treatment Options

Success has been reported with photocoagulation of the nematode; however, careful observation after photocoagulation is required, as reports have documented the persistence of the nematode even after appearing effectively terminated with photocoagulation. In cases with persistent symptoms or inability to photocoagulate the nematode, anthelminthic agents have shown some benefit. Visual recovery is variable, but some have modest improvement after treatment.

63.4.2 Follow-up

In cases of the early disease, it is important to monitor patients for the development of late characteristics, which could signify continued infection even after treatment. In the cases of photocoagulation, it is important to repeat the fundus examination to ensure the death of the nematode.

Suggested Reading

[1] Ávila M, Isaac D. Chapter 86—Helminthic Disease A2—Ryan, Stephen J. In: Sadda SR, Hinton DR, Schachat AP, et al, eds. Retina. 5th ed. London: W.B. Saunders; 2013:1500–1514

[2] Gass JD, Braunstein RA. Further observations concerning the diffuse unilateral subacute neuroretinitis syndrome. Arch Ophthalmol. 1983; 101(11): 1689–1697

[3] de Amorim Garcia Filho CA, Gomes AH, de A Garcia Soares AC, de Amorim Garcia CA. Clinical features of 121 patients with diffuse unilateral subacute neuroretinitis. Am J Ophthalmol. 2012; 153(4):743–749

[4] Vezzola D, Kisma N, Robson AG, Holder GE, Pavesio C. Structural and functional retinal changes in eyes with DUSN. Retina. 2014; 34(8):1675–1682

64 Multifocal Choroiditis and Panuveitis

Rajinder S. Nirwan and Angela P. Bessette

Summary

Multifocal choroiditis and panuveitis (MCP) is a rare, chronic, and recurrent idiopathic condition that predominantly affects young, healthy, myopic women. Typical presenting symptoms include decreased central visual acuity, floaters, photopsias, and visual field defects. On examination, lesions are small and multifocal, and associated with anterior and posterior inflammation. It may be unilateral or bilateral, but significant asymmetry often exists. Characteristic findings are observed on various imaging techniques, including spectral domain optical coherence tomography, fluorescein angiography, indocyanine green angiography, and fundus autofluorescence. The diagnosis of MCP is one of exclusion, and a complete workup should be performed. Treatments are aimed at reversing/controlling the inflammation and the sequelae that may arise.

Keywords: FA, ICGA, multifocal choroiditis and panuveitis, OCT, posterior uveitis

64.1 Features

Multifocal choroiditis and panuveitis (MCP) was first reported in 1973 in two patients who had a chorioretinopathy that resembled the lesions of presumed ocular histoplasmosis syndrome (POHS). In contrast to POHS, however, these patients had associated bilateral anterior chamber and vitreous inflammation. Although classically a panuveitis, MCP is categorized as a white dot syndrome due to its characteristic fundoscopic appearance. It is a rare, chronic, recurrent inflammatory eye disease that has a predilection for healthy individuals, especially young, myopic, women. Though idiopathic, it is presumed to be autoimmune in nature; however, there is no agreed upon etiology. The disease has been reported to appear in a broad age range from 6 to 69 years of age, with the most common occurrence between the third and fifth decades of life. Though MCP is bilateral, it may be asymmetric and is characterized by recurrent bouts of clinically evident inflammation around the sites of previous inflammation. The recurrences may occur unilaterally, bilaterally, separately, or simultaneously.

64.1.1 Common Symptoms

Clinically, most patients present subacutely and may complain of symptoms of posterior uveitis, including decreased central visual acuity (VA), floaters, photopsias, and visual field defects. Anterior segment symptoms such as photophobia may also occur. Initial presenting VA is highly variable from 20/20 to light perception. Vision loss is typically attributed to inflammation or choroidal neovascularization (CNV).

64.1.2 Exam Findings

During the active stage, examination discloses anterior chamber and vitreous inflammation, which is an important

distinguishing feature from POHS. The anterior uveitis associated with MCP is nongranulomatous, may include posterior synechiae, and can range from mild to moderate in severity. The vitritis has a comparable degree of inflammation and can be asymmetric. The classic fundoscopic findings of active lesions are fluffy, yellow–gray chorioretinal lesions with pigmented borders that occur at the level of the retinal pigment epithelium (RPE) and choriocapillaris (▶ Fig. 64.1). These lesions range from 50 to 350 μm in diameter, although some may be larger, and can be distributed in the posterior, midperipheral, or peripheral retina. They may be found singly, arranged in clusters, or in linear streaks. Active disease may be associated with subretinal fluid, optic nerve hyperemia and edema, cystoid macular edema (CME), and macular and peripapillary CNV. Eventually, the older inactive lesions evolve into round, punched-out, atrophic, yellow–white areas with varying degrees of pigmentation. This, in turn, can lead to peripapillary scarring and extensive subretinal fibrosis. The peripapillary scarring resembles that seen in POHS. The recurrent bouts of inflammation make patients more susceptible to cataract formation, CME, and epiretinal membrane.

64.2 Key Diagnostic Tests and Findings

64.2.1 Optical Coherence Tomography

Active lesions appear as deposits of drusen-like homogeneous material and exhibit RPE elevation. These acute lesions

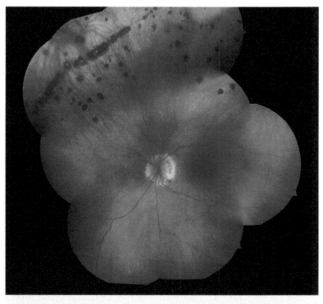

Fig. 64.1 Montage color fundus photograph of inactive multifocal choroiditis and panuveitis, left eye, demonstrating multiple old, discrete, punched-out lesions with varying degrees of hyperpigmentation.

demonstrate moderate reflectivity and are located in the sub-RPE and subretinal spaces (▶ Fig. 64.2). With more widespread involvement, it may incorporate the ellipsoid zone and extend beyond the zone of RPE elevation. In some cases, older lesions demonstrate scarring and loss of tissue, while others resolve without any evidence of anatomical alterations. During the acute phase, the choroid does not appear to be consistently affected by the disease process on optical coherence tomography (OCT). However, newer choroidal imaging techniques, such as enhanced depth imaging OCT and swept-source OCT, may demonstrate a subtle increase in choroidal thickness in the areas of activity.

64.2.2 Fluorescein Angiography or Ultra-Widefield Fluorescein Angiography

Active lesions display early hypofluorescence and show staining and leakage late in the sequence (▶ Fig. 64.3). Where the RPE is dehisced, the leakage is more pronounced. Following treatment, the fluorescein angiography (FA) appearance may demonstrate various patterns: small white scars with early slight hyperfluorescence and late staining, a punched-out lesion of absent RPE with window defect, or no appreciable change (on examination or FA). Furthermore, new areas of CNV will present with early fluorescence and late leakage. Similarly, regressed CNV will also show hyperfluorescence early but demonstrate staining late. Inactive lesions of MCP will show window defects with early hypofluorescence and well-defined borders.

64.2.3 Indocyanine Green Angiography

Indocyanine green angiography may provide additional diagnostic information, highlighting lesions that are in greater quantities than that seen on exam or FA as hypocyanescent spots, representing areas of nonperfused choriocapillaris (▶ Fig. 64.4).

64.2.4 Fundus Autofluorescence

The fundus autofluorescence features, which reflect the structural changes of the RPE, show hyperautofluorescence in areas of active chorioretinitis (▶ Fig. 64.5). Hyperautofluorescent lesions disappear with the institution of immunosuppressive treatment and are replaced by punctate areas of hypoautofluorescence in areas of chorioretinal atrophy.

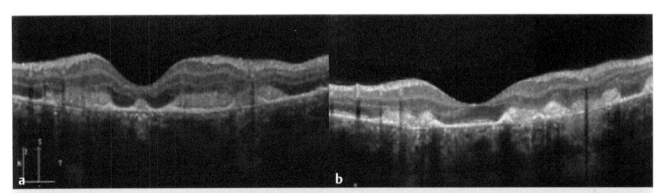

Fig. 64.2 **(a)** Optical coherence tomography (OCT) of the left eye in a patient with multifocal choroiditis and panuveitis at baseline, showing conical lesions involving the outer retina with retinal pigment epithelium (RPE) rupture and hyperreflectivity both above and below the RPE and **(b)** OCT following 1 month of treatment with 60-mg prednisone. Note that the lesions become more consolidated and well defined, as well as the subfoveal improvement with steroid therapy. (Courtesy of Sunil Srivastava, MD.)

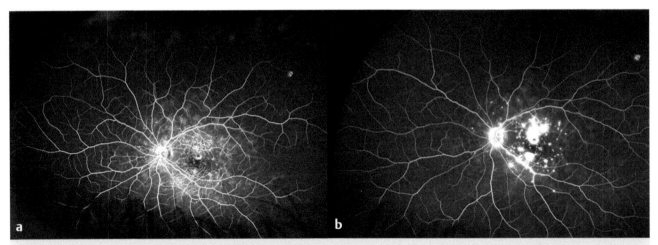

Fig. 64.3 **(a)** Early and **(b)** late phases in ultrawidefield fluorescein angiogram of the left eye in multifocal choroiditis and panuveitis, with areas of staining and leakage. (Courtesy of Sunil Srivastava, MD.)

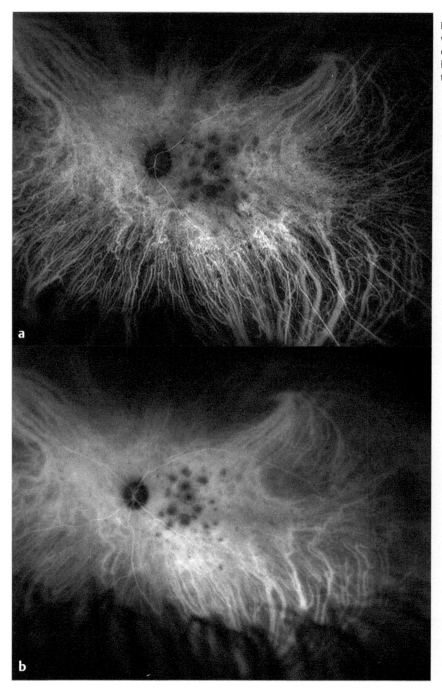

Fig. 64.4 (a) Early and (b) late phases in ultra-widefield ICGA of the left eye in multifocal choroiditis and panuveitis indicating multiple hypocyanescent areas that remain unchanged throughout. (Courtesy of Sunil Srivastava, MD.)

64.3 Critical Work-up

The diagnosis of MCP is one of exclusion, which can be accomplished through a thorough history, in addition to laboratory and diagnostic testing. It is prudent to rule out infectious etiologies prior to initiating immunosuppressive therapy. Workup should include testing for syphilis (nontreponemal and treponemal) serology, tuberculosis (tuberculin skin test or interferon-γ release assays and chest radiographs), and sarcoidosis (serum angiotensin-converting enzyme, lysozyme, and chest radiograph or spiral chest computed tomography scan). Human leukocyte antigen A29 testing can confirm the diagnosis of birdshot retinochoroidopathy in the appropriate clinical setting.

Lyme and West Nile virus titers should be evaluated in endemic areas or if the clinical history and/or symptoms are suggestive of infection with one of these pathogens.

64.4 Management

64.4.1 Treatment Options

Currently, there is no universal standard of treatment. Therapy, however, can be initiated once infectious etiologies are ruled out and is geared at controlling anterior and posterior inflammation along with their sequelae. Systemic corticosteroids (e.g., prednisone) are considered first-line treatment for active

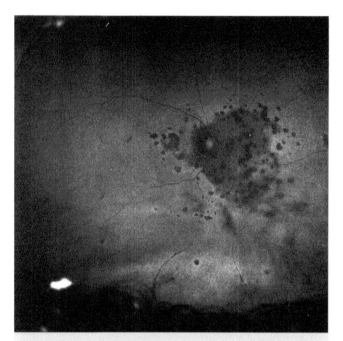

Fig. 64.5 Ultra-widefield fundus autofluorescence of a patient with inactive multifocal choroiditis and panuveitis, right eye, showing multiple hypoautofluorescent lesions in areas of previous inflammation. (Courtesy of Sunil Srivastava, MD.)

posterior inflammation but can be combined with topical steroids for anterior chamber inflammation. Oral prednisone can be tapered when there is evidence of improvement in inflammation. This regimen may be supplemented with more aggressive local therapy, including posterior sub-Tenon Kenalog injections or intravitreal injections of triamcinolone or the dexamethasone implant. Again, it is critical to rule out infection prior to administering periocular or intraocular steroids. Alternatively, immunosuppressive agents, such as antimetabolites and anti-tumor necrosis factor agents, may be used to help facilitate more long-term stability when individuals are refractory to corticosteroids, or in cases where prednisone cannot be tapered without recurrence of inflammation. Historically, CNV, when present, was treated with thermal laser and photodynamic therapy. With the advent of anti-vascular endothelial growth factor (anti-VEGF) therapy, however, the treatment of CNV has shifted toward intravitreal anti-VEGF as the first-line approach for CNV management. In select cases, CNV activity may also more primarily reflect inflammatory activity and may be managed with intraocular or systemic steroids. These therapies may be combined with anti-VEGF therapy.

64.4.2 Follow-up

MCP is a chronic disease that lasts months to years with subsequent recurrent bouts of inflammation. Patients may initially present with CNV or they may develop it late in follow-up. The same is true for CME. Patients on prednisone and/or immunomodulatory therapy should be monitored for side effects that can have life-threatening consequences. Those individuals who develop disciform macular scarring, atrophy, or chronic CME have a poor visual prognosis. For these reasons, close and long-term follow-up along with good compliance is paramount in obtaining control of the disease. Those patients requiring systemic immunomodulatory therapy may also benefit from coordinated follow-up with a rheumatologist for ongoing surveillance of systemic issues.

Suggested Reading

[1] Spaide RF, Goldberg N, Freund KB. Redefining multifocal choroiditis and panuveitis and punctate inner choroidopathy through multimodal imaging. Retina. 2013; 33(7):1315–1324

[2] Raven ML, Ringeisen AL, Yonekawa Y, Stem MS, Faia LJ, Gottlieb JL. Multimodal imaging and anatomic classification of the white dot syndromes. Int J Retina Vitreous. 2017; 3:12

[3] Tavallali A, Yannuzzi LA. Idiopathic multifocal choroiditis. J Ophthalmic Vis Res. 2016; 11(4):429–432

[4] Mirza RG, Jampol LM. White Spot Syndromes and Related Diseases. In: Ryan S, Schachat A, Hinton D, Wilkinson C, Sadda S, Wiedemann P, eds. Ryan's retina. 6th ed. London: Elsevier; 2018:1535–1541

65 Ocular Sarcoidosis

Sruthi Arepalli and Careen Lowder

Summary

Sarcoidosis is a multisystemic, idiopathic, granulomatous inflammatory disease without a cure. Interestingly, ocular manifestations can be the presenting and sometimes sole symptom of systemic sarcoidosis, requiring careful diagnosis and management. Ocular sarcoidosis commonly presents as bilateral, chronic uveitis, but it can involve any ocular or adnexal structure, and mimic other ophthalmic conditions as well. While biopsy is the gold standard for diagnosis, this may be difficult to attain, and ancillary clinical signs and laboratory results can support the diagnosis. Treatment relies on establishing quiescence and preserving vision, usually through corticosteroids and/or immunosuppression.

Keywords: cystoid macular edema, fluorescein angiography, granuloma, indocyanine green angiography, optical coherence tomography, sarcoidosis, uveitis

65.1 Features

Sarcoidosis, a granulomatous inflammatory disorder of unknown etiology, can affect almost every organ, including the eye. Ocular involvement can be the presenting manifestation of the disease, requiring astute ophthalmic diagnosis and careful management. Definitive diagnosis requires noncaseating granulomas on biopsy from involved tissue, but this may be difficult to attain, and other clinical and laboratory findings can support the diagnosis.

Ocular sarcoidosis can involve any eye structure, including the orbit, adnexa, intraocular structures, and the optic nerve. A large percentage of patients develop bilateral, chronic granulomatous uveitis. The prevalence of ocular sarcoidosis is unknown as diagnostic criteria differ. Racial predilection varies; according to some, African Americans are more likely to develop ocular manifestations, while others show a high incidence in Japanese patients. A few studies show no difference between genders, while others reveal a female predominance. Ocular sarcoidosis can present at any age, even in young children. Typically, it is bimodal, with peak incidence at the second and third decades or the fifth and sixth decades. Recently, reports have described the development of systemic as well as ocular sarcoidosis in conjunction with granulomatous inflammation of tattoos. The cause of sarcoidosis remains unknown.

65.1.1 Common Symptoms

Symptoms typically reflect the tissue impacted. Inflammation of the lacrimal gland, eyelids, or conjunctiva results in eye irritation and dryness. In cases of intraocular inflammation, photophobia, pain, and decreased vision occur. With orbital inflammation, diplopia, proptosis, and pain develop. Neurological involvement may result in cranial nerve palsies and meningitis.

65.1.2 Exam Findings

Eyelids, Lacrimal System, Orbit, Conjunctiva, and Sclera

Focal infiltration of granulomas leads to papules or larger nodules, which can mimic tumors. Sarcoid can infiltrate the entire eyelid, creating a pseudocellulitis. The lacrimal gland is the most common orbital structure involved and can enlarge to a palpable mass. Orbital inflammation can involve fat and muscles, leading to proptosis, diplopia, and vision loss. Granulomas may involve the palpebral conjunctiva and chronic inflammation can cause cicatricial changes. If conjunctival granulomas are present, these lesions may be a good option for confirmatory biopsy. Scleral involvement is infrequent but can develop any scleritis.

Intraocular Inflammation

Anterior chamber inflammation is the most common presentation of sarcoid uveitis; however, hypopyon is rare. Patients can develop mutton-fat keratic precipitates (KP) or granulomas of the iris or trabecular meshwork (TM). Intermediate uveitis includes vitreous opacities, snowballs, pars plana exudates, or cystoid macular edema (CME). In posterior uveitis, retinal and choroidal lesions can be small (Dalen-Fuchs-like nodules) or large (granulomas), which may simulate choroidal tumors (▶ Fig. 65.1). Small choroidal lesions may resemble multifocal choroiditis or birdshot chorioretinopathy, with retinal pigment epithelium atrophy. An exudative retinal detachment may overlay large choroidal granulomas (▶ Fig. 65.2). Rarely, the optic disc or peripheral retina become neovascularized, potentially leading to intraretinal or vitreous hemorrhage. Perivascular sheathing may occur. Infrequently, severe cases develop periphlebitis, where yellow–white exudates or "candle wax drippings" develop along retinal veins. Rarely, retinal vein occlusions have been reported.

Ocular Hypertension and Uveitic Glaucoma

Glaucoma may occur secondarily to leukocytes clogging the TM, the development of TM nodules, or inflammatory synechiae. Compression from masses also increases intraocular pressure. Chronic inflammation accelerates the formation of cataracts and epiretinal membrane (ERM).

Optic Nerve and Neuro-Ophthalmic Manifestations

The optic nerve can become swollen from either granulomas or inflammation, or retrobulbar inflammation can develop without intraocular involvement (▶ Fig. 65.3). Sarcoidosis can present with a range of neurological symptoms, including cranial nerves palsies and aseptic meningitis.

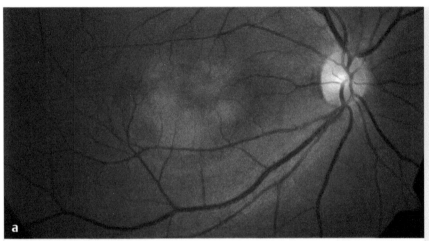

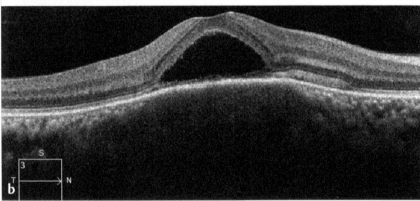

Fig. 65.1 (a) Fundus photograph of a large macular choroidal granuloma with overlying retina fluid in sarcoidosis. (b) Optical coherence tomography through the granuloma, showing choroidal elevation, loss of choroidal vasculature, and overlying subretinal fluid with ellipsoid zone disruption.

65.2 Key Diagnostic Tests and Findings

65.2.1 Optical Coherence Tomography

Detects and monitors CME and ERM. It can also assess the location (e.g., depth) and size of choroidal granulomas, and inflammatory or neovascular changes overlying lesions. Scans of the posterior vitreous can provide an estimate on the amount of vitreous cell.

65.2.2 Fluorescein Angiography or Ultra-Widefield Fluorescein Angiography

Detects CME and peripheral leakage, which may be indicative of disease activity, and highlights areas of occlusive vasculitis and neovascularization (▶ Fig. 65.4). In addition, may identify areas of nonperfusion secondary to vascular occlusions.

65.2.3 Indocyanine Green Angiography

Illuminates areas of hypocyanescence, which can correlate to choroidal granulomas. An increase in total hypocyanescent spots can indicate increased disease burden. Interestingly, these spots do not always correlate to fundus examination (▶ Fig. 65.5).

65.3 Critical Work-up

The gold standard for diagnosis requires a biopsy with noncaseating granulomas. However, given the difficulty of attaining biopsy in sarcoid patients with intraocular manifestations, the International Workshop of Ocular Sarcoidosis established a set of diagnostic criteria based on clinical and laboratory data to classify patients into four categories: definite, presumed, probable, and possible. Definite requires a positive biopsy with concurrent uveitis. Presumed does not require biopsy but has bilateral hilar adenopathy (BHL) with compatible uveitis. Probable does not require biopsy but has BHL, three clinical signs, and two positive laboratory results. Possible has a negative biopsy but with four clinical signs and two positive laboratory results. The clinical signs include mutton-fat KP and/or iris nodules, TM nodules and/or tent-shaped peripheral anterior synechiae, snowballs and/or vitreous opacities, choroidal lesions, periphlebitis and/or macroaneurysms, granulomas of the optic disc and/or choroid, or bilateral uveitis. Laboratory results include a negative tuberculin skin test in a patient with a previously positive skin test or a history of bacille Calmette-Guérin vaccination, BHL on chest radiography or chest CT, elevated angiotensin-converting enzyme and/or serum lysozyme levels, alkaline phosphatase three times higher than the upper limit of normal, or at least two of the following two times higher than the upper limit of normal: alkaline phosphatase, aspartate aminotransferase, alanine aminotransferase, lactic dehydrogenase, or γ-glutamyltransferase.

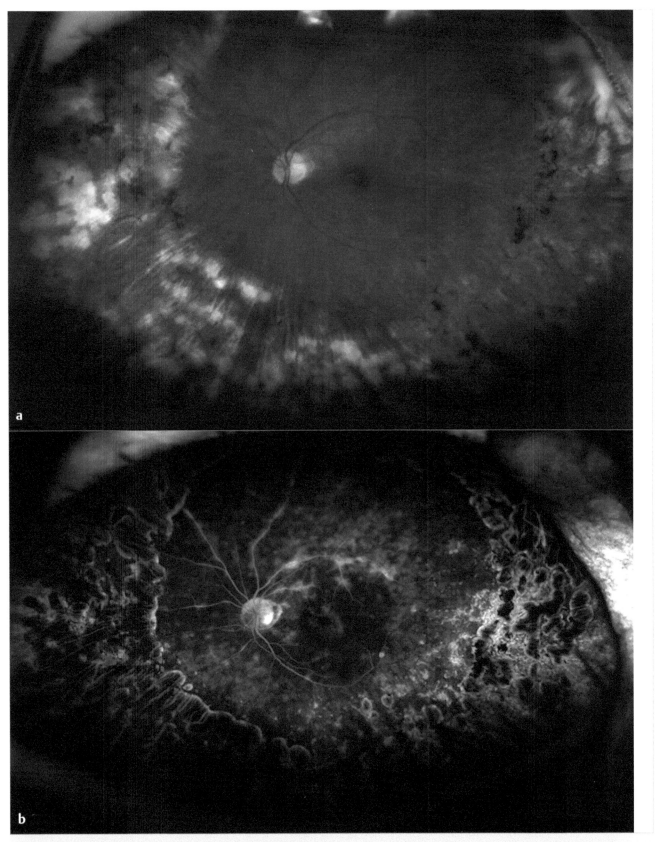

Fig. 65.2 (a) Ultra-widefield fundus photograph showing widespread, confluent peripheral chorioretinal lesions with scarring in sarcoidosis. (b) Fluorescein angiography with impressive window defects corresponding to the chorioretinal scars as well as leakage in the posterior pole.

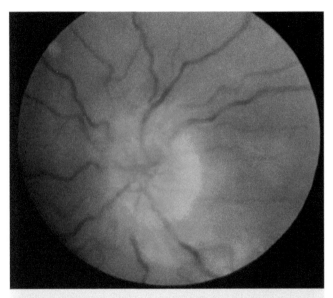

Fig. 65.3 Marked disc edema as a presenting clinical sign in sarcoidosis.

Additionally, chest CT can be useful in elderly patients presenting with uveitis. Even in patients with ocular inflammation and a negative chest radiograph, a chest CT can reveal parenchymal, mediastinal lesions or hilar adenopathy. In a review of 30 elderly women, ranging from ages 61 to 83, who presented with chronic iritis, vitritis, or choroiditis, 17 of the patients had CT chest findings consistent with sarcoid, and of these, 14 were biopsy proven.

65.4 Management

65.4.1 Treatment Options

Treatment is aimed at the preservation of vision and achieving quiescence. If inflammation is localized to the anterior chamber, topical steroids and cycloplegics are employed. If inflammation involves posterior structures, steroids are administered in other forms, including periocular, intravitreal, or systemic. Systemic steroids are also valuable for bilateral or orbital disease. In patients requiring long-term treatment, immunosuppressive agents are utilized.

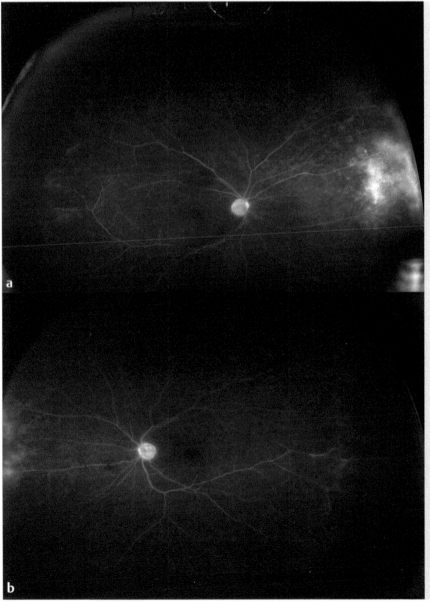

Fig. 65.4 (a) Late ultra-widefield fluorescein angiogram displaying temporal and superior nonperfusion in an eye with active ocular sarcoidosis.

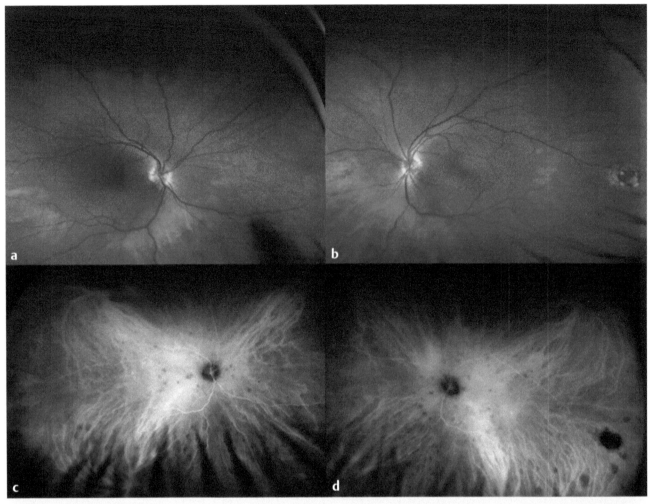

Fig. 65.5 **(a)** Ultra-widefield fundus photograph of the right eye in tattoo-associated sarcoidosis without discernable granulomas on clinical examination. **(b)** Fundus photograph of the left eye with an inactive peripheral chorioretinal scar and no clinically appreciated granulomas. **(c,d)** Ultra-widefield indocyanine green angiography of both eyes reveals choroidal granulomas not observed on examination as hypocyanescent foci on imaging.

65.4.2 Follow-up

It is important to follow patients closely until quiescence. If there is any doubt on the diagnosis, or inadequate response to treatment, referral to a uveitis specialist is warranted. Ongoing intermittent surveillance is important following achievement of quiescence to monitor for any recurrence.

Suggested Reading

[1] Whitcup SM. Sarcoidosis. In Nussenblatt RB, Whitcup SM, (Eds). Uveitis Fundamentals and Clinical Practice. Philadelphia, PA: Mosby 2010:278-288

[2] Acharya NR, Browne EN, Rao N, Mochizuki M. Distinguishing features of ocular sarcoidosis in an international cohort of uveitis patients. Ophthalmology. 2018; 125(1):119–126

[3] Pasadhika S, Rosenbaum JT. Ocular sarcoidosis. Clin Chest Med. 2015; 36(4): 669–683

[4] Herbort CP, Rao NA, Mochizuki M, members of Scientific Committee of First International Workshop on Ocular Sarcoidosis. International criteria for the diagnosis of ocular sarcoidosis: results of the first International Workshop on Ocular Sarcoidosis (IWOS). Ocul Immunol Inflamm. 2009; 17(3):160–169

[5] Kaiser PK, Lowder CY, Sullivan P, et al. Chest computerized tomography in the evaluation of uveitis in elderly women. Am J Ophthalmol. 2002; 133(4): 499–505

66 Serpiginous Choroiditis

Sarina Amin and Ashleigh Levison

Summary

Serpiginous choroiditis is a rare white dot syndrome with inflammation, involving the choriocapillaris, retinal pigment epithelium, and outer retina. Patients typically present with unilateral vision loss but usually have bilateral fundus findings. Recurrence of symptoms is common, usually months to years after the initial onset. Management should not only address active lesions but also prevent recurrence due to the progressive nature of the disease.

Keywords: helicoid, geographic choroidopathy, peripapillary, serpiginous choroiditis, white dot syndrome

66.1 Features

66.1.1 Common Symptoms

Typically presents with unilateral vision loss in fourth to seventh decades of life but usually have bilateral fundus findings as below; paracentral or central scotomas; decreased vision if lesions involve the fovea (75% of patients develop central loss of vision over the course of the disease in at least one eye). The recurrence of symptoms is common, usually months to years after the initial onset.

66.1.2 Exam Findings

Active Classic Variant

Yellow–gray peripapillary lesions with helicoid or serpentine appearance with centrifugal progression. Mild vitritis may be present (reported in 33% of cases).

Macular Variant

Lesions similar to the classic presentation; however, lesions initiate in the macula and therefore portend a poorer prognosis.

Inactive/Chronic

Geographic areas of chorioretinal atrophy, subretinal fibrosis, and retinal pigment epithelial clumping (▶ Fig. 66.1).

Recurrence

New yellow placoid lesions at the edge of old atrophic scars (▶ Fig. 66.2).

Tuberculosis-Related Serpiginous Choroiditis

May present with vitritis and more peripheral lesions.

Other possible ocular findings include choroidal neovascularization (in up to 20% of patients), optic disc edema or neovascularization of the disc, retinal vasculitis (secondary to the extension from underlying inflammation), vascular occlusion (due to inflammation-related obstruction), and cystoid macular edema.

66.2 Key Diagnostic Tests and Findings

66.2.1 Optical Coherence Tomography

Outer retinal atrophy, loss of the inner segment/outer segment junction, and hyperreflectivity of underlying choroidal vasculature. Active lesions may demonstrate increased reflectivity in the outer retina.

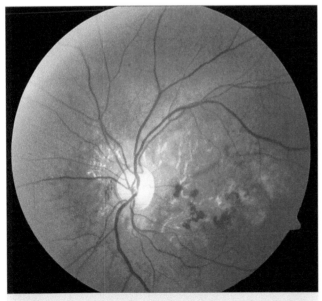

Fig. 66.1 Fundus photograph of inactive serpiginous choroiditis with geographic areas of atrophy in a helicoid pattern, retinal pigment epithelial clumping, and fibrosis.

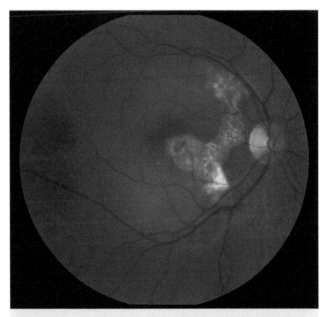

Fig. 66.2 Fundus photograph demonstrating recurrent serpiginous choroiditis with activity at the fovea and inferior border of an area of chorioretinal atrophy.

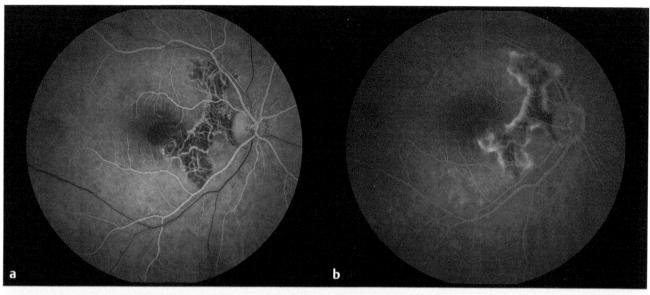

Fig. 66.3 (a) Arterial phase of fluorescein angiogram in serpiginous choroiditis, showing hypofluorescence of the atrophic areas due to choriocapillaris nonperfusion. (b) Late frame of fluorescein angiogram in serpiginous choroiditis, showing continued central hypofluorescence of the atrophic region with hyperfluorescence and staining of the lesion margins consistent with choriocapillaris injury.

66.2.2 Fluorescein Angiography or Ultra-Widefield Fluorescein Angiography

Active, Acute Phase

Early hypofluorescence due to choriocapillaris hypoperfusion and blocking from the edematous outer retina, with late staining of the lesion margins.

Chronic

Early hyperfluorescence from window defects secondary to retinal pigment epithelial atrophy or hypofluorescence from choriocapillaris nonperfusion, with late leakage adjacent to the margins secondary to choriocapillaris injury (▶ Fig. 66.3).

The choroidal neovascular membrane may be noted as late leakage noted from the margin of the lesion.

66.2.3 Indocyanine Green Angiography

Provides more accuracy when determining the extent of activity when compared with fluorescein angiography due to the primary mechanism of choriocapillaris inflammation.

Lesions appear hypofluorescent on indocyanine green angiography in early and late phases due to lack of perfusion, although a slight increase in fluorescence may be noted in later phases due to delayed perfusion and increased choroidal permeability.

66.2.4 Fundus Autofluorescence

Chronic inactive lesions display hypoautofluorescence due to retinal pigment epithelium loss. Active lesions appear hyperautofluorescent. Fundus autofluorescence may be helpful in differentiating serpiginous choroiditis from tuberculosis (TB)-related serpiginous choroiditis (TB-related disease may have more mottled hypoautofluorescence compared with the idiopathic disease).

66.2.5 Optical Coherence Tomography Angiography

Lower vessel density of the choriocapillaris within the borders of the lesion compared with unaffected areas. May be helpful in distinguishing lesions of serpiginous choroiditis from choroidal neovascularization.

66.3 Critical Work-up

66.3.1 Laboratory Evaluation

TB testing (purified protein derivative skin test and Quanti-FERON Gold), angiotensin-converting enzyme and lysozyme, syphilis immunoglobulin G with reflex rapid plasma reagin (RPR) or RPR and fluorescent treponemal antibody absorption, toxoplasma titer, viral screen (aqueous tap with polymerase chain reaction is suggested if anterior chamber cells are present and concern for possible diagnosis of viral retinitis), and complete blood count with differential.

66.3.2 Systemic Imaging

Chest radiography for TB evaluation.

66.4 Management

66.4.1 Treatment Options

Management should not only treat active lesions but also prevent recurrence due to the progressive nature of the disease.

Acute phase treatment options include corticosteroids (oral, intravenous, periocular, and intraocular). Intraocular or periocular steroids can be used in patients that are intolerant to systemically administered corticosteroids, once infectious etiologies have been ruled out. A combination of systemic and periocular/intraocular corticosteroids can be used for fovea-threatening lesions for more aggressive treatment. Immunosuppressive therapy is a maintenance treatment to prevent recurrences. Options can include methotrexate, mycophenolate, cyclosporine, adalimumab, and infliximab. The choroidal neovascular membrane can be treated with intravitreal anti-vascular endothelial growth factor agents or photodynamic therapy (PDT; although PDT may exacerbate inflammation). Cystoid macular edema treatment includes intravitreal steroids.

66.4.2 Follow-up

Initial close follow-up during acute active phases to monitor response to treatment and home monitoring with Amsler grid for recurrences. Monitor for side effects of immunosuppressive therapies in conjunction with a rheumatologist.

Suggested Reading

[1] Mirza R, Jampol L. White spot syndromes and related diseases. In: Ryan S, Schachat A, Wilkinson C, et al, eds. Retina. London: Elsevier; 2018:1346–1350

[2] Freund K, Sarraf D, Mieler W, Yannuzzi L. Inflammation. In: Freund K, Sarraf D, Mieler W, Yannuzzi L, eds. The Retinal Atlas. Philadelphia, PA: Elsevier; 2017:279–398

[3] Montorio D, Guiffrè C, Miserocchi E, et al. Swept-source optical coherence tomography angiography in serpiginous choroiditis. Br J Ophthalmol. 2018; 1; 0; 2(7):991–995

67 Birdshot Retinochoroiditis

Akshay S. Thomas and Glenn Jaffe

Summary

Birdshot retinochoroiditis (BRC), also referred to as birdshot chorioretinopathy, is a form of posterior uveitis, which mainly affects the retina and choroid with characteristic hypopigmented lesions. Classically, there are creamy ovoid lesions, which over time may coalesce into linear streaks. No single imaging modality completely reflects disease activity in BRC. Disease stability or activity is usually ascertained using a combination of imaging modalities and functional tests in addition to patient symptomatology and clinical examination. BRC is usually treated with a combination of systemic corticosteroids, steroid-sparing immunomodulatory therapy, and local corticosteroids.

Keywords: birdshot chorioretinopathy, choroidal neovascularization, cystoid macular edema, birdshot retinochoroiditis

67.1 Features

Birdshot retinochoroiditis (BRC), also referred to as birdshot chorioretinopathy, is a chronic uveitic condition affecting the retina, retinal pigment epithelium (RPE), and choroid. The etiology of BRC is unclear, though there is a strong association with human leukocyte antigen (HLA)-A29, which is positive in over 95% of patients with BRC.

67.1.1 Common Symptoms

Floaters, photopsias, blurry vision, nyctalopia, dyschromatopsia, and/or photophobia.

67.1.2 Exam Findings

Diagnostic criteria for BRC are summarized in ▶ Table 67.1. Typically, there is a variable low-grade anterior chamber inflammation. Findings such as keratic precipitates or posterior synechiae should prompt suspicion for an alternate diagnosis. Additional findings include anterior vitreous cells, mild to moderate vitreous haze, and bilateral cream-colored ovoid choroidal lesions with indistinct borders (▶ Fig. 67.1). The choroidal lesions are usually about 500 to 1,500 μm in diameter and their long axes are oriented radial from the optic nerve head. The choroidal lesions are most often located in the peripapillary retina and tend to be more numerous nasally and inferiorly. With time, these lesions may coalesce in a linear pattern along retinal veins. Additional variably present findings include optic nerve swelling, epiretinal membrane (ERM), cystoid macular edema (CME), choroidal neovascularization (CNV), perivenous sheathing, and retinal neovascularization. Late changes include optic atrophy, vascular attenuation, macular scar formation, and chorioretinal atrophy (▶ Fig. 67.2). Patients may have symptoms for years prior to the development of typical birdshot lesions. In such cases, ancillary testing may be critical for diagnosing BRC.

67.2 Key Diagnostic Tests and Findings

67.2.1 Optical Coherence Tomography

Possible findings on optical coherence tomography (OCT) include CME, ERM, and/or changes associated with CNV formation such as intraretinal fluid, subretinal fluid, and subretinal hyperreflective material. Advanced cases may show outer retinal layer disruption and/or chorioretinal atrophy. Enhanced depth imaging OCT can help identify choroidal lesions, which may appear as focal or diffuse areas of hyporeflectivity.

67.2.2 Fluorescein Angiography or Ultra-Widefield Fluorescein Angiography

Venous leakage, papillitis, CME, CNV, and rarely retinal neovascularization can be identified based on leakage patterns (▶ Fig. 67.3). Birdshot lesions are not usually highlighted on fluorescein angiography, although advanced lesions may be hyperfluorescent secondary to a window defect or staining. "Quenching" may appear wherein dye disappears from the retinal circulation more rapidly than normal.

67.2.3 Indocyanine Green Angiography and Ultra-Widefield Indocyanine Green Angiography

Indocyanine green angiography (ICGA) testing will often reveal a greater number of birdshot lesions than readily evident on

Table 67.1 Diagnostic criteria for birdshot retinochoroiditis based on 2006 UCLA international workshop

Required characteristics	• Bilateral disease • ≥ 3 peripapillary birdshot lesions nasal or inferior to the optic disc in at least one eye • ≤ 1 + cells in the anterior chamber • ≤ 2 + vitreous haze
Supportive findings	• HLA-A29 positivity • Retinal vasculitis • Cystoid macular edema
Exclusion criteria	• Keratic precipitates • Posterior synechiae • Presence of infectious, neoplastic, or alternate inflammatory disease that can produce multifocal choroidal lesions

Abbreviations: HLA, human leukocyte antigen; UCLA, University of California, Los Angeles.

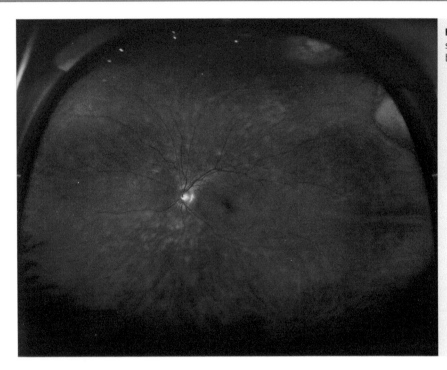

Fig. 67.1 Ultra-widefield color photograph showing widespread depigmented lesions in birdshot retinochoroiditis.

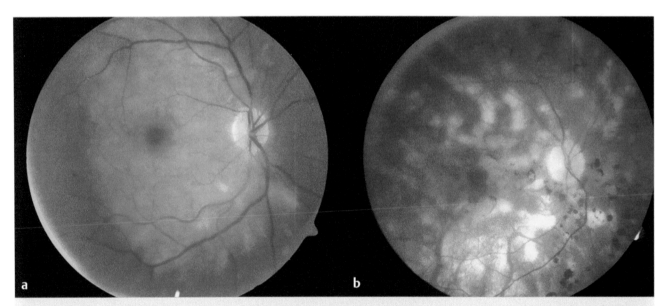

Fig. 67.2 (a) Color fundus photograph of birdshot retinochoroiditis at presentation and (b) 8 years later, showing interval development of numerous additional depigmented lesions in the macula and areas of chorioretinal atrophy nasal to the disc.

ophthalmoscopy and appear as hypocyanescent spots (▶ Fig. 67.4). These spots may fade or resolve with therapy.

67.2.4 Fundus Autofluorescence

May show changes not readily apparent on clinical examination. Patterns vary widely and include confluent peripapillary hypoautofluorescence, macular and/or peripheral hyper- and hypoautofluorescence, and perivascular hyper- and hypoautofluorescence. Hypoautofluorescence may be stippled earlier in the disease process and progress to patches of confluent hypoautofluorescence with progressive RPE loss.

67.2.5 Full-Field Electroretinography

A delayed 30-Hz flicker implicit time is an early and sensitive sign of retinal dysfunction in BRC. The dim-scotopic b-wave amplitude appears to correlate well with overall disease activity and nyctalopia. A decline in electroretinography (ERG) parameters should prompt the escalation of therapy. Typically, performed every 6 to 12 months.

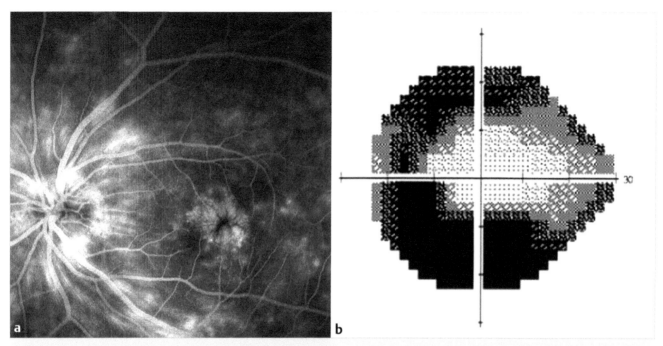

Fig. 67.3 Multimodal imaging and functional testing to assess disease activity in birdshot retinochoroiditis. **(a)** Fluorescein angiography in an eye with birdshot, showing hyperfluorescence/leakage at the disc and along the vessels and petaloid leakage in the macula. **(b)** Humphrey visual field of the left eye of a patient with birdshot, showing peripheral visual field loss.

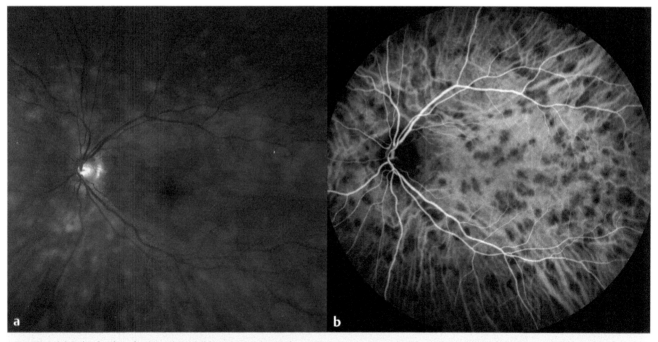

Fig. 67.4 (a) Color fundus photograph and **(b)** corresponding indocyanine green angiogram of an eye with birdshot retinochoroiditis. The birdshot lesions correspond to areas of hypocyanescence on indocyanine green angiography (ICGA). More lesions are readily evident on ICGA than on ophthalmoscopy.

67.2.6 Visual Fields

May reveal patchy peripheral scotomas. Typically, performed every 6 to 12 months and used to assess midperipheral visual function. Special attention needs to be paid to the mean deviation and pattern standard deviation values on automated Humphrey visual fields to help assess the stability or quantify progression.

67.2.7 Optical Coherence Tomography Angiography

Vascular abnormalities such as hypoperfusion of the choriocapillaris, telangiectatic capillaries, and increased perifoveal intercapillary spaces have been observed.

67.3 Critical Work-up

Other causes of posterior uveitis that are associated with depigmented fundus lesions such as sarcoidosis, tuberculosis, and syphilis should be evaluated with antitreponemal antibodies, QuantiFERON Gold testing, and a chest X-ray. When clinical suspicion is high, testing for HLA-A29 positivity is appropriate. Approximately 6 to 8% of the general population is positive for HLA-A29. Thus, a negative HLA-A29 is helpful to rule against the diagnosis of BRC but a positive HLA-A29 in the absence of classic funduscopic findings is not diagnostic of BRC.

67.4 Management

67.4.1 Treatment Options

BRC is usually treated with a combination of systemic corticosteroids, steroid-sparing immunomodulatory therapy (IMT), and local corticosteroids.

Systemic Corticosteroids

Typically, employed as initial therapy and during acute disease exacerbations as a bridge until steroid-sparing IMT levels become therapeutic. Systemic corticosteroids are not usually used as monotherapy. Initially, a prolonged corticosteroid taper may be required. When it is not possible to reduce oral corticosteroids to a reasonable dose (≤ 5.0–7.5 mg/d), IMT or local therapy should be initiated.

Immunomodulatory Therapy

Antimetabolites and biologic agents can effectively control disease activity. Mycophenolate mofetil, azathioprine, and adalimumab are commonly employed (either individually or in combination). Although IMT may achieve stability as measured by ERG, visual fields, and ICGA, it is variably efficacious in the management of uveitic CME. Biological agents may be more effective than antimetabolites in this regard. Appropriate laboratory work to screen for side effects related to the IMT is mandatory.

Local Corticosteroids

Periocular and intravitreal corticosteroids are often effective to manage CME, the most common cause of vision loss in eyes with BRC. A long-acting delivery system such as a fluocinolone acetonide intravitreal implant or a shorter term implant such as a dexamethasone delivery system can be used to treat eyes responsive to local corticosteroid injection or oral corticosteroids. Sustained intraocular implants are especially useful in patients with recurrent or recalcitrant CME, in patients for whom oral steroids cannot be effectively tapered, or in those who cannot tolerate immunomodulatory agents.

67.4.2 Follow-up

Typically, every 2 to 3 months until disease control is noted at which time clinic visits can be spaced out further.

Suggested Reading

[1] Böni C, Thorne JE, Spaide RF, et al. Fundus autofluorescence findings in eyes with birdshot chorioretinitis. Invest Ophthalmol Vis Sci. 2017; 58(10):4015–4025

[2] Böni C, Thorne JE, Spaide RF, et al. Choroidal findings in eyes with birdshot chorioretinitis using enhanced-depth optical coherence tomography. Invest Ophthalmol Vis Sci. 2016; 57(9):OCT591–OCT599

[3] Pichi F, Sarraf D, Arepalli S, et al. The application of optical coherence tomography angiography in uveitis and inflammatory eye diseases. Prog Retin Eye Res. 2017; 59:178–201

[4] Calvo-Río V, Blanco R, Santos-Gómez M, et al. Efficacy of anti-IL6-receptor tocilizumab in refractory cystoid macular edema of birdshot retinochoroidopathy report of two cases and literature review. Ocul Immunol Inflamm. 2017; 25(5):604–609

68 Multiple Evanescent White Dot Syndrome

Geraldine R. Slean and Rahul N. Khurana

Summary

Multiple evanescent white dot syndrome (MEWDS) is a rare condition that was first described in 1984. Patients are typically young, myopic women who present with acute, unilateral, painless blurry vision. Patients can also experience photopsias and an enlarged blind spot. White spots are visible on dilated exam in the posterior pole and midperiphery, and the fovea may appear granular. Fluorescein angiography (FA) shows early punctate hyperfluorescence and late staining. Fundus autofluorescence reveals more hyperautofluorescent spots than are seen on FA or with ophthalmoscopy. MEWDS is typically self-limiting with recovery in weeks to months.

Keywords: white dot syndrome, photopsias, dyschromatopsia

68.1 Features

Multiple evanescent white dot syndrome (MEWDS) is unilateral, multifocal retinitis that affects young, myopic women aged 12 to 57 years, with a mean age of 27 years. Females are affected three to five times more often than males. There are few reports of bilateral or asymmetric presentation. There is no apparent ethnic preponderance.

68.1.1 Common Symptoms

Acute, painless, unilateral blurry vision common; photopsias, dyschromatopsia, and an enlarged blind spot or central/para-central scotoma are often present. About one-third to one-half of patients generally report a flu-like prodrome 1 to 2 weeks prior to presentation.

68.1.2 Exam Findings

Multiple discrete nummular white spots from 100 to 750 μm are seen in the posterior pole and midperipheral retina at the level of the outer retina, retinal pigment epithelium, and inner choroid (▶ Fig. 68.1). Each spot is actually composed of a cluster of smaller lesions. The fovea may appear granular with white, yellow, or orange specks. Other less common findings include a mild vitritis, retinal vasculitis, disc edema and hyperemia, and relative afferent pupillary defect. External and anterior segment examinations are typically normal. Ophthalmoscopy typically confirms the diagnosis, but additional imaging can be supportive.

68.2 Key Diagnostic Tests and Findings

68.2.1 Optical Coherence Tomography

A dome-shaped hyperreflective lesion in the subretinal space with increased choroidal reflectivity corresponds to the white dots. Inner segment/outer segment (i.e., ellipsoid zone) disruption can also be seen, often in both eyes.

68.2.2 Fluorescein Angiography or Ultra-Widefield Fluorescein Angiography

White spots exhibit early punctate hyperfluorescence with a wreath-like appearance. Late staining of the spots and late leakage of the disc are also visible (▶ Fig. 68.2). Window defects may correlate with macular granularity. Fluorescein angiography (FA) can continue to show lesions even after clinical resolution of spots.

68.2.3 Indocyanine Green Angiography

Multiple hypocyanescent spots are visible which correspond to white dots. More spots are seen with indocyanine green angiography (ICGA) than are detected with ophthalmoscopy or FA. A hypocyanescent annular area encircling the optic nerve is associated with the enlarged blind spot. Spots may persist for many months after resolution of visual symptoms and inflammation. Spots are sometimes present in the other, asymptomatic eye.

68.2.4 Fundus Autofluorescence

Hyperautofluorescence corresponds to the white dots, which may be more easily visualized with fundus autofluorescence

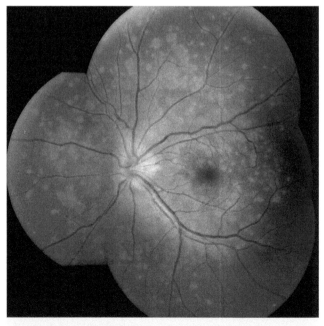

Fig. 68.1 Multiple white lesions at the level of the outer retina and retinal pigment epithelium are seen in the posterior pole and the midperiphery in multiple evanescent white dot syndrome.

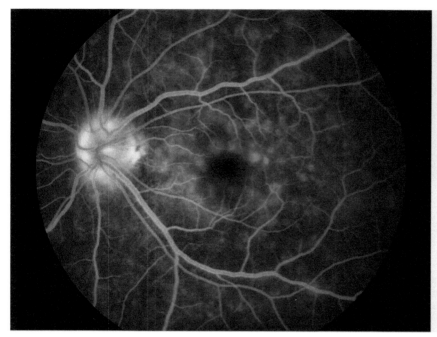

Fig. 68.2 Fluorescein angiography shows disk leakage, mild vascular staining, and wreath-like staining of the white lesions in the posterior pole in the late phase.

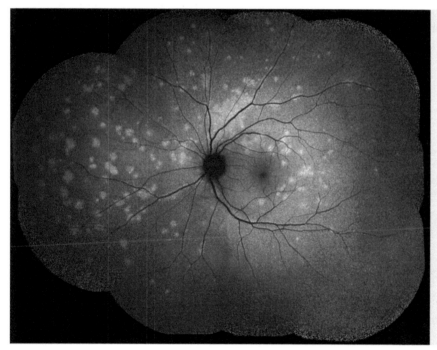

Fig. 68.3 Montage fundus autofluorescence demonstrates hyperautofluorescent dots that correlate with the white dots observed on funduscopy.

(FAF; ▸ Fig. 68.3). Even in the absence of white dots on funduscopic examination, FAF can reveal the characteristic lesions. FAF lesions can persist even after FA and ICGA lesions appear resolved.

68.2.5 Electroretinography

Electroretinography (ERG) shows a decreased a-wave and reduced early receptor potential amplitudes. Multifocal ERG demonstrates areas of depression that correlate with the scotoma or enlarged blind spot. These changes typically resolve after 6 weeks.

68.3 Critical Work-up

The differential for MEWDS includes acute posterior multifocal placoid pigment epitheliopathy, acute zonal occult outer retinopathy (AZOOR), birdshot chorioretinopathy, ocular infiltration by lymphoma, multifocal choroiditis, sarcoidosis, and syphilis. If a patient presents with atypical findings or delayed recovery with suspected MEWDS, the differential should be further explored and appropriately worked up with additional laboratory evaluation. Standardized visual field testing with a Humphrey visual field 24–2 test can also be performed to better document a scotoma.

Table 68.1 Summary of MEWDS symptoms, findings, and treatment

MEWDS	Symptoms	Exam	OCT	FA	ICGA	Treatment
	• Acute, unilateral blurry vision • Photopsias • Enlarged blind spot	• Nummular white spots in midperiphery • Granular fovea	• IS/OS disruption • Subretinal hyperreflectivity	• Early hyperfluorescence, late staining	• More hypocyanescent spots than visible by ophthalmoscopy	• Self-resolving

Abbreviations: FA, fluorescein angiography; ICGA, indocyanine green angiography; IS/OS, inner segment/outer segment; MEWDS, multiple evanescent white dot syndrome; OCT, optical coherence tomography.

68.4 Management

68.4.1 Treatment Options

MEWDS is self-limiting with visual recovery in 3 to 10 weeks (▶ Table 68.1). However, retina sequelae such as chorioretinal scars, peripapillary atrophy, and choroidal neovascularization can occur.

68.4.2 Follow-up

MEWDS can in rare cases recur or progress to bilateral involvement. Patients can also develop secondary inflammation (such as multifocal choroiditis, panuveitis, acute macular neuroretinopathy, AZOOR, and autoimmune retinopathy). As such, patients should have regular long-term follow-up.

Suggested Reading

[1] Mirza RG, Jampol LM. White Spot Syndromes and Related Diseases. In: Ryan SJ, ed. Retina. 5th ed. Philadelphia, PA: Elsevier; 2013: 1337–1380

[2] dell'Omo R, Pavesio CE. Multiple evanescent white dot syndrome (MEWDS). Int Ophthalmol Clin. 2012; 52(4):221–228

[3] Jampol LM, Wiredu A. MEWDS, MFC, PIC, AMN, AIBSE, and AZOOR: one disease or many? Retina. 1995; 15(5):373–378

[4] Barile GR, Harmon SA. Multiple evanescent white dot syndrome with central visual loss. Retin Cases Brief Rep. 2017; 11 Suppl 1:S219–S225

69 Acute Posterior Multifocal Placoid Pigment Epitheliopathy

David Xu and David Sarraf

Summary

Acute posterior multifocal placoid pigment epitheliopathy (APMPPE) is an idiopathic bilateral inflammatory condition, which presents with painless, rapid-onset vision loss and may be associated with antecedent flu-like symptoms reported in about half of patients. The visual prognosis is favorable with most patients retaining near-normal central vision, although most report residual deficits or persistent scotomas. Severe vision loss may occur in some cases. The evaluation and management of APMPPE is guided by multimodal imaging. Patients should be questioned for neurological symptoms and be urgently referred for the evaluation if they develop.

Keywords: APMPPE, central nervous system vasculitis, retinal pigment epithelium

69.1 Features

Acute posterior multifocal placoid pigment epitheliopathy (APMPPE) is an idiopathic bilateral inflammatory condition most often affecting young individuals aged 20 to 40 years with equal sex predilection. The disease presents with painless, rapid-onset vision loss, and about half of patients report antecedent flu-like symptoms. Uncommonly, central nervous system (CNS) vasculitis has been reported with serious complications, including parenchymal and basal ganglia stroke, intracranial hemorrhage, and small-vessel vasculopathy. While APMPPE is a self-limited disease, there are other forms of this disorder that have a more unfavorable course and prognosis. Persistent placoid maculopathy is remarkable for persistent choroidal ischemia that may last weeks or months and is often complicated by choroidal neovascularization (CNV). Relentless placoid chorioretinitis may be associated with multiple recurrent lesions in the posterior pole and periphery. Serpiginous choroidopathy may also have a relentless course with the development of lesions in a helicoid pattern around the disc and toward the fovea. These variants fall on a spectrum that can be difficult to specifically categorize some cases.

The exact mechanism of APMPPE is unknown; however, a primary inflammatory process involving the choriocapillaris or the retinal pigment epithelium (RPE) has been proposed. Recently, optical coherence tomography (OCT) angiography (OCTA) and indocyanine green angiography (ICGA) have identified flow reduction in the choriocapillaris, suggesting this layer is the primary site of disease. The underlying etiology may be an immune-driven reaction triggered by viral illness or vaccination rather than direct infection. APMPPE has also been reported after vaccination against meningococcus C, mumps, influenza, and hepatitis B. The disease has been grouped into the so-called uveocerebral vasculitic syndromes along with Vogt–Koyanagi–Harada (VKH) disease, Susac syndrome, and Eales disease. Occlusive choroidal vasculitis along with systemic vasculitis and neurologic complications may be linked. An association has also been identified with infectious and inflammatory conditions caused by delayed-type hypersensitivity reactions, including sarcoidosis, tuberculosis (TB), ulcerative colitis, and group A *Streptococcus* infection. APMPPE has also been observed in antineutrophil cytoplasmic antibody (ANCA)-associated vasculitis and syphilis. Approximately 40 to 50% of patients show positivity for human leukocyte antigen (HLA)-DR2 and HLA-B7, which suggests a common susceptibility to abnormal immune activation.

69.1.1 Common Symptoms

Ocular

Typically, patients note acute-onset vision loss, metamorphopsia, and scotomas; at least 75% of patients have bilateral disease or experience sequential onset of symptoms affecting the fellow eye within days or weeks.

Systemic (Nonneurologic)

About 50% of patients report an antecedent flu-like illness. Other symptoms include erythema nodosum, thyroiditis, nephritis, and systemic vasculitis.

Neurologic

Headache is common. Patients may experience hearing loss, seizure, stroke symptoms, cranial nerve palsies, meningoencephalitis, and cavernous sinus thrombosis. Neurologic complications are important to exclude because APMPPE-associated CNS vasculitis can have serious consequences, including death in rare circumstances.

69.1.2 Exam Findings

In the acute stage, multifocal, plaque-like, creamy yellow–white lesions at the level of the RPE are present that mask the underlying choroidal features (▶ Fig. 69.1). Lesions are localized to the posterior pole and may extend to the midperiphery. There may be mild to moderate vitreous inflammation, although the anterior chamber is typically quiet. New lesions may arise over days or weeks and existing lesions may enlarge. A temporal dissociation of lesions is characteristic. Retinal findings differ in the acute versus the chronic stage.

69.2 Key Diagnostic Tests and Findings

69.2.1 Optical Coherence Tomography

Acute

Multifocal, discrete hyperreflective lesions extend from the ellipsoid zone (EZ) to the outer plexiform layer and along the Henle fiber layer (▶ Fig. 69.2). There may be dome-shaped

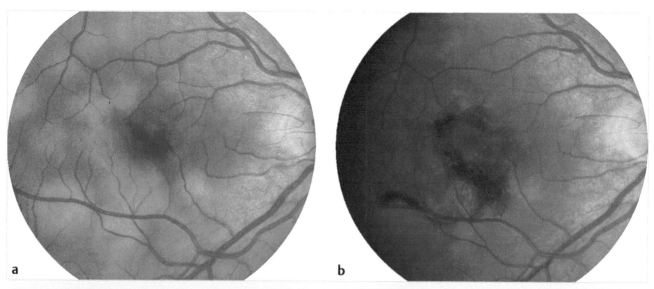

Fig. 69.1 **(a)** The fundus photograph shows multiple creamy yellow lesions at the level of the retinal pigment epithelium **(b)** that eventually resolve with variable degrees of hyperpigmentation.

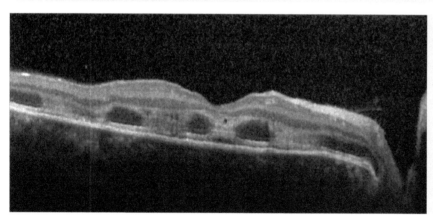

Fig. 69.2 Optical coherence tomography demonstrates hyperreflective lesions spanning the outer nuclear layer and coursing along the Henle fiber layer, characteristic of acute posterior multifocal placoid pigment epitheliopathy.

separation of the EZ and RPE, and intraretinal or subretinal fluid. Thickening and widening of the choriocapillaris band underscore the importance of the inner choroid in this disease.

Chronic

Disruption of the EZ, loss of the external limiting membrane, and RPE atrophy may be present.

69.2.2 Fluorescein Angiography or Ultra-Widefield Fluorescein Angiography

Early hypofluorescence (due to choroidal ischemia) and late staining of the lesions are characteristic in APMPPE and other placoid-related disorders (▶ Fig. 69.3). Widefield fluorescein angiography (FA) will often reveal subclinical peripheral lesions that block early and stain late.

69.2.3 Indocyanine Green Angiography

Multifocal hypofluorescent areas (more numerous than those identified clinically) are present early in the study and may be associated with choroidal filling delay and choroidal nonperfusion (▶ Fig. 69.4).

69.2.4 Fundus Autofluorescence

Acute lesions are typically hyperautofluorescent due to RPE disruption, while chronic lesions are hypoautofluorescent due to RPE atrophy. Fundus autofluorescence provides a simple and noninvasive tool to assess lesion resolution.

69.2.5 Optical Coherence Tomography Angiography

Remarkable patches of flow deficit and nonperfusion of the choriocapillaris and inner choroid are identified and colocalize with the hypofluorescent areas on FA and ICGA. OCTA provides a simple, fast, and noninvasive tool to diagnose choroidal ischemia and to assess lesions for progression and treatment response.

69.3 Critical Work-up

The evaluation and management of APMPPE is guided by multi-modal imaging. The classic FA and ICGA patterns described

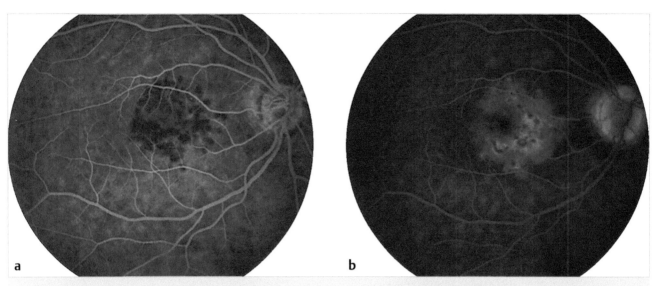

Fig. 69.3 (a) Fluorescein angiography demonstrates early hypoautofluorescence and (b) late staining of the lesions.

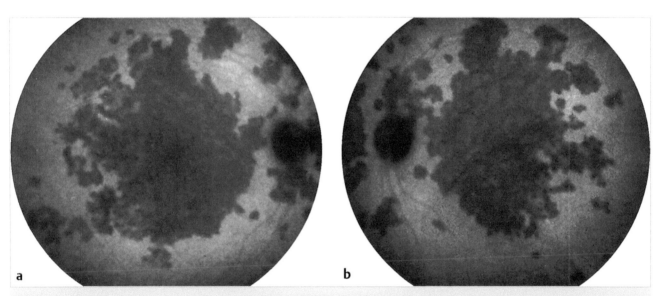

Fig. 69.4 (a,b) Indocyanine green angiography discloses diffuse, multifocal filling defects in the choroid. OCT angiography has localized the ischemia to the choriocapillaris.

above are typically diagnostic, especially in association with the characteristic OCT and OCTA findings. In the era of advanced retinal imaging, OCT and OCTA may be employed to monitor recovery of placoid lesions and response to therapy, if instituted. Infectious and inflammatory masquerades of APMPPE and the other white dot syndromes include VKH disease, sarcoidosis, ocular syphilis, and ocular TB. Systemic workup for vasculitis should be performed, including erythrocyte sedimentation rate, C-reactive protein, cytoplasmic ANCA, as well as testing for sarcoidosis, syphilis, and TB.

Importantly, patients should be questioned for neurological symptoms. Any signs of neurologic involvement should prompt urgent evaluation for CNS vasculitis or stroke, which have serious, potentially life-threatening consequences. While APMPPE may affect men and women equally, the majority of patients with CNS vasculitis are men. Urgent neurological consultation

should be arranged to consider magnetic resonance imaging (MRI), cerebral angiography, computed tomography angiography, and lumbar puncture (LP) when CNS vasculitis is suspected. MRI may reveal white matter infarcts, parenchymal or basal ganglia strokes, or intracerebral hemorrhage. Cerebral angiography may illustrate small-vessel vasculitis or cerebral artery occlusion. LP may show cerebrospinal fluid pleocytosis.

69.4 Management

Lesions resolve over the course of weeks or months beginning with central clearing and progressive hypopigmentation, leaving a legacy of scattered patches of RPE atrophy and pigment hyperplasia in the chronic stage. The visual prognosis is favorable with most patients retaining near-normal central vision, although most report residual deficits or persistent scotomas. Uncommonly, severe vision loss may occur due to foveal atrophy and/or scarring. The recurrence of acute APMPPE is rare but occurs in a minority of patients associated with new placoid lesions. Recurrent CNS vasculitis and recurrent stroke have also been reported and may be triggered by rapid taper of corticosteroid after the initial event. Late-onset complications such as CNV may occur even years after the resolution of acute disease.

69.4.1 Treatment Options

APMPPE is generally a self-limited disease that can be observed without treatment. Macula-threatening or recurrent APMPPE can be treated with corticosteroid therapy. CNS vasculitis should be treated with high-dose corticosteroids with a slow taper or bridged to another immunosuppressant such as aza-thioprine or mycophenylate or cyclophosphamide and should be typically managed with a multidisciplinary team.

69.4.2 Follow-up

Patients should be observed for resolution of acute disease and subsequently followed at intervals to check for progression of atrophy and pigmentary changes and for the development of CNV. Patients should be urgently referred for evaluation if they develop neurologic symptoms.

Suggested Reading

[1] Case D, Seinfeld J, Kumpe D, et al. Acute posterior multifocal placoid pigment epitheliopathy associated with stroke: a case report and review of the literature. J Stroke Cerebrovasc Dis. 2015; 24(10):e295–e302

[2] Raven ML, Ringeisen AL, Yonekawa Y, Stem MS, Faia LJ, Gottlieb JL. Multi-modal imaging and anatomic classification of the white dot syndromes. Int J Retina Vitreous. 2017; 3:12

[3] Mrejen S, Sarraf D, Chexal S, Wald K, Freund KB. Choroidal involvement in acute posterior multifocal placoid pigment epitheliopathy. Ophthalmic Surg Lasers Imaging Retina. 2016; 47(1):20–26

[4] Klufas S, Phasukkijwatana D, Iafe S, et al. Optical Coherence Tomography Angiography Reveals Choriocapillaris Flow Reduction in Placoid Chorioretinitis. Ophthalmol Retina. 2017 Jan-Feb; 1(1):77–91

70 Behçet Disease

Sarina Amin and Ashleigh Levison

Summary

Behçet disease is a chronic and relapsing-remitting disorder characterized by obliterative vasculitis affecting multiple organ systems. Visual prognosis is related to the location and severity of uveitis, with severe posterior occlusive vasculitis resulting in a worse prognosis. There is a high mortality rate if central nervous system involvement is present. Various imaging modalities are useful in determining disease activity level, monitoring disease progression, and evaluating response to treatment.

Keywords: Behçet disease, Iridocyclitis, panuveitis, uveitis

70.1 Features

70.1.1 Common Symptoms

Ocular complaints (noted in up to 50% of Behçet patients) are usually bilateral; symptoms include photophobia, eye pain, decreased vision, red eye, and floaters. Systemic manifestations, including oral and genital ulcers, usually precede ocular manifestations (▶ Table 70.1).

70.1.2 Exam Findings

Patients develop recurrent, nongranulomatous uveitis (anterior, intermediate, posterior, or most commonly panuveitis). Anterior segment findings include cell, flare, keratic precipitates, cyclitic membranes, posterior synechiae, and/or anterior synechiae. Other possible anterior segment findings include hypopyon (12%) with or without conjunctival injection; cataracts (cortical secondary to inflammation and posterior subcapsular secondary to corticosteroid treatment); episcleritis or ciliary flush; neovascularization of the iris; seclusio pupillae

(with the associated risk of secondary pupillary block glaucoma); and uncommonly conjunctival ulcer. Posterior segment findings vary (▶ Table 70.2) but often include vitritis, retinal vasculitis, retinal hemorrhage, and areas of retinitis (▶ Fig. 70.1▶ Fig. 70.2). Phthisis bulbi may be observed in end-stage disease.

70.2 Key Diagnostic Tests and Findings

70.2.1 Optical Coherence Tomography

Optical coherence tomography (OCT) findings include inner retinal hyperreflectivity in regions of occlusive vasculitis, thinning/atrophy in areas of previous vascular occlusion, cystoid macular edema, and/or epiretinal membrane (▶ Fig. 70.1). OCT is useful in diagnosing macular pathology and monitoring response to treatment.

70.2.2 Fluorescein Angiography or Ultra-Widefield Fluorescein Angiography

Fluorescein angiography (FA) commonly reveals leakage from retinal vessels in cases with retinal vasculitis and petaloid leakage in the macula in a patient with cystoid macular edema. Hypofluorescent regions may signify areas of capillary nonperfusion. Disc or retinal neovascularization may be noted as increase and expansion of hyperfluorescence from early to later phases of the FA. FA is useful in determining disease activity level and response to treatment and may show retinal vascular alterations in up to 6% of the patient despite lack of clinical exam findings.

Table 70.1 Behçet's Disease Research Committee of Japan diagnostic criteria (92% sensitivity and 89% specificity). All four major criteria are required for the diagnosis of complete-type Behçet disease. An incomplete-type diagnosis consists of the presence of three major criteria, two major and two minor criteria, ocular disease plus one major criterion, or ocular disease plus two minor criteria. (Data from Lehner et al. 1979; Behçet's Disease Research Committee of Japan, 1987.)

Major criteria	Minor criteria
• Recurrent oral aphthous ulcers (nearly all patients; must have three recurrences over 12-mo period) • Skin lesions (seen in up to 80%; erythema nodosum-like lesions, folliculitis, acneiform lesions, thrombophlebitis, and cutaneous hypersensitivity) • Genital ulcers • Ocular disease (Iridocyclitis and posterior uveitis)	• Arthritis (50%; affects knees, ankles, wrists, and elbows) • Epididymitis • Intestinal symptoms attributed to ileocecal ulcerations • Vascular symptoms • Neurologic symptoms (headache, cranial nerve palsies, seizures, stroke, meningitis, etc.)

Source: Adapted from Lehner et al. 1979; Behçet's Disease Research Committee of Japan, 1987.

Table 70.2 Posterior segment findings in Behçet disease

Vitreous	• Vitreous cell or haze • Vitreous hemorrhage • Vitreous snowbanking/snowballs
Optic nerve	• Disc edema • Neovascularization of the disc (▶ Fig. 70.1) • Pallor • Disc hyperemia
Retina	• Retinal vasculitis (affecting arterioles and venules) • Retinitis • Cystoid macular edema • Intraretinal hemorrhage • Neovascularization • Chorioretinitis • Epiretinal membrane • Macular hole • Retinal vascular occlusion (secondary to obliterative vasculitis) • Exudative or tractional retinal detachment • Retinal pigment epithelial atrophy

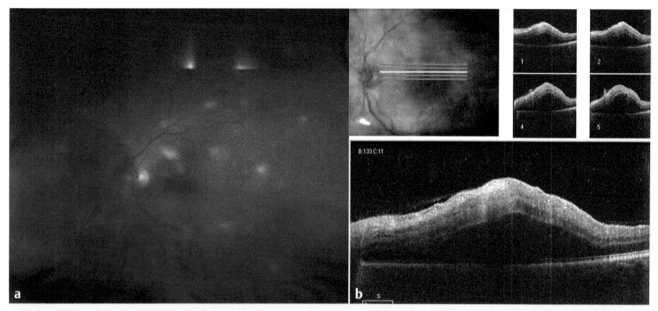

Fig. 70.1 **(a)** Ultra-widefield fundus photograph and **(b)** optical coherence tomography (OCT) of active Behçet disease. The fundus photograph demonstrates multiple cotton wool spots from an active flare. The corresponding OCT on the right shows inner retinal hyperreflectivity and retinal thickening consistent with retinal ischemia and ongoing inflammation.

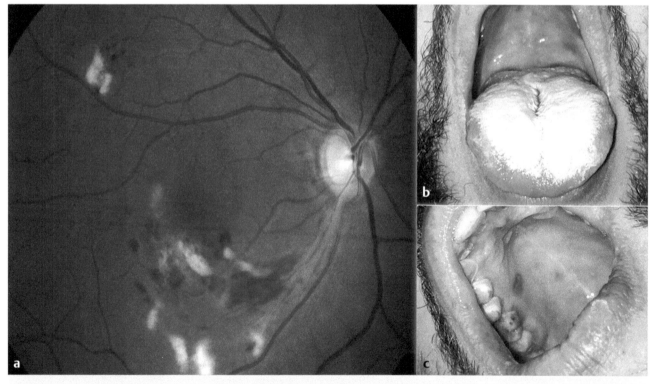

Fig. 70.2 Acute vascular occlusion with systemic findings of Behçet disease. **(a)** Fundus photograph of the right eye demonstrates retinal hemorrhage and retinal ischemia in Behçet disease consistent with vascular occlusion. **(b,c)** The external photographs show oral involvement, including classic aphthous ulcers on the roof of his mouth.

70.2.3 Indocyanine Green Angiography

Hyperfluorescence secondary to choroidal hyperpermeability or hypofluorescence secondary to choroidal hypoperfusion may be noted. Typically, not used for monitoring disease progression as pathophysiology primarily involves inflammation of the retina and its vasculature.

70.2.4 Optical Coherence Tomography Angiography

Emerging technology that provides depth-encoded information related to vascular flow. Enables visualization of retinal flow voids representing nonperfusion and ischemia. Current technology is primarily useful for macular assessment; however, faster systems, such as swept-source OCT, enable wider field visualization.

70.3 Critical Work-up

Laboratory evaluation includes human leukocyte antigen B51 (negative result does not exclude diagnosis); tuberculosis (TB) testing (purified protein derivative skin test, QuantiFERON Gold); angiotensin-converting enzyme; syphilis immunoglobulin G with reflex rapid plasma reagin (RPR) or RPR and fluorescent treponemal antibody absorption; antineutrophil cytoplasmic antibodies; lupus testing (ANA with anti-double-stranded DNA); and viral screen (aqueous tap with polymerase chain reaction is suggested if anterior chamber cells are present and concern for possible diagnosis of viral retinitis). Imaging should include chest radiography for sarcoid and TB evaluation. Visual prognosis is related to the location and severity of uveitis; severe posterior occlusive vasculitis portends a worse prognosis. There is a high mortality rate if central nervous system involvement is present.

70.4 Management

70.4.1 Treatment Options

Acute-Phase

Corticosteroids (oral, intravenous, periocular, and intraocular). Topical therapy with cycloplegics and corticosteroids can be used for isolated anterior segment inflammation. Intraocular or periocular steroids can be used for posterior segment inflammation, possibly in conjunction with systemic corticosteroids.

Maintenance to Prevent Recurrences

Immunosuppressive therapy, such as mycophenolate, azathioprine, cyclosporine or tacrolimus, infliximab, and adalimumab, may all be considered. If severe occlusive vasculitis is present, patients are typically started on anti-tumor necrosis factor. Cyclophosphamide or chlorambucil is often reserved for more severe cases and those with neurologic manifestations.

Cystoid Macular Edema

Intravitreal steroids.

Disc or Retinal Neovascularization

Laser photocoagulation to areas of peripheral capillary nonperfusion and anti-vascular endothelial growth factor agents.

Surgical Intervention

May be required for cataract, pupillary block, uveitic glaucoma, macular hole, epiretinal membrane, nonresolving vitreous hemorrhage, or tractional retinal detachment.

70.4.2 Follow-up

Follow-up closely during acute active phases to monitor response to treatment and monitor for side effects of immunosuppressive therapies in conjunction with a rheumatologist.

Suggested Reading

[1] Atmaca-Somez P, Atmaca L. Posterior pole manifestations of Behçet's disease. In: Arevalo, JF, ed. Retinal and choroidal manifestations of selected systemic diseases. New York, NY: Springer; 2013:225–245

[2] Özyazgan Y, Bodaghi B. Eye disease in Behçet's syndrome. In: Yazici Y and Yazici H, eds. Behçet's syndrome. New York, NY: Springer; 2010:73–9

71 Pars Planitis

Aniruddha Agarwal, Peter H. Tang, Kanika Aggarwal, and Quan Dong Nguyen

Summary

Pars planitis is a subset of intermediate uveitis where the cause is idiopathic. Depending on the severity of vitreous inflammation, some patients may develop blinding sequelae and complications such as tractional retinal detachment and optic disc edema. Given the potentially severe and debilitating nature of pars planitis, patients should be thoroughly evaluated for other causes of intermediate uveitis such as multiple sclerosis, and prompt management with corticosteroids, immunosuppressive agents, or biological agents should be initiated when indicated. Multimodal imaging is employed in the management of these patients to understand and determine the exact extent of tissue damage in eyes with pars planitis. In general, the disease prognosis is worse in patients diagnosed at a younger age. While pars planitis has a variable natural history and prognosis, most cases show progressive worsening of inflammation and tissue damage in the absence of therapy. It is therefore imperative to strategically initiate a system of escalating anti-inflammatory therapy with/without immunosuppressive agents based on the clinical findings and disease response.

Keywords: intermediate uveitis, pars planitis, snowballs, snow-banking

71.1 Features

Intermediate uveitis is the general terminology for inflammation localized predominantly in the vitreous, ciliary body, and peripheral retina that may or may not be associated with an infectious agent or systemic disease. Pars planitis is a subset of intermediate uveitis where the cause is idiopathic, and clinical findings include snowbank or snowball formation. Such nomenclature is an important distinction, as pars planitis is a diagnosis of exclusion that is made only after a thorough investigation into potential infectious or autoimmune causes has been conducted. Pars planitis is a nongranulomatous bilateral uveitis occurring in young individuals (e.g., 15–35 years old). As the majority of pediatric patients with uveitis have an indeterminate cause, pars planitis is most often diagnosed in this patient population. Due to the wide spectrum of clinical findings, the reported incidence and prevalence of this disease is highly variable with an incidence of between 1.5 and 2.0 per 100,000 people. Studies have suggested a genetic predisposition, and various haplotypes such as HLA-DR2, -DR15, -B51, and -DRB1*0802 have been associated with the disease. There is a strong association with the development of multiple sclerosis in patients with pars planitis, and individuals with either the HLA-DR2 or -DR15 haplotype showed the highest association.

71.1.1 Common Symptoms

Blurred vision (74%) and floaters (61%) may be present in the majority of patients at the time of diagnosis. Other less common symptoms include pain (6.5%), photophobia (6.5%), and red eye (4.3%).

71.1.2 Exam Findings

This disease usually occurs bilaterally; however, there can be asymmetric involvements. Often, the inflammation may be limited to only a few anterior vitreous cells with or without cystoid macular edema (CME). Common clinical findings include vitritis, snowballs, snow-banking (i.e., confluent deposits of snowballs inferiorly that appears as a whitish thickened area), peripheral retinal vasculitis, and CME. The peripheral retinal vasculitis may be present for 360 degrees. In addition, there may also be associated papillitis. Anterior segment inflammation, band keratopathy, peripheral corneal opacification, and posterior synechiae are observed more often in children as compared to adults.

Vitreous snowball and snowbank formation in pars planitis is common with over 65 and 95%, respectively (▶ Fig. 71.1, ▶ Fig. 71.2). Vitreous snowballs are yellow-white inflammatory aggregates that are usually found in the mid- and inferior peripheral vitreous. The frequency of retinal vasculitis is variable. Optic disc edema is also a common finding in more than 50% of cases. The presence of retinochoroidal lesions rules out the diagnosis of pars planitis.

71.2 Key Diagnostic Tests and Findings

71.2.1 Optical Coherence Tomography

Optical coherence tomography (OCT) is valuable in detecting CME and other sequelae such as epiretinal membrane (ERM), macular hole, and atrophy (▶ Fig. 71.3). It is useful in tracking therapeutic response and may provide prognostic information based on foveal thickness as well as other factors such as outer retinal and photoreceptor abnormalities. Eyes with abnormal ellipsoid zones on OCT may show poor prognosis and irreversible vision loss.

71.2.2 Fluorescein Angiography or Ultra-Widefield Fluorescein Angiography

Ultra-widefield fluorescein angiography (UWFA) and fluorescein angiography (FA) may demonstrate the presence of retinal vascular inflammation, papillitis, and CME. In the area of snow-banking with active inflammation, there is early hyperfluorescence with late leakage, signifying the presence of inflammation (▶ Fig. 71.4). UWFA may detect subclinical disease activity through identification of peripheral vascular leakage. The leakage may be followed as a marker of disease activity and treatment response with serial UWFA.

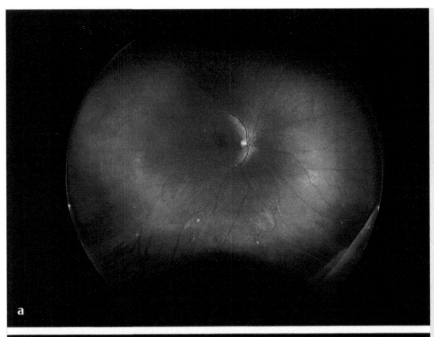

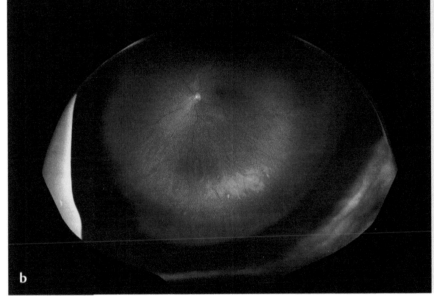

Fig. 71.1 (a,b) Bilateral pars planitis. Ultra-widefield fundus photographs demonstrate bilateral inferior snowballs.

71.2.3 Optical Coherence Tomography Angiography

Optical coherence tomography angiography may provide macular perfusion status in eyes affected by pars planitis.

71.2.4 Ultrasonography

In eyes with media opacity preventing posterior segment exam, ultrasonography can help detect vitritis, posterior segment complications such as retinal detachment (RD), vitreous hemorrhage (VH), and other vitreoretinal abnormalities. Ultrasound biomicroscopy (UBM) is particularly useful in the detection of cyclitic membranes and ciliary body atrophy. UBM can also detect peripheral snowballs and peripheral vitreous traction.

71.2.5 Fundus Photography

Color fundus photography provides documentation of vitreous haze, vitreous snowballs, and visible vascular changes consistent with vasculitis. With ultra-widefield imaging, snow-banking may also be visualized (▶ Fig. 71.1, ▶ Fig. 71.2).

71.3 Critical Work-up

The diagnosis of pars planitis is established in the absence of other causes of intermediate uveitis and must be rechallenged over the patient's course of disease since its clinical findings can predate other manifestations of systemic conditions. It is imperative to rule out other causes such as multiple sclerosis, an entity whose diagnosis may be established later during the

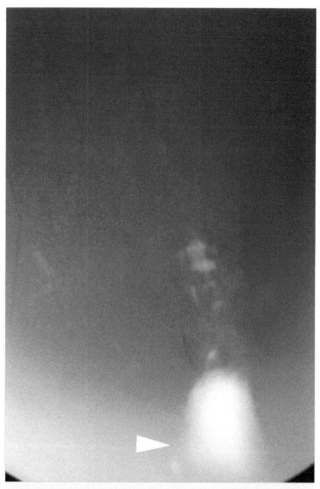

Fig. 71.2 Fundus photograph demonstrating an inferior snowbank (*arrowhead*).

course of the disease. Baseline neuroimaging is performed to rule out white matter lesions of the central nervous system. It is also important to rule out other common causes of intermediate uveitis such as sarcoidosis and infectious etiologies such as tuberculosis. The evaluations can be performed through laboratory testing (e.g., angiotensin-converting enzyme levels, interferon gamma assays) and imaging studies (e.g., chest X-ray or chest computed tomographic scan). Additional causes of chronic ocular inflammation such as juvenile idiopathic arthritis must be kept in the differential diagnosis. In the elderly, intraocular lymphoma may present as intermediate uveitis. The majority of these conditions can be differentiated from pars planitis by a thorough clinical history and laboratory tests.

71.4 Management

71.4.1 Treatment Options

Observation

Many pars planitis patients can be managed through observation as long as symptoms are minimal and there is no significant involvement of the macula/optic nerve. Dense vitreous debris from previous active inflammation leading to persistent floaters may be present. Therefore, it is imperative to assess the level of inflammation, using imaging techniques such as UWFA to provide baseline information and to better gauge the need for intervention.

Pharmacotherapy

The first-line treatment typically consists of local (sub-Tenon) periocular corticosteroids such as triamcinolone acetonide. Intravitreal injections of corticosteroids are also used in patients with pars planitis; however, intravitreal use of steroids

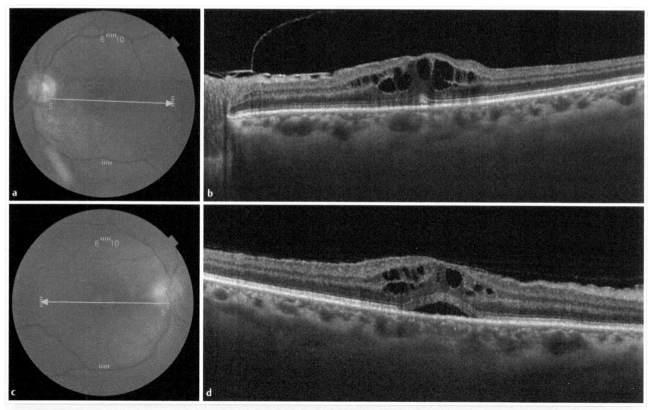

Fig. 71.3 Optical coherence tomography and corresponding fundus images of the **(a,b)** right and **(c,d)** left eyes of the same patient show presence of multiple cystoid spaces in both eyes along with subfoveal serous detachment in the right eye indicating cystoid macular edema.

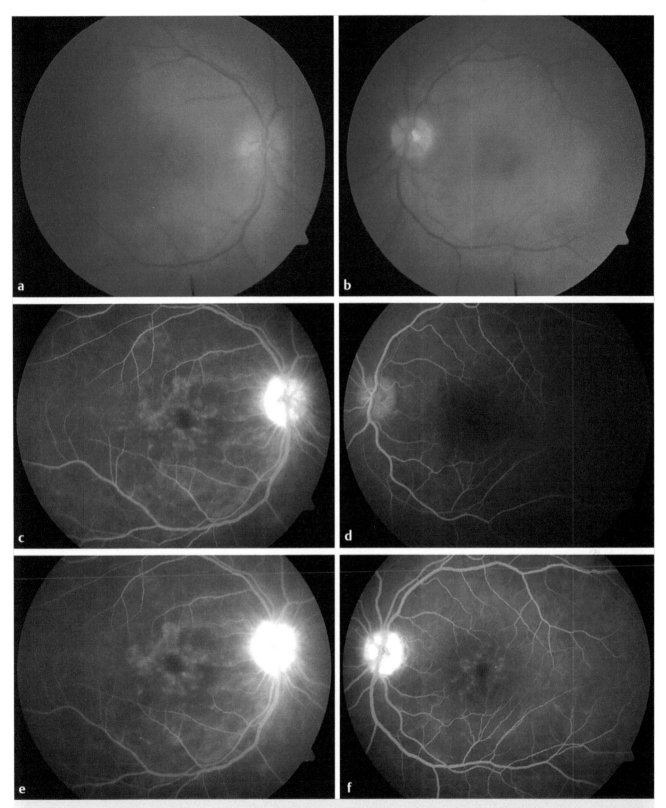

Fig. 71.4 Bilateral pars planitis. (a) The fundus photographs of the right and (b) left eye show presence of vitritis, mild disc swelling (especially in the right eye), and dull foveal reflex. (c,d) Fluorescein angiography in the early phase shows presence of early disc hyperfluorescence and perifoveal hyperfluorescence especially in the right eye indicative of cystoid macular edema. (e,f) The late frames show presence of significant disc hyperfluorescence in both eyes and macular leakage suggestive of cystoid macular edema in both eyes.

may be associated with a higher rate of cataract and increased intraocular pressure compared to periocular steroids. In severe cases of pars planitis or in patients with significant bilateral involvements, systemic steroids and/or immunosuppressants may be indicated. Various immunosuppressive agents such as azathioprine, mycophenolate mofetil, and biological agents such as anti-tumor necrosis factor (anti-TNF)-α have been used in severe or refractory cases of pars planitis.

Surgery

Surgical intervention with pars plana vitrectomy (PPV) is reserved for patients with severe ocular complications such as VH, extensive vitreous opacity, RD, and ERM. Rarely, PPV may be performed to reduce the burden of inflammation in the vitreous cavity by clearing all the inflammatory mediators. However, careful case selection is mandated as PPV can have its own set of complications such as choroidal hemorrhage, cataract formation, and retinal tears or RD.

71.4.2 Follow-up

Long-term uncontrolled pars planitis can lead to severe ocular complications (e.g., cataract, CME, VH), especially within the pediatric population where delayed diagnosis and treatment are prevalent. These ocular complications place children with pars planitis at a very high risk for developing amblyopia if diagnosis and treatment are not initiated early. Patient should be followed up closely while the disease is active and therapeutic modifications are being made. Once the inflammation is quiescent, the follow-up interval is extended, but ongoing follow-up for recurrence is important.

Suggested Reading

[1] de Boer J, Berendschot TT, van der Does P, Rothova A. Long-term follow-up of intermediate uveitis in children. Am J Ophthalmol. 2006; 141(4):616–621

[2] Donaldson MJ, Pulido JS, Herman DC, Diehl N, Hodge D. Pars planitis: a 20-year study of incidence, clinical features, and outcomes. Am J Ophthalmol. 2007; 144(6):812–817

[3] Smith JA, Mackensen F, Sen HN, et al. Epidemiology and course of disease in childhood uveitis. Ophthalmology. 2009; 116(8):1544–1551, 1551.e1

[4] Smith JA, Mackensen F, Sen HN, et al. Epidemiology and course of disease in childhood uveitis. Ophthalmology. 2009; 116(8):1544–1551, 1551.e1

[5] Ozdal PC, Berker N, Tugal-Tutkun I. Pars planitis: epidemiology, clinical characteristics, management and visual prognosis. J Ophthalmic Vis Res. 2015; 10 (4):469–480

[6] Lai WW, Pulido JS. Intermediate uveitis. Ophthalmol Clin North Am. 2002; 15 (3):309–317

[7] Campbell JP, Leder HA, Sepah YJ, et al. Wide-field retinal imaging in the management of noninfectious posterior uveitis. Am J Ophthalmol. 2012; 154(5): 908–911.e2

[8] Thomas AS, Redd T, Campbell JP, et al. The impact and implication of peripheral vascular leakage on ultra-widefield fluorescein angiography in uveitis. Ocul Immunol Inflamm. 2017 Oct; 16:1–7. doi: 10.1080/09273948.2017.1367406. [Epub ahead of print]

[9] Agarwal A, Afridi R, Agrawal R, Do DV, Gupta V, Nguyen QD. Multimodal imaging in retinal vasculitis. Ocul Immunol Inflamm. 2017; 25(3):424–433

[10] Quinones K, Choi JY, Yilmaz T, Kafkala C, Letko E, Foster CS. Pars plana vitrectomy versus immunomodulatory therapy for intermediate uveitis: a prospective, randomized pilot study. Ocul Immunol Inflamm. 2010; 18(5):411–417

72 Vogt-Koyanagi-Harada Syndrome

Nima Justin Bencohen, Benjamin Kambiz Ghiam, and Pouya Nachshon Dayani

Summary

Vogt-Koyanagi-Harada (VKH) syndrome is an aggressive, bilateral granulomatous panuveitis associated with serous retinal detachments. The extraocular manifestations of the condition are variable, and can include headaches, meningismus, hearing loss, alopecia, poliosis, and vitiligo. Prompt initiation of systemic therapy with high-dose corticosteroids is important to minimize secondary complications and vision loss. Steroid-sparing immunosuppressive therapy is typically needed for long-term management to reduce disease recurrence and steroid-related side effects.

Keywords: panuveitis, sunset glow fundus, serous retinal detachment, Vogt-Koyanagi-Harada syndrome

72.1 Features

Vogt-Koyanagi-Harada (VKH) syndrome is a multisystem inflammatory condition affecting the eye, skin, inner ear, and meninges. The condition is characterized by ocular inflammation in association with patchy depigmentation of the skin (▶ Fig. 72.1), patchy hair loss, and whitening of hair (in particular the eyelashes). VKH syndrome more commonly affects those with pigmented skin and of certain genetic predisposition. The prevalence varies and is more common in Asia, Latin America, and the Middle East. In the United States, VKH accounts for approximately 3 to 7% of uveitis referrals and Hispanics are most frequently affected. The mean age at presentation is 32 to 35 years of age, though it has been reported in children as young as 3 years.

Immunological and histopathological studies suggest that CD4+T cells targeting melanocytes may be the primary factor initiating the inflammatory process seen in VKH. Genetic susceptibility in patients expressing HLA DRB1*0405 may also predispose some patients, possibly in combination with a viral trigger.

VKH is a systemic disorder and the extraocular manifestations are critical in the diagnosis. The revised criteria for the diagnosis of VKH categorized the disease into definite (complete and incomplete) and probable diagnosis. The syndrome evolves through four distinct phases, including prodromal, uveitic, convalescent, and chronic recurrent phase.

72.1.1 Common Symptoms

Prodromal

Nonspecific symptoms, typically lasting 3 to 5 days; most commonly headaches and meningismus. Photophobia, orbital pain, vertigo, nausea, weakness, and flulike symptoms (including fever) are frequently reported. Hearing disturbances such as tinnitus and sensory hearing loss are common (typically involving the higher frequencies). Dysacousia may persist for years; focal neurologic deficits, including cranial nerve palsies and optic neuritis, have been reported; pleocytosis of cerebrospinal fluid can be seen in more than 80% of patients and can last up to 8 weeks; some patients report sensitivity of hair and skin to touch.

Uveitic

This phase lasts for several weeks; although some patients may experience a delay before the onset of symptoms in the second eye, most patients present with bilateral vision loss as the most common presenting symptom.

72.1.2 Exam Findings

Uveitic

Ocular presentation is an acute, bilateral granulomatous panuveitis in up to 70% of patients characterized by diffuse, increased choroidal thickening, multifocal detachments of the sensory retinal, and optic nerve edema (▶ Fig. 72.2, ▶ Fig. 72.3, ▶ Fig. 72.4, ▶ Fig. 72.5). Inferior pooling of subretinal fluid can be seen. Early in the disease, shallowing of the anterior chamber with an increased intraocular pressure may result from edema of the ciliary processes. Anterior segment findings may include mutton-fat keratic precipitates, iris nodules, pupillary membranes, or diffuse iris thickening.

Convalescent

The third stage, termed the "convalescent stage" lasts for months to years and is characterized by depigmentation of the uvea and integument. Sugiura sign, perilimbal vitiligo, is the earliest finding in this stage. Although this finding is common

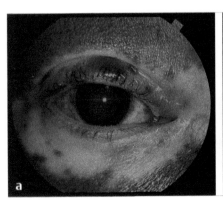
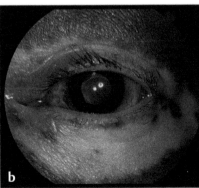

Fig. 72.1 (a,b) Vitiligo with a symmetric distribution.

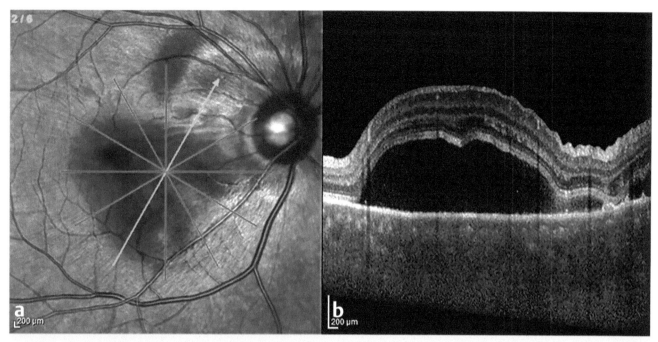

Fig. 72.2 (a,b) Optical coherence tomography in acute Vogt-Koyanagi-Harada uveitis demonstrating multifocal subretinal fluid.

in Japanese patients (up to 85% of patients), it is rarely seen in North America. Twenty-two percent of patients can develop vitiligo, often with a symmetric distribution (▶ Fig. 72.1). "Sunset glow" fundus describes the characteristic bright, orange appearance of the fundus associated with depigmentation of the choroid and retinal pigment epithelium (RPE; ▶ Fig. 72.6, ▶ Fig. 72.7). Multiple well-circumscribed areas of chorioretinal atrophy can be seen in the periphery.

Chronic Recurrent Phase

The final stage presents with granulomatous anterior uveitis and often results from suboptimal therapy. This phase usually develops 6 to 9 months following initial presentation. Posterior segment inflammation and serous detachments are less commonly observed. Choroidal neovascularization, subretinal fibrosis, and reactive proliferation of the RPE may be seen during this stage (▶ Fig. 72.7). Epiretinal membrane, cataract formation, and secondary glaucoma are also common.

72.2 Key Diagnostic Tests and Findings

72.2.1 Optical Coherence Tomography

In the acute phase, optical coherence tomography (OCT) is most helpful in detecting choroidal thickening and presence of subretinal fluid. Common findings include subretinal septae associated with serous retinal detachment, subretinal fibrinoid deposits, hyperreflective dots, loss of choroidal vasculature lacunae, and chorioretinal and retinal folds (▶ Fig. 72.2, ▶ Fig. 72.5). Enhanced-depth imaging with OCT during the chronic recurrent stage of the disease can be useful in guiding

therapy by detecting subclinical disease recurrence manifested by increased choroidal thickening (▶ Fig. 72.4). In the convalescent stage of the disease, OCT can detect choroidal thinning (▶ Fig. 72.6).

72.2.2 Fluorescein Angiography or Ultra-Widefield Fluorescein Angiography

During the acute stage of the disease, fluorescein angiography (FA) demonstrates multifocal hyperfluorescent pinpoint leaks at the level of the RPE with late pooling of subretinal dye (▶ Fig. 72.3). Optic disc and peripapillary hyperfluorescence, delayed choroidal filling, and areas of choroidal hyperfluorescence are also frequently observed (▶ Fig. 72.3, ▶ Fig. 72.5). In patients with chronic disease, FA shows a "moth-eaten" appearance with numerous areas of window defect from RPE loss and blockage from pigment migration (▶ Fig. 72.7).

72.2.3 Indocyanine Green Angiography

Indocyanine green (ICG) angiography shows delayed perfusion of the choriocapillaris and early choroidal stromal hypercyanescence in the acute stage of the disease. Hypocyanescence dark spots and fuzzy or lost pattern of large stromal vessels are also commonly seen (▶ Fig. 72.3). Diffuse choroidal and disk hypercyanescence are observed in later frames. Choroidal vascular inflammation tends to show a rapid response to therapy, whereas the hypocyanescence dark spots show a more variable response and resolve more slowly. ICG angiography can also be effective in monitoring the response to therapy and to detect subclinical therapy.

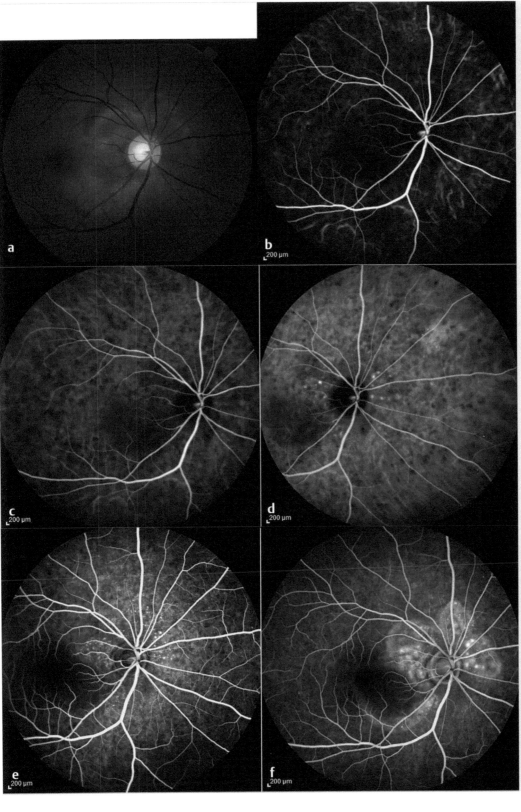

Fig. 72.3 Acute Vogt-Koyanagi-Harada (VKH) angiographic and fundus imaging. **(a)** Fundus photography. **(b–d)** Characteristic indocyanine green angiography findings during acute VKH. **(e,f)** Fluorescein angiography showing pinpoint areas of hyperfluorescence with late pooling.

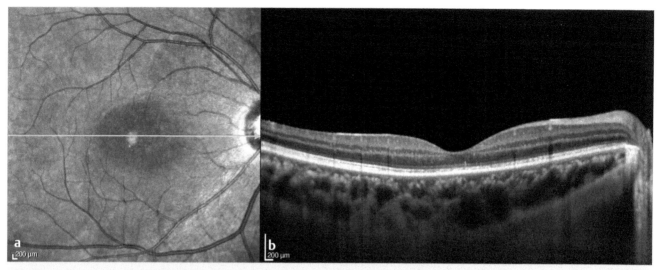

Fig. 72.4 (a,b) Enhanced-depth imaging optical coherence tomography (OCT) in Vogt-Koyanagi-Harada. Imaging demonstrates increased choroidal thickening without fluid on enhanced-depth OCT in chronic, recurrent subclinical disease.

72.2.4 Fundus Autofluorescence

Fundus autofluorescence (FAF), in particular wide-field FAF, can be helpful in assessing early damage to the RPE. In the acute phase, diffuse hyper-autofluorescence is seen with areas of blockage from subretinal fluid. In the chronic stage, a mixed pattern of hyper-autofluorescent and hypo-autofluorescent areas can be seen (▶ Fig. 72.6). Nummular and peripapillary hypo-autofluorescent areas are also observed corresponding to areas of atrophy.

72.2.5 Ultrasonography

Can be particularly useful in patients with media opacities and an obscured view to the posterior segment. Typical findings include diffuse, low to medium reflective choroidal thickening, serous retinal detachment (most prominent inferiorly), and vitreous opacities.

72.3 Critical Work-up

VKH is a clinical diagnosis based on a constellation of signs and symptoms, and no confirmatory testing is available. Differential diagnoses include sympathetic ophthalmia, sarcoidosis, posterior scleritis, central serous chorioretinopathy, uveal effusion syndrome, eclampsia, primary intraocular lymphoma, diffuse uveal lymphoid hyperplasia, metastatic choroidal cancer, and infectious etiologies such as tuberculosis and syphilis. Laboratory work-up for infectious and other inflammatory etiologies should be strongly considered, particularly to rule out syphilis, sarcoid, and tuberculosis. Other laboratory work-up can be tailored to the clinical presentation.

72.4 Management

72.4.1 Treatment Options

Initial medical management is typically with high-dose systemic corticosteroids. An initial dose of 1 mg/kg is frequently used, though some patients with more aggressive disease may benefit from an intravenous high-dose pulse of steroids. With systemic corticosteroid therapy, subretinal fluid improves by roughly 50% in the first week, and fully by 2 to 4 weeks. Similarly, choroidal thickness can return to normal levels by 4 weeks. Early and aggressive initiation of appropriate therapy has been shown to result in fewer recurrences, less pigment degeneration, and a reduced incidence of sunset glow fundus. Improved clinical course has been observed with longer duration of corticosteroid therapy, lasting greater than 6 months. Given the chronic nature of the condition, the American Uveitis Society and the International Uveitis Study Group recommend steroid-sparing agents to minimize the side effects associated with chronic corticosteroid therapy and to reduce the risk of recurrence. Antimetabolites, alkylating agents, calcineurin inhibitors, and biologics have all shown efficacy in treating VKH.

Topical corticosteroids and cycloplegics are used during the acute phase of the disease to manage the anterior segment inflammation. Periocular or intraocular corticosteroids injections can be used during the acute stage as adjunctive therapy in patients showing an incomplete response to systemic therapy and can be used in chronic VKH in those intolerant of systemic therapy. During the acute phase, however, local therapy alone is not recommended given the need to manage the extraocular manifestations of the condition. Ocular complications of

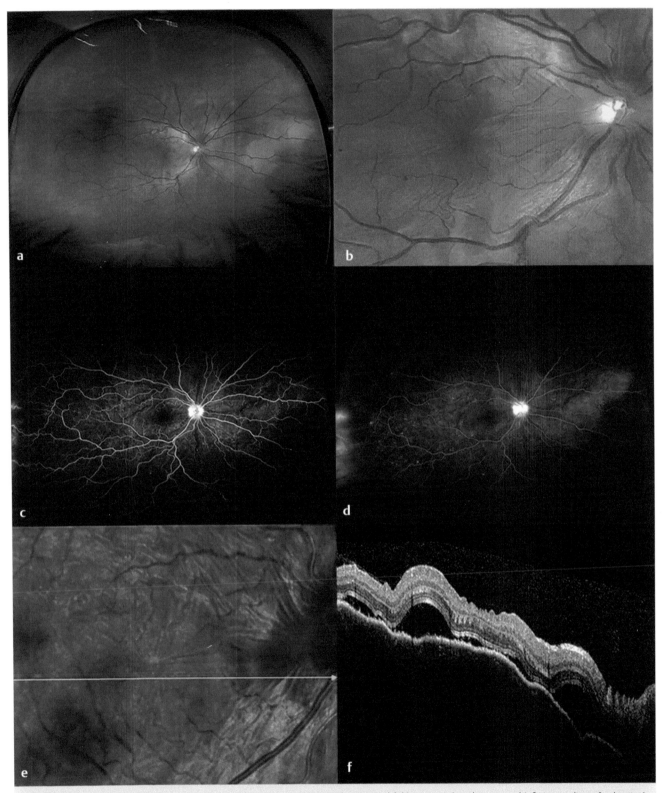

Fig. 72.5 Multimodal imaging in active Vogt-Koyanagi-Harada (VKH). **(a)** Chorioretinal folds, serous detachment, and inferior pooling of subretinal fluid with serous detachment on ultra-widefield imaging. **(b)** Chorioretinal folds are more visible on macular view. **(c,d)** Wide-field fluorescein angiography shows numerous pinpoint areas of leakage with multifocal late pooling of subretinal dye in acute VKH—"starry sky" appearance. **(e,f)** Subretinal fluid and chorioretinal folds on optical coherence tomography.

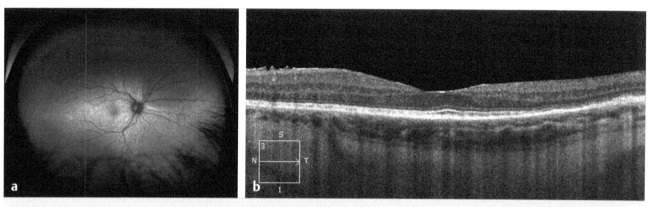

Fig. 72.6 Chronic Vogt-Koyanagi-Harada (VKH) imaging with fundus autofluorescence and optical coherence tomography (OCT). **(a)** VKH fundus autofluorescence imaging and **(b)** OCT in chronic convalescent VKH without active fluid.

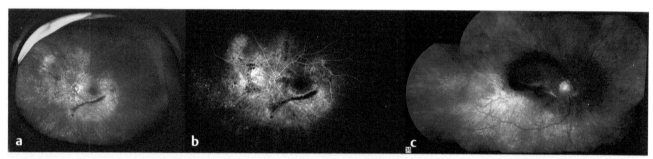

Fig. 72.7 Chronic Vogt-Koyanagi-Harada (VKH) imaging. **(a)** Sunset glow fundus with peripheral depigmented lesions and subretinal fibrosis. **(b)** Ultra-widefield angiography window defects and blocking from pigment atrophy and migration. **(c)** Dense subretinal fibrosis involving the macula.

VKH include cataract formation, glaucoma, synechiae formation, subretinal fibrosis, and choroidal neovascularization. Formal auditory testing is recommended for patients with suggestive symptoms.

72.4.2 Follow-up

Follow-up is based on level of disease activity. More frequent follow-up is needed during periods of acute exacerbations and while stabilizing the therapeutic regimen.

Suggested Reading

[1] O'Keefe GA, Rao NA. Vogt-Koyanagi-Harada disease. Surv Ophthalmol. 2017; 62(1):1–25

[2] Baltmr A, Lightman S, Tomkins-Netzer O. Vogt-Koyanagi-Harada syndrome - current perspectives. Clin Ophthalmol. 2016; 10:2345–2361

[3] Read RW, Holland GN, Rao NA, et al. Revised diagnostic criteria for Vogt-Koyanagi-Harada disease: report of an international committee on nomenclature. Am J Ophthalmol. 2001; 131(5):647–652

[4] Bouchenaki N, Herbort CP. The contribution of indocyanine green angiography to the appraisal and management of Vogt-Koyanagi-Harada disease. Ophthalmology. 2001; 108(1):54–64

73 Sympathetic Ophthalmia

Rahul Kapoor and Jayanth Sridhar

Summary

Sympathetic ophthalmia (SO) is a rare, bilateral, diffuse granu-lomatous uveitis that generally presents several months after a penetrating injury or trauma to one eye. Although 90% of cases present within 1 year of trauma, the range of presentation widely varies between days to decades. The diagnosis of SO is based primarily on history and clinical examination. Further-more, there are clinical features revealed through several imag-ing modalities that are useful in confirming the diagnosis of SO.

Keywords: intraocular surgery, ocular injury, panuveitis, sympa-thetic ophthalmia

73.1 Features

73.1.1 Common Symptoms

Clinical symptoms are typically consistent with uveitis, includ-ing blurry vision, conjunctival injection, and ocular irritation. Other symptoms of sympathetic ophthalmia (SO) include pho-tophobia in the sympathizing (nontraumatic) eye, epiphora, floaters, loss of accommodation, bilateral eye pain, and decreased vision. On rare occasions, patients may report extra-ocular symptoms such as hearing loss, headache, vitiligo, and meningeal irritation.

73.1.2 Exam Findings

Anterior segment exam may demonstrate mutton-fat keratic precipitates on the corneal endothelium (▶ Fig. 73.1), conjuncti-val injection, and thickened iris due to anterior inflammation possibly leading to posterior synechiae. Intraocular pressure can be increased due to blockage of trabecular meshwork or decreased due to impaired ciliary body function. The extent of inflammation in the posterior segment varies. Patients may present with vitritis, retinal vasculitis, and choroiditis. Serous retinal detachments, papilledema, and classic Dalen-Fuchs nod-ules, characterized as yellowish white choroidal lesions, may also be present on posterior examination (▶ Fig. 73.2).

73.2 Key Diagnostic Tests and Findings

73.2.1 Optical Coherence Tomography

Optical coherence tomography (OCT) frequently demonstrates choroidal and retinal pigment epithelium (RPE) thickening; may also reveal retinal detachment, intraretinal edema, disinte-gration of RPE and choriocapillaris, and thinning and disorgani-zation of the inner retina (▶ Fig. 73.3).

73.2.2 Fluorescein Angiography or Ultra-Widefield Fluorescein Angiography

Angiography often reveals multiple hyperfluorescent sites of leakage at the level of the RPE during the venous phase (▶ Fig. 73.4). Possible hypofluorescent areas may correspond to Dalen-Fuchs nodules. In the chronic phase, the nodules become atrophic and appear as window defects. Retinal vasculitis may also be visualized in late staining.

73.2.3 Indocyanine Green Angiography

May be used as an adjunct to fluorescein angiography (FA) for diagnosis and evaluation of the response to treatment in SO. In the intermediate and late stages of the study, hypofluorescent areas correspond to the hyperfluorescent areas on FA and may correlate with choroidal atrophy (▶ Fig. 73.4). However, hypo-fluorescent areas on indocyanine green angiography that are present only in the intermediate stage may represent areas of active choroiditis.

73.2.4 Fundus Autofluorescence

Can be used to distinguish between the acute and chronic phases of SO. In the acute phase, fundus autofluorescence (FAF) may reveal vitritis, Dalen-Fuchs nodules, papilledema,

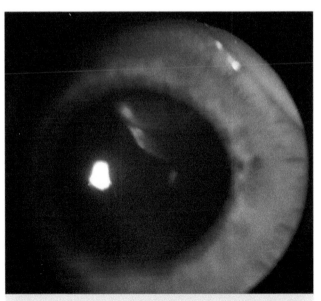

Fig. 73.1 Mutton-fat keratic precipitates on the corneal endothelium may be noted in the setting of sympathetic ophthalmia. (Courtesy of Derek Kunimoto.)

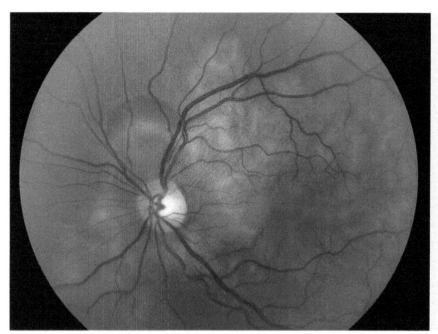

Fig. 73.2 Fundus examination of sympathetic ophthalmia may reveal multifocal serous retinal detachments. (Courtesy of Michael Dollin and Rajiv Shah.)

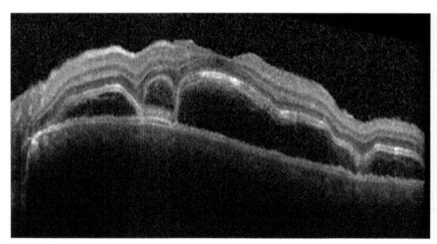

Fig. 73.3 Optical coherence tomography may demonstrate multifocal retinal detachment with thickening of the outer retina and intraretinal fluid. Increased hyperreflectivity is also noted in the outer retina. (Courtesy of Michael Dollin and Rajiv Shah.)

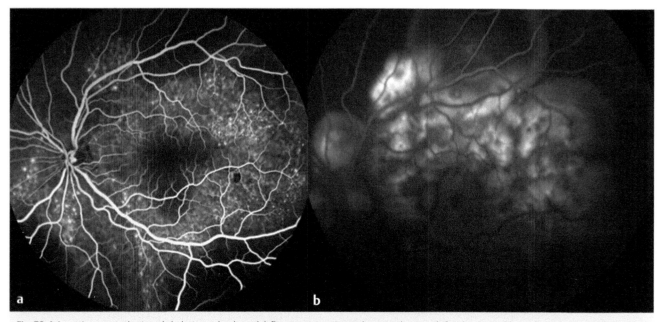

a b

Fig. 73.4 In active sympathetic ophthalmia, early-phase **(a)** fluorescein angiography may show multifocal points of hyperfluorescence with larger areas of hypofluorescence. **(b)** Late fluorescein angiography phases may reveal leakage and pooling. (Courtesy of Michael Dollin and Rajiv Shah.)

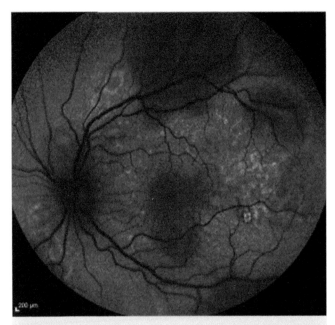

Fig. 73.5 Fundus autofluorescence may reveal hypo-autofluorescent areas corresponding to Dalen-Fuchs nodules and hyper-autofluorescent spots corresponding to areas of leakage seen on fluorescein angiography (Courtesy of Michael Dollin and Rajiv Shah.)

choroidal lesions, macular edema, retinal detachments, subretinal hemorrhages, and vasculitis (▶ Fig. 73.5). During the chronic phase, FAF may reveal retinal, choroidal, disk atrophy, subretinal fibrosis, chorioretinal scars, and subretinal fibrosis.

73.2.5 Ultrasonography

B-scan ultrasonography may demonstrate choroidal thickening and retinal detachment. Therefore, B-scan can be useful for differentiating SO from bilateral phacoanaphylactic uveitis, which lacks these findings.

73.3 Critical Work-up

The diagnosis of SO is based primarily on history and clinical exam. Since SO cannot be diagnosed based on any specific laboratory studies, the differential diagnosis of SO includes diseases that commonly present with panuveitis. Therefore, work-up includes ruling out diseases in addition to a history that reveals previous ocular injury or intraocular surgery with corresponding imaging that confirms the diagnosis. Vogt-Koyanagi-Harada (VKH) disease is a bilateral granulomatous panuveitis that has a very similar presentation to SO. However, VKH patients present with a prominent choroidal involvement that is not characteristic of SO and have optic nerve involvement and serous retinal detachments that are not commonly seen in SO. Cerebrospinal fluid from patients with VKH may reveal pleocytosis and is another feature of VKH that can be used to differentiate it from SO.

Syphilis may also cause bilateral granulomatous panuveitis and should be excluded with serum rapid plasmin reagin and fluorescent treponemal antibody absorption. Tuberculosis and sarcoidosis should be ruled out requiring purified protein derivative (PPD) skin testing, chest radiographs, and serum angiotensin-converting enzyme levels. Finally, if lymphoma is suspected, systemic work-up and neurological testing might be necessary. A vitreous sample may also be obtained if diagnosis of lymphoma remains unclear.

73.4 Management

73.4.1 Treatment Options

Prevention

Enucleation of the exciting (traumatic) eye within 2 weeks is thought to prevent the development of SO in the sympathizing (nontraumatic) eye. Controversy between enucleation and evisceration still exists, but enucleation is the preferred form of prevention, according to literature, because uveal tissue might remain in the scleral emissary channels during evisceration that can eventually lead to SO.

Immunomodulatory Therapy

Enucleation after the development of SO is still a controversial topic. Immunomodulatory therapy is the mainstay of treatment. Initial therapy with systemic corticosteroids with addition of corticosteroid-sparing agents later in therapy is the common protocol. Corticosteroids may be given topically, periocularly, or systemically. High-dose oral prednisone (1–2 mg/kg/day) is the most commonly employed initial treatment and slowly tapered over 3 to 4 months. Intravenous therapy with methylprednisolone can be used for severe cases. A dosing schedule of at least a year is required to control SO in most cases. Once a significant decrease in inflammation is noted, oral corticosteroids may be tapered. Acute anterior uveitis associated with SO can be treated with topical corticosteroids in combination with cycloplegic or mydriatic agents. Additional immunosuppressive agents such as chlorambucil, cyclophosphamide, and azathioprine may be used to manage SO. Mycophenolate is recommended for treatment of refractory uveitis unresponsive to high-dose steroids (> 15 mg/day) or if significant steroid toxicity develops. Moreover, cyclosporine (5 mg/kg/day) can be used as a long-term immunomodulatory agent, especially if the patient is steroid resistant or develops toxic side-effects. Once the disease is in remission for at least 3 months, a slow taper (0.5 mg/kg/day) may be considered.

73.4.2 Follow-up

SO rarely resolves spontaneously, and the relapsing nature in addition to the potential toxicity of the treatment modalities warrants careful follow-up of patients with SO. Patients should be followed up every few days initially in order to monitor the effectiveness of therapy and side-effects of treatments (e.g., intraocular pressure). Once the condition improves, follow-up can be extended. When all signs of inflammation have resolved, corticosteroids should be maintained for 3 to 6 months in order to prevent relapse. Then, periodic checkups are necessary to check for recurrence of SO.

Suggested Reading

[1] Arevalo JF, Garcia RA, Al-Dhibi HA, Sanchez JG, Suarez-Tata L. Update on sympathetic ophthalmia. Middle East Afr J Ophthalmol. 2012; 19(1):13–21

[2] Chu XK, Chan C-C. Sympathetic ophthalmia: to the twenty-first century and beyond. J Ophthalmic Inflamm Infect. 2013; 3(1):49

[3] Castiblanco C, Adelman RA. Imaging for sympathetic ophthalmia: impact on the diagnosis and management. Int Ophthalmol Clin. 2012; 52(4):173–181

[4] Aziz HA, Flynn HW, Jr, Young RC, Davis JL, Dubovy SR. SYMPATHETIC OPHTHALMIA: Clinicopathologic correlation in a consecutive case series. Retina. 2015; 35(8):1696–1703

74 Susac Syndrome

Jawad I. Arshad and Sunil K. Srivastava

Summary

Susac syndrome is an immune-mediated disease of the brain, retina, and inner ear that produces ischemia, pauci-inflammation, and occlusive microvascular endotheliopathy. The three common manifestations of Susac syndrome are encephalopathy, branch retinal artery occlusion, and low-to-medium frequency sensorineural hearing loss. The classic finding seen on MRI includes supratentorial "snowball" lesions in the central corpus callosum. Susac syndrome often affects more women than men (3:1 ratio) with age ranging between 20 and 40 years. Less than 20% of all patients present with all the aforementioned triad of clinical symptoms. Initially only one of the symptoms may present with the other components presenting weeks or up to months later. This, in turn, can delay the diagnosis and subsequent treatment of the disease.

Keywords: branch retinal artery occlusion, encephalopathy, hearing loss, Susac syndrome

74.1 Features

Susac syndrome is an immune-mediated disease of the brain, retina, and inner ear that produces ischemia, pauci-inflammation, and occlusive microvascular endotheliopathy.

The three common manifestations of Susac syndrome are encephalopathy, branch retinal artery occlusion (BRAO), and low-to-medium frequency sensorineural hearing loss. The classic finding seen on MRI includes supratentorial "snowball" lesions in the central corpus callosum. Susac syndrome often affects more women than men (3:1 ratio) with age ranging between 20 and 40 years. Less than 20% of all patients present with all the aforementioned triad of clinical symptoms. Initially, only one of the symptoms may present with the other components presenting weeks or up to months later. This, in turn, can delay the diagnosis and subsequent treatment of the disease.

74.1.1 Symptoms

Possible loss of peripheral vision and/or central scotomas is often described. Review of systems can reveal signs of auditory involvement including tinnitus and hearing loss. Neurologic symptoms indicative of encephalopathy includes mood changes, headaches, emotional lability, and motor and sensory loss.

74.1.2 Exam Findings

Ophthalmic findings in Susac syndrome are consequences of acute BRAOs or evidence of previous occlusion(s). In the acute setting, branch retinal artery thinning, cotton wool spots, and retinal whitening are seen on clinical exam. In those presenting with previous BRAO, sclerotic and thinned vessels may be seen. Additional evidence of retinal capillary remodeling (telangiectasias and microaneurysms) can also be observed.

74.2 Key Diagnostic Tests and Findings

74.2.1 Optical Coherence Tomography

Thinning of the inner retina in areas of previous BRAOs will be found (▶ Fig. 74.1). In an acute BRAO, inner retinal hyperreflectance is seen. More mild areas of ischemia may demonstrate middle retinal hyperreflectances (e.g., PAMM-like lesions).

74.2.2 Fluorescein Angiography or Ultra-Widefield Fluorescein Angiography

Ultra-widefield fluorescein angiography (UWFA) is a key diagnostic for Susac syndrome. Loss of retinal artery perfusion and associated capillary nonperfusion consistent with BRAO can be

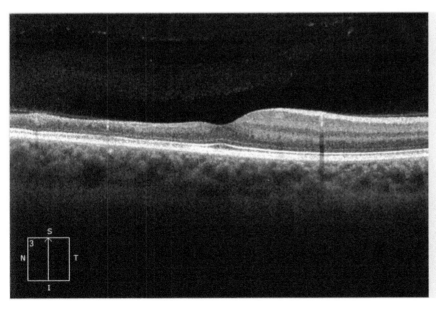

Fig. 74.1 Optical coherence tomography B-scan demonstrating focal inner retinal atrophy consistent with previous branch retinal artery occlusion.

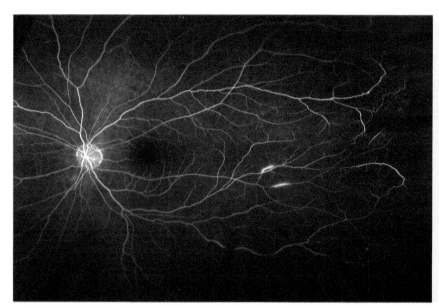

Fig. 74.2 Ultra-widefield fluorescein angiography demonstrating segmental vascular leakage and multifocal areas of nonperfusion.

seen in one or both eyes. Often, evidence of previous BRAOs can be seen as evidenced by multifocal peripheral capillary nonperfusion and/or posterior capillary remodeling. In the acute setting, segmental retinal vessel wall hyperfluorescence can be seen (▶ Fig. 74.2).

74.2.3 Optical Coherence Tomography Angiography

Optical coherence tomography angiography can be useful in some cases to identify previous artery occlusions with loss of inner retinal perfusion (▶ Fig. 74.3).

74.3 Critical Work-up

Suspected Susac syndrome work-up can be extensive. The critical ophthalmic feature is a BRAO or multiple BRAO. The presence of BRAO or multiple BRAO in combination with encephalopathy and low-to-medium frequency sensorineural hearing loss establishes the diagnosis of the Susac syndrome. Audiometry is required and will reveal low-to-mid frequency sensorineural hearing loss. An MRI of the brain will show multiple hyperdense lesions in the central corpus callosum and are considered pathognomonic in the setting of recurrent BRAOs and hearing loss. Ruling out other systemic inflammatory diseases is required; thus, laboratory testings are often obtained in a setting of a careful review of systems.

74.4 Management

74.4.1 Treatment Options

The retinal vasculopathy in Susac syndrome can precede, accompany, or follow the central nervous system (CNS) manifestations. Treatment of CNS manifestations takes priority. The treatment regimen will be more targeted and less aggressive for primarily ophthalmic manifestations compared to CNS disease.

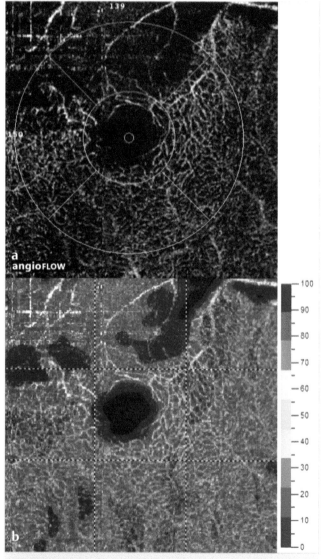

Fig. 74.3 (a) Optical coherence tomography angiography exhibiting significant superior flow void and nonperfusion in the retinal circulation. (b) Perfusion density map confirming significant reduction in flow density in superior macula.

Pharmacotherapy

Recommended pharmacotherapy for non-CNS Susac syndrome includes intravenous immunoglobulin (IVIG), mycophenolate mofetil, and pulse steroids. UWFA should be conducted serially to guide subsequent treatment decisions and for subclinical vascular disease activity. Monitoring for new or worsening brain and inner ear involvement is also important. Brain involvement can sometimes develop quickly and management of CNS disease will take precedence. IVIG can be tapered and halted in cases where there is no recurrence of active retinal disease for several months in the context of no inner ear of brain involvement. Mycophenolate mofetil may be able to be stopped after 6 to 12 months.

74.4.2 Follow-up

In addition to providing immunosuppressive therapy that is aggressive, sustained, and anticipatory at an appropriate level, it is vitally important to adaptively monitor patient status. MRIs, UWFAs, and audiograms should be used at regular intervals to provide optimal surveillance for disease activity.

Suggested Reading

[1] Rennebohm RM, Asdaghi N, Srivastava S, Gertner E. Guidelines for treatment of Susac syndrome - an update. Int J Stroke. 2018;1747493017751737

[2] Dörr J, Krautwald S, Wildemann B, et al. Characteristics of Susac syndrome: a review of all reported cases. Nat Rev Neurol. 2013; 9(6):307–316

[3] Rennebohm R, Susac JO, Egan RA, Daroff RB. Susac's syndrome–update. J Neurol Sci. 2010; 299(1–2):86–91

[4] Jarius S, Kleffner I, Dörr JM, et al. Clinical, paraclinical and serological findings in Susac syndrome: an international multicenter study. J Neuroinflammation. 2014; 11:46

[5] Kleffner I, Dörr J, Ringelstein M, et al. European Susac Consortium (EuSaC). Diagnostic criteria for Susac syndrome. J Neurol Neurosurg Psychiatry. 2016; 87(12):1287–1295

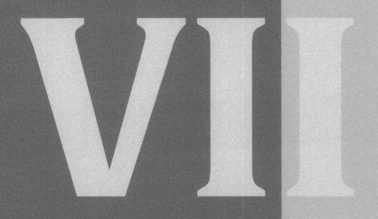

75 Traumatic Macular Hole

Robert B. Garoon and Jorge Fortun

Summary

A macular hole is a full-thickness loss of the neurosensory retina, traditionally in the fovea, leading to decreased visual acuity and central visual distortion. Traumatic macular holes occur most often after blunt force trauma to the eye, but the mechanism of formation of the hole is still not clear. Optical coherence tomography is a vital imaging technique in traumatic macular holes to facilitate diagnosis and guide management. Evaluate for concurrent traumatic ocular injuries, including commotio retinae. Pars plana vitrectomy with removal of posterior hyaloid and ILM tissue and intraocular gas tamponade is the treatment of choice for persistent traumatic macular holes, although spontaneous resolution is not uncommon and select cases should be carefully observed.

Keywords: blunt trauma, macular hole, traumatic macular hole

75.1 Features

A macular hole is a full-thickness loss of the neurosensory retina, traditionally at the fovea, leading to decreased visual acuity and central visual distortion. Idiopathic macular holes caused by vitreous traction are more common than traumatic macular holes, but both types may result in significant vision loss. Traumatic macular holes, as compared to idiopathic holes, are more commonly seen in younger patients, males, and may have worse vision on presentation. Traumatic macular holes occur most often after blunt force trauma to the eye, but the mechanism of formation of the hole is still not clear. One possible hypothesis for the pathogenesis of a traumatic macular hole is the concept that with blunt trauma to the eye flattening of the cornea is seen, followed by an expansion of the globe in an anteroposterior direction. Upon recoil of the globe, there is a rapid posterior movement of the posterior pole leading to dynamic horizontal forces and a splitting of the retinal layers of the fovea. An alternate theory centers around the role of the vitreous in traumatic macular holes, such that sudden vitreous separation caused by blunt trauma leads to an excessive pulling by the vitreous and hole formation in the fovea. A final potential mechanism is that energy from the traumatic blow itself is transmitted through the globe and causes a rupture of the fovea. Despite the exact pathogenesis of a traumatic macular hole, there are certain characteristics which are common on exam of traumatic macular holes and a range of treatment options exist depending on the clinical scenario.

75.1.1 Common Symptoms

Patients generally present with sudden vision loss immediately after the traumatic event, though cases of delayed vision loss up to several days after trauma have been reported.

75.1.2 Exam Findings

On examination, patients present with a macular hole that may appear more ellipsoid in nature as compared to idiopathic macular holes which generally have a circular appearance with mildly elevated appearance to the edges of the hole. In addition, other sequelae of significant blunt trauma may be present, including vitreous hemorrhage, subretinal hemorrhage, choroidal rupture, and commotio retinae (▶ Fig. 75.1, ▶ Fig. 75.2, ▶ Fig. 75.3).

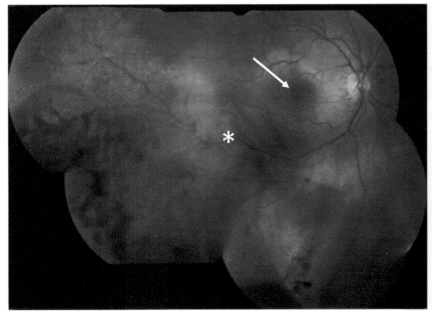

Fig. 75.1 Montage fundus photograph following high-speed projectile injury with a paintball. Examination revealed vitreous hemorrhage, choroidal rupture (*) and a full-thickness macular hole (*arrow*).

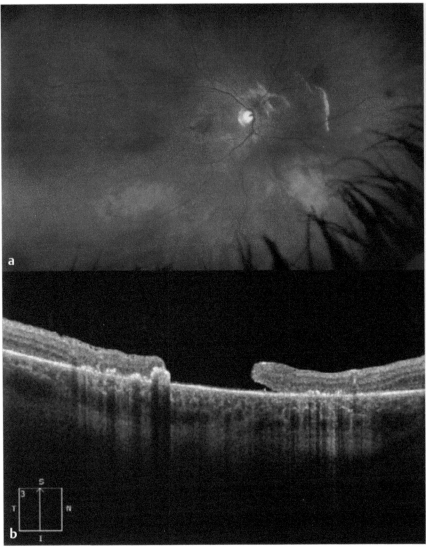

Fig. 75.2 Ultra-widefield fundus photo of chronic large macular hole. **(a)** Nasal subretinal fibrosis and multiple choroidal rupture sites are noted nasally. Optical coherence tomography demonstrating large persistent full-thickness macular hole without associated retinal edema and minimal subretinal fluid. **(b)** Extensive retinal pigment epithelium abnormalities are noted and outer retinal atrophy extends significantly past the edge of macular hole.

75.2 Key Diagnostic Tests and Findings

75.2.1 Optical Coherence Tomography

Optical coherence tomography (OCT) enables visualization of the foveal anatomy and confirmation of a full-thickness hole. OCT also identifies any additional major anatomic alterations, including photoreceptor loss, choroidal rupture, and any alterations to the vitreoretinal relationship (▶ Fig. 75.2, ▶ Fig. 75.3, ▶ Fig. 75.4).

75.2.2 Fundus Photography

Color fundus photographs may be used for documentation of macular hole and other concurrent injuries (▶ Fig. 75.1, ▶ Fig. 75.2, ▶ Fig. 75.3).

75.3 Critical Work-up

A thorough ophthalmic examination is critical as patients who present after trauma can present with a variety of clinical findings including hyphema, vitreous hemorrhage, commotio retinae, choroidal rupture, retinal tears/dialyses, photoreceptor or RPE damage, or even open globe injury.

75.4 Management

75.4.1 Treatment Options

Observation

Reports of visual improvement and documented spontaneous closure have been noted anywhere from 2 weeks up to 12 months after the initial trauma. The rate of spontaneous closure

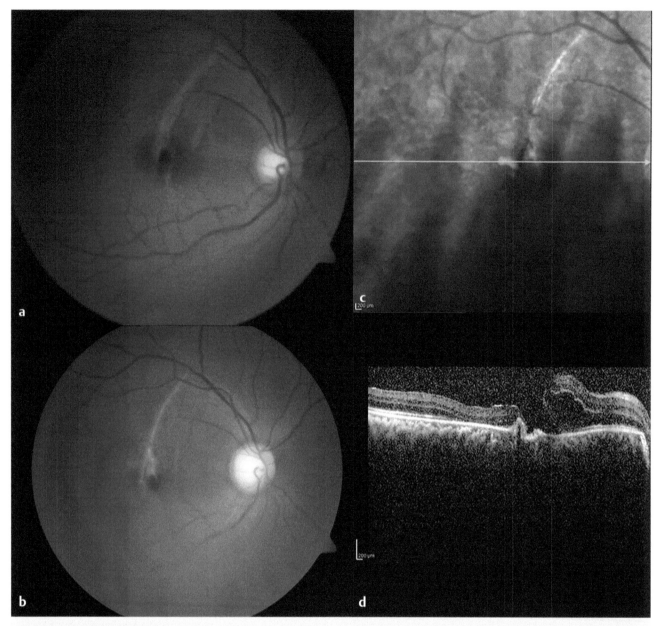

Fig. 75.3 (a) Fundus photograph of subacute presentation of traumatic macular hole with submacular hemorrhage and associated choroidal ruptures. (b) Fundus photograph 8 weeks later with more extensive subretinal fibrosis noted at area of rupture. Persistent full-thickness macular hole is present with choroidal rupture bisecting the fovea, and media opacity is present due to formation of cataract. (c,d) Optical coherence tomography demonstrates persistent traumatic full-thickness macular hole with subfoveal retinal pigment epithelium disruption due to choroidal rupture.

is significantly higher than in primary full-thickness macular hole (FTMH) and an initial short period (e.g., 2–4 weeks) of observation is often reasonable.

Pars Plana Vitrectomy

Pars plana vitrectomy has a high rate of anatomic success and is typically performed similarly to primary FTMH with elevation/removal of the posterior hyaloid, peeling of the internal limiting membrane, and gas tamponade. A technique for particularly large macular holes or traumatic macular holes which has failed a previous vitrectomy to facilitate closure is to create a flap of ILM which is then laid over the macular hole intraoperatively. This ILM scaffold is thought to aid in the migration of glial cells to the fovea to promote hole closure. Varying concentrations of sulfur hexafluoride and perfluorocarbon gas have been used to provide adequate surface tension that acts as a seal at the site of the hole to prevent fluid reaccumulation during hole closure. It is imperative that the patient's ability to position face-down after this type of procedure is taken into account when choosing the intraocular tamponade. Care must be taken to limit peripheral retinal traction during hyaloid elevation/vitrectomy, as retinal tears in this population may illicit a very strong proliferative vitreoretinopathy which can affect long-term visual outcomes.

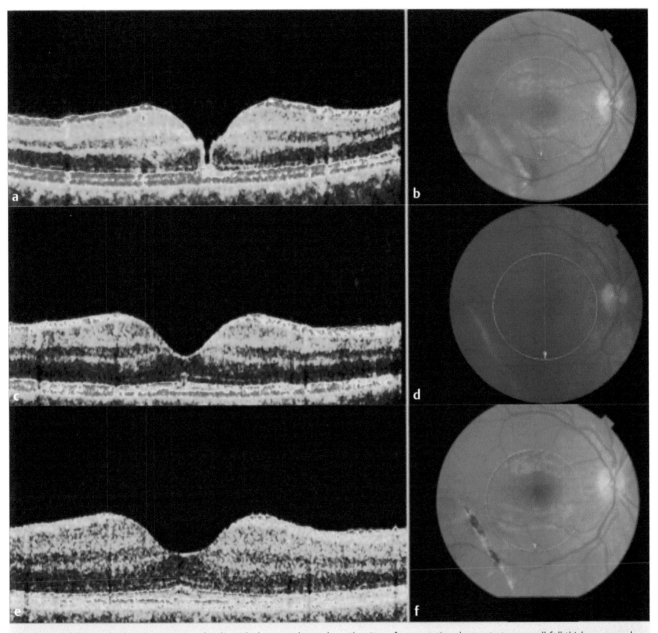

Fig. 75.4 (a,b) Optical coherence tomography through the central macula at the time of presentation demonstrates a small full-thickness macular hole. **(c,d)** Ten days after presentation, there is a near-total resolution of the macular hole with a small residual outer retinal disruption/separation. **(e, f)** Seven months after presentation with complete resolution of the macular hole. (Courtesy of Charles W. Mango, MD.)

75.4.2 Follow-up

Follow-up is determined based on treatment plan and other concurrent traumatic injuries. If observation is elected, the patient is typically followed up every 2 to 4 weeks for the first month. If spontaneous closure does not occur, vitrectomy is typically indicated unless the prognosis for visual recovery even with hole closure is quite guarded due to other concurrent traumatic injuries (e.g., outer retinal atrophy, traumatic optic neuropathy, subfoveal choroidal rupture). If a patient undergoes vitrectomy, follow-up is typically dictated by a surgeon's standard postoperative regimen. Once the gas bubble meniscus has passed the center of the macula, OCT should be used to confirm hole closure.

Suggested Reading

[1] Liu W, Grzybowski A. Current management of traumatic macular hole. J Ophthalmol. 2017; 2017:1748135

[2] Johnson RN, McDonald HR, Lewis H, et al. Traumatic macular hole: observations, pathogenesis, and results of vitrectomy surgery. Ophthalmology. 2001; 108(5):853–857

[3] Miller JB, Yonekawa Y, Eliott D, Vavvas DG. A review of traumatic macular hole: diagnosis and treatment. Int Ophthalmol Clin. 2013; 53(4): 59–67

[4] Chen H, Chen W, Zheng K, Peng K, Xia H, Zhu L. Prediction of spontaneous closure of traumatic macular hole with spectral domain optical coherence tomography. Sci Rep. 2015; 5:12343

76 Commotio Retinae

Alexander C. Barnes and Justis P. Ehlers

Summary

Commotio retinae (also known as Berlin's edema when confined to the posterior pole) is a common condition involving damage to the outer layers of the retina following blunt force injury to the eye. Declines in visual acuity range in longevity and severity. Optical coherence tomography can be used to detect hyperreflectivity of the retina and to predict visual and anatomic outcomes. Although cases are often self-resolving, continued observation is important to assess for other traumatic sequelae.

Keywords: Berlin's edema, commotio retinae, sequelae

76.1 Features

76.1.1 Common Symptoms

Asymptomatic. Decreased vision may be experienced if macula is involved. Mild/transient to severe/permanent declines in visual acuity depending on the degree/location of photoreceptor damage; associated with blunt trauma/contrecoup injuries.

76.1.2 Exam Findings

Retinal whitening/opacification occurs rapidly following injury (▶ Fig. 76.1, ▶ Fig. 76.2). Commotio retinae is associated with disruption of the outer retina and RPE and can be associated with other traumatic sequelae (retinal hemorrhage, macular hole, choroidal rupture, etc.). Severe cases are associated with pigmentary changes and retinal atrophy, and cases confined to the posterior pole are known as Berlin's edema.

76.2 Key Diagnostic Tests and Findings

76.2.1 Optical Coherence Tomography

Transient hyperreflective changes of the outer retina in mild cases; acute disruption of the ellipsoid zone with overlying hyperreflectivity in more severe cases is noted (▶ Fig. 76.1, ▶ Fig. 76.2). Other findings of traumatic sequelae include increased reflectivity/shadowing from hemorrhage or RPE disruption in choroidal rupture.

76.3 Critical Work-up

Conduct comprehensive ophthalmic examination including dilated fundus examination with scleral depression unless otherwise contraindicated. Optical coherence tomography (OCT) may be helpful in evaluating extent of anatomic disruption.

76.4 Management

76.4.1 Treatment Options

Observation. There are no known treatment modalities. Many cases are self-resolving without long-term retinal defects.

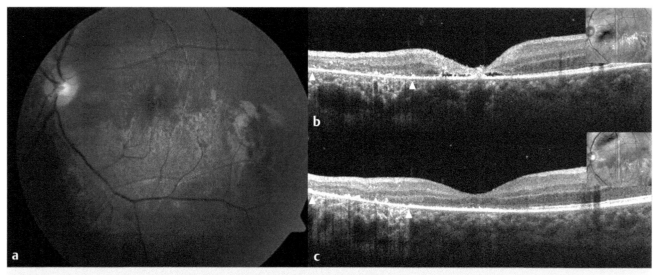

Fig. 76.1 Commotio retinae of the inferior macula following blunt trauma. **(a)** Fundus photograph demonstrating resolving commotio retinae involving the inferior macula. Other notable findings include a resolving macular lamellar hole and temporal intraretinal/subretinal hemorrhages. **(b)** Optical coherence tomography (OCT) images showing ellipsoid zone disruption (*arrowheads*) corresponding to areas of commotio retinae at the time of fundus photo with associated subfoveal fluid and foveal thinning. **(c)** Two weeks later, OCT demonstrates notable improvement in the subfoveal fluid and foveal architecture. Outer retinal disruption/loss is still present.

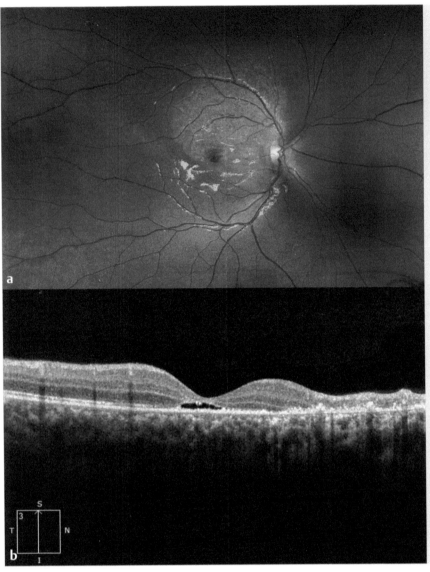

Fig. 76.2 Commotio retinae following blunt trauma with a soccer ball. **(a)** Fundus photograph reveals superior macular circular area of retinal whitening consistent with commotio, approximately 6 days after the injury. **(b)** Optical coherence tomography confirms severity of retinal injury given presence of significant outer retinal disruption and ellipsoid zone loss (*arrowheads*).

76.4.2 Follow-up

Follow-up within several weeks of presentation to assess for other traumatic sequelae. The follow-up interval often may be dictated by other associated injuries (e.g., hyphema). Examination may include gonioscopy to evaluate for angle recession and dilated fundus examination to monitor for the resolution of commotio retinae, the development of atrophic or pigmentary changes, and the presence of other retinal pathology (e.g., retinal detachment, dialysis). Serial OCTs may also be helpful for evaluating photoreceptor repopulation and prognostication regarding visual acuity.

Suggested Reading

[1] Ahn SJ, Woo SJ, Kim KE, Jo DH, Ahn J, Park KH. Optical coherence tomography morphologic grading of macular commotio retinae and its association with anatomic and visual outcomes. Am J Ophthalmol. 2013; 156 (5):994–1001.e1

[2] Souza-Santos F, Lavinsky D, Moraes NS, Castro AR, Cardillo JA, Farah ME. Spectral-domain optical coherence tomography in patients with commotio retinae. Retina. 2012; 32(4):711–718

[3] Mansour AM, Green WR, Hogge C. Histopathology of commotio retinae. Retina. 1992; 12(1):24–28

[4] Sipperley JO, Quigley HA, Gass DM. Traumatic retinopathy in primates. The explanation of commotio retinae. Arch Ophthalmol. 1978; 96(12): 2267–2273

77 Choroidal Rupture

Lucy T. Xu and Alex Yuan

Summary

Choroidal ruptures result from blunt force trauma causing a contrecoup injury which results in a break of the choriocapillaris, Bruch's membrane, and retinal pigment epithelium. Clinically, it presents as a yellow crescent concentric to the optic nerve. Initially, the choroidal rupture may be visually obscured by subretinal hemorrhage. Choroidal neovascularization (CNV) is a late complication of choroidal ruptures. CNV can be treated with intravitreal anti-vascular endothelial growth factor injections.

Keywords: choroidal rupture, blunt trauma, subretinal hemorrhage, choroidal neovascularization, Bruch's membrane, retinal pigment epithelium

77.1 Features

A choroidal rupture is defined as a break in the choriocapillaris, Bruch's membrane, and retinal pigment epithelium. Choroidal ruptures occur after 5 to 10% of blunt force trauma. They may be direct ruptures that occur anteriorly at the site of impact or, more commonly, indirect ruptures that occur in the posterior globe away from the site of impact (contrecoup force).

Indirect choroidal ruptures are often seen after nonpenetrating, closed-globe blunt trauma that causes anteroposterior compression of the globe. The elasticity of the retina and tensile strength of the sclera protect these structures from rupture, while Bruch's membrane is most susceptible to rupture (▶ Fig. 77.1). The mechanism of rupture also explains why patients with underlying weakness of Bruch's membrane, such as those with angioid streaks, are more susceptible to choroidal rupture.

A choroidal rupture differs from sclopetaria in that sclopetaria is defined as a rupture of both the choroid and retina after the transmission of shock waves through the eye wall. Sclopetaria typically occurs after a high-speed concussion-type, nonpenetrating injury (e.g., bullet in orbit). While the sclera is intact, the injury heals with a white proliferative scar tissue over the site.

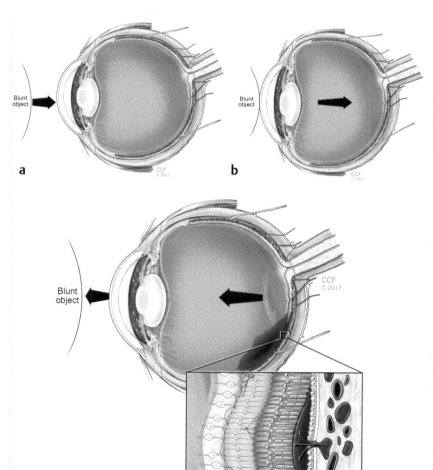

Fig. 77.1 Mechanism of choroidal rupture. **(a,b)** Blunt trauma results in sudden compression of the globe. **(c)** As the eye abruptly relaxes, a tear of the choriocapillaris, Bruch's membrane, and retinal pigment epithelium occurs forming the choroidal rupture which often results in subretinal hemorrhage. (Reprinted with permission, Cleveland Clinic Center for Medical Art and Photography © 2017. All Rights Reserved.)

77.1.1 Common Symptoms

Most often decreased visual acuity, scotoma, or floaters; may be completely asymptomatic if the rupture site and associated hemorrhage does not involve the macula.

77.1.2 Exam Findings

Choroidal ruptures are often associated with subretinal hemorrhage due to trauma to the choriocapillaris. Often during the initial presentation, this subretinal hemorrhage could obscure visualization of the choroidal rupture and thus choroidal ruptures should be suspected with subretinal hemorrhages that present after trauma (▶ Fig. 77.2). The choroidal rupture appears as a yellow, curvilinear line often concentric to the disc (▶ Fig. 77.3). Choroidal neovascular membrane can also develop after a rupture due to a break in Bruch's membrane. Rate of CNV development ranges between 11 and 37.5%. CNV associated with choroidal ruptures usually presents late (a median time of 8 months later in one study) and underscores the importance of follow-up in these patients.

77.2 Key Diagnostic Tests and Findings

77.2.1 Optical Coherence Tomography

Disruption/break in Bruch's membrane and the retinal pigment epithelium (RPE) may be visualized on optical coherence tomography (OCT). Additionally, OCT may facilitate confirmation of hemorrhage location during the acute phase. OCT is also useful in detecting secondary CNV (▶ Fig. 77.4).

77.2.2 Fluorescein Angiography or Ultra-Widefield Fluorescein Angiography

There is typically early hypofluorescence due to disruption of the choroid and underlying choriocapillaris; the adjacent choriocapillaris may leak into the rupture site and become hyperfluorescent due to staining.

77.2.3 Indocyanine Green Angiography

ICG offers better visualization of the rupture compared to fluorescein angiography due to less leakage of dye from the adjacent choriocapillaris and less blockage from overlying hemorrhage. Choroidal ruptures appear as hypocyanescent during all phases of indocyanine green.

77.2.4 Fundus Autofluorescence

The rupture is delineated by hyper-autofluorescence due to RPE hyperplasia at the margins of the rupture.

77.3 Critical Work-up

Due to the traumatic etiology of choroidal ruptures, other injuries associated with trauma should be ruled out including ruptured globe, hyphema, commotio retinae, sclopetaria, iris tears, angle recession, corneal abrasion, lens subluxation or dislocation, retinal dialysis, and vitreous hemorrhage. A thorough examination should be performed to look for evidence of these associated ocular defects. Presence of hyphema or dense vitreous hemorrhage may initially obscure visualization of the choroidal rupture.

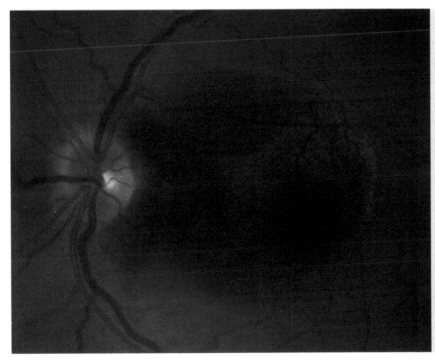

Fig. 77.2 Fundus image of subretinal hemorrhage that obscures a choroidal rupture. Choroidal ruptures should be suspected with subretinal hemorrhage after trauma.

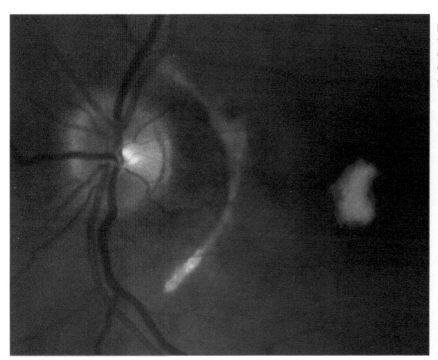

Fig. 77.3 The same patient from ▶ Fig. 77.2 after the subretinal hemorrhage cleared. A yellow crescent line (choroidal rupture) concentric to the optic disc is seen. A small amount of dehemoglobinized blood remains in the fovea.

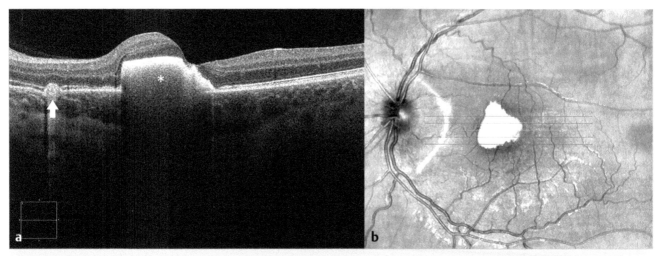

Fig. 77.4 (a) Optical coherence tomography of choroidal rupture showing a break in Bruch's membrane and retinal pigment epithelium (RPE; *arrow*) with sub-RPE hyperreflective material in between. There is also subretinal hemorrhage (*star*). (b) En face image.

77.4 Management

77.4.1 Treatment Options

There is no treatment for isolated choroidal ruptures. In cases where there is subretinal hemorrhage associated with an underlying rupture, the hemorrhage is most often observed to clear on its own. In select cases, extensive submacular hemorrhages can be treated with vitrectomy and pneumatic displacement, but the benefit of this procedure over observation has not been thoroughly examined. CNV from choroidal ruptures can be treated with anti-vascular endothelial growth factor therapy.

77.4.2 Follow-up

Patients who present with subretinal hemorrhage suspicious for choroidal rupture should be followed up closely every 1 to 2 weeks to document clearing of the hemorrhage and visualization of the choroidal rupture. Following the acute phase, patients should be followed up every 6 to 12 months for development of CNV. There is also a risk of angle recession associated with choroidal rupture, so patients should have a gonioscopy exam and if angle recession is suspected, ongoing surveillance of increased intraocular pressure is needed. Visual prognosis after choroidal rupture varies and poor outcome is associated with macular rupture and baseline vision less than 20/40.

Suggested Reading

[1] Patel MM, Chee YE, Eliott D. Choroidal rupture: a review. Int Ophthalmol Clin. 2013; 53(4):69–78

[2] Raman SV, Desai UR, Anderson S, Samuel MA. Visual prognosis in patients with traumatic choroidal rupture. Can J Ophthalmol. 2004; 39(3):260–266

[3] Ament CS, Zacks DN, Lane AM, et al. Predictors of visual outcome and choroidal neovascular membrane formation after traumatic choroidal rupture. Arch Ophthalmol. 2006; 124(7):957–966

[4] Williams DF, Mieler WF, Williams GA. Posterior segment manifestations of ocular trauma. Retina. 1990; 10 Suppl 1:S35–S44

[5] Doi S, Kimura S, Morizane Y, et al. Successful displacement of a traumatic submacular hemorrhage in a 13-year-old boy treated by vitrectomy, subretinal injection of tissue plasminogen activator and intravitreal air tamponade: a case report. BMC Ophthalmol. 2015; 15:94

78 Chorioretinitis Sclopetaria

Nitish Mehta and Yasha S. Modi

Summary

Chorioretinitis sclopetaria is a rare but characteristic simultaneous rupture of the choroid and retina. It is seen in the setting of a high-speed missile or bullet injury without rupturing of the sclera. Damage is believed to be from direct deformation of the globe from the course of the bullet and via an indirect shockwave injury to the globe from the high-speed bullet that enters the orbit. Due to reparative gliosis and dense chorioretinal adhesion at the margin of the chorioretinal defect, retinal detachment is rare and observation is recommended.

Keywords: choroid, chorioretinitis, missile, projectile, retina, sclopetaria, trauma

78.1 Features

78.1.1 Common Symptoms

A history of orbital bullet injury with associated signs and symptoms of orbital trauma. Visual acuity is variably affected based on the presence of associated trauma including maculopathy and/or neurologic injury. Visual field defect is present in areas of chorioretinal rupture. Pathology may be identified incidentally during routine examination in patients with a history of remote trauma.

78.1.2 Exam Findings

Acute exam often has extensive patch of choroidal and retinal hemorrhages. Late examination shows full-thickness chorioretinal defect with white fibrous proliferation and surrounding pigmentary changes (▶ Fig. 78.1). Rare association with early retinal detachment.

78.2 Key Diagnostic Tests and Findings

78.2.1 Optical Coherence Tomography

Optical coherence tomography demonstrates full-thickness hyperreflectivity and disorganization consistent with chorioretinal disruption and subsequent reparative gliotic proliferation.

78.2.2 Fluorescein Angiography or Ultra-Widefield Fluorescein Angiography

Early chorioretinitis sclopetaria displays hypofluorescence due to blocking from fibrous proliferation and loss of chorioretinal tissue. Late imaging has hyperfluorescent staining at lesion edges and bed of sclera (▶ Fig. 78.2).

78.2.3 Indocyanine Green Angiography or Ultra-Widefield Indocyanine Green Angiography

Lack of choroidal flow within the lesion throughout the study.

78.2.4 Fundus Autofluorescence

Complete hypo-autofluorescence of lesion due to lack of any chorioretinal structures.

78.2.5 Computed Tomography

May reveal a retained orbital foreign body and/or bony defects.

78.3 Critical Work-up

Complete ophthalmic and neurologic exam to assess for globe trauma, optic nerve damage, and central nervous system injury. Computed tomographic (CT) scan can assess for globe integrity, optic nerve status, bony injury, cranial injury, and projectile location.

78.4 Management

78.4.1 Treatment Options

Observe and manage associated orbital and/or ocular trauma as appropriate.

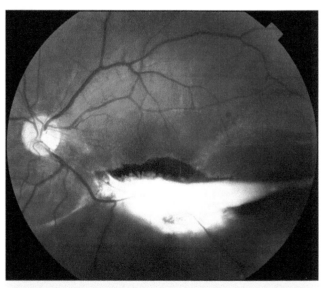

Fig. 78.1 Color fundus photo of the left eye with remote history of orbital missile injury demonstrating an area of macular fibrosis along inferior arcade with pigment superiorly consistent with chorioretinitis sclopetaria.

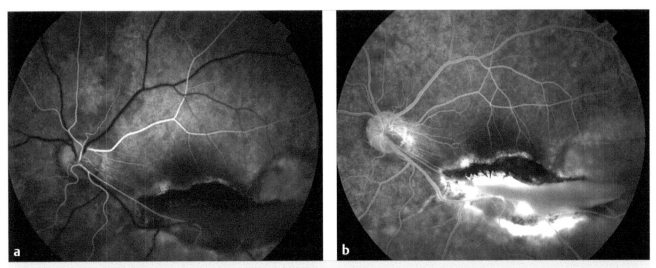

Fig. 78.2 (a) Early fluorescein angiography demonstrating lack of choroidal circulation due to loss of tissue. (b) Late fluorescein angiography demonstrating staining of the sclera and at the lesion's margins.

78.4.2 Follow-up

Weekly fundus examinations until stability of reparative fibrosis is established, and then routinely. Low chance of delayed retinal detachment despite full-thickness retinal defect due to strong fibrous chorioretinal adhesions at the margins of the lesion.

Suggested Reading

[1] Martin DF, Awh CC, McCuen BW, II, Jaffe GJ, Slott JH, Machemer R. Treatment and pathogenesis of traumatic chorioretinal rupture (sclopetaria). Am J Ophthalmol. 1994; 117(2):190–200

[2] Papakostas TD, Yonekawa Y, Wu D, et al. Retinal detachment associated with traumatic chorioretinal rupture. Ophthalmic Surg Lasers Imaging Retina. 2014; 45(5):451–455

[3] Rayess N, Rahimy E, Ho AC. Spectral-domain optical coherence tomography features of bilateral chorioretinitis sclopetaria. Ophthalmic Surg Lasers Imaging Retina. 2015; 46(2):253–255

[4] Richards RD, West CE, Meisels AA. Chorioretinitis sclopetaria. Am J Ophthalmol. 1968; 66(5):852–860

79 Dislocated Lens

Katherine E. Talcott and Omesh P. Gupta

Summary

Dislocated lenses, including both crystalline and intraocular lens implants (IOLs), are typically related to weakening or damage to the capsular support. It is often related to complicated surgeries, trauma, or zonular weakness due to intrinsic causes. These cases can be both interesting and challenging to manage surgically, both with regard to lens removal/rescue and implantation of a secondary IOL. While surgical options were previously limited to anterior chamber IOLs, multiple new techniques have been described including iris fixation, scleral suturing, and sutureless scleral fixation. These techniques show promise in minimizing complications, including corneal decompensation, pigment dispersion, optical aberration, and suture erosion and breakage. Future studies are needed to further elucidate long-term results.

Keywords: anterior chamber intraocular lens, dislocated lens, lens subluxation, intraocular lens implant, scleral fixated

79.1 Features

Dislocated lenses, including both crystalline lenses and intraocular lens implants (IOL), can prove to be interesting cases for which there are a variety of options for surgical management. They are typically caused by weakening of capsular support, especially zonular weakness/loss or posterior capsule defects. Lens dislocation can occur due to insufficient capsular-zonular support after cataract surgery or following traumatic injury. Other predisposing factors include prior retinal surgery, high myopia, pseudoexfoliation syndrome, hypermature cataracts, and uveitis (▶ Fig. 79.1). Subluxed lenses can also be due to hereditary causes with systemic associations (e.g., Marfan syndrome, homocystinuria, Weill-Marchesani syndrome, Ehlers-Danlos syndrome) and those without systemic associations (familial ectopia lentis, ectopia lentis et pupillae, and aniridia; ▶ Fig. 79.2, ▶ Fig. 79.3). Defects in genes causing microfibril assembly are thought to underlie a majority of these syndromes associated with subluxed lenses and ectopia lentis.

79.1.1 Common Symptoms

Impact on vision depends on the severity of the dislocation; possible decreased vision, monocular diplopia, glare, and seeing the edge of the lens implant. Symptoms may be intermittent depending on the mobility of the lens or IOL.

79.1.2 Exam Findings

In the setting of lens subluxation and dislocation, it is important to assess capsular support and structures as this can help guide surgical management. Key questions to address that impact decisions for surgical approach include the following: (1) Where is the lens or IOL located? (2) What type of IOL is present and what material is it made of? (3) Is the anterior or posterior capsule intact? The presence of phacodonesis should

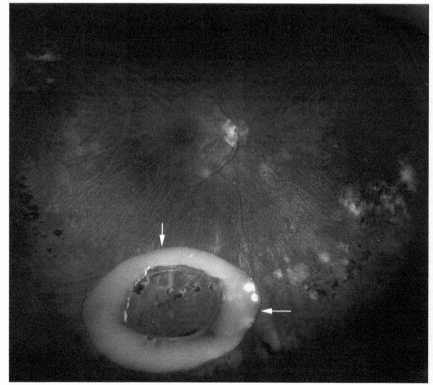

Fig. 79.1 Ultra-widefield fundus photograph of a dislocated intraocular lens implant in capsular bag (*arrows*) likely related to previous vitrectomy.

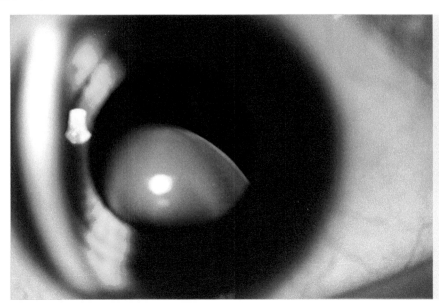

Fig. 79.2 Subluxed crystalline lens in a patient with Marfan syndrome.

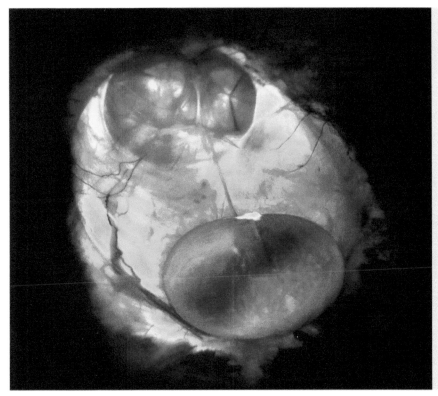

Fig. 79.3 Subluxed crystalline lens in a patient with optic nerve coloboma. (Courtesy of William Benson.)

be noted. Phacodonesis can be detected by having the patient look from side to side or jarring the slit lamp. Presence of vitreous in the anterior chamber or to any surgical wounds should also be noted.

Dislocated lenses can also be associated with other ocular complications: pupillary block glaucoma, uveitis, lens-corneal touch leading to corneal decompensation, vitreous hemorrhage, retinal breaks, and amblyopia in children. These should be evaluated at the time of exam.

79.2 Key Diagnostic Tests and Findings

79.2.1 Ultrasonography

B-scan can be helpful to evaluate for retinal pathology if vitreous hemorrhage, cataract, corneal edema, or other pathology is present. In some cases, the dislocated IOL obstructs the visual axis and impairs view of the fundus.

79.2.2 Keratometry

If surgical management is planned, it is critical to get good quality IOL measurements, including corneal keratometry and A-scan.

79.3 Critical Work-up

In addition to those mentioned earlier, it is imperative to consider systemic associations particularly if a hereditary cause is suspected. Connective tissue disorders such as Marfan syndrome can be associated with life-threatening complications including aortic root aneurysms. These patients should be referred to appropriate specialists for further evaluation and monitoring.

79.4 Management

79.4.1 Treatment Options

There are many surgical approaches available for the management of dislocated lenses. The surgical risk profile should be considered when weighing which approach to use for a specific patient.

Nonsurgical Management

If the lens dislocation is minimal or minimally symptomatic, one could observe so long as there are no associated complications including glaucoma or corneal edema. If the lens is dislocated outside of the visual axis, nonsurgical management with aphakic correction (often with a contact lens) could be considered. This may be a preferable option in pediatric patients or those for whom vitreoretinal surgery would have increased risks of complications, like Marfan patients.

Removal of Lens

If surgical removal is necessitated, care must be taken to avoid vitreous traction through performing an anterior or posterior vitrectomy. For patients with minimal lens instability, traditional phacoemulsification techniques can be used with care taken to avoid stressing the zonules and using adjuvants such as a capsular tension ring. If there is enough capsular support, a sulcus IOL could be considered. Similarly, hooks, scissors, or forceps can be used to remove minimally dislocated IOLs through a clear corneal wound. A pars plana approach to lens removal enables more complete vitrectomy and reduces the vitreoretinal risks associated with limbal extraction. Care should first be taken to remove vitreous traction and zonules if needed using a vitrector and possibly dislocating the lens posteriorly before attempting removal. In children and young adults, the vitrector can be used to perform the lensectomy, but denser lenses will require phacofragmentation. Dislocated IOLs can be brought anteriorly using forceps before removal through a corneal wound.

Anterior Chamber Intraocular Lens

If there is not enough capsular-zonular support for a secondary sulcus IOL, one could consider an anterior chamber intraocular lens (ACIOL). Traditional closed-loop ACIOLs were associated with a high incidence of pseudophakic bullous keratopathy, pigment dispersion, and chronic iritis. However, open-loop newer-generation ACIOLs have decreased contact with ocular tissues with lower haptic erosion into the angle with less damage to the corneal endothelium. A review by the American Academy of Ophthalmology supported them as safe and effective, finding insufficient evidence to demonstrate the superiority of scleral-sutured or iris-sutured IOLs compared to them. The relative ease of inserting them compared with scleral-fixated IOLs make them an attractive option.

Iris-Fixated Intraocular Lens

Sutureless iris-claw lenses are fixated by a small knuckle of iris tissues on either side of the iris. They can be used with an anterior or retropupillary implantation. Sutured iris fixation has also been described and involves directly suturing an IOL to the iris with one of a variety of strategies, including the McCannel suture, Siepser knot, and girth-hitch knot. Potential complications of iris fixation include pupillary distortion, synechia, pigment dispersion, and chronic iritis.

Scleral-Sutured Intraocular Lens

Scleral-sutured intraocular lens (SSIOL) is a widely used option in the management of dislocated lenses. They can be used in eyes that have abnormal anterior segment structures or insufficient capsular support and are placed in the correct anatomic location reducing optical aberrations and complications related to pigment dispersion and abnormal pupillary movement. Vitreous management during IOL placement can be performed from either an anterior or posterior approach. Potential complications from SSIOL include suture breakage, erosion, and exposure potentially leading to bleeding or endophthalmitis. Different techniques have been described to minimize these complications, including the creation of triangular scleral flaps or pockets as well as suture knot rotation into the eye.

More recently, the use of expandable polytetrafluoroethylene (Gore-Tex; WL Gore & Associates, Inc. Elkton, MD) suture has been described for the scleral fixation of Bausch and Lomb Akreos AO60 or Alcon CZ7OBD IOLs, as these sutures may have less risk of degrading or breaking with time. Outcomes have been promising. The foldable nature of the AO60 lens, simplified surgical technique, and often excellent surgical results provide significant appeal (▶ Fig. 79.4). However, the AO60 lens is hydrophilic and IOL opacification has been described with the use of an air or gas tamponade (▶ Fig. 79.5). Use of the Bausch and Lomb EnVista MX60 hydrophobic acrylic lens in conjunction with Gore-Tex sutures has been described without opacification with air or gas tamponade, though long-term data have not yet been gathered (▶ Fig. 79.6).

Sutureless Scleral-Fixated Intraocular Lens

To avoid sutures and their complications, sutureless techniques have been described including using cannulas to create sclerotomy tunnels through which the haptics of a three-piece IOL are subsequently pulled through. Others have modified this technique with posterior segment instruments and the use of

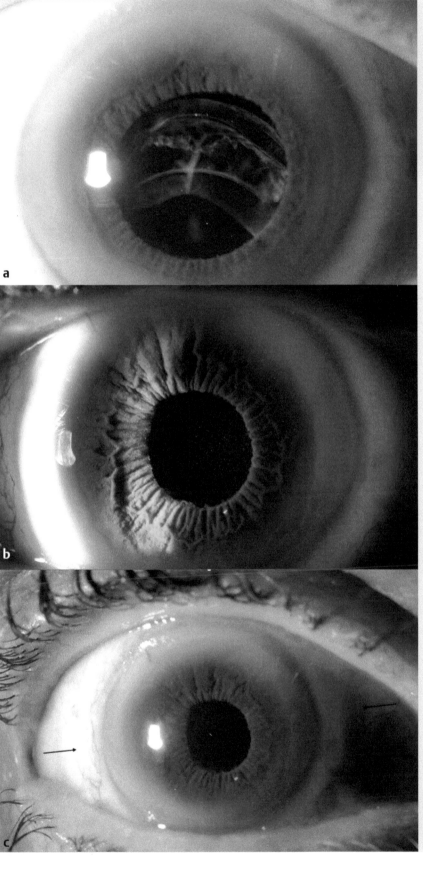

Fig. 79.4 (a) Preoperative slit-lamp photo demonstrating in-the-bag subluxation of single-piece acrylic lens from pseudoexfoliation with haptic in the visual axis. **(b,c)** Postoperative slit-lamp photo following placement of Akreos AO60 implant with excellent centration. Gore-Tex sutures are visible under the conjunctiva (*black arrows*).

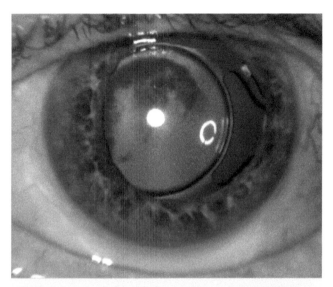

Fig. 79.5 Opacified hydrophilic Akreos AO60 acrylic lens implant.

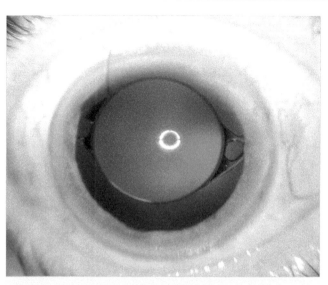

Fig. 79.6 Well-centered Gore-Tex scleral-sutured EnVista MX60 hydrophobic acrylic.

transconjunctival trocars. Complications including broken haptics intraoperatively can be minimized by using forceps through the cannula to grasp the haptic but removing the cannula before withdrawing the haptic. These techniques appear to decrease specific complications related to suture degradation, which may be useful to younger patients.

Sutureless Scleral Fixation Using Fibrin Glue

Another technique to avoid sutures is scleral fixation of IOLs using fibrin glue. A single-stage simultaneous rescue of dislocated three-piece IOLs and sutureless intrascleral fixation using fibrin glue has been described. Partial-thickness limbal-based scleral flaps are created and needles are used to create sclerotomies before fibrin glue is used to fixate the haptics and close the flaps. It avoids the need for an incision for IOL explanation but has only been described in dislocated three-piece IOLs.

Intraocular Sutured Rescue

In select cases, the dislocated IOL can be rescued without removal. Techniques that have been described include scleral fixation of the IOL or IOL/bag complex, iris fixation of a three-piece IOL, or sutureless scleral fixation as described earlier. These surgeries may be technically challenging, but provide the benefit of avoiding corneal incisions for IOL removal.

79.4.2 Follow-up

Close follow-up is needed postoperatively in these patients to monitor for potential complications including elevated intraocular pressure, hypotony, corneal edema, hyphema, vitreous hemorrhage, suture breakage/exposure, and infection. Due to other factors leading to a dislocated lens, these eyes tend to have other pathology that can increase these risks. In general, patients with dislocated lenses and extracapsular IOL fixation have improved visual outcomes. However, predisposing factors often limit best-corrected visual acuity and outcomes. While many studies describe a specific surgical technique or outcomes related to that technique, less is known on how these techniques directly compare. Further studies are needed to further elucidate long-term results as well as compare techniques.

Suggested Reading

[1] Sadiq MA, Vanderveen D. Genetics of ectopia lentis. Semin Ophthalmol. 2013; 28(5–6):313–320
[2] Wagoner MD, Cox TA, Ariyasu RG, Jacobs DS, Karp CL, American Academy of Ophthalmology. Intraocular lens implantation in the absence of capsular support: a report by the American Academy of Ophthalmology. Ophthalmology. 2003; 110(4):840–859
[3] Dajee KP, Abbey AM, Williams GA. Management of dislocated intraocular lenses in eyes with insufficient capsular support. Curr Opin Ophthalmol. 2016; 27(3):191–195
[4] Khan MA, Samara WA, Gerstenblith AT, et al. Combined pars plana vitrectomy and scleral fixation of an intraocular lens using gore-text suture: one-year outcomes. Retina. 2018; 38(7):1377–1384

80 Intraocular Foreign Body

Rahul Kapoor and Jayanth Sridhar

Summary

Diagnosis and management of an intraocular foreign body (IOFB) is complex and depends on the size, shape, location, material, nature, and momentum upon impact of the foreign body. Patients' knowledge of the mechanism of injury can help identify the nature and location of the IOFB. However, history of trauma may be remote and patients might not recall the injury. Therefore, diagnostic imaging modalities, along with proper history and clinical examination, are crucial in the diagnosis and management of IOFB.

Keywords: chalcosis, endophthalmitis, metallosis, siderosis bulbi, trauma, vitrectomy

80.1 Features

80.1.1 Common Symptoms

Presentation is highly variable and depends on the nature, size, and location of the intraocular foreign body (IOFB). Patients might be asymptomatic or complain of decreased vision, pain, floaters, and diplopia.

80.1.2 Exam Findings

Anterior segment examination may reveal conjunctival injection, subconjunctival hemorrhage, scleral laceration, focal lens opacities/capsular defects, self-sealing corneal or scleral wounds, and uveal prolapse. Iris transillumination defects and heterochromia, anisocoria, and a positive Seidel test may also be noted. Corneal deposits, anterior subcapsular cataracts, lens dislocation, and optic atrophy could be present especially with chronic iron-containing IOFBs. Gonioscopy can reveal occult IOFB in the angle and scleral depression may reveal in occult IOFB in the pars plana/anterior retina. Patient with occult IOFB and developing endophthalmitis may present with cells in the anterior chamber, hypopyon, and vitritis (▶ Fig. 80.1). Posterior examination can reveal retinal tears or detachments, commotio retinae, choroid rupture or detachment, sclopetaria, vitreous hemorrhage, or a posterior exit wound.

80.2 Key Diagnostic Tests and Findings

80.2.1 Plain X-Rays

Plain films are a quick and effective screening tool used to detect and localize radiopaque foreign bodies (▶ Fig. 80.2). Plain films can reveal small IOFBs that are sometimes missed by CT scans.

80.2.2 Ultrasonography

Can be used to visualize IOFBs in real time and from various angles. Ultrasonography may demonstrate radiolucent foreign bodies that are not seen on CT scans. High-resolution ultrasound biomicroscopy is useful for locating small, nonmetallic bodies in the angle, ciliary body, ciliary processes, and retrolental space (▶ Fig. 80.3, ▶ Fig. 80.4). Extreme care should be taken with the ultrasound probe in order to prevent extrusion of intraocular materials in case of a ruptured globe.

80.2.3 Computed Tomography

Computed tomographic (CT) scan of the orbits is the primary modality used to survey the globes, orbital bones, and the retrobulbar space in cases of suspected IOFB (▶ Fig. 80.5). Moreover, the amount of attenuation can help determine the type of

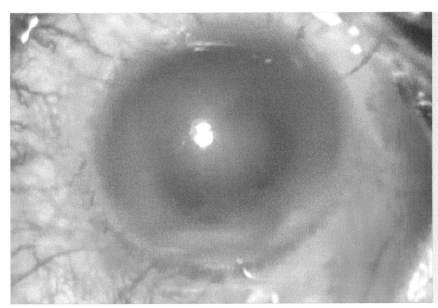

Fig. 80.1 Mixed hypopyon and hyphema in an eye noted to have pain after hammering without eye protection is suspicious for occult intraocular foreign body and associated endophthalmitis.

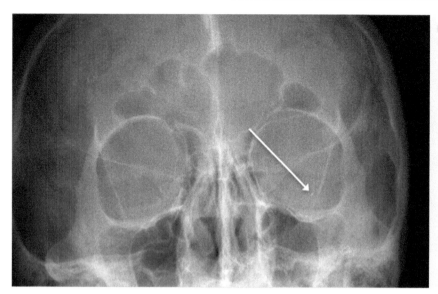

Fig. 80.2 Plain film X-ray may detect even a small metallic intraocular foreign body (*arrow*).

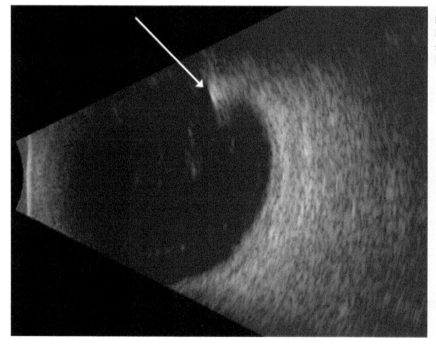

Fig. 80.3 B-scan ultrasound with a focal hyperechoic body (*arrow*) with associated shadowing is characteristic for metallic intraocular foreign bodies.

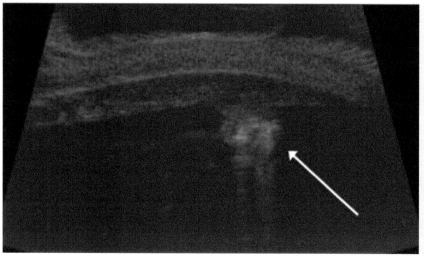

Fig. 80.4 High-resolution ultrasound biomicroscopy can detect intraocular foreign bodies hidden behind the iris in the iridolenticular recess (*arrow*).

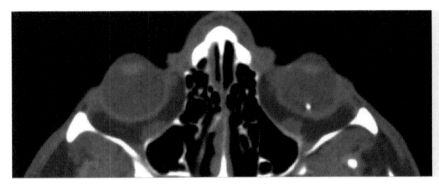

Fig. 80.5 Metallic intraocular foreign bodies appear hyperintense on CT scan, as seen in the left eye here.

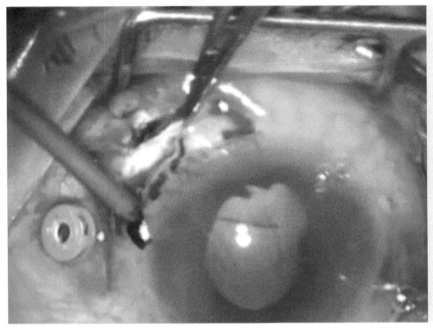

Fig. 80.6 Definitive removal of intraocular foreign bodies may be undertaken via pars plana approach when the lens posterior capsule and/or posterior segment is involved.

foreign body. However, CT scans may miss IOFBs composed of plastic, glass, wood, and ceramic materials. Spiral CT with multiplanar reconstruction is the most effective way to visualize glass IOFBs.

80.2.4 Magnetic Resonance Imaging

Magnetic resonance imaging (MRI) can be useful in visualizing nonmetallic IOFB, such as wood, but is contraindicated in metallic IOFBs because magnetic forces on the metallic body can lead to further intraocular damage. MRI can also detect small IOFBs that are missed by CT scans, ultrasound, and plain films.

80.3 Critical Work-up

Definitive treatment includes surgical removal of the IOFB. Therefore, patients are generally admitted to the hospital and kept NPO to prepare for surgery. A protective shield is placed over the involved eye. Broad spectrum intravenous antibiotics, such as vancomycin and ceftazidime, are started and tetanus immunoglobulin or toxoid is administered as needed. The location, size, and nature of the IOFB determine the urgency and surgical approaches to remove the IOFB. Vegetable matter poses

a higher risk for endophthalmitis and should be removed urgently. Inert substances may be removed at a later time upon closure of the initial wound.

80.4 Management

80.4.1 Treatment Options

Location of the IOFB (anterior or posterior to the iris plane) and lenticular involvement determine the surgical approach necessary to remove the IOFB. Anterior IOFBs without involvement of the crystalline lens are generally removed via limbal incisions through forceps with viscoelastic used to maintain the chamber depth and protect the corneal endothelium and lens. Lenticular IOFBs generally require IOFB removal with phacoemulsification or a pars plana lensectomy with vitrectomy if the posterior capsule is involved. Posterior IOFBs generally require pars plana vitrectomy and removal of the IOFBs via the corneal or scleral wound (▶ Fig. 80.6). In case of a small magnetic IOFB near the pars plana, an electromagnet can be placed over the sclerotomy site to help remove the IOFB. Intravitreal antibiotics, such as vancomycin and ceftazidime, may be considered for endophthalmitis prophylaxis.

80.4.2 Follow-up

Follow-up depends on the nature and extent of injury. Postoperative imaging is important if there is suspicion for only partial removal of the IOFB. Observation for clinical signs of infection and inflammation is necessary, and patients should be followed up routinely for a year. Electroretinogram (ERG) should be performed if a chronic retained IOFB is suspected to look for signs of metallosis, toxicity resulting from intraocular metallic bodies. Specifically, siderosis bulbi results from iron deposition and can lead to iris heterochromia, mydriasis, glaucoma, cataracts, and retinal pigment degeneration. Chalcosis is toxicity from copper containing IOFBs and causes intraocular damage likely through free radical formation. Serial ERGs can be used to follow the resolution of symptoms from metallosis after removal of the IOFB.

Suggested Reading

[1] Loporchio D, Mukkamala L, Gorukanti K, Zarbin M, Langer P, Bhagat N. Intraocular foreign bodies: a review. Surv Ophthalmol. 2016; 61(5):582–596

[2] Yeh S, Colyer MH, Weichel ED. Current trends in the management of intraocular foreign bodies. Curr Opin Ophthalmol. 2008; 19(3):225–233

[3] Mahmoud A, Messaoud R, Abid F, Ksiaa I, Bouzayene M, Khairallah M. Anterior segment optical coherence tomography and retained vegetal intraocular foreign body masquerading as chronic anterior uveitis. J Ophthalmic Inflamm Infect. 2017; 7(1):13

[4] Greven CM, Engelbrecht NE, Slusher MM, Nagy SS. Intraocular foreign bodies: management, prognostic factors, and visual outcomes. Ophthalmology. 2000; 107(3):608–612

81 Terson Syndrome

Atsuro Uchida and Justis P. Ehlers

Summary

Terson syndrome is the occurrence of any intraocular hemorrhage in patients suffering from cerebral diseases with raised intracranial pressure, classically subarachnoid hemorrhage. Vitreous hemorrhage and sub-internal limiting membrane hemorrhage are common, but intraocular hemorrhage may occur in various locations and multiple layers of the retina. The mechanism of intraocular hemorrhage remains controversial. The most accepted hypothesis is that congestion of the central retinal vein at the level of lamina cribrosa resulting in rupture of the retinal vessel caused by a rapid elevation of intracranial pressure transmitted along the optic nerve sheath (i.e., subarachnoid space). Visual symptoms include decreased vision, floaters, and visual field defects, which is often reported after brain surgery or when a patient regains consciousness. For eyes with a limited amount of intraocular hemorrhage sparing the fovea, careful observation is the first choice of treatment. In eyes with persistent intraocular hemorrhage, vitrectomy can promote the recovery of vision, and may also prevent permanent visual loss from severe complications. In patients with bilateral visual impairment and without spontaneous resorption precluding rehabilitation, vitrectomy should be considered in at least one eye under the condition that the patient is systemically stable.

Keywords: Terson syndrome, subarachnoid hemorrhage, sub-internal limiting membrane hemorrhage, vitreous hemorrhage, vitrectomy

81.1 Features

Terson syndrome is generally defined as the occurrence of any intraocular hemorrhage in patients suffering from cerebral diseases with raised intracranial pressure, classically subarachnoid hemorrhage (SAH). It usually develops within a couple of hours after the onset of SAH, but it can rarely develop as late as 6 weeks. Less frequently, it may be caused by intracerebral hemorrhage, epidural/subdural hematoma, severe brain injury, spinal SAH, intraventricular hemorrhage, or endoscopic third ventriculostomy. Terson syndrome can occur at any age, but most commonly affects adults between the age of 30 and 60. SAH patients with a low Glasgow Coma Scale (GCS) and high Hunt & Hess scale (H&H) have a higher reported incidence of Terson syndrome. The presence of Terson syndrome following SAH is associated with a higher mortality rate of up to 50–60%.

81.1.1 Common Symptoms

Common symptoms are decreased vision, floaters, visual field defects or blindness, with a history of SAH. Intraocular hemorrhage that involves the macular or visual axis significantly impacts visual acuity. Accompanying conditions such as epiretinal membrane formation, secondary macular holes, retinal detachment, retinal hemosiderosis, or optic neuropathy may exacerbate visual impairment and final visual outcomes.

Visual symptoms are often reported after brain surgery or when patients regain consciousness.

81.1.2 Exam Findings

Terson syndrome develops in 20 to 40% of acute aneurysmal SAH, and vitreous hemorrhage (VH) occurs in 3 to 5% of cases, but actual incidence may be higher due to the high early mortality rate hindering accurate diagnosis. Approximately 60% of cases are bilateral. Intraocular hemorrhage may involve various locations and multiple layers of the retina. These include the vitreous, subhyaloid, sub-internal limiting membrane (ILM), intraretinal, and subretinal spaces.

81.2 Key Diagnostic Tests and Findings

81.2.1 Optical Coherence Tomography

Optical coherence tomography (OCT) helps identify the precise location of premacular, submacular, and intraretinal hemorrhage when performance is feasible (► Fig. 81.1, ► Fig. 81.2).

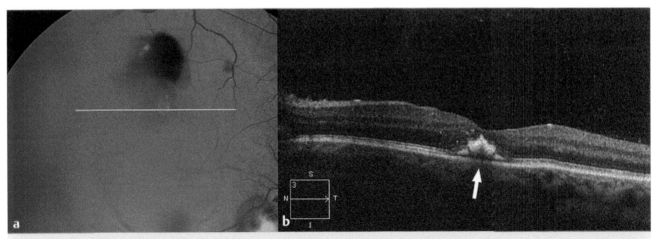

Fig. 81.1 (a) Fundus photo and **(b)** optical coherence tomography (OCT) performed 2 weeks after the onset of subarachnoid hemorrhage. The horizontal B-scan reveals a small amount of subretinal hemorrhage at the fovea (*arrow*).

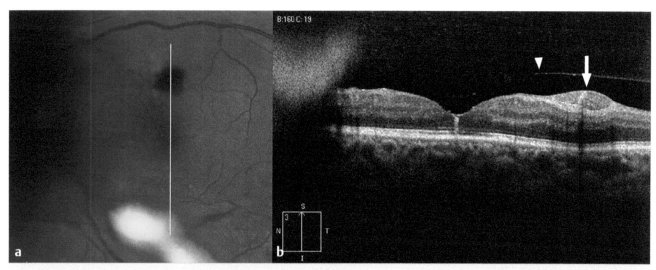

Fig. 81.2 (a) Fundus photos and **(b)** optical coherence tomography performed 2 months after the onset of subarachnoid hemorrhage. The vertical B-scan illustrates the existence of sub-internal limiting membrane hemorrhage (*arrow*) and incomplete separation of the posterior hyaloid (*arrowhead*). The OCT beam is partially blocked by vitreous hemorrhage.

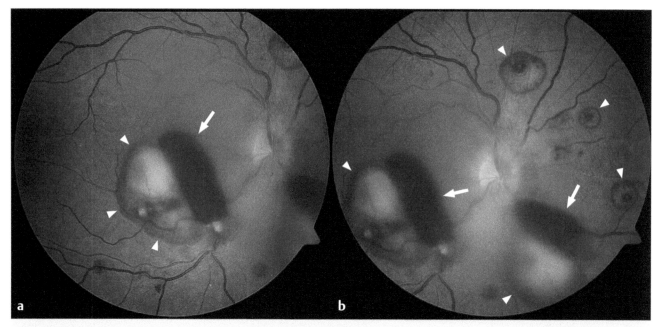

Fig. 81.3 Color fundus image of right eye obtained 2 weeks after the onset of subarachnoid hemorrhage due to aneurysmal rupture in the anterior communicating cerebral artery. Imaging illustrates intraocular hemorrhage in various locations and retinal layers. Optic disc and surrounding area are slightly obscured by the presence of mild vitreous hemorrhage. Preretinal hemorrhage (*arrow*) involving the **(a)** macula and **(b)** periphery and subretinal hemorrhage (*arrowhead*) are observed.

81.2.2 Fundus Photography

Vitreous, sub-ILM, subhyaloid, intraretinal, and/or subretinal hemorrhage may be documented with fundus photography (▶ Fig. 81.3).

81.2.3 B-Scan Ultrasonography

Increased hyperechoic material within the vitreous may be visualized in cases of VH. Preretinal hemorrhage appears as dome-shaped formation on the retinal surface (▶ Fig. 81.4). Subretinal hemorrhage may also be identified.

81.2.4 Computed Tomography

Computed tomography may illustrate preretinal hemorrhage as a crescent or nodule-shaped hyperdensity on the retinal surface adjacent to the optic nerve (▶ Fig. 81.5). In a rare instance, the patient may present to the eye care provider due to visual symptoms prior to the diagnosis of SAH. Patients who present

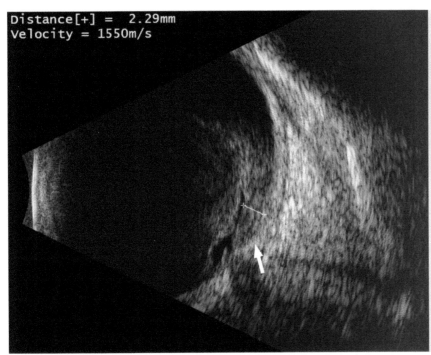

Fig. 81.4 Ocular B-mode ultrasonography demonstrates increased reflectivity of the vitreous suggestive of vitreous hemorrhage and macular thickening (*arrow*) presumably due to preretinal hemorrhage, 3 weeks after the onset of subarachnoid hemorrhage. Posterior vitreous detachment is absent. The B-mode scan confirms no retinal tears or retinal detachment.

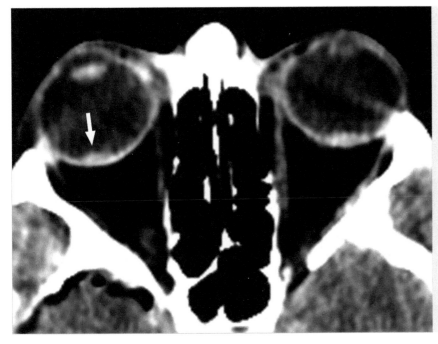

Fig. 81.5 A computed tomography scan obtained 2 days after an intracranial hemorrhage reveals a hyperdense crescent on the central retinal surface (*arrow*) suggestive of intraocular hemorrhage.

with findings consistent with Terson syndrome and associated neurologic symptoms should be sent for urgent neuroimaging and evaluation.

81.3 Critical Work-up

Diagnosis is usually straightforward with the coexistence of cerebral diseases/hemorrhage and new onset of symptoms.

81.4 Management

For eyes with a limited amount of intraocular hemorrhage sparing the fovea, careful observation without active treatment is recommended. Small localized retinal hemorrhages spontaneously clear within a few weeks. In patients with premacular hemorrhages (subhyaloid or sub-ILM), spontaneous resorption can be slow and result in prolonged visual impairment. In patients with VH, spontaneous resorption may take several months depending on the amount of bleeding.

81.4.1 Treatment Options

Nonclearing Vitreous/Premacular Hemorrhage

Vitrectomy can promote rapid recovery of vision. No consensus guidelines exist regarding the timing of ophthalmological surgical interventions. However, in patients with bilateral visual impairment and without spontaneous resorption precluding rehabilitation, vitrectomy should be considered in at least one eye once the patient becomes systemically stable for surgery.

Premacular Hemorrhage

In large premacular hemorrhages, disruption of the posterior hyaloid membrane or ILM utilizing the neodymium:yttrium aluminum garnet (Nd-YAG) laser may be an alternative vitrectomy.

81.4.2 Follow-up

Patients should be followed up closely until resolution of the hemorrhage is achieved.

Suggested Reading

[1] Skevas C, Czorlich P, Knospe V, et al. Terson's syndrome–rate and surgical approach in patients with subarachnoid hemorrhage: a prospective interdisciplinary study. Ophthalmology. 2014; 121(8):1628–1633

[2] Bäuerle J, Gross NJ, Egger K, et al. Terson's syndrome: diagnostic comparison of ocular sonography and CT. J Neuroimaging. 2016; 26(2):247–252

[3] Sung W, Arnaldo B, Sergio C, Juliana S, Michel F. Terson's syndrome as a prognostic factor for mortality of spontaneous subarachnoid haemorrhage. Acta Ophthalmol. 2011; 89(6):544–547

[4] Garweg JG, Koerner F. Outcome indicators for vitrectomy in Terson syndrome. Acta Ophthalmol. 2009; 87(2):222–226

82 Purtscher and Purtscher-Like Retinopathy

Charles C. Wykoff and Harris Sultan

Summary

Purtscher and Purtscher-like retinopathies are a group of retinal vascular diseases secondary to trauma or other disease processes with characteristic retinal findings, including polygonal inner retinal whitening, cotton wool spots, and intraretinal hemorrhages. The most common cause is trauma; however, cases have been reported secondary to numerous other pathologies including acute pancreatitis, valsalva, thrombotic thrombocytopenic purpura, hemolytic uremic syndrome, cryoglobulinemia, pregnancy, and connective tissue disorders. Impact on vision may range from asymptomatic to hand-motions vision, and may be delayed 24 to 48 hours following the instigating event. Purtscher retinopathy is most commonly bilateral, but unilateral cases have been described. Optical coherence tomography may demonstrate increased inner retinal reflectivity consistent with cotton-wool spots and subretinal and intraretinal fluid accumulation. Fluorescein angiography may show areas of retinal nonperfusion, delayed transit, and peripapillary leakage. Approximately half of patients experience two lines of visual improvement with observation.

Keywords: Purtscher, Purtscher-like, retinal vascular disease

82.1 Features

Purtscher and Purtscher-like retinopathies are a group of retinal vascular diseases secondary to trauma or other disease processes with characteristic retinal findings, including polygonal inner retinal whitening, cotton wool spots, and intraretinal hemorrhages. The most common cause is trauma; however, cases have been reported secondary to numerous other pathologies including acute pancreatitis, valsalva, thrombotic thrombocytopenic purpura, hemolytic uremic syndrome, cryoglobulinemia, pregnancy, and connective tissue disorders. Impact on vision may range from asymptomatic to hand-motions vision, and may be delayed 24 to 48 hours following the instigating event. Purtscher retinopathy is most commonly bilateral, but unilateral cases have been described.

82.1.1 Common Symptoms

Variable vision loss ranges from none to hand-motion level visual acuity. Vision loss may be delayed 24 to 48 hours following the instigating event. Central, paracentral, or arcuate scotomata may be present with preservation of peripheral visual field.

82.1.2 Exam Findings

Most common findings are cotton wool spots, retinal hemorrhages, and Purtscher Flecken (i.e., areas of polygonal, retinal whitening in the superficial, inner retina, with a clear demarcating line, with 50 μm between the affected retina and retinal vasculature, ▶ Fig. 82.1). These typically present in the posterior pole and area immediately nasal to the optic disc. Pseudo-

cherry red spot with surrounding retinal whitening and optic disc edema may be present. Most cases are bilateral. Retinal vessels appear healthy.

82.2 Key Diagnostic Tests and Findings

82.2.1 Optical Coherence Tomography

Subretinal and intraretinal fluid with resolution in most cases after 1 month (▶ Fig. 82.2). Inner retinal hyperreflectivity corresponding to cotton-wool spots and areas of retinal whitening. Cases with severe edema may result in retinal atrophy.

82.2.2 Fluorescein Angiography or Ultra-Widefield Fluorescein Angiography

Angiographic findings include areas of nonperfusion and retinal ischemia, variable early hypofluorescence and late leakage, delayed AV transit, and peripapillary staining (▶ Fig. 82.3).

82.3 Critical Work-up

Purtscher retinopathy is secondary to severe head trauma or crush injury. Purtscher-like retinopathy includes similar retinal

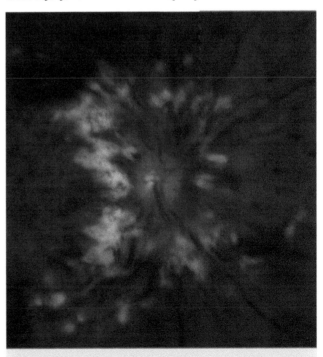

Fig. 82.1 Fundus photograph of optic nerve and peripapillary retina demonstrating extensive cotton wool spots with associated retinal hemorrhage in a Purtscher-like presentation related to an exacerbation of pemphigus vulgaris.

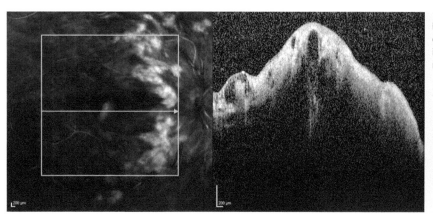

Fig. 82.2 Optical coherence tomography of same eye demonstrating significant subretinal and intraretinal fluid with significant increased inner retinal hyperreflectivity related to ischemia.

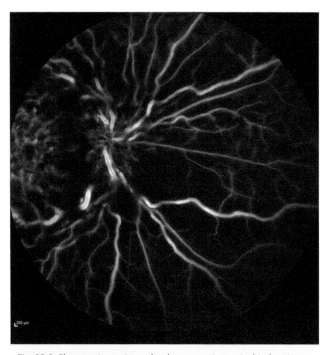

Fig. 82.3 Fluorescein angiography demonstrating retinal ischemia, extensive retinal nonperfusion, and capillary leakage.

findings but without antecedent trauma. Without trauma history, patient should be evaluated for systemic disease processes associated with the ocular findings. Associations for Purtscher or Purtscher-like retinopathy include long bone fracture, orthopaedic surgery, chest compression, shaken baby syndrome, acute pancreatitis, chronic renal failure, thrombotic thrombocy-topenic purpura, hemolytic uremic syndrome, connective tissue disorders (lupus, scleroderma, and dermatomyositis), cryoglobulinemia, air embolization, and amniotic fluid embolization.

82.4 Management

82.4.1 Treatment Options

There is no definitive, evidence-based data for benefit of interventional treatment. If a causative nontraumatic disease process is identified, the underlying disease should be managed appropriately. Visual acuity improves in approximately half of patients. High-dose systemic steroids have been evaluated without clear evidence of efficacy. Steroids may have a clearer role in patients with underlying inflammatory etiologies.

82.4.2 Follow-up

Regular follow-up is recommended to confirm expected resolution of retinal findings and documentation of visual acuity. Normalization of retinal appearance occurs frequently, but optic atrophy and RPE mottling are also common findings.

Suggested Reading

[1] Eliott D, Papakostas T. In: Ryan SJ, Sadda SR, Hinton DR, et al., eds. Retina. Sixth Edition. London: W.B. Saunders; 2018

[2] Agrawal A, McKibbin MA. Purtscher's and Purtscher-like retinopathies: a review. Surv Ophthalmol. 2006; 51(2):129–136

[3] Miguel AI, Henriques F, Azevedo LF, Loureiro AJ, Maberley DA. Systematic review of Purtscher's and Purtscher-like retinopathies. Eye (Lond). 2013; 27 (1):1–13

[4] Agrawal A, McKibbin M. Purtscher's retinopathy: epidemiology, clinical features and outcome. Br J Ophthalmol. 2007; 91(11):1456–1459

83 Laser Maculopathy

Dilsher S. Dhoot and John D. Pitcher, III

Summary

Laser light is commonly used for a variety of applications including entertainment, medicine, research, industry, and for military purposes. Laser retinal exposure is an infrequent but potentially blinding injury and numerous cases are documented in the literature. Inadvertent or malicious exposure to laser can result in immediate retinal injury that is often irreversible. The responsible use of lasers helps prevent such injuries. The manifestations of laser injury vary and depend on the type and power of laser and exposure time and location.

Keywords: chorioretinal scarring, laser maculopathy, photocoagulation

83.1 Features

In the United States, the Food and Drug Administration (FDA) regulates laser products. The FDA classifies lasers as class 1 through 4 based on type of light emitted and the hazard posed by this light. The laser radiation in class 1 lasers is typically confined to the product and considered to be low hazard, an example would be laser printers or CD players. Class 2 products emit less than 1 mW of power of visible laser light, an example would be a bar code scanner. The majority of commercially available laser pointers fall under class 3a and have a limit of 5 mW of power. Both class 2 and 3a lasers are considered relatively safe because eye exposure leads to the blink reflex which helps prevent damage by limiting the exposure time of laser to 0.15 to 0.25 seconds. It is important to note, however, that injuries with class 3a lasers have been reported when these lasers are not used in a responsible fashion. Class 3b (maximum output power: 5–500 mW) and Class 4 (maximum output power: > 500 mW) laser devices serve industrial or specialized purposes and are extremely dangerous because they can cause severe injury with minimal exposure times. The blink reflex is ineffective in preventing retinal damage with such lasers. Moreover, the cornea and lens focus laser radiation onto a small spot on the retina, increasing the exposure risk. High-powered lasers are used for research, industrial, and medical purposes. Laser safety precautions including laser eyeglasses, protective housings, and safety training help limit occupational exposure. Nonetheless, there are many reports of hazardous laser use by laypersons, improperly trained operators, and malicious users. Use of lasers in lighting shows has been reported to cause ocular injury. Children are an especially vulnerable population and may be the victim of laser accidents because they are unaware of laser safety and find laser pointers curious and attractive (▶ Fig. 83.1**a**). Low-cost, high-powered lasers (up to 1,200 mW) have become popular in recent years and have been relatively easy to obtain via the internet; these lasers have potential for retinal injury and cases of such have been reported. Photocoagulation, photodisruption, and photochemical interaction are all possible mechanisms of damage to the retina. Damage varies depending on the wavelength, exposure time, power, and the location of exposure. Blue light lasers are considered relatively more dangerous than green or red light laser given their shorter wavelengths which are more readily absorbed by the retinal pigment epithelium (RPE), though retinal damage and injury can occur at all wavelengths of light.

83.1.1 Common Symptoms

Typically causes a sudden, painless loss of vision, in some cases with an audible "pop." Vision of 20/200 or worse and visual field defects may be present. Notably, the anterior segment is unaffected in most cases. In many cases, improvement in vision occurs as hemorrhage and inflammation resolve, though sustained vision loss can also occur depending on the injury location and exposure. Chorioretinal scarring is the most common complication of laser exposure and can result in sustained vision loss.

83.1.2 Exam Findings

The manifestations of laser retinal exposure are typically immediate and can lead to permanent changes. Retinal damage from lasers invariably results in retinal or vitreous bleeding with single or multiple lesions of retinal edema, holes, or burns, most frequently in the macula (▶ Fig. 83.1**b,c**). Macular holes, epiretinal membranes, and macular cysts have also been reported following laser exposure. Finally, choroidal neovascularization (CNV), a known complication of retinal photocoagulation for various diseases, has also been reported in the setting of accidental laser exposure.

83.2 Key Diagnostic Tests and Findings

83.2.1 Optical Coherence Tomography

Spectral domain optical coherence tomography has been used to aid in diagnosis of laser maculopathy. Findings vary depending on the severity of the injury. Mild acute cases may have minimal focal discontinuation of the photoreceptor ellipsoid layer and/or retinal pigment epithelium, while severe acute cases may have frank disruption of the outer retina, subretinal hemorrhage, macula edema, or even full-thickness macular hole (▶ Fig. 83.1**d**). Later in the clinical course, mild case may show spontaneous improvement, while more extensive injuries may have persistent atrophy or fibrosis.

83.2.2 Fluorescein Angiography or Ultra-Widefield Fluorescein Angiography

Fluorescein angiography may demonstrate early hyperfluorescence from window defects in cases of RPE abnormalities, or hypofluorescence due to blocking from hemorrhage. Late staining would be expected with the development of a chronic

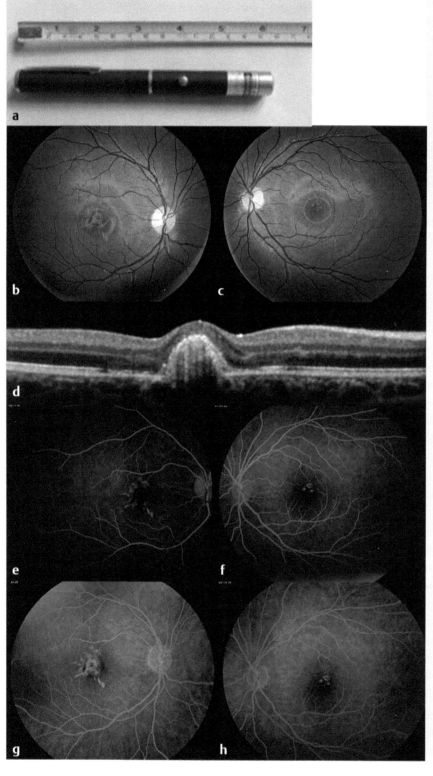

Fig. 83.1 Laser maculopathy. **(a)** Handheld laser point responsible for the injury following reflection off of a mirror. **(b,c)** Color fundus photographs demonstrate central yellow lesions in both foveas, with a ring of surrounding subretinal hemorrhage in the right eye. **(d)** Optical coherence tomography of the right eye showed subfoveal elevated hyperreflective lesion with disruption of the outer retinal layers while the left eye showed a small focal area of attenuation of the photoreceptor–retinal pigment epithelium complex. **(e–h)** Fluorescein angiography was remarkable for focal early hyperfluorescence with late staining in the foveal region of both eyes.

scar, while frank leakage may indicate development of CNV
(▶ Fig. 83.1**e–h**).

83.3 Management

83.3.1 Treatment Options

Treatment

Treatment of laser exposure can be medical or surgical depending on the type of injury. Systemic corticosteroids have been used, although randomized clinical trials are lacking. Anecdotal reports have shown variable results. Vasodilator drugs and antioxidants have also been utilized for laser injury, though again these reports are anecdotal. Surgical intervention with vitrectomy has been reported in cases of vitreous or preretinal hemorrhage, as well as laser-induced macular hole repair.

Prevention

Prevention of laser injuries can be achieved with the use of wavelength-specific filters, which block a specific wavelength of light yet allow sufficient unfiltered light of other wavelengths to be transmitted. Glasses with wavelength-specific filters are widely employed in research and medical settings to prevent occupational exposure. The use of these filters requires knowledge of the specific wavelength desired to be blocked. In certain settings, such as the battlefield, these filter goggles have limited use, as the wavelength of enemy laser may be unknown and it is impractical to block multiple wavelengths as this would limit vision. Incidental laser exposure has been reported in the literature. Industrial or research employees have been found to have incidental lesions most consistent with prior laser injuries; in many cases, the patient has no recollection of the injury given the peripheral location and typically asymptomatic nature of these injuries. Consequently, the overall incidence of laser injuries in these individuals is difficult to estimate given likely underreporting.

Suggested Reading

[1] FDA. Available at: https://www.fda.gov/radiation-emittingproducts/radiatio-nemittingproductsandprocedures/homebusinessandentertainment/laserpro-ductsandinstruments/ucm116373.html. Accessed April 12, 2019

[2] Ajudua S, Mello MJ. Shedding some light on laser pointer eye injuries. Pediatr Emerg Care. 2007; 23(9):669–672

[3] Barkana Y, Belkin M. Laser eye injuries. Surv Ophthalmol. 2000; 44(6):459–478

[4] Marshall J. Lasers in ophthalmology: the basic principles. Eye (Lond). 1988; 2 Suppl:S98–S112

[5] Ham WT, Jr, Ruffolo JJ, Jr, Mueller HA, Clarke AM, Moon ME. Histologic analysis of photochemical lesions produced in rhesus retina by short-wave-length light. Invest Ophthalmol Vis Sci. 1978; 17(10):1029–1035

84 Solar Retinopathy

Alexander R. Bottini, Michael A. Klufas, and Yasha S. Modi

Summary

Solar retinopathy is a type of photic maculopathy that results in central macular (i.e., foveal) damage following intense light exposure. It characteristically follows direct sun-gazing, commonly eclipse viewing. Symptoms include blurred vision, scotoma, and metamorphopsia. The degree of damage is related to the intensity and duration of light exposure. Fundus examination reveals a focal macular lesion or lesions. Optical coherence tomography imaging reveals focal discontinuity of the ellipsoid zone with or without retinal pigment epithelium transmission defects. While there is no proven therapy, the visual prognosis is good in many cases.

Keywords: eclipse, eclipse retinopathy, solar retinitis, solar retinopathy, sun-gazing

84.1 Features

Solar retinopathy describes a focal retinal injury occurring in the setting of intense light exposure, characteristically associated with sun-gazing. It is also known as eclipse retinopathy, eclipse burn, solar retinitis, and solar chorioretinal burn. Historical anecdotes linking direct sun-gazing to ocular damage date back to the time of Plato. Case reports began in the 17th century, and the first fundus findings were described with the advent of ophthalmoscopy in the early 20th century.

The primary mechanism implicated in solar retinopathy is a photochemical retinal injury from intense light exposure. Early studies reported thermal damage from light exposure leading to heat absorption and subsequent protein denaturation. Later studies have articulated the role of photochemical damage inciting free radical formation, DNA injury, and metabolic damage.

The degree of injury in solar retinopathy is determined by the intensity and duration of light exposure. Patients with emmetropia and low hyperopia are at increased risk given the sharp focus of light on the macula. Greater pupillary size at the time of exposure increases risk of retinal damage. Aphakic and young patients are also at greater risk as age-related lens changes yield progressive protective absorption of ultraviolet (UV) light not filtered by the cornea. The dominant eye is also at greater risk given the tendency to squint in the nondominant eye when sun-gazing. Thus, although solar retinopathy is a bilateral process, the damage can be asymmetric between the two eyes.

84.1.1 Common Symptoms

Common symptoms are blurred vision (usually 20/30 to 20/100), central or paracentral scotoma, dyschromatopsia, metamorphopsia, photophobia, and headache. Events preceding the onset of solar retinopathy include eclipse viewing without protective eyewear and protracted sun-gazing. Risk factors include psychiatric predisposition (e.g., schizophrenia), hallucinogenic drug use, or select religious rituals. Occurrence among sunbathers and aviation military personnel has been reported. Patients with direct exposure to visible-light laser pointers may present with similar symptoms. Patients may not readily connect the exposure event to the subsequent symptoms.

84.1.2 Exam Findings

In the acute phase (e.g., 1–7 days after exposure), fundus examination reveals a yellowish-gray spot or spots at or near the fovea (► Fig. 84.1, ► Fig. 84.2). Approximately 2 weeks

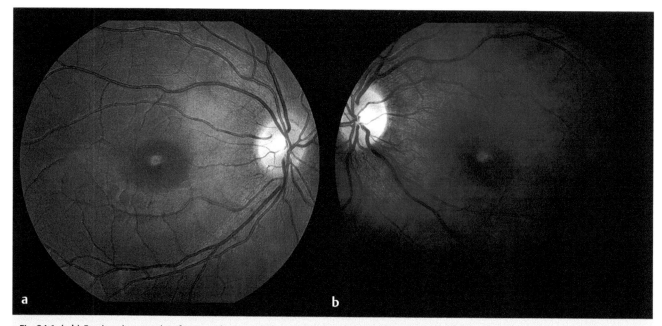

Fig. 84.1 (a,b) Fundus photographs of acute solar retinopathy with characteristic yellowish-gray foveal lesion.

after exposure, an oval-shaped outer lamellar defect is evident in the fovea, or juxtafoveal area. There may be associated pigmentary changes if the retinal pigment epithelium (RPE) is involved. In the chronic phase, pigmentary changes may abate, but cystoid or cavitary spaces remain (▶ Fig. 84.3, ▶ Fig. 84.4).

84.2 Key Diagnostic Tests and Findings

84.2.1 Optical Coherence Tomography

Optical coherence tomography may reveal outer retinal or full-thickness focal hyperreflectivity in the acute phase (▶ Fig. 84.2).

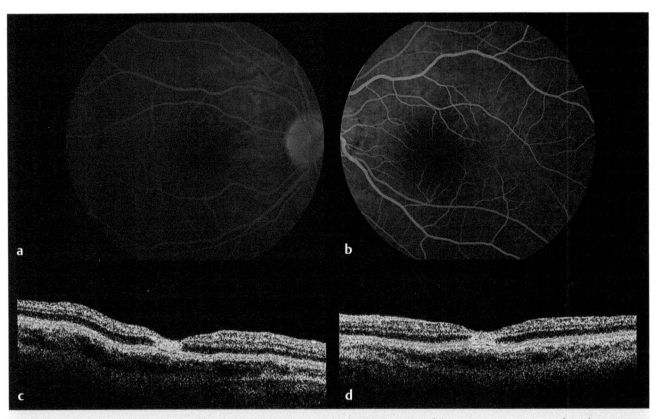

Fig. 84.2 (a–d) Fluorescein angiography (FA) and optical coherence tomography (OCT) imaging of the same acute presentation from the patient in ▶ Fig. 84.1. Late-phase FA is unremarkable bilaterally. OCT reveals full-thickness hyperreflectivity in the fovea.

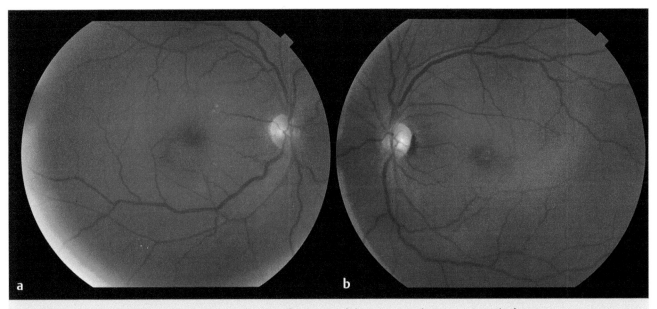

Fig. 84.3 (a,b) Fundus photography of solar retinopathy years after injury. Subtle pigmentary changes persist in the foveae.

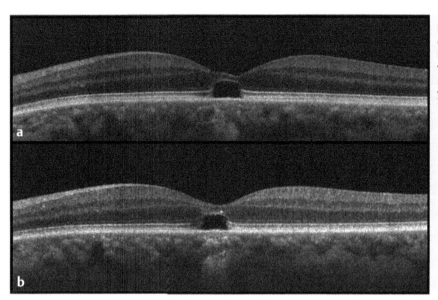

Fig. 84.4 **(a,b)** Longitudinal spectral-domain optical coherence tomography in chronic solar retinopathy demonstrating a stable foveal lesion with focal retinal pigment epithelium and outer retinal discontinuity over 6 years. **(a)** Taken 6 years prior to that shown in **(b)**.

Focal discontinuity of the ellipsoid zone may be observed at the level of the fovea with or without RPE transmission defects (▶ Fig. 84.4). Cavitary lesions involving the outer retina are possible in more severe cases. Late findings may demonstrate RPE migration into the outer retina if the RPE was damaged at initial presentation. The foveal contour typically remains preserved.

84.2.2 Fluorescein Angiography or Ultra-Widefield Fluorescein Angiography

Fluorescein angiography may demonstrate early hyperfluorescence (i.e., window defect) in cases of RPE damage; however, it is unremarkable in the absence of RPE disruption (▶ Fig. 84.1**b**).

84.2.3 Fundus Autofluorescence

Fundus autofluorescence may reveal a hypofluorescent spot surrounded by a hyper-autofluorescent ring within the context of the larger hypo-autofluorescent macula in acute phase and remaining hypo-autofluorescent spot in chronic phase (contingent on RPE attenuation and loss from thermal injury).

84.3 Management

84.3.1 Treatment Options

No proven therapy. The majority of patients have a good prognosis. Vision in most cases may return to 20/20 to 20/30 within 3 to 9 months of exposure. A small central scotoma and/or metamorphopsia may persist. Prevention, including safe eclipse viewing, is critical. The International Organization for Standardization has developed a standard, ISO 12312–2, that applies to all afocal (plano power) products intended for direct viewing of the sun.

Suggested Reading

[1] Yannuzzi LA, Fisher YL, Krueger A, Slakter J. Solar retinopathy: a photobiological and geophysical analysis. Trans Am Ophthalmol Soc. 1987; 85: 120–158
[2] Jain A, Desai RU, Charalel RA, Quiram P, Yannuzzi L, Sarraf D. Solar retinopathy: comparison of optical coherence tomography (OCT) and fluorescein angiography (FA). Retina. 2009; 29(9):1340–1345
[3] Michaelides M, Rajendram R, Marshall J, Keightley S. Eclipse retinopathy. Eye (Lond). 2001; 15(Pt 2):148–151

85 Choroidal Detachments

Ankur Mehra and Nathan Steinle

Summary

Choroidal detachments are the result of fluid collections in the suprachoroidal space between the choroid and sclera. Serous choroidal is most often due to causes that lead to hypotony of the eye and/or inflammation resulting in exudation of fluid into the space. Small serous choroidals may be asymptomatic and self-resolving. Hemorrhagic choroidal detachments are more often devastating with potentially severe vision loss. Choroidal hemorrhages most commonly occur in trauma or during/following intraocular surgery. Diagnosis is usually made based on clinical history, fundus exam, and ultrasonography. Treatment options include observation, removal of inciting factors, medical therapy (primarily anti-inflammatory such as steroids), or surgical drainage.

Keywords: choroidal detachment, choroidal effusion, expulsive hemorrhage, hypotony, sclerotomy, ultrasound

85.1 Features

A choroidal detachment is a collection of serous fluid or blood that forms in the space separating the choroid and sclera (the suprachoroidal space). Other common terms for choroidal detachments include choroidal effusion, ciliochoroidal effusion, ciliochoroidal detachment, choroidal hemorrhage, suprachoroidal hemorrhage, uveal effusion, and the colloquial term "choroidals." Though they may be asymptomatic and can resolve with time, choroidal detachments can also be severe, leading to significant and/or permanent changes in vision in the affected eye. This is particularly true of choroidal detachments either caused by or leading to suprachoroidal hemorrhages, which tend to have worse outcomes.

The most frequent cause of this combination is glaucoma surgery, particularly if overfiltration or leakage occurs postoperatively, leading to chronic hypotony. All forms of intraocular surgery, however, can be associated with hypotony and inflammation. Laser surgery has also been known to lead to choroidal detachments, including both retinal and anterior segment procedures. Advancing age, hypertension, prior vitrectomy, nanophthalmos, and certain conditions such as Sturge-Weber are associated with increased risk for developing choroidal detachments after surgeries. If choroidal hemangiomas are present with Sturge-Weber, the risk is increased even further.

Idiopathic chronic detachment, uveal effusion syndrome (UES), is rare, but is usually chronic in nature and can lead to significant visual loss. UES is a diagnosis of exclusion and tends to occur with intraocular pressures in the normal range, compared to classic choroidal detachment.

Hemorrhagic choroidal detachments, known as suprachoroidal hemorrhages, occur due to disruption of the choroidal blood vessels that pass through the space. While this may occasionally occur with no inciting factors, they are more often associated with trauma or during acute hypotony with choroidal detachments from another cause, usually intraocular surgery, which can lead to stretching and possible rupture of these blood vessels. The subsequent bleeding into the suprachoroidal space can lead to rapid development or worsening of a choroidal detachment. One dreaded potential complication of suprachoroidal hemorrhage during intraocular surgery is expulsive hemorrhage, as the rapidly enlarging hemorrhagic detachment leads to expulsion of intraocular contents out of the surgical wound (s). Previous ocular surgery is a risk factor for spontaneous suprachoroidal hemorrhages, as is a history of glaucoma, advancing age, and extremes of axial length.

85.1.1 Common Symptoms

Variable symptoms depending on the size, location, and nature of the detachment. Serous detachments are likely to be smaller; most postsurgical detachments are small, peripheral, self-limited, and often subclinical, with minimal to no pain or vision changes. Larger or more central effusions are likely to affect vision; decreased acuity or scotoma at the areas of detachment, or through refractive changes due to pressure and displacement of the lens and iris. Compared to serous detachments, hemorrhagic detachments most often present with acute, severe pain in the affected eye; more likely to cause vision changes.

85.1.2 Exam Findings

Choroidal detachments are most often noted during physical exam, but appearance and ease of visualization may vary. They usually appear as smooth, orange, or light brown, dome-shaped elevations. If large, the elevations may have a lobulated appearance, due to the fibrous attachments between the choroid and the vortex veins as they pass through the sclera. If the detachments are large, the lobes may come into appositional contact with each other ("kissing choroidals"). In severe cases, they may even come into contact with the posterior surface of the lens. With the chronic, relapsing-remitting choroidal detachments of UES, diffuse pigmented spots can develop, often described as "leopard skin" spots. On slit lamp examination, detachments may cause narrowing of the peripheral anterior chamber and angles, shallowing of the entire anterior chamber, and/or anterior rotation of the ciliary body. Acute, rapidly progressing choroidal detachments during intraocular surgery at risk of leading to expulsive hemorrhage may first present as loss of the red reflex during surgery.

85.2 Key Diagnostic Tests and Findings

85.2.1 Optical Coherence Tomography

When exam is limited, optical coherence tomography may also be useful in differentiating choroidal detachment from other causes of postoperative posterior pole elevation (e.g., retinal detachment).

85.2.2 Ultrasonography

B-scan ultrasonography of the eye can be valuable in identifying and differentiating choroidal detachments (▶ Table 85.1), may locate detachments not visible or noted on the clinical exam, and can differentiate between a hemorrhagic choroidal detachment (in which the suprachoroidal space is filled with hyperechoic blood) and a serous choroidal detachment (in which the suprachoroidal space is filled with hypoechoic transudate). Ultrasonography can be critical for preoperative planning for choroidal drainage.

85.3 Critical Work-up

Differentiate choroidal detachments from other similarly presenting conditions, particularly retinal detachments (▶ Table 85.1). Compared to retinal detachments, choroidal detachments have a more fixed, lobulated, or hourglass appearance on ultrasound. Also common on the differential are choroidal masses, but these typically present less acutely.

Table 85.1 Acoustic criteria for differentiating choroidal detachment and retinal detachment

Ultrasound technique	Choroidal detachment	Retinal detachment
Topographic	Smooth, dome, or flat shaped. Inserts at the ciliary body with no disc insertion	Corrugated, open, or closed funnel with disc insertion, inserts at the ora. Chronic retinal detachments may have associated cysts
Kinetic	Mild to none	Moderate to none

85.4 Management

85.4.1 Treatment Options

Observation

The majority of choroidal detachments are self-limited and resolve slowly with time; observe smaller, nonvisually significant detachments, particularly if any underlying or contributing factors have been alleviated. Addressing the inciting cause (e.g., hypotony) is critical.

Medication

If the choroidal detachments are thought to be medication related, those medications can be decreased or halted as tolerated in order to promote resolution. Topical or oral steroid treatments are also often used to treat underlying inflammation. Cycloplegic agents are also often started in order to counteract the anterior rotation of the ciliary body, as well as deepen the anterior chamber. There may occasionally be elevations of intraocular pressure as the detachment develops, which may necessitate temporary use of medications to lower ocular pressure instead.

Surgical Treatment

In cases of large choroidal detachments and "kissing choroidals," surgical drainage is often indicated. For hemorrhagic detachments, it is often necessary to wait 7 to 14 days to allow the blood to liquefy, which is usually evaluated with ultrasonography. While exact techniques can differ, surgical drainage usually involves creation of one or more sclerotomies with maintenance of the anterior chamber during the surgery to express fluid/hemorrhage through the sclerotomies posteriorly. The sclerotomies may be left open following the surgery for continuing drainage. Vitrectomy and/or gas exchange may also be indicated, depending on the exact circumstances of the case.

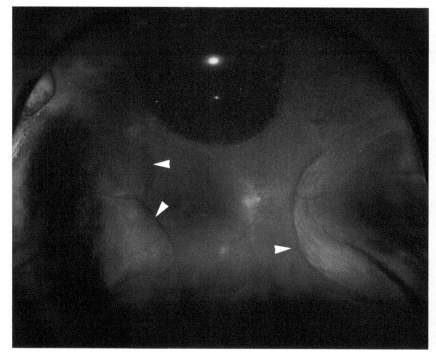

Fig. 85.1 Ultra-widefield fundus photography of choroidal detachments (*arrowheads*) following vitrectomy surgery.

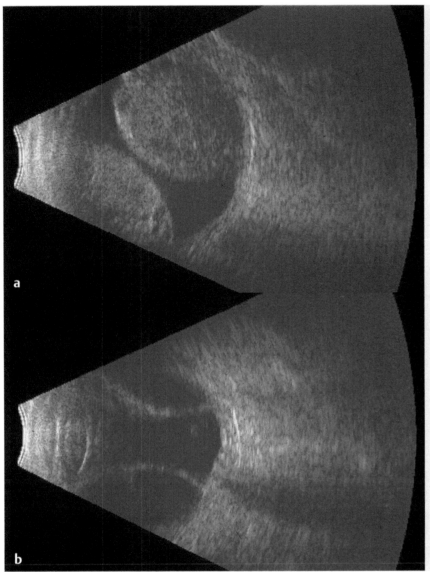

Fig. 85.2 (a,b) B-scan ultrasonography demonstrating choroidal detachment. **(a)** shows a hemorrhagic choroidal detachment (with the suprachoroidal space filed with hyperechoic blood) while **(b)** shows a serous choroidal detachment (in which the suprachoroidal space is filled with hypoechoic transudate).

Prevention

Steps that may help prevent choroidal detachment development include the decreased use of pressure-reducing medications peri- and postoperatively, avoidance of overfiltration or leak, cessation of anticoagulants in the perioperative period, and judicious use of antimetabolites.

85.4.2 Follow-up

Close monitoring in the acute period around the time of choroidal development is necessary. Serial ultrasounds or serial wide-field photography (if the media is clear) can be helpful in monitoring the slow resolution process (▶ Fig. 85.1, ▶ Fig. 85.2).

Suggested Reading

[1] Reddy AC, Salim S. Diagnosis and management of choroidal effusions. Eyenet 2012:47–49

[2] Kahook MY, Noecker RJ. Why do choroidals form, and how do you treat them? Glaucoma Today 2007:36–38

[3] Elagouz M, Stanescu-Segall D, Jackson TL. Uveal effusion syndrome. Surv Ophthalmol. 2010; 55(2):134–145

[4] Bakir B, Pasquale LR. Causes and treatment of choroidal effusion after glaucoma surgery. Semin Ophthalmol. 2014; 29(5–6):409–413

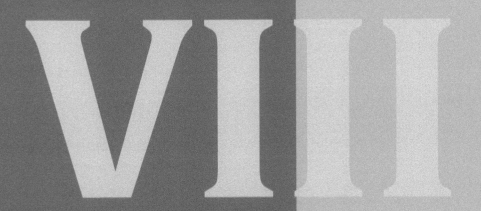

86 Hydroxychloroquine Retinopathy

Vishal S. Parikh and Rishi P. Singh

Summary

Hydroxychloroquine (HCQ) retinopathy can result in permanent vision loss. It is most influenced by daily dose, length of use, and cumulative dose over time. In early stages of HCQ retinopathy, patients are usually asymptomatic with preservation of visual acuity. A baseline HCQ retinopathy screening followed by ongoing regular screening with spectral-domain optical coherence tomography (OCT) and visual field testing is important. No diet or medical therapy has proven effective at preventing, treating, or reducing risk from HCQ retinopathy other than cessation of HCQ, and cessation of HCQ does not necessarily prevent progression of HCQ retinopathy.

Keywords: hydroxychloroquine, spectral-domain optical coherence tomography, vision loss

86.1 Features

86.1.1 Common Symptoms

Patients are often asymptomatic when hydroxychloroquine (HCQ) retinopathy is found during screening given the initial decrease in vision is paracentral to fixation. Sometimes patients may notice changes in vision at near instead of at distance given the decrease in paracentral visual field.

Symptomatic loss of vision usually presents when severe retinal damage from HCQ retinopathy has already occurred and the paracentral field loss has progressed to a central scotoma in severe disease. Photopsia, metamorphopsia, reduced color vision, and peripheral field loss are reported to be found in later stages of the disease.

86.1.2 Exam Findings

Retinal pigment epithelium (RPE) stippling and loss of the foveal reflex in the macula in early disease.

Bull's eye maculopathy with parafoveal RPE depigmentation in late disease (▶ Fig. 86.1).

86.2 Key Diagnostic Tests and Findings

86.2.1 Optical Coherence Tomography

Early

Initially with thinning of inner retinal layers followed by loss of parafoveal photoreceptor inner segment/outer segment junction leading to parafoveal thinning of outer nuclear layer leading to outer displacement of inner retinal structures toward RPE resulting in the "flying saucer sign" on spectral-domain optical coherence tomography (SD-OCT; ▶ Fig. 86.2).

Late

Atrophy of outer retinal layers with parafoveal RPE irregularities on SD-OCT (▶ Fig. 86.2). *En face* visualization of outer retinal loss may facilitate visualization of subtle annular/parafoveal loss. Rarely, intraretinal fluid may be present.

86.2.2 Fundus Autofluorescence

Early

Parafoveal ring of increased autofluorescence from photoreceptor loss (▶ Fig. 86.3).

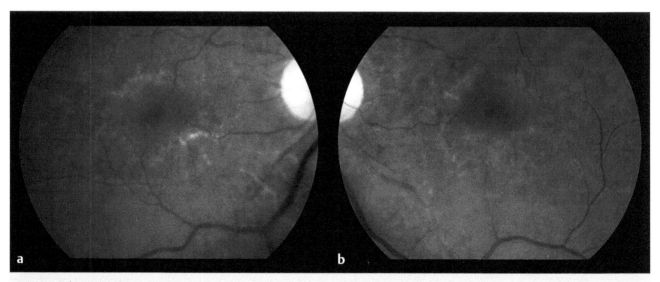

Fig. 86.1 (a,b) Fundus photos with bilateral bull's eye maculopathy with parafoveal depigmentation of the retinal pigment epithelium in hydroxychloroquine toxicity.

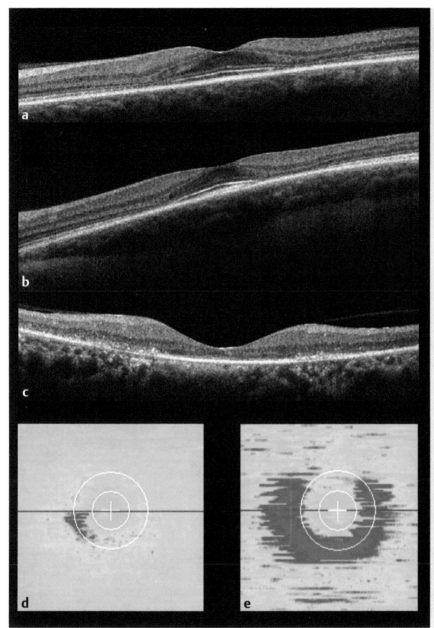

Fig. 86.2 Progression of optical coherence tomography (OCT) findings in hydroxychloroquine toxicity. **(a)** OCT showing loss of parafoveal photoreceptor inner segment/outer segment junction (i.e., ellipsoid zone [EZ]). **(b)** The "flying saucer sign" with parafoveal thinning of outer nuclear layer leading to outer displacement of inner retinal structures toward retinal pigment epithelium (RPE). **(c)** Advanced disease demonstrating loss/atrophy of outer retinal layers with parafoveal RPE irregularities. EZ-RPE thickness maps demonstrating **(d)** *en face* visualization of early atrophy parafoveal EZ loss and **(e)** bull's eye configuration of EZ-RPE thinning; courtesy of Justis P. Ehlers.

Late

Generalized loss of pigment epithelium manifested as absent autofluorescence.

86.2.3 Fluorescein Angiography or Ultra-Widefield Fluorescein Angiography

In more advanced cases, window defect may be present and may occasionally have macular edema that has minimal leakage (▶ Fig. 86.4).

86.2.4 Humphrey Visual Field 10–2 White Stimulus

Paracentral scotomas (▶ Fig. 86.5).

86.3 Critical Work-up

Frequency for HCQ retinopathy screening includes a baseline screening within the first year of HCQ use followed by annual screening after 5 years of HCQ use with SD-OCT and Humphrey visual field with a 10–2 white stimulus for non-Asian patients and 24–2 for Asian patients. Fundus autofluorescence or multifocal electroretinogram can be considered for adjunct testing. Annual screening upon starting HCQ is recommended if patients have major risk factors such as HCQ daily dosage of greater than 5.0 mg/kg real weight, renal disease, tamoxifen use, or concurrent macular disease that could confound screening.

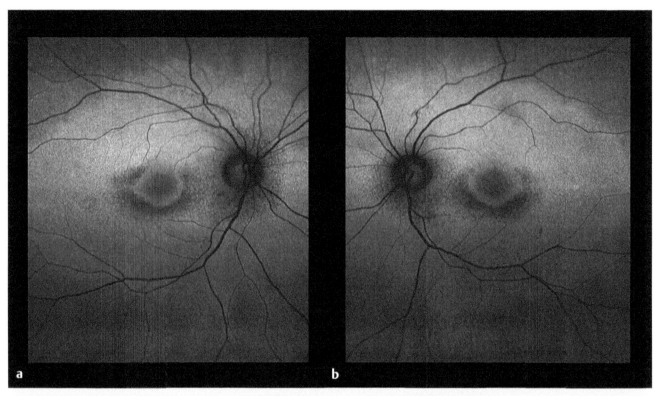

Fig. 86.3 (a,b) Fundus autofluorescence with bilateral parafoveal ring of hyper-autofluorescence surrounded by a ring of hypo-autofluorescence.

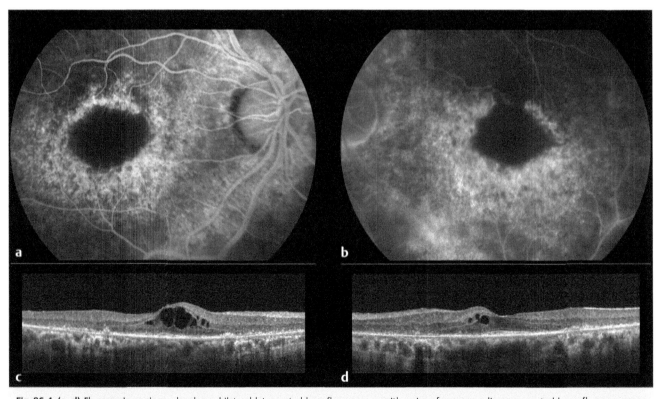

Fig. 86.4 (a–d) Fluorescein angiography shows bilateral late central hypofluorescence with a rim of nonexpanding paracentral hyperfluorescence consistent with window defect corresponding with optical coherence tomography findings of bilateral parafoveal outer retinal atrophy and retinal pigment epithelium disruption. Nonleaking cystoid macular edema is present.

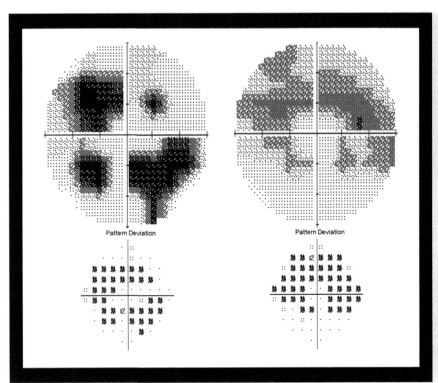

Fig. 86.5 Humphrey visual field 10–2 with white stimulus showing bilateral parafoveal scotomas.

86.4 Management

86.4.1 Treatment Options

No diet or medical therapy has proven effective at preventing, treating, or reducing risk from HCQ retinopathy other than cessation of HCQ. Once HCQ retinopathy is detected, a discussion between the examining ophthalmologist and prescribing rheumatologist should take place to discuss the risk and benefits of discontinuing HCQ so that the patient receives the best care possible.

86.4.2 Follow-up

Cessation of HCQ does not necessarily prevent progression of HCQ retinopathy. Risk of progression is minimal with early detection. However, if bull's eye maculopathy is present, progression of HCQ retinopathy could continue for a couple of years after cessation before plateauing.

Suggested Reading

[1] Ding HJ, Denniston AK, Rao VK, Gordon C. Hydroxychloroquine-related retinal toxicity. Rheumatology (Oxford). 2016; 55(6):957–967

[2] Yusuf IH, Sharma S, Luqmani R, Downes SM. Hydroxychloroquine retinopathy. Eye (Lond). 2017; 31(6):828–845

[3] Marmor MF, Kellner U, Lai TY, Melles RB, Mieler WF, American Academy of Ophthalmology. Recommendations on screening for chloroquine and hydroxychloroquine retinopathy (2016 revision). Ophthalmology. 2016; 123(6):1386–1394

[4] Parikh VS, Modi YS, Au A, et al. Nonleaking cystoid macular edema as a presentation of hydroxychloroquine retinal toxicity. Ophthalmology. 2016; 123(3):664–666

87 Ocriplasmin Retinopathy

Merina Thomas and Mark W. Johnson

Summary

Ocriplasmin is a recombinant truncated form of plasmin that is FDA-approved for the treatment of symptomatic vitreomacular adhesion. The potential advantages of a vitreolytic agent like ocriplasmin include the induction of posterior vitreous detachment with less vitreoschisis, avoidance of surgical risk, and ease of use in clinic. However, acute visual symptoms after intravitreal ocriplasmin injection have included acute reduction in visual acuity, atypical photopsias, nyctalopia, dyschromatopsia, and visual field loss. Most commonly, these are transient and self-limiting, but in a small subset of eyes there may be permanent sequelae. Examination findings may include anisocoria, relative afferent pupillary defect, retinal vessel attenuation, macular hole enlargement, macular detachment, and even diffuse pigmentary changes in severe cases. The key diagnostic tests for ocriplasmin retinopathy are spectral-domain optical coherence tomography (SD-OCT) and electroretinography (ERG). SD-OCT reveals outer retinal disruption/thinning, most commonly involving the ellipsoid and interdigitation zones, and variable amounts of subretinal fluid. ERG may reveal panretinal dysfunction, with reduced responses in every parameter, and affecting rods more than cones. In rare severe cases, fundus autofluorescence photography may show diffuse alterations. There are currently no known treatment options for ocriplasmin retinopathy. Although the acute symptoms and signs spontaneously resolve in most patients, long-term retinal dysfunction is apparent in a minority, and further studies are needed to evaluate the frequency and severity of chronic retinal damage from ocriplasmin.

Keywords: macular hole, ocriplasmin, vitreomacular adhesion, vitreomacular traction, vitreolysis

87.1 Features

Ocriplasmin is a recombinant truncated form of plasmin approved by the FDA in 2012 for the treatment of symptomatic vitreomacular adhesion. The enzyme has nonspecific proteolytic activity against multiple proteins, including laminin and fibronectin which are constituents of vitreous. Phase 3 randomized clinical trials showed that an intravitreal injection of ocriplasmin resolved vitreomacular adhesion in 26.5% of patients versus 10.1% of controls injected with placebo. The potential advantages of ocriplasmin compared with vitrectomy include the ease of a simple office-based procedure, avoidance of surgical risk, and faster visual and procedure-related recovery. Following more widespread use, it is clear that ocriplasmin may be associated with acute transient panretinal dysfunction in a significant portion of treated eyes. While the retinal alterations are reversible in the majority of eyes, retinal dysfunction and visual compromise persist indefinitely in a small minority of eyes.

Although the intended targets for ocriplasmin are laminin and fibronectin at the vitreoretinal interface, laminin is also found in many other ocular structures, including the zonules and multiple layers of the retina. Because the adverse effects of ocriplasmin correlate well with the distribution of laminin within the eye, enzymatic degradation of laminin is a plausible hypothesis for the primary pathogenic mechanism of ocriplasmin retinopathy. However, ocriplasmin is a nonspecific protease and cleavage of more than one protein may be responsible for its various potential transient adverse effects in the eye.

87.1.1 Common Symptoms

Acute ocriplasmin retinopathy symptoms vary; patients may have atypical photopsias not related to PVD formation (e.g., sparkles, continuous kaleidoscopic lines, white floaters), dyschromatopsias (e.g., black and white or "negative" vision, yellow tint), nyctalopia, acute reduction in visual acuity (rarely to as low as light perception), fragmented or pixilated vision, and/or visual field defect.

87.1.2 Exam Findings

Signs of acute ocriplasmin retinopathy include relative afferent pupillary defect, anisocoria, lens subluxation or phacodonesis, retinal vessel attenuation, macular hole enlargement, macular detachment, and rarely diffuse fundus pigmentary changes (▶ Fig. 87.1, ▶ Fig. 87.2).

87.2 Key Diagnostic Tests and Findings

87.2.1 Optical Coherence Tomography (OCT)

Spectral Domain OCT (SD-OCT) typically shows disruption of the outer retina, most commonly the ellipsoid zone (EZ) and interdigitization zone (▶ Fig. 87.1). Ocriplasmin-associated structural changes in the outer retina have been seen in 40–50% of treated eyes and are usually accompanied by acute reduction of visual acuity and other visual symptoms. Varying amounts of subretinal fluid are also commonly seen after ocriplasmin treatment (▶ Fig. 87.2). These changes typically occur rapidly after initial treatment and improve/resolve over 4–12 weeks following injection.

87.2.2 Fundus Autofluorescence

In rare severe cases, fundus autofluorescence photography may show diffuse alterations.

87.2.3 Electroretinography

Affected eyes have varying degrees of panretinal dysfunction, sometimes resulting in flat ERG tracings. ERG abnormalities are seen in 33 to 69% of tested eyes. B-wave amplitudes may be

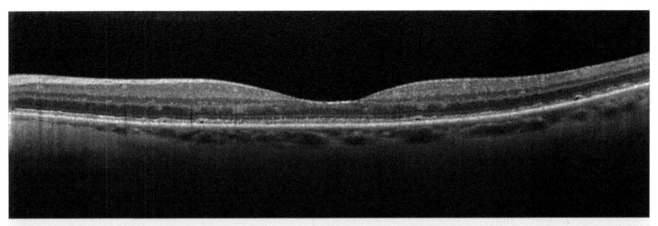

Fig. 87.1 Ocriplasmin retinopathy. Horizontal spectral domain optical coherence tomography imaging of the left eye 1 month after ocriplasmin injection. The patient complained bitterly of dyschromatopsia and poor quality vision in the left eye. There is irregular attenuation of the outer retinal signals, including the external limiting membrane, ellipsoid layer, and interdigitation zone. Note also the multifocal microblebs of subretinal fluid, suggesting reduced adhesion between the photoreceptors and retinal pigment epithelium.

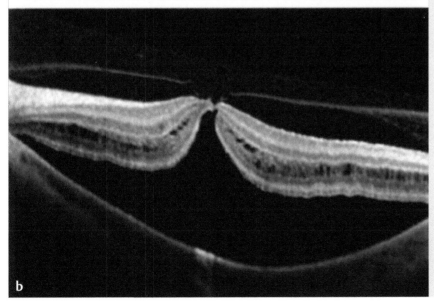
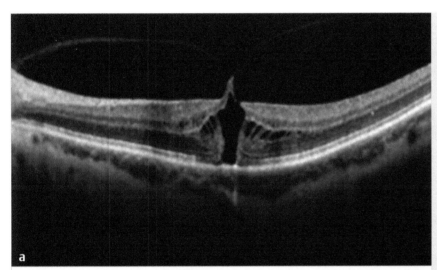

Fig. 87.2 Macular detachment. Spectral domain optical coherence tomography **(a)** before and **(b)** after ocriplasmin injection. Before treatment, there is vitreomacular traction and a likely small full-thickness macular hole. Following treatment, there is persistent vitreomacular adhesion with extensive macular detachment and attenuation of the ellipsoid layer. (Courtesy of David Saperstein, MD.)

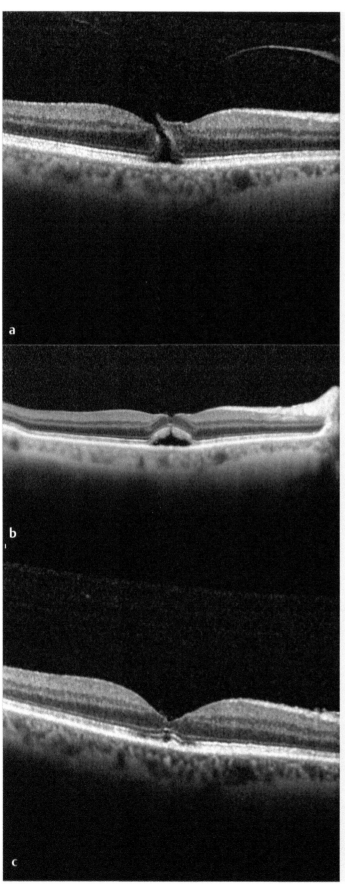

Fig. 87.3 Longitudinal optical coherence tomography (OCT) imaging in ocriplasmin retinopathy. **(a)** Spectral-domain OCT (SD-OCT) before ocriplasmin injection shows a small full-thickness macular hole with vitreomacular traction to the inner layer flap. **(b)** Three months after ocriplasmin injection, SD-OCT demonstrates vitreomacular traction release and hole closure, but also demonstrates new and persisting subretinal fluid with mild attenuation of the outer retinal signals elsewhere in the macula. **(c)** Ten months after ocriplasmin injection, SD-OCT demonstrates resolution of the subretinal fluid but persistent attenuation of the ellipsoid layer in the subfoveal area with a small amount of subfoveal pseudo-vitelliform material.

reduced more than A-wave amplitudes, suggesting decreased activity in both photoreceptor and bipolar cells, and rod function is typically more affected than cone function.

87.3 Management

87.3.1 Treatment Options

There are currently no known treatment options for ocriplasmin retinopathy. Most cases have been reported to be transient and at least partially reversible, usually within 2 to 3 months of the injection. Even cases of profound visual acuity and visual field loss have been reported to resolve completely over 4 to 36 months. Rare reports have demonstrated visual acuity loss, nyctalopia, SD-OCT, and ERG changes that persisted beyond 6 months and up to 2 years, suggesting potential permanent retinal damage in a minority of eyes (▶ Fig. 87.3). Further studies

are needed to evaluate the effect of ocriplasmin on long-term visual function.

Suggested Reading

[1] Stalmans P, Benz MS, Gandorfer A, et al. MIVI-TRUST Study Group. Enzymatic vitreolysis with ocriplasmin for vitreomacular traction and macular holes. N Engl J Med. 2012; 367(7):606–615

[2] Hahn P, Chung MM, Flynn HW, Jr, et al. Safety profile of ocriplasmin for symptomatic vitreomacular adhesion: a comprehensive analysis of premarketing and postmarketing experiences. Retina. 2015; 35(6):1128–1134

[3] Fahim AT, Khan NW, Johnson MW. Acute panretinal structural and functional abnormalities after intravitreous ocriplasmin injection. JAMA Ophthalmol. 2014; 132(4):484–486

[4] Itoh Y, Kaiser PK, Singh RP, Srivastava SK, Ehlers JP. Assessment of retinal alterations after intravitreal ocriplasmin with spectral-domain optical coherence tomography. Ophthalmology. 2014; 121(12):2506–2507.e2

[5] Johnson MW, Fahim AT, Rao RC. Acute ocriplasmin retinopathy. Retina. 2015; 35(6):1055–1058

88 Hemorrhagic Occlusive Retinal Vasculitis Secondary to Drug Exposure

Michael N. Cohen and Andre J. Witkin

Summary

Since 2014, there have been a number of reports describing hemorrhagic occlusive retinal vasculitis (HORV), whose only common link was the use of intracameral vancomycin during an otherwise routine cataract surgery. Frustratingly, the presentation of this disease often had a delayed onset, and the U.S. FDA now suggests avoiding intracameral vancomycin for endophthalmitis prophylaxis during cataract surgery. Optical coherence tomography and fluorescein angiography are useful imaging modalities. Work-up is essential to differentiate HORV from other sight-threatening conditions including acute postoperative endophthalmitis, toxic anterior segment syndrome, viral retinitis, and central retinal vein occlusion.

Keywords: endophthalmitis, hemorrhagic occlusive retinal vasculitis, vancomycin

88.1 Features

After the release of a large, randomized, multicentered, prospective trial by the European Society of Cataract and Refractive Surgeons, which showed a fivefold decrease in the rates of postoperative endophthalmitis after prophylactic intracameral cefuroxime injection, there has been a steady increase in the number of ophthalmologists who routinely use prophylactic intracameral antibiotics after cataract surgery. Up until recently, the most common choice in the United States has been vancomycin, selected by 52% of providers of those who use intracameral antibiotics. Its low cost, broad coverage, ease of availability, and previously reported safety profile all contributed to its popularity. However, since 2014, there have been a number of reports describing a rare and devastating retinal condition, termed "hemorrhagic occlusive retinal vasculitis (HORV)," whose only common link was the use of intracameral vancomycin during an otherwise routine cataract surgery. Frustratingly, the presentation of this disease often had a delayed onset. Therefore, in the most devastating cases of HORV, individuals did not develop any symptoms until both eyes had already undergone bilateral sequential cataract surgery, and some of these patients went on to develop bilateral severe visual loss. Because of the severity of this disease, the U.S. FDA now suggests avoiding intracameral vancomycin for endophthalmitis prophylaxis during cataract surgery.

Due in part to the delated presentation, the underlying pathophysiology of HORV is theorized to be immune-mediated, as opposed to a direct toxic effect of vancomycin. The time course of presentation and appearance of the disease is consistent with a type III hypersensitivity reaction, which has a peak onset of 1 to 2 weeks after initial antigen introduction, and primarily affects the postcapillary venules. Type III hypersensitivity responses are driven by antigen–antibody complex deposition within the walls of the blood vessels, leading to activation of macrophages, complement, and other inflammatory mediators. HORV may be similar to a known rare type III hypersensitivity reaction to vancomycin that occurs in the skin: leukocytoclastic vasculitis. However, a recent clinical–pathologic correlation suggested that the inflammatory response in this disease was a T-cell–mediated response which primarily affects the choroid, rather than an antibody-mediated response that affects the retina, and future studies may shed light on the specific pathogenesis of this disease.

88.1.1 Common Symptoms

Symptoms typically begin 1 to 21 days (mean = 8 days) postoperatively with painless peripheral scotomas or blurred vision; patients with less severe findings may be asymptomatic.

88.1.2 Examination Findings

Typical findings include mild to moderate anterior chamber reaction without a hypopyon, and mild to moderate vitreous inflammation, with a relatively clear view to the posterior pole (which may help distinguish this disease from postoperative endophthalmitis). Most notably, patients often have large, sectoral areas of retinal vascular occlusion, with intraretinal hemorrhages localized to areas of retinal vascular occlusion. Hemorrhages are usually large or confluent, but occasionally appear as smaller dot hemorrhages (▶ Fig. 88.1, ▶ Fig. 88.2). Rarely, peripheral retinal vascular occlusion without retinal hemorrhage has been seen. Venules may be sheathed and surrounded by particularly dense clusters of hemorrhages. The peripheral retina appears to be nearly always involved, but severe cases may also demonstrate macular ischemia and whitening.

88.2 Key Diagnostic Tests and Findings

88.2.1 Optical Coherence Tomography

If the macula is involved, OCT often shows thickening and hyperreflectivity of the inner retinal layers, consistent with inner retinal ischemia (▶ Fig. 88.1, ▶ Fig. 88.2). Although present in some cases, cystoid macular edema was not common. OCT can be normal in cases where only the peripheral retina is involved.

88.2.2 Fluorescein Angiography or Ultra-Widefield Fluorescein Angiography

Can be useful in highlighting the full extent of retinal vascular compromise/occlusion, which frequently coincides with sectoral areas of retinal hemorrhages. There may be hyperfluorescence of

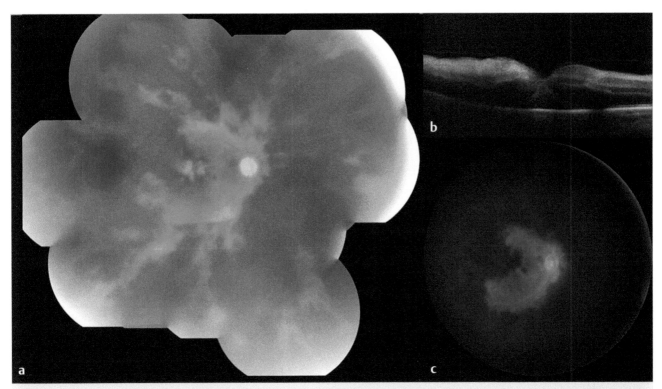

Fig. 88.1 Hemorrhagic occlusive retinal vasculitis (HORV) secondary to drug exposure. **(a)** Color mosaic photograph of the right eye of a patient with HORV. The disease developed 1 week after otherwise uncomplicated cataract surgery, which was performed using intracameral vancomycin 1 mg/ 0.1 mL. The right eye surgery was performed first, followed by the left eye surgery 1 week later. The photo demonstrates extensive confluent retinal hemorrhages in regions of retinal nonperfusion, as well as macular whitening. **(b)** Optical coherence tomography of the macula demonstrates inner retinal thickening and hyperreflectivity (consistent with macular ischemia), as well as a small pocket of subfoveal fluid. **(c)** Widefield fluorescein angiography demonstrates extensive peripheral retinal nonperfusion which co-localize with areas of retinal hemorrhage.

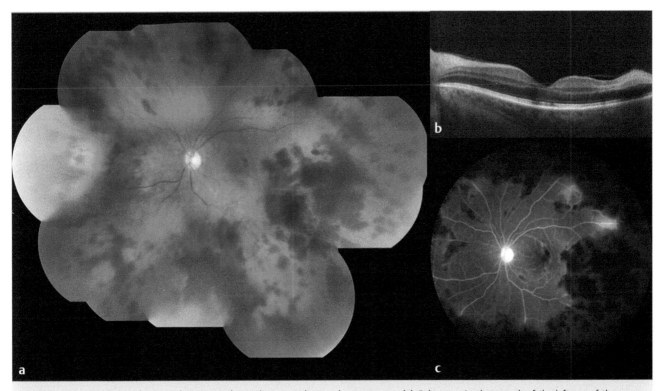

Fig. 88.2 Sequential hemorrhagic occlusive retinal vasculitis secondary to drug exposure. **(a)** Color mosaic photograph of the left eye of the same patient as in ▶ Fig. 88.1. The disease developed 1 week after otherwise uncomplicated cataract surgery, which was performed using intracameral vancomycin 1 mg/0.1 mL. The left eye surgery was performed 1 week after the right eye surgery. The photo demonstrates extensive confluent retinal hemorrhages in regions of retinal nonperfusion. **(b)** Optical coherence tomography of the macula demonstrates some foci of inner retinal thinning (consistent with previous macular ischemia). **(c)** Widefield fluorescein angiography demonstrates extensive peripheral retinal nonperfusion which co-localize with areas of retinal hemorrhage. Also evident are hyperfluorescence of the optic disc, as well as staining of some of the retinal venules.

the optic nerve and vascular staining, particularly of the retinal venules.

88.3 Critical Work-up

All of the known cases of HORV received intraocular vancomycin prior to presentation (usually 1 mg/0.1 mL); therefore, a key part of the history is determining whether the patient received this particular medication prior to presentation. It is essential to differentiate HORV from other sight-threatening conditions including acute postoperative endophthalmitis, toxic anterior segment syndrome (TASS), viral retinitis, and central retinal vein occlusion. TASS features that help distinguish it include acute onset, severe inflammation of the anterior segment, corneal edema, and lack of posterior findings. Key distinguishing features of infectious endophthalmitis include lack of pain, lack of anterior segment and vitreous inflammation, and characteristic sectoral retinal hemorrhages in regions of vascular occlusion and with a predilection to clustering along venules. It is important to distinguish HORV from postoperative endophthalmitis, as a repeat bolus of intravitreal vancomycin for treatment of presumed endophthalmitis has been associated with worse outcomes in eyes with HORV. Most commonly, viral retinitis presents as acute retinal necrosis (ARN), secondary to a virus in the Herpesviridae family (herpes simplex virus, varicella zoster virus). Distinguishing features of ARN are rapid, progressing segments of retinal whitening with significant vitreous inflammation. Although cytomegalovirus retinitis can present with marked intraretinal hemorrhages when contrasted to ARN, it is characteristically slow to progress and almost always found in the immunosuppressed. There is also no association of viral retinitis with ocular surgery. However, if there are characteristic features of viral retinitis, a work-up for this etiology should be considered.

88.4 Management

The prevention of this disease must be emphasized. If intracameral antibiotics are desired by the surgeon, antibiotics other than vancomycin (such as moxifloxacin or cefuroxime) should be considered. If intracameral vancomycin is used, consider waiting for 2 to 3 weeks before operating on the fellow eye and performing a dilated fundus examination to ensure there are no unexpected retinal findings that would suggest HORV.

88.4.1 Treatment Options

If HORV occurs, there seems to be two phases to the disease. The initial phase involves a dramatic inflammatory response. This is often followed by a rapidly progressive neovascular proliferative response. Over 50% of eyes have been reported to develop neovascular glaucoma, which often occurred 1 to 2 months after the disease onset.

Treatment for the initial inflammatory response includes aggressive topical and systemic corticosteroids with possible addition of intraocular or periocular corticosteroids. To prevent neovascular glaucoma, anti-vascular endothelial growth factor therapy and panretinal photocoagulation (applied to the areas of ischemia) in the subacute phase may be prudent.

88.4.2 Follow-up

Patients should be followed up closely in the initial phase to assure that inflammation improves and neovascular glaucoma is avoided. Visual outcomes in these cases have been quite poor, including over 20% with no light perception vision and over 60% with 20/200 or worse.

Suggested Reading

[1] Braga-Mele R, Chang DF, Henderson BA, Mamalis N, Talley-Rostov A, Vasavada A, ASCRS Clinical Cataract Committee. Intracameral antibiotics: safety, efficacy, and preparation. J Cataract Refract Surg. 2014; 40(12):2134–2142

[2] Witkin AJ, Shah AR, Engstrom RE, et al. Postoperative hemorrhagic occlusive retinal vasculitis: expanding the clinical spectrum and possible association with vancomycin. Ophthalmology. 2015; 122(7):1438–1451

[3] Witkin AJ, Chang DF, Jumper JM, et al. Vancomycin-associated hemorrhagic occlusive retinal vasculitis: clinical characteristics of 36 eyes. Ophthalmology. 2017; 124(5):583–595

[4] A case of hemorrhagic occlusive retinal vasculitis (HORV) following intraocular injections of a compounded triamcinolone, moxifloxacin, and vancomycin formulation. October 3, 2017. Available at: https://www.fda.gov/Drugs/GuidanceComplianceRegulatoryInformation/PharmacyCompounding/ucm578514.htm. Accessed April 12, 2019

[5] Todorich B. New insights in vancomycin-associated hemorrhagic occlusive retinal vasculopathy (HORV). Retina Society Annual Meeting. Boston MA. October 5, 2017

89 Talc Retinopathy

Sai Chavala

Summary

Talc (magnesium silicate) serves as a common vehicle for many intravenous medications used for recreational use such as heroin, codeine, meperidine, pentazocine, methadone, and methylphenidate hydrochloride (Ritalin). Intravenous injection of talc embolizes to the lung, leading to pulmonary hypertension. Eventually, this leads to the development of collateral vessels, which allows the talc to enter into the systemic circulation. Optical coherence tomography and fluorescein angiography may be helpful diagnostic tests. Panretinal photocoagulation and anti-vascular endothelial growth factor are treatment options for retinal neovascularization along with cessation of intravenous drug use.

Keywords: neovascularization, ischemia, talc emboli

89.1 Features

Talc (magnesium silicate) serves as a common vehicle for many intravenous medications used for recreational use such as heroin, codeine, meperidine, pentazocine, methadone, and methylphenidate hydrochloride (Ritalin). Intravenous injection of talc embolizes to the lung, leading to pulmonary hypertension. Eventually, this leads to the development of collateral vessels, which allows the talc to enter into the systemic circulation.

89.1.1 Common Symptoms

Blurry vision, floaters, asymptomatic.

89.1.2 Exam Findings

Glistening yellow crystals in the small arterioles of the posterior pole; talc emboli possible in the nerve fiber layer capillaries and choriocapillaris; microaneurysmal dots and venous loops have been reported.

89.2 Key Diagnostic Tests and Findings

89.2.1 Optical Coherence Tomography

Multiple hyperreflective dots and thinning of the inner retinal layers (▶ Fig. 89.1).

89.2.2 Fluorescein Angiography or Ultra-Widefield Fluorescein Angiography

Macular ischemia, irregular foveal avascular zone (FAZ), and vascular leakage. Retinal neovascularization may occur at the borders of nonperfusion and perfusion zones.

89.2.3 Optical Coherence Tomography Angiography

Emerging technology that may demonstrate focal flow voids, areas of retinal ischemia, and FAZ enlargement.

89.3 Critical Work-up

Obtain history of intravenous drug use. Differential diagnoses to consider include Bietti crystalline corneal dystrophy, oxalosis, cystinosis, and drusen.

89.4 Management

89.4.1 Treatment Options

Panretinal photocoagulation or anti-vascular endothelial growth factor may be necessary to treat retinal neovascularization. Intravenous drug use should be ceased.

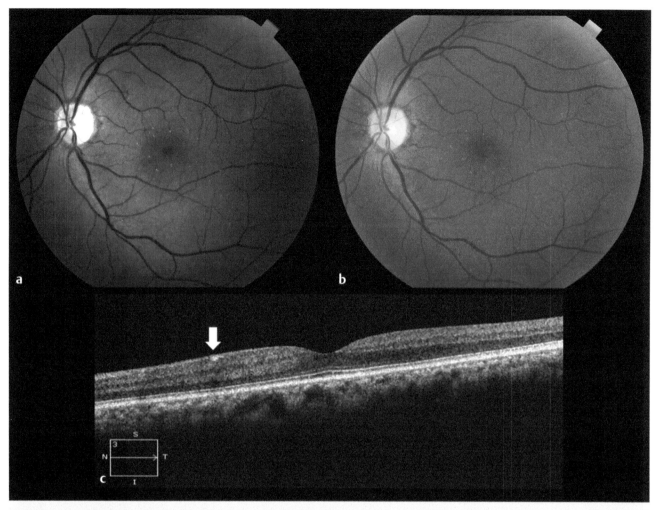

Fig. 89.1 Talc retinopathy. **(a)** Red free and **(b)** color fundus photograph demonstrate punctate crystals/dots in the macula in a patient with history of cocaine use and intravenous methylphenidate hydrochloride (Ritalin) use. **(c)** Optical coherence tomography confirms localization of punctate dots to the inner retina. (Images courtesy of Pouya Dayani.)

89.4.2 Follow-up

Regular follow-up is recommended to assess for retinal ischemia and development of neovascularization.

Suggested Reading

[1] McLane NJ, Carroll DM. Ocular manifestations of drug abuse. Surv Ophthalmol. 1986; 30(5):298–313
[2] Shah VA, Cassell M, Poulose A, Sabates NR. Talc retinopathy. Ophthalmology. 2008; 115(4):755–755.e2

90 Tamoxifen Retinopathy

Daniel G. Cherfan and Justis P. Ehlers

Summary

Tamoxifen is a commonly used antiestrogen oral medication that has been used in the management of breast cancer since the 1970s. This medication is particularly effective as an adjuvant therapy in postsurgical advanced estrogen-receptor positive breast cancer. Though this medication is relatively well tolerated, it has rarely been known to cause ocular toxicity including a crystalline retinopathy with long-term use. Tamoxifen ocular toxicity was initially attributed to the higher dosing of this agent that ranged from 60 to 100 mg/day with an accumulative dosing of greater than 100 g over a period of 12 months. More recently, there have been reports of tamoxifen ocular toxicity even with the low-dose therapy of 20 to 40 mg/day and a cumulative dose of as low as 8 g. Tamoxifen toxicity can manifest in different structures of the eye such as a crystalline keratopathy, crystalline lens opacities or cataract, inner retinal deposits with or without edema, and less commonly as an optic neuropathy.

Keywords: crystalline keratopathy, crystalline retinopathy, tamoxifen

90.1 Features

Tamoxifen is a commonly used antiestrogen oral medication that has been used in the management of breast cancer since the 1970s. This medication is particularly effective as an adjuvant therapy in postsurgical advanced estrogen-receptor positive breast cancer. Though this medication is relatively well tolerated, it has rarely been known to cause ocular toxicity including a crystalline retinopathy with long-term use. Tamoxifen ocular toxicity was initially attributed to the higher dosing of this agent that ranged from 60 to 100 mg/day with an accumulative dosing of greater than 100 g over a period of 12 months. More recently, there have been reports of tamoxifen ocular toxicity even with the low-dose therapy of 20 to 40 mg/day and a cumulative dose of as low as 8 g. Tamoxifen toxicity can manifest in different structures of the eye such as a crystalline keratopathy, crystalline lens opacities or cataract, inner retinal deposits with or without edema, and less commonly as an optic neuropathy.

90.1.1 Common Symptoms

It may be asymptomatic. Progressive decline in visual acuity with or without distortion may occur; may manifest as color vision deficiency.

90.1.2 Exam Findings

Tamoxifen toxicity can be detected in various types of ocular tissue causing a crystalline keratopathy, cataract formation, crystalline retinopathy, and optic neuropathy. Toxic retinopathy or maculopathy presents as small retractile yellow or white deposits, predominantly located in the paramacular region and do tend to increase in number with worsening toxicity (▶ Fig. 90.1). The crystalline deposits may also be associated with underlying retinal pigmentary changes as well as macular edema with a blunted foveal light reflex.

90.2 Key Diagnostic Tests and Findings

90.2.1 Optical Coherence Tomography

Parafoveal pseudocystic changes, hyperreflective inner retinal deposits, and outer retinal/ellipsoid zone cavitation/atrophy (▶ Fig. 90.2).

90.2.2 Fluorescein Angiography or Ultra-Widefield Fluorescein Angiography

Macular hyperfluorescence without leakage may be present; window defect seen in cases with outer retinal atrophy.

90.2.3 Optical Coherence Tomography Angiography

This is an emerging technology that may demonstrate normal retinal vasculature (▶ Fig. 90.3). Subtle flow voids may be present depending on severity. It may be particularly helpful in discriminating between other similar presenting conditions that may have distinct optical coherence tomography angiography features (e.g., MacTel).

90.2.4 Fundus Autofluorescence

Mild hyper-autofluorescence in areas that correspond to crystalline deposits may be seen.

90.2.5 Electroretinography

Decreased photopic and scotopic A- and B-wave amplitude may be present.

90.3 Management

90.3.1 Treatment Options

Discontinuation of tamoxifen leads to reversal of mild retinopathy, but more severe cases can be irreversible. Cystoid macular edema may reverse with discontinuation of the drug. Treatment with anti-vascular endothelial growth factor therapy for persistent cystoid macular edema has been reported. Coordination and communication with patient's oncologist is critical when recommending discontinuation of tamoxifen.

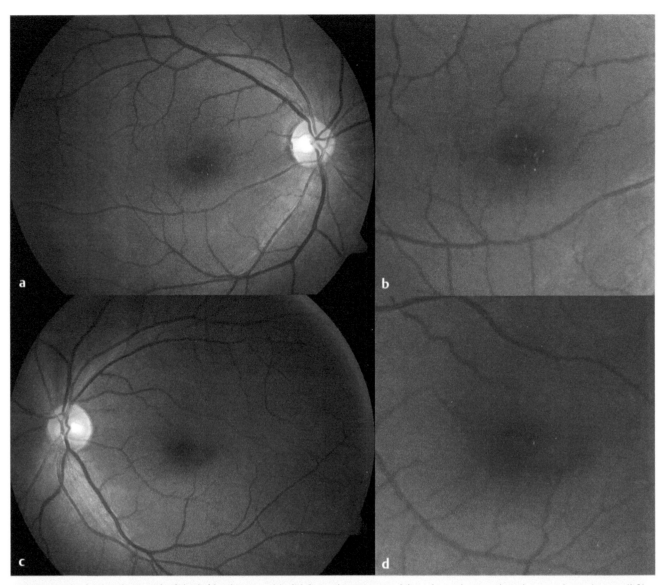

Fig. 90.1 Color fundus photograph of the **(a,b)** right eye and **(c,d)** left eye demonstrating bilateral macular crystals in the central macular area (*left*), more visible on the high magnification view (*right*).

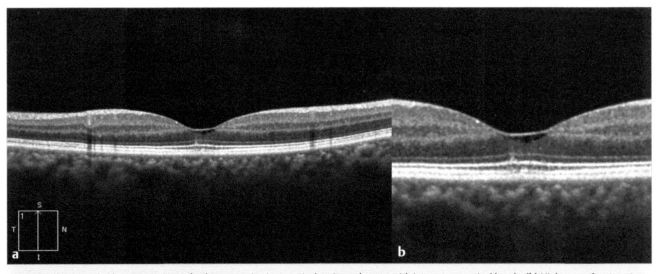

Fig. 90.2 **(a)** Optical coherence tomography demonstrating inner retinal cavitary changes with intact outer retinal bands. **(b)** High-magnification view of fovea enables visualization of hyporeflective spaces.

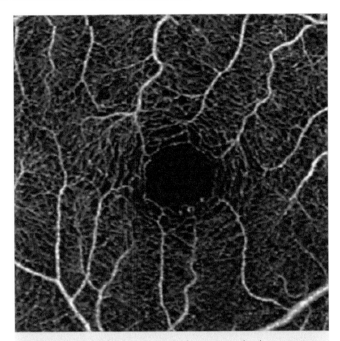

Fig. 90.3 Optical coherence tomography angiography demonstrates intact retinal vascular flow with minimal to no flow voids. No evidence of significant vascular telangiectasia.

90.3.2 Follow-up

There are no specific recommendations for screening examinations for patients on tamoxifen. Any patient on tamoxifen therapy who experiences any visual symptoms be referred for a comprehensive ophthalmologic examination. Ongoing regular follow-up for patients with evidence of toxicity is recommended.

Suggested Reading

[1] Mittra RA, Mieler WF. Drug toxicity of the posterior segment. In: Ryan SJ, Schachat AP, SriniVas SR, eds. Retina. Elsevier; 2013:1532–1554

[2] Nayfield SG, Gorin MB. Tamoxifen-associated eye disease. A review. J Clin Oncol. 1996; 14(3):1018–1026

[3] Kaiser-Kupfer MI, Kupfer C, Rodrigues MM. Tamoxifen retinopathy. A clinico-pathologic report. Ophthalmology. 1981; 88(1):89–93

[4] Doshi RR, Fortun JA, Kim BT, Dubovy SR, Rosenfeld PJ. Pseudocystic foveal cavitation in tamoxifen retinopathy. Am J Ophthalmol. 2014; 157(6):1291–1298.e3

[5] Todorich B, Yonekawa Y, Thanos A, Randawa S. OCT angiography findings in tamoxifen maculopathy. Ophthalmol Retina. 2017; 1(5):450–452

91 Retinopathy Secondary to Targeted Cancer Therapies

Priya Patel, Edmund Tsui, and Yasha S. Modi

Summary

Cancer therapy drugs for the treatment of metastatic melanoma have shown great advances in recent years and, although rare, ocular side effects from these therapies certainly have clinical significance. While differing immunomodulators have varying mechanisms of action, the ocular consequences are largely similar, with the hallmark being multifocal serous retinal detachment without leakage on fluorescein angiography. Treatment should be tailored to each specific case and, in conjunction with the oncologist's preference, may involve observation, cessation of the inciting agent, or, in some cases, steroid therapy. As more therapies with promising data emerge for the treatment of these cancers, it is important for the clinician to be aware of the possible toxicities of these medications and the appropriate management.

Keywords: checkpoint inhibition, metastatic melanoma, retinopathy, serous retinal detachment, uveitis

91.1 Features

Despite the increasing prevalence of melanoma worldwide, the mortality from this disease entity continues to decline due to improved and targeted therapies. Specifically in the case of metastatic disease, the use of novel immunomodulatory therapies has shown great promise, significantly improving progression-free survival.

Immune checkpoint inhibitors, which serve to "release the brakes" on the immune system and enzyme inhibitors that have specific molecular targets, have been reported to have significant systemic side effects. Ocular immune-related adverse events, although less common, have also been reported.
Immune checkpoint inhibitors:
- Anti-CTLA-4 monoclonal antibody: ipilimumab.
- Anti-PD-1 antibodies: nivolumab and pembrolizumab.
- Anti-PDL-1 antibodies: atezolizumab, avelumab, and durvalumab.

Enzyme inhibitors:
- BRaf enzyme inhibitors: vemurafenib and dabrafenib.
- MEK pathway inhibitors: binimetinib, trametinib, and cobimetinib.

The imaging features of retinopathy from these immune modulators are similar given they all reflect the hallmark feature of subretinal fluid with or without inflammation. However, the pathophysiology is postulated to be different. The immune checkpoint inhibitor antibody drugs likely act via an increase in inflammation as they lead to T-cell activation and secretion of proinflammatory molecules, which is believed to cause leakage of vessels from the choroidal circulation. In contrast, the BRAF and MEK inhibitors disrupt the FGFR-MAPK pathway, which is responsible for maintaining the integrity of the retinal pigment epithelium (RPE) cells, affecting their ability to maintain fluid

balance as well as deal with oxidative stress, thus resulting in fluid accumulation and possible retinal vein occlusions.

91.1.1 Common Symptoms

Common symptoms are blurred vision (usually bilateral), photophobia, and eye pain or foreign body sensation.

91.1.2 Exam Findings

Inflammation may range from none to mild anterior chamber and/or vitreous cell. Blunted foveal reflexes indicate subretinal or intraretinal fluid. Multifocal serous retinal detachments are possible. In rare cases associated with combined ipilimumab and nivolumab, concurrent choroidal detachment with secondary angle closure was observed. Retinal vein occlusion is seen particularly with MEK pathway and BRaf inhibitors.

91.2 Key Diagnostic Tests and Findings

91.2.1 Optical Coherence Tomography

Optical coherence tomography demonstrates multifocal areas of neurosensory retinal detachment with or without intraretinal edema and possible undulation of the RPE if there are associated choroidal detachments (▶ Fig. 91.1).

91.2.2 Fluorescein Angiography or Ultra-Widefield Fluorescein Angiography

Demonstrates normal vasculature without early or late hyperfluorescence (▶ Fig. 91.2). The hallmark feature is "nonleaking" neurosensory detachments. Additionally, there is no leakage from the disc or vessels; in some cases, there may be slight pooling centrally in the area of serous retinal detachment.

91.2.3 Fundus Autofluorescence

There may be possible hyper-autofluorescent changes corresponding to the areas of serous retinal detachment. Chronically, there may be areas of hypo-autofluorescence corresponding to RPE atrophy. The late stages may ultimately mimic the fundus autofluorescence appearance of uveal melanocytic proliferation, which is associated with metastatic melanoma.

91.3 Critical Work-up

Work-up should include complete medical history including exact timings of initiation of immunomodulatory medications. A thorough review of systems to assess for any other systemic medication toxicities, and depending on the clinical picture

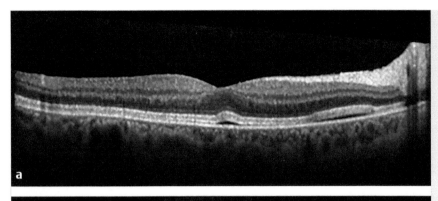

Fig. 91.1 (a) Right and (b) left eyes of a patient on MEK inhibitor therapy with small pockets of subretinal fluid. (Images courtesy of Jasmine Francis, MD and Irina Belinsky, MD)

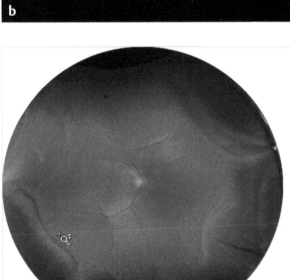
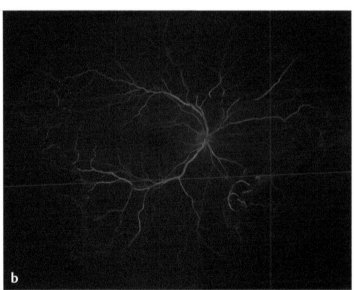

Fig. 91.2 (a) Ultra-widefield fundus photograph and (b) ultra-widefield fluorescein angiography from a patient treated with both ipilimumab (anti-CTLA-4 antibody) and nivolumab (anti-PD-1 antibody). Fundus photography demonstrates multiple serous retinal detachments and choroidal effusions without significant hyperfluorescence or leakage on fluorescein angiography.

additional lab work may be considered to rule out other causes (e.g., RPR, FTA-ABS, c-ANCA, p-ANCA, Quantiferon Gold, Toxoplasma gondii IgG, antiproteinase 3, ACE, lysozyme, and serum protein electrophoresis [SPEP]).

91.4 Management

91.4.1 Treatment Options

While the hallmark of immunomodulatory therapy–associated retinopathy is multifocal serous retinal detachments, diagnosis is dependent on the history as well as other negative studies (no leakage on fluorescein angiography and possibly a negative lab work-up) to rule out other entities. Management of this condition requires a multidisciplinary approach and close contact with the patient and his/her oncologist to achieve the delicate balance between minimizing side effects while adequately treating the patient's disease. Options include observation with regular follow-up to assess for resolution or worsening of symptoms, reduced dosage or cessation of immune-modulating therapy in conjunction with the oncologist, and systemic (oral or intravenous) steroid therapy and/or topical cortical steroids for treatment of uveitis.

Suggested Reading

[1] Larkin J, Chiarion-Sileni V, Gonzalez R, et al. Combined nivolumab and ipilimumab or monotherapy in untreated melanoma. N Engl J Med. 2015; 373(1): 23–34

[2] Stjepanovic N, Velazquez-Martin JP, Bedard PL. Ocular toxicities of MEK inhibitors and other targeted therapies. Ann Oncol. 2016; 27(6):998–1005

[3] van der Noll R, Leijen S, Neuteboom GH, Beijnen JH, Schellens JH. Effect of inhibition of the FGFR-MAPK signaling pathway on the development of ocular toxicities. Cancer Treat Rev. 2013; 39(6):664–672

[4] Wong RK, Lee JK, Huang JJ. Bilateral drug (ipilimumab)-induced vitritis, choroiditis, and serous retinal detachments suggestive of Vogt-Koyanagi-Harada syndrome. Retin Cases Brief Rep. 2012; 6(4):423–426

[5] Niro A, Strippoli S, Alessio G, Sborgia L, Recchimurzo N, Guida M. Ocular toxicity in metastatic melanoma patients treated with mitogen-activated protein kinase inhibitors: a case series. Am J Ophthalmol. 2015; 160(5):959–967.e1

Part IX

Posterior Segment Tumors

IX

92 Choroidal Nevus

Carol L. Shields and Jerry A. Shields

Summary

Choroidal nevus is a benign, stable, asymptomatic intraocular tumor appearing as a chronic pigmented lesion. The estimated prevalence is approximately 5% in U.S. adults. Several clinical features allow identification of nevus and differentiation from melanoma. Nevus carries risk for vision loss, especially if subfoveal, and risk for transformation into melanoma, especially if manifesting three or more risk factors. Risk factors are remembered by the mnemonic "To Find Small Ocular Melanoma – Using Helpful Hints Daily" representing Thickness > 2 mm (T), subretinal Fluid (F), Symptoms (S) of flashes/floaters and blurred vision, Orange pigment (O), Margin less ≤ 3 mm from optic disc (M), Ultrasonographic Hollowness (UH), Halo absent (H), and Drusen absent (D). Choroidal nevus is monitored with dilated fundus evaluation and possible fundus photography once or twice yearly.

Keywords: choroid, nevus, melanoma, risk factors, tumor

92.1 Features

Choroidal nevus is the most common benign intraocular tumor, found predominantly in Caucasian patients. The estimated prevalence is approximately 5% in U.S. adults. Several clinical features allow identification of nevus and differentiation from melanoma. This tumor carries risk for visual acuity loss, especially if near the foveola, and risk for transformation into malignant melanoma.

92.1.1 Common Symptoms

Typically asymptomatic; fluid leakage and neovascularization can result in photopsias and/or loss of vision.

92.1.2 Exam Findings

Flat or minimally elevated mass with brown pigmentation (melanotic; pigmented) or without pigmentation (amelanotic; nonpigmented), generally in the postequatorial fundus (91%) and pigmented (77%), equivalent distribution in all quadrants, and most likely extrafoveolar (94%) compared to subfoveolar (6%). Overlying drusen common, particularly as the patient ages (▶ Fig. 92.1). Tumor size varies depending on the study, but one ocular oncology clinic-based center found mean basal tumor diameter was 5 mm and thickness was 1.5 mm, compared to a population-based study where choroidal nevus was found to have mean basal diameter of 1.25 mm. Choroidal nevus can be categorized into low or high risk for transformation into melanoma.

Low-Risk Choroidal Nevus

Thickness ≤ 2 mm, absence of subretinal fluid, orange pigment and symptoms. These lesions classically appear echodense on ultrasonography and demonstrate overlying retinal pigment epithelium (RPE) alterations such as drusen, RPE atrophy, dependent RPE trough from previous subretinal fluid, RPE hyperplasia, RPE detachment, RPE fibrous metaplasia, and RPE osseous metaplasia (▶ Fig. 92.2). Rarely, choroid nevus can produce chronic RPE damage that leads to the development of choroidal neovascular membrane (CNVM).

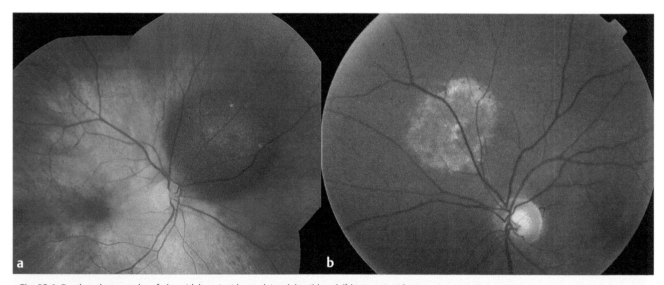

Fig. 92.1 Fundus photographs of choroidal nevi with overlying (a) mild and (b) extensive drusen.

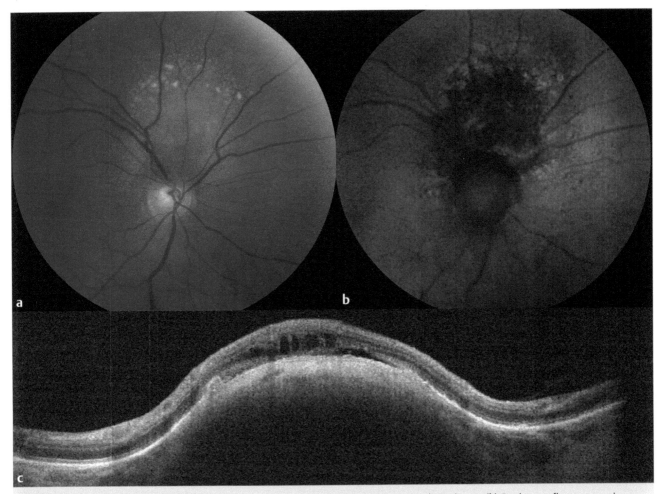

Fig. 92.2 Multimodal imaging of a choroidal nevus. **(a)** Fundus photography demonstrates overlying drusen. **(b)** Fundus autofluorescence shows retinal pigment epithelium (RPE) atrophy centrally and mild ring-shaped hyper-autofluorescence of drusen in the periphery. **(c)** Optical coherence tomography documents overlying drusen, RPE thinning, focal RPE detachment, retinal edema, outer retinal disorganization and retraction, and choroidal mass with compression of the choriocapillaris and loss of normal choroidal vasculature.

High-Risk Choroidal Nevus

Carries high likelihood for transformation into melanoma with features including thickness greater than 2 mm, presence of subretinal fluid, orange pigment and/or symptoms, acoustic hollowness on ultrasonography, and absence of chronic features such as drusen or surrounding halo (▶ Fig. 92.3). High-risk nevus should be evaluated by an ocular oncologist. These risk factors can be remembered with the mnemonic "To Find Small Ocular Melanoma – Using Helpful Hints Daily" representing Thickness > 2 mm (T), subretinal Fluid (F), Symptoms (S) of flashes/floaters and blurred vision, Orange pigment (O), Margin less ≤ 3 mm from optic disc (M), Ultrasonographic Hollowness (UH), Halo absent (H), and Drusen absent (D) (▶ Table 92.1).

Halo Nevus

Central pigmented nevus with surrounding depigmented halo, most often found in young patients and believed to represent an immune response (▶ Fig. 92.4). These represent 5% of all choroidal nevi and are felt to be low risk. Halo nevus has been linked to a previous history of skin melanoma ($p < 0.001$) and no association with autoimmune dysfunction or vitiligo.

Giant Nevus

Giant nevus is defined as a nevus with basal diameter ≥ 10 mm and represents 8% of all choroidal nevi from an ocular oncology practice (▶ Fig. 92.5). Due to its large basal dimension, this can be mistaken for choroidal melanoma. Transformation rate has been reported as high as 18% at 10 years. The features predictive of transformation included close proximity to the foveola ($p = 0.02$) and ultrasonographic acoustic hollowness ($p = 0.05$).

92.2 Key Diagnostic Tests and Findings

92.2.1 Optical Coherence Tomography

Highly valuable for evaluation of choroidal nevus, particularly for the status of the overlying retina and RPE. Most nevi show

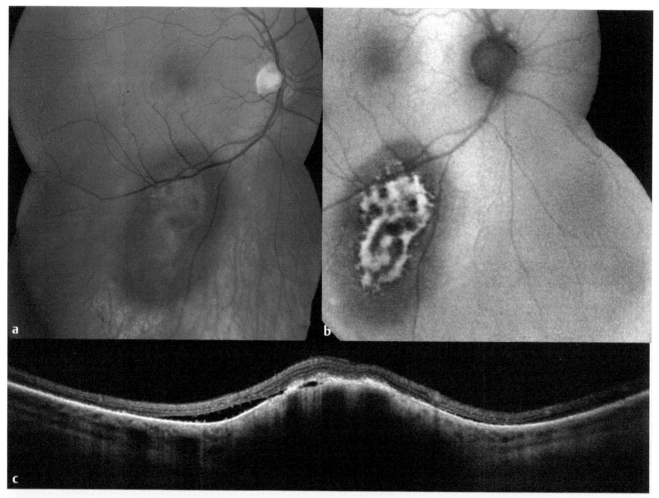

Fig. 92.3 High-risk choroidal "nevus" suggestive of small melanoma. **(a)** Fundus photograph demonstrates overlying orange pigment which is confirmed with **(b)** fundus autofluorescence documenting hyper-autofluorescence of lipofuscin. **(c)** Optical coherence tomography documents subretinal fluid with minimal shaggy photoreceptors over the tumor apex, and choroidal mass impression of the choriocapillaris and loss of normal choroidal vasculature.

Table 92.1 Risk factors for choroidal nevus growth to melanoma

Mnemonic	Initial	Variable	Hazard ratio	p-Value
To	T	Thickness > 2 mm	2	< 0.001
Find	F	Subretinal Fluid	3	0.002
Small	S	Symptoms Decreased vision Flashes/floaters	2 2	0.02 0.002
Ocular	O	Orange pigment	3	< 0.001
Melanoma	M	Margin distance to optic nerve ≤ 3 mm	2	0.001
Using Helpful	UH	Ultrasonographic Hollowness	3	< 0.001
Hints	H	Halo absent	6	0.009
Daily	D	Drusen absent	na	na

Abbreviation: na, not available.

Source: Data from Shields CL, Furuta M, Berman EL, et al. Choroidal nevus transformation into melanoma: analysis of 2514 consecutive cases. Arch Ophthalmol 2009;127:981–987.

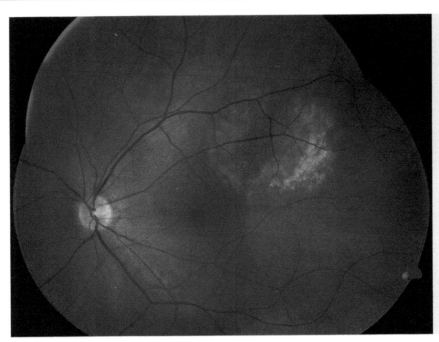

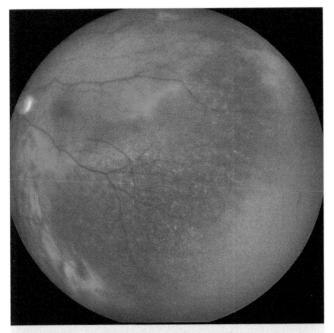

Fig. 92.5 Giant choroidal nevus measuring 16 mm in diameter and with overlying drusen. There was no subretinal fluid or orange pigment.

choriocapillaris thinning over the nevus apex (94%), partial (59%) or complete (35%) choroidal shadowing deep to the nevus, depending on nevus pigmentation, RPE atrophy (43%), and photoreceptor loss (43%) (▶ Fig. 92.1, ▶ Fig. 92.2). Subretinal fluid overlying nevus (16%) is generally minimal and usually located over the apex of the mass. Concerning optical coherence tomography (OCT) findings for melanoma include greater tumor thickness, larger amount of subretinal fluid remote from

the mass, and more significant preservation of "shaggy" photoreceptors. "Shaggy" photoreceptors might represent subretinal macrophages aligned on the posterior retinal surface. A large study on OCT of choroidal melanocytic tumors revealed "shaggy" photoreceptors in 49% of small melanoma and in 0% of nevus.

92.2.2 Fluorescein Angiography or Ultra-Widefield Fluorescein Angiography

Not often necessary, but if there is subretinal fluid, hemorrhage, or exudation it can identify pinpoint RPE leaks or CNVM.

92.2.3 Indocyanine Green Angiography

Thin choroidal nevus and melanoma typically show hypocyanescence. It may be useful in delineating overlying CNVM related to nevus.

92.2.4 Fundus Autofluorescence

Reliable marker of nevus versus melanoma as nevus tends to show overlying RPE hypo-FAF, whereas small melanoma shows overlying hyper-FAF, representing lipofuscin (orange pigment) (▶ Fig. 92.2, ▶ Fig. 92.3, ▶ Fig. 92.6).

92.2.5 Optical Coherence Tomography Angiography

A comparative analysis of choroidal nevus versus small melanoma using OCT angiography revealed eyes with nevus showed no effect on central macular thickness, foveal avascular zone area, and capillary vascular density (superficial and deep

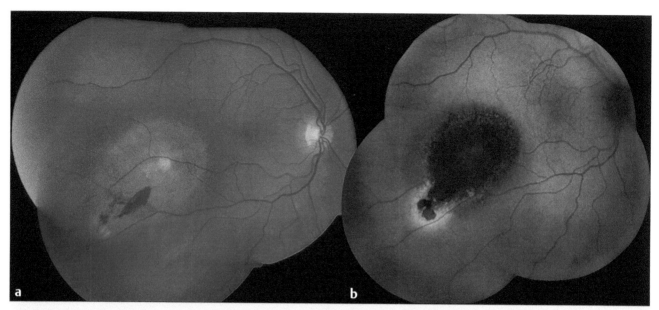

Fig. 92.6 Fundus photography (**a**) demonstrating choroidal nevus with retinal pigment epithelium (RPE) atrophy, hyperplasia, and fibrosis. Fundus autofluorescence (**b**) shows hypo-autofluorescence centrally, indicating RPE loss.

plexuses), whereas eyes with small melanoma showed macular microischemia with significantly increased central macular thickness, enlarged foveal avascular zone, and reduction of capillary vascular density (superficial and deep plexuses). This microischemic environment is likely related to elevated vascular endothelial growth factor (VEGF) levels in eyes with melanoma. Visualization of choriocapillaris and choroidal flow may also be impacted by a nevus.

92.2.6 Ultrasonography

Employed for tumor thickness measurement as well as intrinsic tumor echogenicity. Most choroidal nevi are nearly flat as a single echo and baseline tumor thickness is measured, often recorded as ≤ 2 mm. Nevus tends to demonstrate high internal reflectivity on A-scan and echodensity on B-scan. In contrast, melanoma demonstrates low to medium internal reflectivity on A-scan and echolucency on B-scan.

92.3 Management

92.3.1 Treatment Options

Subretinal Fluid

Choroidal nevus demonstrates overlying subretinal fluid in approximately 10% of patients. If asymptomatic, observation is typically the treatment of choice. Photodynamic therapy has demonstrated fluid resolution in nearly 90% of eyes with visual acuity improvement in over 50% and should be considered in eyes that have symptomatic fluid. Other treatment options include anti-VEGF and oral/topical carbonic anhydrase inhibitors.

Choroidal Neovascularization

Choroidal nevus may have associated CNVM in approximately 1% of patients. Management of CNVM secondary to nevus typically involves anti-VEGF therapy with functional and anatomical improvements in most cases. Peripheral CNVM that are asymptomatic may also be observed closely.

Growth into Melanoma

Choroidal nevus growth into melanoma is confirmed by imaging modalities, and treatment is instituted with plaque radiotherapy, proton beam radiotherapy, transpupillary thermotherapy, Aura-011 nanoparticle therapy, transscleral resection, or enucleation.

92.3.2 Follow-up

Most choroidal nevi are managed with periodic observation (every 6–12 months). Fundus photography, ultrasonography, OCT, and autofluorescence are useful imaging modalities at each examination. Eyes with a subfoveal choroidal nevus are at highest risk for vision loss (▶ Fig. 92.7). Choroidal nevus should be routinely monitored for potential malignant transformation into melanoma. Some demonstrate slow, minimal growth of less than 0.06 mm/year over long period of time (10 years) and represents slow nevus enlargement without malignant transformation. Transformation to melanoma is suspected with rapid growth over a short period of time (1–2 years or less). Early identification of transformation is important for prompt treatment at a time when the melanoma is small and systemic prognosis is favorable. Tumors with three or more risk factors likely represent small melanoma, with malignant transformation in more than 50% of cases at 5 years and treatment should be considered early.

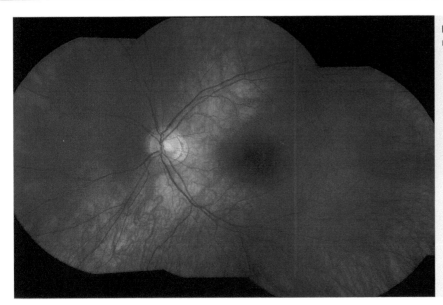

Fig. 92.7 Fundus photo of subfoveal choroidal nevus which is a risk factor for vision loss.

Suggested Reading

[1] Qiu M, Shields CL. Choroidal nevus in the United States adult population: racial disparities and associated factors in the National Health and Nutrition Examination Survey. Ophthalmology. 2015; 122(10):2071–2083

[2] Chien JL, Sioufi K, Surakiatchanukul T, Shields JA, Shields CL. Choroidal nevus: a review of prevalence, features, genetics, risks, and outcomes. Curr Opin Ophthalmol. 2017; 28(3):228–237

[3] Shields CL, Furuta M, Mashayekhi A, et al. Clinical spectrum of choroidal nevi based on age at presentation in 3422 consecutive eyes. Ophthalmology. 2008; 115(3):546–552.e2

[4] Shields CL, Furuta M, Berman EL, et al. Choroidal nevus transformation into melanoma: analysis of 2514 consecutive cases. Arch Ophthalmol. 2009; 127 (8):981–987

[5] Shields CL, Dalvin LA, Ancona-Lezama D, et al. Choroidal nevus imaging features in 3806 cases and risk factors for transformation into melanoma in 2355 cases. The 2020 Taylor R. Smith and Victor T. Curtin Lecture. Retina. 2018 Dec 31. doi: 10.1097/IAE.0000000000002440. [Epub ahead of print]

[6] Shields JA, Shields CL. Management of posterior uveal melanoma: past, present, and future: the 2014 Charles L. Schepens lecture. Ophthalmology. 2015; 122(2):414–428

93 Choroidal Melanoma

Claudine Bellerive and Arun D. Singh

Summary

Choroidal melanoma is a primary cancer of the eye arising from the pigmented cells of the choroid. Small tumors are typically asymptomatic, but at advanced stages, flashes, floaters, variable vision or visual field loss, and, rarely, pain secondary to neovascular glaucoma are possible. Choroidal melanomas are chemoresistant tumors and are life-threatening due to their metastatic potential. They are commonly unifocal and unilateral, and lesions appear as brown dome-shaped or mushroom-shaped masses arising from choroid, but may occasionally be amelanotic. Treatment options include transpupillary thermotherapy for small tumors and radiotherapy or enucleation for medium and large tumors.

Keywords: choroidal melanoma, neovascularization, transpupillary thermotherapy

93.1 Features

Choroidal melanoma is a primary cancer of the eye arising from the pigmented cells of the choroid. Choroidal melanomas are chemoresistant tumors and are life-threatening due to their metastatic potential. They are commonly unifocal and unilateral, and lesions appear as brown dome-shaped or mushroom-shaped masses arising from choroid, but may occasionally be amelanotic.

93.1.1 Common Symptoms

Small tumors are typically asymptomatic. At advanced stages, flashes and floaters, variable vision or visual field loss, and, rarely, pain secondary to neovascular glaucoma are possible.

93.1.2 Exam Findings

Choroidal melanomas are classified as small, medium, or large according to their largest basal diameter and height at the time of diagnosis (▶ Table 93.1). These are commonly unifocal and unilateral. Lesions appear as brown dome-shaped or mushroom-shaped masses arising from choroid, but may occasionally be amelanotic. Some have subretinal fluid or orange pigmentation (lipofuscin accumulation) overlying their surface (▶ Fig. 93.1). Choroidal melanomas may be associated with exudative retinal detachment, anterior segment neovascularization and secondary neovascular glaucoma, and episcleral sentinel

Table 93.1 Classification of choroidal melanoma: COMS criteria

Size	LBD	Height
Small	5–16 mm	1.5–2.4 mm
Medium	≤16 mm	2.5–10 mm[a]
Large	>16 mm	>10 mm

Abbreviation: LBD, largest basal diameter.
[a]Changed from 3.1 to 8 mm (November 1990).

vessels in the same quadrant when the tumor extends into the ciliary body.

93.2 Key Diagnostic Tests and Findings

93.2.1 Optical Coherence Tomography

Optical coherence tomography (OCT) may demonstrate subretinal fluid overlying the lesion. Choroidal elevation is noted with obliteration of the overlying choroidal vessels and choriocapillaris. Alterations in retinal pigment epithelium structure may also be noted. Choroidal pathology may be best visualized with enhanced depth imaging or swept source optical coherence tomography.

93.2.2 Fluorescein Angiography or Ultra-Widefield Fluorescein Angiography

"Double-circulation" pattern (simultaneous fluorescence of retinal and tumor vessels) in venous phase.

93.2.3 Indocyanine Green Angiography

Hypofluorescence lesions (for smaller tumors) or presence of hyperfluorescent intrinsic choroidal vasculature (for larger tumors) in early phases (▶ Fig. 93.2), with variable leakage from the tumoral blood vessels in late phases.

93.2.4 Fundus Autofluorescence

Hyper-autofluorescence may be noted in cases with significant orange pigment. Subretinal fluid often produces hyper-autofluorescence, if present. Areas of "guttering" may be observed due to the gravity with chronic subretinal fluid.

93.2.5 Ultrasonography

A-scan ultrasonography characteristically demonstrates medium to low internal reflectivity, positive angle kappa (decrease in height of the inner tumor spikes due to irregular internal structure), and fast and continuous low-amplitude flickering consistent with internal vascular flow. B-scan ultrasonography provides information about the tumor shape and dimension. A mushroom-shaped tumor corresponds generally to a break in Bruch's membrane and is very characteristic of choroidal melanoma (▶ Fig. 93.3). Acoustic hollowing, choroidal excavation, and shadowing of the orbital fat are also common on B-scan.

93.2.6 Transillumination

A shadow will be cast on the sclera in cases of melanocytic tumors.

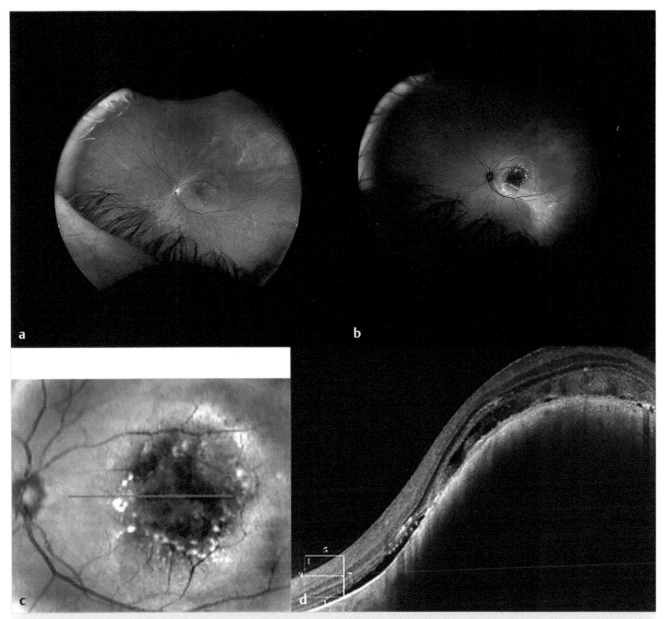

Fig. 93.1 Small choroidal melanoma. **(a)** Ultra-widefield fundus photograph of a small choroidal melanoma with overlying orange pigment. **(b)** Ultra-widefield fundus autofluorescence demonstrates both hyper-autofluorescence associated with areas of orange pigment and previous subretinal fluid and hypo-autofluorescence in the area of the nevus. **(c,d)** Optical coherence tomography demonstrates minimal subretinal fluid, lack of shaggy photoreceptors, outer retinal integrity disruption, choroidal elevation, and obliteration of the choroidal vasculature.

93.2.7 Magnetic Resonance Imaging

Choroidal melanomas appear bright on T1 and dark on T2.

93.2.8 Genetic Profiling and/or Chromosomal Analysis

The genetic makeup of the tumor appears to be predictive of metastatic risk. Different groups have proposed various tests for evaluating tumor profile, including gene profiling with classification (e.g., class I vs. class II [higher risk]) and chromosomal assessment (e.g., monosomy 3 [higher risk]). This is an active area of research but may be helpful in prognostication in the future. It may also be useful for stratifying risk for future clinical trials and characterizing indeterminate lesions following biopsy.

93.3 Critical Work-up

While choroidal melanomas have a sporadic occurrence in most cases, higher risk is observed in patients with oculodermal melanocytosis. For this reason, annual dilated examination is indicated for these patients. Genetic testing should be considered in individuals with history of cutaneous melanoma (to rule out

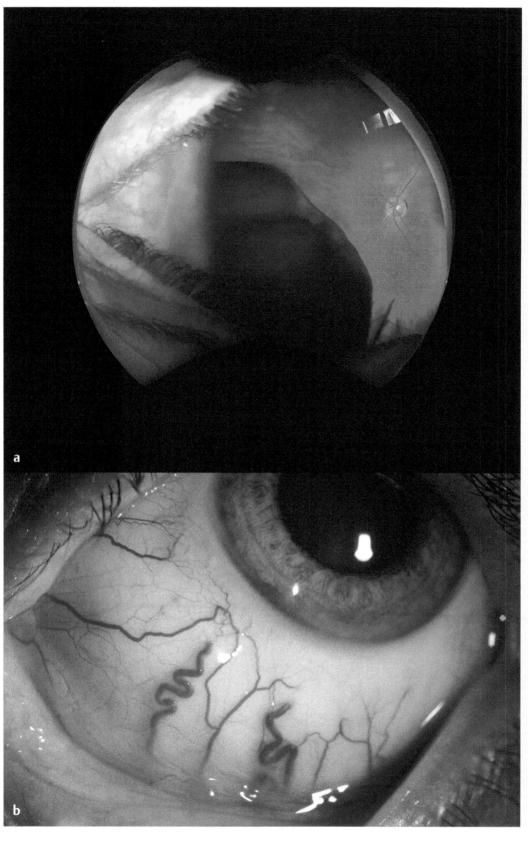

Fig. 93.2 Large ciliochoroidal melanoma. **(a)** Ultra-widefield photograph demonstrating large ciliochoroidal melanoma obscuring view to the nasal retina. The ora serrata is visible at the apex of the tumor. **(b)** An external photograph documents its association with episcleral feeder vessels.

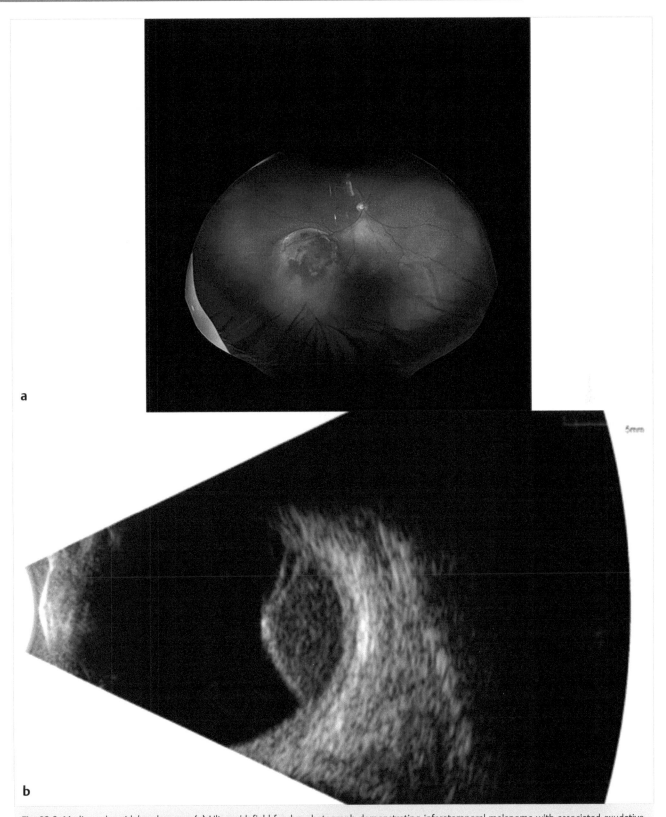

Fig. 93.3 Medium choroidal melanoma. **(a)** Ultra-widefield fundus photograph demonstrating inferotemporal melanoma with associated exudative retinal detachment that extends inferonasally. **(b)** B-scan ultrasonography confirms presence of elevation and enables measurements and assessment of echogenicity. Area of shallow subretinal fluid is also visualized.

familial atypical multiple mole melanoma syndrome—mutation CDKN2A) or familial history of cancer including cutaneous and/or ocular melanoma, renal cell carcinoma, and mesothelioma (to rule out hereditary cancer predisposition syndrome—germline mutations of BAP1).

93.4 Management

93.4.1 Treatment Options

Transpupillary thermotherapy (TTT) may be considered for small tumors (≤ 3 mm in height and ≤ 10 mm in largest basal diameter). TTT may also be helpful as adjuvant therapy in combination with brachytherapy for juxtapapillary tumors. For medium and large tumors, radiotherapy or enucleation can be proposed without affecting the long-term risk of metastasis. Multiple types of radiation therapy frequently used in choroidal melanoma treatment include episcleral plaque brachytherapy, proton beam therapy, and stereotactic radiosurgery (gamma knife, cyber knife, or linear accelerator). Choice of treatment is often center dependent. Local tumor control is most often achieved with iodine-125 or ruthenium-106 (which is reserved for tumors < 5 mm thickness) episcleral plaques. Choroidal melanomas are chemoresistant tumors.

93.4.2 Follow-up

Choroidal melanomas are life-threatening disease according to their metastatic potential. Pretreatment systemic staging is recommended. Long-term surveillance for metastases includes liver imaging (ultrasonography, CT, or MRI) at 6-month intervals for the first 5 years after diagnosis, and then annually. Liver function tests (serum markers) appear not to be helpful for early detection of metastasis.

Suggested Reading

[1] Singh AD, De Potter P, Fijal BA, Shields CL, Shields JA, Elston RC. Lifetime prevalence of uveal melanoma in white patients with oculo(dermal) melanocytosis. Ophthalmology. 1998; 105(1):195–198

[2] Abdel-Rahman MH, Pilarski R, Cebulla CM, et al. Germline BAP1 mutation predisposes to uveal melanoma, lung adenocarcinoma, meningioma, and other cancers. J Med Genet. 2011; 48(12):856–859

[3] Cheung M, Talarchek J, Schindeler K, et al. Further evidence for germline BAP1 mutations predisposing to melanoma and malignant mesothelioma. Cancer Genet. 2013; 206(5):206–210

[4] Bataille V, Sasieni P, Cuzick J, Hungerford JL, Swerdlow A, Bishop JA. Risk of ocular melanoma in relation to cutaneous and iris naevi. Int J Cancer. 1995; 60(5):622–626

[5] Choudhary MM, Gupta A, Bena J, Emch T, Singh AD. Hepatic ultrasonography for surveillance in patients with uveal melanoma. JAMA Ophthalmol. 2016; 134(2):174–180

94 Choroidal and Retinal Metastasis

Carol L. Shields and Jerry A. Shields

Summary

Metastases to the eye can involve the choroid (88%), iris (9%), or ciliary body (2%), and rarely the retina (< 1%). Intraocular metastases most commonly originate from primary cancers in the breast (47%), lung (21%), gastrointestinal tract (4%), kidney (2%), skin (melanoma) (2%), prostate gland (2%), and other sites (4%). Most metastases are often unilateral (76%) and fewer are bilateral (24%). Patient prognosis is poor, and those with metastatic skin melanoma or lung carcinoma typically show poorest survival.

Keywords: breast cancer, choroid, lung cancer, metastasis, retina, tumor

94.1 Features

In a recent report to the nation on the status of cancer in America, it was documented that the incidence and death rates from all cancers combined have decreased significantly. Systemic cancers can metastasize to the eye, the most common of which being breast and lung cancer. The decreasing cancer rates could impact the frequency of ocular metastasis. Metastases to the eye can involve the choroid (88%), iris (9%), or ciliary body (2%), and rarely the retina (< 1%). Intraocular metastases most commonly originate from primary cancers in the breast (47%), lung (21%), gastrointestinal tract (4%), kidney (2%), skin (melanoma) (2%), prostate gland (2%), and other sites (4%). Most metastases are often unilateral (76%) and fewer are bilateral (24%). Patient prognosis is poor, and those with metastatic skin melanoma or lung carcinoma typically show poorest survival.

Several conditions can simulate choroidal metastasis including amelanotic nevus, amelanotic melanoma, hemangioma, osteoma, posterior scleritis, retinitis and choroiditis, rhegmatogenous retinal detachment, Harada disease, uveal effusion syndrome, and central serous chorioretinopathy. A detailed history is often helpful in making the differentiation, but the ophthalmoscopic differences are also important.

94.1.1 Common Symptoms

Can be asymptomatic or might experience painless blurred vision, photopsia, floaters, visual field loss, or low-grade ocular pain. Often there is a history of previous systemic cancer, but in approximately 25% of cases, the patient is unaware of underlying cancer.

94.1.2 Exam Findings

Intraocular metastases show a strong tendency to involve choroid, less commonly affect the iris and ciliary body, and rarely involve the retina or optic disc. Metastases can occur in more than one ocular location; most choroidal metastases show multifocality and/or bilaterality (▶ Fig. 94.1, ▶ Fig. 94.2). In an analysis of 520 eyes with uveal metastases, the mean number of tumors per eye was 1.6. In that large analysis, the tumor demonstrated 1 site (71%), 2 sites (12%), and 3 or more sites (17%), up to a maximum number of 13 sites in one eye.

Choroidal metastasis characteristically appears as a homogeneous, creamy-yellow placoid lesion in the postequatorial region. Most metastases produce a serous detachment of the retina and alterations in the retinal pigment epithelium (RPE). When the detachment is extensive, dramatic shifting of the subretinal fluid can be demonstrated with movements of the patient's head. The RPE changes can be marked, appearing as well-delineated clumps of lipofuscin on the surface of the tumor.

Retinal metastasis often appears with inflammatory-like features along the inner retina and with overlying vitreous seeding (▶ Fig. 94.3). Commonly, the diagnosis is not suspected as the tumor appears like inflammation or infection.

94.2 Key Diagnostic Tests and Findings

94.2.1 Optical Coherence Tomography

Optical coherence tomography (OCT) can easily detect related subretinal fluid, retinal edema, and RPE changes associated with choroidal metastases. Choroidal metastasis demonstrates a "lumpy bumpy" surface, in contrast to choroidal melanoma and hemangioma that appear smooth (▶ Fig. 94.4, ▶ Fig. 94.5). Enhanced depth imaging spectral-domain OCT (SD-OCT) and swept source OCT provide greater details of the choroidal features of these tumors.

94.2.2 Fluorescein Angiography or Ultra-Widefield Fluorescein Angiography

Fluorescein angiography or ultra-widefield fluorescein angiography reveals the tumor as hypofluorescent in the arterial and early venous phases and with progressive hyperfluorescence in the subsequent phases. Pinpoint foci of hyperfluorescence appear over the tumor in the venous phase and persist into the late angiograms, correlating with serous subretinal fluid.

94.2.3 Indocyanine Green Angiography

Indocyanine green angiography reveals mild hypocyanescence throughout the angiography; rarely does a metastasis show hypercyanescence. By contrast, choroidal melanoma shows gradual hypercyanescence over 5 to 10 minutes and choroidal hemangioma shows bright hypercyanescence within 1 minute.

94.2.4 Fundus Autofluorescence

Important for documentation of overlying RPE abnormalities, particularly lipofuscin hyper-autofluorescence (▶ Fig. 94.4, ▶ Fig. 94.5).

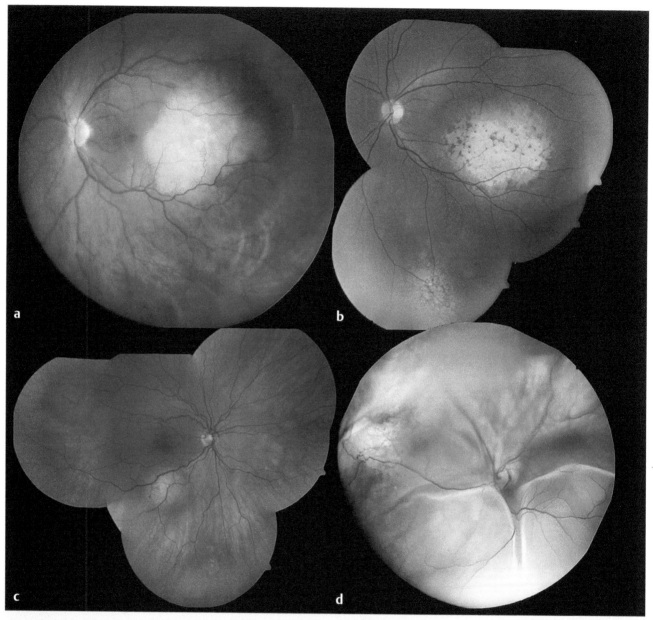

Fig. 94.1 Multifocality of choroidal metastasis. Fundus photography documenting **(a)** solitary, **(b)** bifocal, **(c)** trifocal, and **(d)** hidden choroidal metastasis.

94.2.5 Fundus Photography

Facilitates documentation of tumor growth, resolution, and the appearance of new tumors.

94.2.6 Ultrasonography

Demonstrates a sharp initial spike and moderate internal reflectivity on A-scan and a choroidal mass pattern with moderate to high acoustic solidity, overlying subretinal fluid, and no choroidal excavation on B-scan in contrast to malignant melanoma, which usually shows relatively low internal reflectivity and acoustic hollowness (▶ Fig. 94.4, ▶ Fig. 94.5).

94.2.7 Computed Tomography

Can demonstrate the anatomic location and configuration of choroidal metastasis as well as related disease posterior to the globe. It is important to evaluate the brain in all patients with ocular metastasis as one series found breast cancer with choroidal metastasis showed additional brain metastasis in 30% of patients.

94.2.8 Magnetic Resonance Imaging

It is useful in delineating the anatomic location, configuration, and internal tissue qualities of choroidal metastases and the resolution is far superior to computed tomography for soft

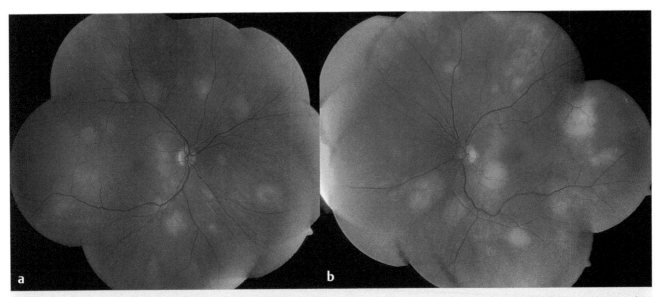

Fig. 94.2 Bilateral multifocal choroidal metastasis from lung cancer. Montage fundus photography demonstrating multifocal lesions in the **(a)** right and **(b)** left eye.

tissue features. In general, uveal metastases are slightly hyperintense to vitreous on T1-weighted images, hypointense to vitreous on T2-weighted images, and contrast enhancement with gadolinium. The associated retinal detachment is hyperintense to vitreous on T1 and isointense to vitreous on T2-weighted images.

94.2.9 Fine Needle Aspiration Biopsy

When the diagnosis of an ocular lesion is particularly difficult to establish, fine needle aspiration biopsy (FNAB) may be employed. This technique requires exceptional skill to retrieve cells from within the eye, using indirect ophthalmoscopy to guide the needle through the pars plana into the solid mass. This is especially useful for patients who present with no previous cancer and systemic evaluation is unrevealing.

94.2.10 Surgical Biopsy

Open surgical biopsy is rarely used for intraocular metastases. If used, complete resection is performed for circumscribed tumors and incisional biopsy for ill-defined tumors. The biopsy is performed microscopically via a scleral flap.

94.3 Critical Work-up

The patient's history might reveal an underlying malignancy, but many patients give no history of cancer. A detailed systemic evaluation is important for any patient with choroidal metastasis, with special focus on breast, lung, and colorectal cancer. Other sites to keep in mind include cancers of the kidney, thyroid, pancreas, prostate, and other organs.

94.4 Management

94.4.1 Treatment Options

In general, the life prognosis for patients with metastatic tumors to the ocular structures is poor. Patients with breast carcinoma metastatic to the uvea have a more favorable survival rate compared to those with lung cancer or cutaneous melanoma. Survival estimates for patients with uveal metastasis from breast cancer are 65% at 1 year, 34% at 3 years, and 24% at 5 years. Treatment for choroidal or retinal metastasis depends on tumor location, extent, activity, and symptoms, as well as the patient's systemic status.

Observation

Some metastatic tumors to the eye are inactive and require no treatment. They may have regressed spontaneously or they may have regressed following systemic treatment of the primary cancer months or years previously. Inactive metastases are typically flat with RPE clumping (leopard spots) on the tumor surface and without retinal detachment.

Chemotherapy, Hormone Therapy, Anti-VEGF Therapy

Active tumors that respond to chemotherapy or hormone therapy that is being used to treat the systemic disease do not need additional intervention. The patient should be followed up at 2- to 4-month intervals for documentation of tumor and visual status (▶ Fig. 94.6). In some cases, intravitreal injection of anti-VEGF medications can resolve the choroidal tumor and/or subretinal fluid.

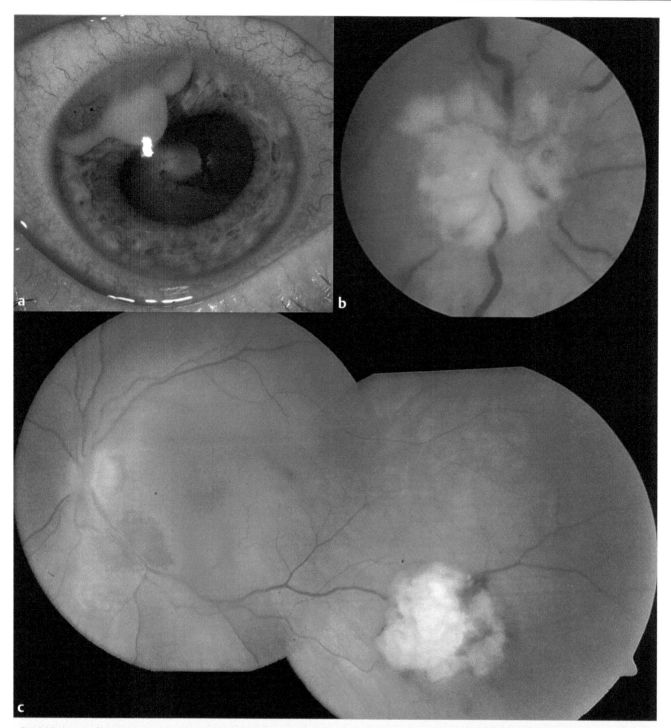

Fig. 94.3 Intraocular metastatic sites. Photographic images of metastatic tumors to the **(a)** iris, **(b)** optic disc, and **(c)** retina in three different patients.

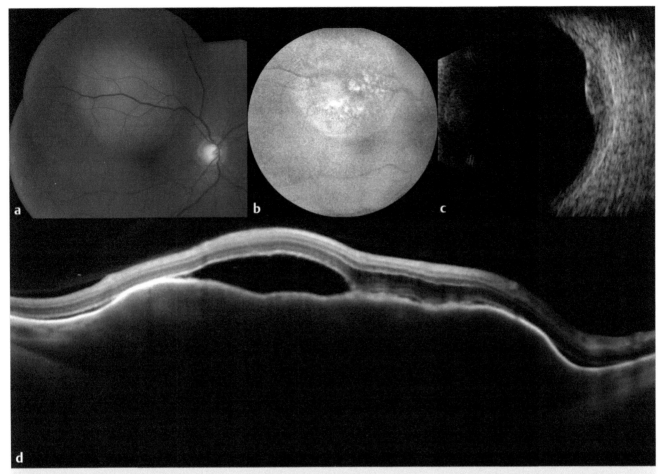

Fig. 94.4 Multimodal imaging of breast cancer metastasis. (a) Fundus photograph demonstrates a creamy-yellow deep lesion. (b) Fundus autofluorescence with hyper-autofluorescence of lipofuscin within the retinal pigment epithelium. (c) B-scan ultrasonography demonstrates elevation. (d) Optical coherence tomography demonstrates lumpy bumpy surface with subretinal fluid and loss of choroidal vasculature.

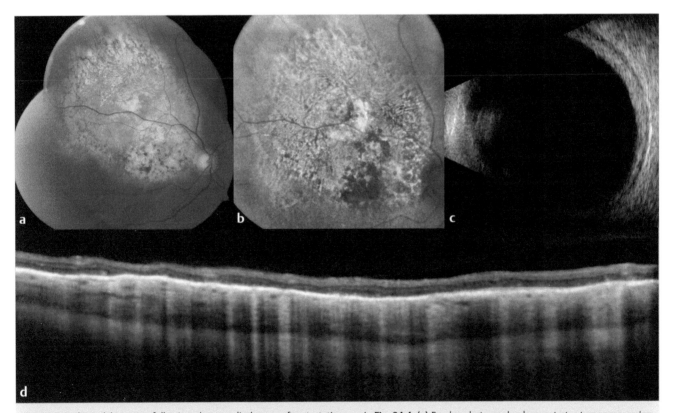

Fig. 94.5 Multimodal imaging following plaque radiotherapy of metastatic mass in Fig. 94.4. (a) Fundus photography demonstrates tumor regression with (b) persistent hyper-autofluorescence of the retinal pigment epithelium on fundus autofluorescence. (c) Ultrasonography confirms tumor flattening and (d) optical coherence tomography is also nearly flat surface with resolution of subretinal fluid.

375

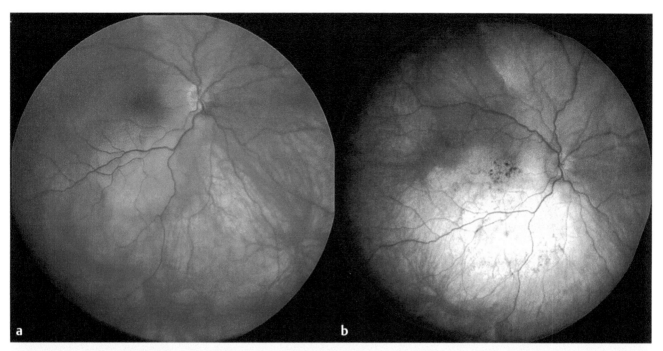

Fig. 94.6 Management of choroidal metastasis from breast carcinoma with chemotherapy. **(a)** Fundus photography before demonstrating yellow choroidal lesion and **(b)** after therapy with subsequent atrophy and retinal pigment epithelium changes.

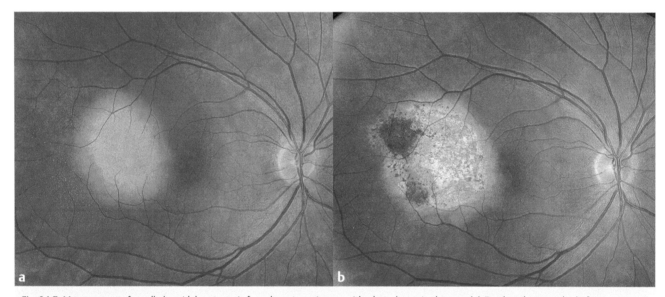

Fig. 94.7 Management of small choroidal metastasis from breast carcinoma with photodynamic therapy. **(a)** Fundus photography before demonstrating temporal yellow choroidal lesion and **(b)** after therapy with subsequent atrophy and retinal pigment epithelium changes.

Photodynamic Therapy

Small to medium size choroidal metastases may be treated with photodynamic therapy. This therapy employs verteporfin followed by treatment with a 689 laser device. Most tumors respond within 1 to 2 months showing regression and resolution of retinal detachment (▶ Fig. 94.7, ▶ Fig. 94.8).

Radiotherapy

Medium to large size choroidal metastases may be treated with plaque radiotherapy, using an apex dose of 35 Gray (▶ Fig. 94.4, ▶ Fig. 94.5). Plaque brachytherapy takes 4 days to deliver the treatment and is much faster than external beam radiotherapy (EBRT) that takes 4 weeks. Large, multifocal, and bilateral metastases are often treated with EBRT.

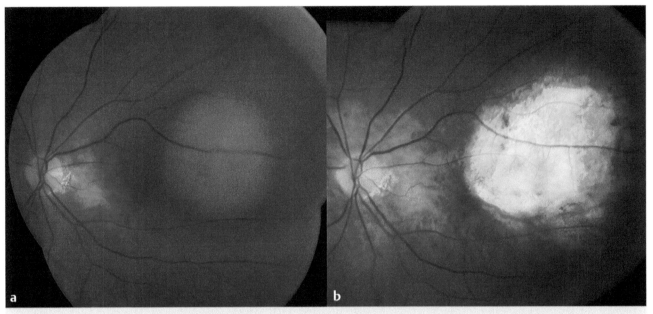

Fig. 94.8 Management of small choroidal metastasis from lung carcinoma with photodynamic therapy. **(a)** Fundus photography before demonstrating superotemporal yellow choroidal lesion and **(b)** after therapy with subsequent atrophy and retinal pigment epithelium changes.

Surgery

In some instances, enucleation or local surgical excision of an intraocular metastasis may be justified. Large tumors with intractable pain generally require enucleation. However, chemotherapy or radiotherapy can be considered first for pain and tumor control.

Suggested Reading

[1] Shields CL, Welch RJ, Malik K, et al. Uveal metastasis: clinical features and survival outcome of 2214 tumors in 1111 patients based on primary tumor origin. Middle East Afr J Ophthalmol. 2018; 25(2):81–90

[2] Shields CL, Shields JA, Gross NE, Schwartz GP, Lally SE. Survey of 520 eyes with uveal metastases. Ophthalmology. 1997; 104(8):1265–1276

[3] Shields CL, Kaliki S, Crabtree GS, et al. Iris metastasis from systemic cancer in 104 patients: the 2014 Jerry A. Shields Lecture. Cornea. 2015; 34(1):42–48

[4] Shields JA, Shields CL, Singh AD. Metastatic neoplasms in the optic disc: the 1999 Bjerrum Lecture: part 2. Arch Ophthalmol. 2000; 118(2):217–224

[5] Demirci H, Shields CL, Chao AN, Shields JA. Uveal metastasis from breast cancer in 264 patients. Am J Ophthalmol. 2003; 136(2):264–271

95 Intraocular Lymphoma

Manuel Alejandro Paez-Escamilla, Michael T. Andreoli, and James William Harbour

Summary

There are various types of intraocular lymphoma, including primary vitreoretinal lymphoma (PVRL), primary uveal lymphoma, and secondary uveal lymphoma. This chapter focuses on PVRL, which is the most common intraocular lymphoma. PVRL is a large B-cell non-Hodgkin lymphoma that frequently involves the central nervous system as well as the eye. PVRL most commonly presents in the fifth to seventh decades in immunocompetent patients, and earlier in immunocompromised patients. PVRL often masquerades as uveitis or other benign conditions, which frequently leads to a delay in diagnosis. This chapter reviews the patient characteristics, clinical features, diagnostic methods, and a summary of treatment options.

Keywords: cancer, intraocular lymphoma, malignancy, ocular oncology, vitreoretinal lymphoma

95.1 Features

There are various types of intraocular lymphoma, including primary vitreoretinal lymphoma (PVRL), primary uveal lymphoma, and secondary uveal lymphoma. This chapter focuses on PVRL, which is the most common intraocular lymphoma. PVRL is a subtype of primary central nervous system large B-cell non-Hodgkin lymphoma (PCNSL). PVRL is usually diagnosed in the fifth to seventh decades of life, although it may present earlier, particularly in immunocompromised patients. About 300 cases are diagnosed per year in the United States. About two-thirds of patients with PVRL will present with bilateral involvement, and the vast majority will eventually exhibit bilateral disease. About 80% of patients with PVRL will develop PCNSL at some point during the course of the disease. In contrast, only 5 to 15% of patients with PCSNL will develop intraocular involvement.

95.1.1 Common Symptoms

May present with floaters, blurred vision, or be asymptomatic.

95.1.2 Exam Findings

The most characteristic clinical features include vitreous infiltration by white cells and creamy yellow sub-retinal pigment epithelium (sub-RPE) deposits (▶ Fig. 95.1). The vitreous cells often appear larger on slit lamp biomicroscopy than are typical of benign forms of vitritis. Less common clinical features include anterior chamber cells, keratic precipitates, pseudo-hypopyon, iris nodules, intra- or subretinal infiltrates, and choroidal infiltration. Rarely, PVRL can masquerade as an infectious retinitis.

95.2 Key Diagnostic Tests and Findings

95.2.1 Optical Coherence Tomography

Optical coherence tomography (OCT) may aid in visualizing subretinal lesions and verifying anatomic location. Most OCT abnormalities are seen at the subretinal or RPE level. Characteristic small hyperreflective nodules at the RPE level are seen in some patients, which may dissipate with treatment.

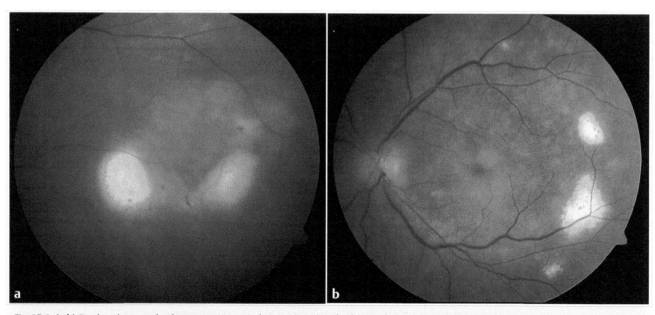

Fig. 95.1 (a,b) Fundus photographs demonstrating typical vitritis (A > B) and sub-retinal pigment epithelium creamy yellow deposits of lymphoma cells that are characteristic of primary vitreoretinal lymphoma.

95.2.2 Fluorescein Angiography or Ultra-Widefield Fluorescein Angiography

Fluorescein angiography (FA) or ultra-widefield fluorescein angiography findings are rarely diagnostic but can provide helpful confirmatory evidence to support the diagnosis of PVRL. The most common findings are diffuse granular RPE changes characterized by patchy hypofluorescence interspersed with pinpoint hyperfluorescence (▶ Fig. 95.2, ▶ Fig. 95.3). These are often out of proportion with the degree of RPE abnormality that is evidenced on ophthalmoscopic examination and color fundus photos. FA can also provide useful diagnostic information, often highlighting diffuse RPE changes that are less obvious clinically.

Classic "leopard spot" hypofluorescent areas are perhaps the most characteristic finding.

95.2.3 Fundus Autofluorescence

Fundus autofluorescence may reveal diffuse granular pin-point hyper-autofluorescence reflecting diffuse subtle RPE abnormalities.

95.2.4 Magnetic Resonance Imaging

In the setting of suspected PVRL, MRI is helpful and important to assess for the presence of PCNSL.

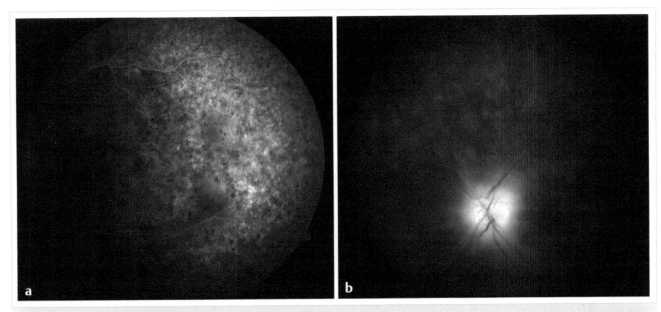

Fig. 95.2 (a) Fluorescein angiography (FA) in an eye with primary vitreoretinal lymphoma (PVRL) showing diffuse granular retinal pigment epithelium changes characterized by patchy hypofluorescence interspersed with pinpoint hyperfluorescence. (b) FA in an eye with PVRL showing optic disc hyperfluorescence and leakage.

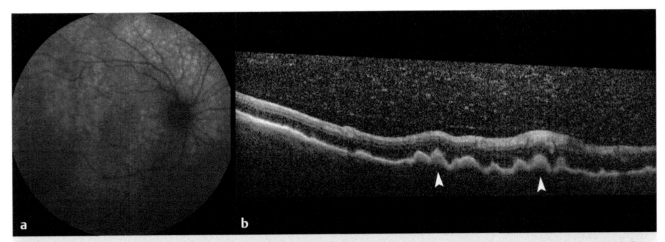

Fig. 95.3 (a) Autofluorescence image of the right eye showing patchy multiple punctuate hyper-autofluorescent areas of retinal pigment epithelium (RPE) damage. (b) Corresponding optical coherence tomography scan through inferior macula showing sub-RPE lymphoma deposits (*arrowheads*) with overlying vitreous opacities consistent with vitritis.

95.3 Critical Work-up

Despite increased awareness of PVRL, the diagnosis is still frequently delayed due to the overlap in clinical presentation with uveitis and other benign conditions, and technical challenges in establishing a laboratory diagnosis.

95.3.1 Cytopathologic Diagnostic Testing

The gold standard for diagnosis is cytopathologic analysis of a vitreous sample or from a localized deposit of lymphoma cells within the eye. Cytopathologic examination of PVRL reveals scattered enlarged lymphoma cells with high nuclear/cytoplasmic ratio, prominent nucleoli, irregular nuclear contours, and fine-to-coarse chromatin pattern, scattered within a background of benign reactive lymphocytes. Immunohistochemistry staining for CD45, CD20, CD45RO, CD68, λ light chains, and κ light chains may also be useful. Flow cytometry is less helpful than many other forms of lymphoma due to the small sample size, but it may be of value as an adjunctive test to assess clonality. Recently, it was discovered that the gene *MYD88* is mutated in about 75% of PVRL and, as such, could represent a powerful new diagnostic tool. Rearrangement of the immunoglobulin heavy chain (IgH) gene is present in most PVRL, but can also be seen in chronic inflammatory conditions. An increased ratio of IL-10 relative to IL-6 from the aqueous or vitreous fluid is suggestive of PVRL rather than an inflammatory process.

95.3.2 Specimen Collection

Common sources of inadequate diagnostic yield for cytopathology include the use of a high vitrectomy cut rate and failure to obtain an undiluted vitreous specimen. This problem can be overcome by obtaining an initial undiluted specimen by manual aspiration into a small syringe using a low cut rate of 300 cuts per minute. It is also critical that the samples be placed on ice and taken immediately to the cytopathology lab for preparation. Subsequently, the cut rate can be increased and a thorough vitrectomy performed. The contents of the vitrectomy cassette can be used for MYD88 mutation, IgH rearrangement, and IL-10/IL-6 testing.

95.3.3 Systemic Work-up

When PVRL is suspected, a systemic work-up to rule out CNS lymphoma is warranted. At a minimum, this work-up should include an MRI of the brain. Lumbar puncture for cytopathologic analysis and MYD88 mutation testing of the cerebrospinal fluid can be helpful when positive, but do not rule out CNS disease when negative.

95.4 Management

95.4.1 Treatment Options

The systemic prognosis for PVRL is guarded, although there is some evidence to suggest that aggressive management and adjuvant CNS treatment may prolong survival.

Systemic chemotherapy alone is rarely effective for PVRL but is often used for concurrent PCNSL or as adjunctive therapy. Thus, local treatment to the affected eye(s) is generally recommended. Local treatment options for PVRL include external beam radiotherapy (EBRT) and intravitreal chemotherapy. EBRT with a relatively low dose of 35 to 40 Gy is highly effective and is associated with a low rate of radiation retinopathy. Local chemotherapy by intravitreal injection of methotrexate is also highly effective, especially if preceded by vitrectomy to debulk the disease burden. Intravitreal rituximab has also shown promise in PVRL. Intrathecal chemotherapy may be required for patients with advanced CNS disease, particularly with meningeal involvement.

Suggested Reading

[1] Chan CC, Rubenstein JL, Coupland SE, et al. Primary vitreoretinal lymphoma: a report from an International Primary Central Nervous System Lymphoma Collaborative Group symposium. Oncologist. 2011; 16(11): 1589–1599

[2] Farkas T, Harbour JW, Dávila RM. Cytologic diagnosis of intraocular lymphoma in vitreous aspirates. Acta Cytol. 2004; 48(4):487–491

[3] Berenbom A, Davila RM, Lin HS, Harbour JW. Treatment outcomes for primary intraocular lymphoma: implications for external beam radiotherapy. Eye (Lond). 2007; 21(9):1198–1201

[4] Smith JR, Rosenbaum JT, Wilson DJ, et al. Role of intravitreal methotrexate in the management of primary central nervous system lymphoma with ocular involvement. Ophthalmology. 2002; 109(9):1709–1716

96 Retinal Vascular Tumors

Jerry A. Shields and Carol L. Shields

Summary

There are several vascular tumors (hemangiomas) that can occur in the retina including retinal hemangioblastoma, cavernous hemangioma, racemose hemangioma, and vasoproliferative tumor. Each has distinct funduscopic and imaging features, as well as systemic findings. Some of these conditions have underlying genetic mutation and are associated with the oculoneurocutaneous syndromes (phakomatoses).

Keywords: Capillary hemangioma, cavernous hemangioma, hemangioblastoma, racemose hemangioma

96.1 Features

There are several vascular tumors (hemangiomas) that can occur in the retina including retinal hemangioblastoma, cavernous hemangioma, racemose hemangioma, and vasoproliferative tumor (VPT). Each has distinct funduscopic and imaging features, as well as systemic findings. Some of these conditions have underlying genetic mutation and are associated with the oculoneurocutaneous syndromes (phakomatoses). These conditions are listed on Online Mendelian Inheritance in Man (OMIM.com) and ocular genetic testing (www.genetests.org) is available to direct the clinician to relevant laboratories for provision of genetic testing.

96.1.1 Retinal Hemangioblastoma

This lesion is a benign vascular hamartoma that has clinical onset in the first two decades of life. This tumor has been termed "retinal capillary hemangioma" or "retinal angiomatosis," but the current term is "retinal hemangioblastoma." Bilateral or multiple retinal hemangioblastomas are associated with von Hippel-Lindau (VHL) syndrome and patients should be evaluated for this condition with brain, renal, and adrenal imaging, as well as genetic testing (▶ Table 96.1). There are three types of mutation in the VHL gene including type1 with deletion or nonsense mutation that manifests mainly hemangioblastomas only;

Table 96.1 Criteria for the diagnosis of von Hippel-Lindau disease

If family history is	Feature
Positive	Any one of the following: • Retinal hemangioblastoma • Brain hemangioblastoma • Visceral lesion
Negative	Any one of the following: • Two or more retinal hemangioblastomas • Two or more brain hemangioblastomas • Single retinal or brain hemangioblastoma with a visceral lesion

Notes: Family history of retinal or brain hemangioma or visceral lesion Visceral lesions include renal cysts, renal carcinoma, pheochromocytoma, pancreatic cysts, islet cell tumors, epididymal cystadenoma, and endolymphatic sac tumor.

type 2 with missense mutation that can manifest hemangioblastomas and pheochromocytomas (type 2A) or additional renal cell carcinoma (type 2B) or only pheochromocytoma (type 2C); and type 3 with risk for polycythemia.

96.1.2 Retinal Cavernous Hemangioma

This tumor is a slow-flow venous vascular mass, occasionally associated with skin and central nervous system hemangiomas. It can occur with cerebral cavernous malformations as a sporadic or familial autosomal dominant disorder. There are three cerebral cavernous malformation (CCM) genes: CCM/KRIT1, CCM2/MGC4607, and CCM3/PDCD10.

96.1.3 Retinal Racemose Hemangioma

This lesion is not a true neoplasm but rather a simple or complex arteriovenous communication. This can be a solitary lesion or it can be part of Wyburn-Mason syndrome (also termed "Bonnet-Dechaume-Blanc syndrome"), anatomically referencing retinoencephalofacial angiomatosis. This nonhereditary arteriovenous malformation can affect the retina, visual pathways, midbrain, and facial bones including the mandible and maxilla. Some evidence implies that genetic or developmental factors early in gestation could lead to dysgenesis of the embryologic vascular plexus, and the time of insult determines the location and extent of manifestations.

96.1.4 Vasoproliferative Tumor

A VPT of the ocular fundus is a vascular mass that can occur as a primary or secondary condition. Secondary tumors result from intermediate uveitis, retinitis pigmentosa, Coats disease, or chronic retinal detachment (▶ Table 96.2). There are no genetic abnormalities associated with this condition, but those with secondary tumors should undergo evaluation for underlying retinal conditions. This lesion is not associated with VHL but can be rarely associated with neurofibromatosis type 1.

96.1.5 Common Symptoms

Retinal Hemangioblastoma

Mostly asymptomatic; commonly diagnosed incidentally; regardless of tumor location, accumulation of subretinal fluid and exudation can lead to profound visual loss.

Retinal Cavernous Hemangioma

May be asymptomatic, or may present with decreased visual acuity depending on the location of the tumor, presence of macular fibrosis, or vitreous hemorrhage.

Racemose Hemangioma

Mostly asymptomatic; visual disturbances may occur depending on the size and location of retinal arterial-venous malformations.

Table 96.2 Tumors in the von Hippel-Lindau syndrome

Tumor	Age (most common) (y) at diagnosis	Frequency of tumor
Head and neck		
Retinal hemangioblastoma	12–25	25–60%
Cerebellar hemangioblastoma	18–25	44–72%
Brainstem hemangioblastoma	24–35	10–25%
Spinal cord hemangioblastoma	24–35	13–50%
Endolymphatic sac tumor	16–28	11–16%
Trunk		
Renal cell carcinoma/cyst	25–50	25–60%
Pheochromocytoma	12–25	10–20%
Pancreatic tumor/cyst	24–35	35–70%
Epididymal cystadenoma	14–40	25–60% males
Broad ligament cystadenoma	16–46	10% females

Source: Data compiled from a survey of papers from 1976 to 2004, including data from the VHL Family Alliance (VHLFA) and adapted from the VHLFA Handbook (http://www.vhl.org/; http://www.chop.edu/service/hereditary-cancer-predisposition-program/genetic-syndromes-with-cancer-risks/von-hippel-lindau-syndrome.html).

Vasoproliferative Tumor

Possible blurriness, floaters, photopsia, or vision loss.

96.1.6 Exam Findings

Retinal Hemangioblastoma

Appears clinically as a nodular, red-orange mass, located randomly in the fundus and notably with prominent dilated and tortuous retinal vessels feeding and draining the tumor (▶ Fig. 96.1). In some cases, the tumor is not visible and only the feeding vessels are seen (▶ Fig. 96.2). When located at the optic disc, the mass can masquerade as optic disc inflammation or papillitis, and feeder vessels are typically not seen. This tumor can produce subretinal fluid, subretinal and intraretinal exudation, and vitreoretinal fibrosis with epiretinal membrane and traction retinal detachment (▶ Fig. 96.3). The exudation often accumulates in the macular region as a macular star.

Retinal Cavernous Hemangioma

This nonprogressive tumor appears as a cluster of dark intraretinal venous aneurysms, sometimes referred to as a "bunch of concord grapes" and can show minimal enlargement over time (▶ Fig. 96.4). There is no feeding artery, but it might display a slightly dilated retinal vein. Occasionally this lesion is on the

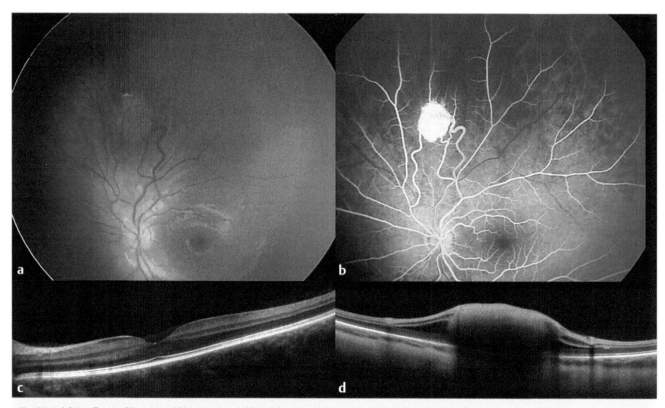

Fig. 96.1 (a) Small retinal hemangioblastoma in a child with known von Hippel-Lindau disease showing dilated vessels leading to an orange-colored intraretinal mass that shows (b) hyperfluorescence on angiography, (c) intact macula on optical coherence tomography (OCT), and (d) with solid intraretinal tumor with surrounding retinal edema on OCT at the tumor site.

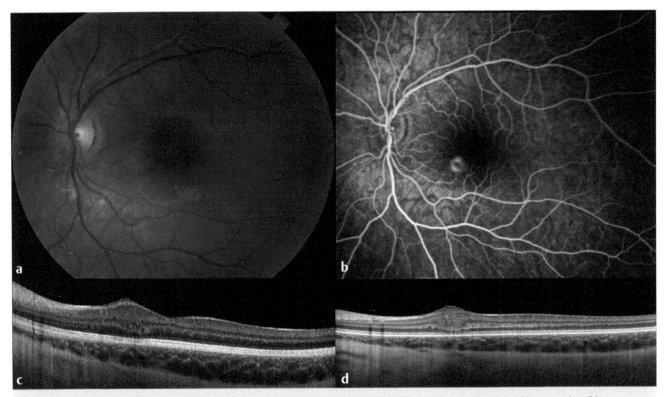

Fig. 96.2 (a) Invisible retinal hemangioblastoma in a child with known von Hippel-Lindau disease but no clinically visible tumor, but (b) hyperfluorescence on angiography reveals the small tumor in the macular region with (c) intact macula on optical coherence tomography (OCT), and (d) solid intraretinal mass on OCT at the tumor site.

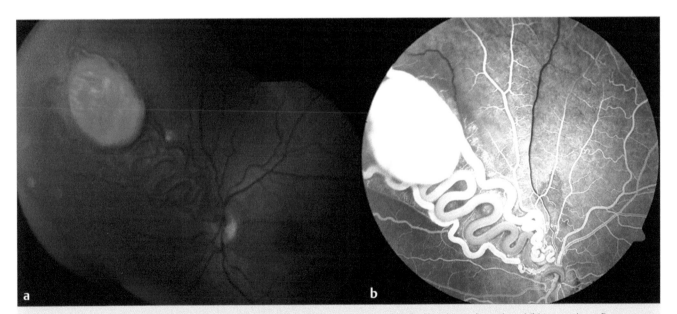

Fig. 96.3 (a) Large retinal hemangioblastoma in a child with von Hippel-Lindau with markedly dilated retinal vessels and (b) intense hyperfluorescence on angiography.

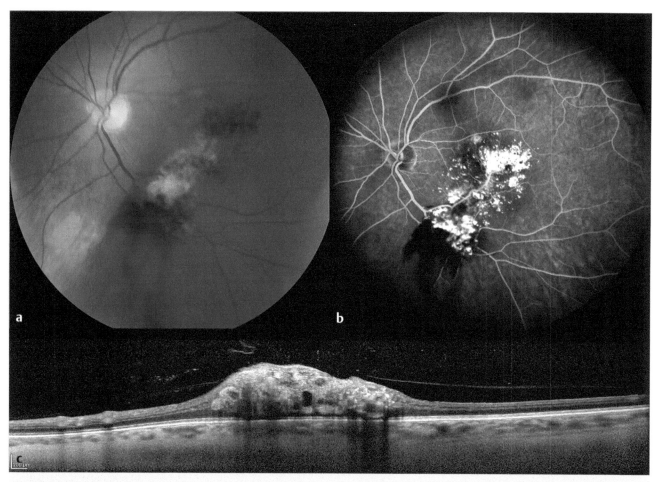

Fig. 96.4 (a) Retinal cavernous hemangioma in the macular region with overlying preretinal fibrosis, showing **(b)** late hyperfluorescence on angiography and **(c)** optical coherence tomography with intraretinal cystic mass.

optic disc. The most common complication is vitreous hemorrhage with later development of overlying white fibroglial scarring on the tumor surface.

Racemose Hemangioma

Clinically, it displays a dilated, tortuous retinal artery that passes from the optic disc into the retina then looping back without capillary formation (▶ Fig. 96.5). The vascular anomaly can be simple or complex in design, and there is usually no exudation or hemorrhage. The Archer classification provides grouping according to size and location of the vascular malformation (▶ Table 96.3).

Vasoproliferative Tumor

Ophthalmoscopically, VPT appears as an ill-defined sessile or dome-shaped yellow-orange retinal mass, typically located in the peripheral inferotemporal region. Minimally dilated retinal feeding artery and draining vein can be found, but not as markedly dilated or tortuous as seen with retinal hemangioblastoma (▶ Fig. 96.6). The tumor can produce findings of intraretinal and subretinal exudation, subretinal fluid, remote epiretinal membrane, cystoid macular edema, retinal hemorrhage, and vitreous

hemorrhage. The retinal exudation generally begins at the tumor margin and gradually marches posteriorly into the macula.

96.2 Key Diagnostic Tests and Findings

96.2.1 Optical Coherence Tomography

Retinal Hemangioblastoma

Optical coherence tomography (OCT) is helpful for evaluating treatment response; intraretinal optically dense tumor within full-thickness retina with related subretinal fluid, exudation, intraretinal edema, and epiretinal membrane may be seen.

Retinal Cavernous Hemangioma

Markedly irregular retinal surface with numerous cavernous spaces.

Vasoproliferative Tumor

Remote macular edema or epiretinal membrane may be present; in most cases, the peripheral location of this tumor precludes adequate OCT of the mass.

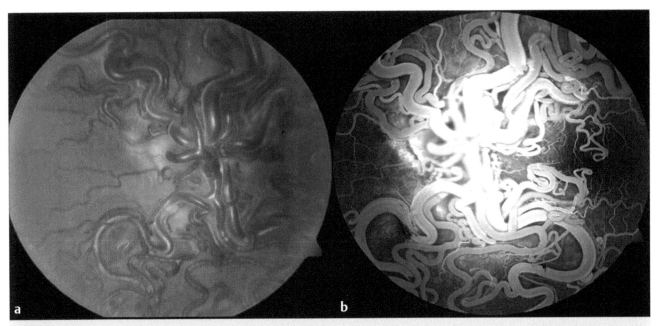

Fig. 96.5 (a) Retinal racemose hemangioma with dramatic large retinal vessels and no intervening capillary system showing (b) early hyperfluorescence on angiography and no capillaries.

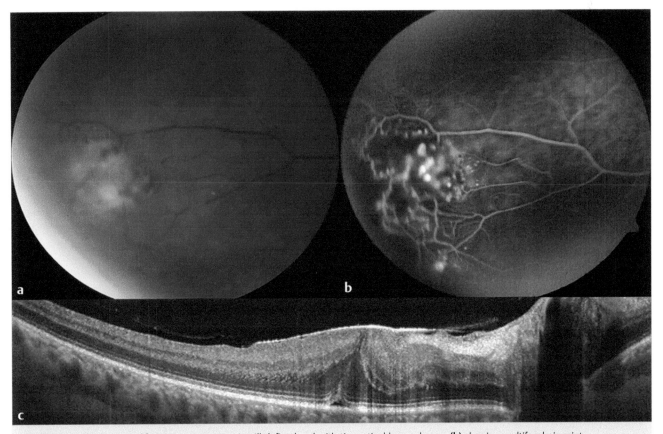

Fig. 96.6 (a) Retinal vasoproliferative tumor appearing ill-defined and with tiny retinal hemorrhages, (b) showing multifocal pinpoint hyperfluorescence on angiography and (c) optical coherence tomography with epiretinal membrane and retinal traction.

96.2.2 Fluorescein Angiography or Ultra-Widefield Fluorescein Angiography

Retinal Hemangioblastoma

It is one of the best modalities for detection and confirmation of retinal hemangioblastoma through early vascular fluorescence of the mass, late staining, and occasional leakage into the vitreous cavity (▶ Fig. 96.1). Fluorescein angiography (FA) shows rapid filling of the feeding artery, then the tumor, and then rapid exit through the draining vein. Subclinical pinpoint tumors can be detected before they become symptomatic. Large tumors can display leakage from the mass into the adjacent retina and vitreous cavity, leading to remote macular edema and epiretinal membrane.

Retinal Cavernous Hemangioma

Shows classic findings of arterial phase hypofluorescence with slow accumulation of fluorescein in the venous aneurysms in the late frames. Within the aneurysmal space, the red blood cells deposit in the inferior portion and plasma in the superior region, without leakage and create the "fluorescein–erythrocyte interface" characteristic of this tumor.

Racemose Hemangioma

Reveals rapid filling of the dilated artery and vein, without capillary channels and without leakage.

Vasoproliferative Tumor

Demonstrates filling of the mass through a slightly dilated and minimally tortuous retinal artery and draining vein. There is commonly leakage from the tumor into the surrounding retina and vitreous cavity. Remote macular edema or epiretinal membrane may present if found on both FA and OCT.

96.2.3 Ultrasonography

Retinal Hemangioblastoma

Can depict the intraocular mass as acoustically solid and with surrounding subretinal fluid.

Retinal Cavernous Hemangioma

Larger tumors can develop vitreous hemorrhage. A-scan ultrasonography demonstrates high initial spike and high internal reflectivity, while B-scan shows irregular dense mass.

96.2.4 Magnetic Resonance Imaging and/or Computed Tomography

Retinal Hemangioblastoma

Can provide information in eyes with extensive retinal detachment, demonstrating an enhancing retinal mass. Brain and systemic imaging is essential for monitoring related central nervous system and systemic neoplasms in VHL disease (▶ Table 96.4).

Table 96.3 Archer classification for Wyburn Mason syndrome

Group	Feature	Comments
I	Abnormal capillary plexus between the major vessels of the arteriovenous malformations	Such lesions tend to be small, patients asymptomatic, and intracranial involvement uncommon
II	Arteriovenous malformations lack any intervening capillary bed between the artery and vein	Risk of retinal decompensation resulting in retina edema, hemorrhage, and vision loss. Low risk for intracranial arteriovenous malformations
III	Extensive arteriovenous malformations with dilated and tortuous vessels and no distinction between artery and vein	High risk for visual loss due to retinal decompensation or retinal compression of nerve fiber layer, optic nerve, or other vessels. High risk for intracranial arteriovenous malformations

Source: Adapted from Archer DM, Deutman A, Ernest JT, Krill AE. Arteriovenous communications of the retina. Am J Ophthalmol 1973;75:224–241.

Retinal Cavernous Hemangioma

Systemic evaluation with brain magnetic resonance imaging (MRI) for related cerebral cavernomas and genetic testing for the CCM genes is advised, especially if there is a positive family history.

Retinal Racemose Hemangioma

Brain imaging should be performed to assess for similar vascular abnormalities.

96.3 Critical Work-up

96.3.1 Retinal Hemangioblastoma

Dilated funduscopic examination, FA, and OCT are all critical for detection of subclinical retinal tumors that might only be visualized by angiography or OCT. Genetically positive patients or at-risk relatives should be routinely monitored for systemic neoplasia. Retinal hemangioblastoma is often the first finding of VHL disease, presenting between 12 and 25 years of age, then other VHL-related tumors tend to occur later, including brain hemangioblastoma and renal cell carcinoma. Solitary retinal hemangioblastoma may or may not be associated with VHL syndrome.

96.3.2 Racemose Hemangioblastoma

Retinal racemose hemangioma is established with ophthalmoscopy and confirmed on FA.

96.4 Management

96.4.1 Treatment Options

Retinal Hemangioblastoma

Management includes both systemic and ophthalmic evaluation. Systemic evaluation should be performed by VHL specialists

Table 96.4 Associated ocular conditions in 56 patients with secondary vasoproliferative tumor

Associated ocular condition	Secondary VPT n = 56 patients n (%)
Retinitis pigmentosa	10 (18)
Pars planitis	11 (20)
Coats disease	11 (20)
Previous retinal detachment repair	8 (14)
Idiopathic peripheral retinal vasculitis	3 (5)
Familial exudative vitreoretinopathy	3 (5)
Toxoplasmosis	3 (5)
Aniridia	1 (2)
Congenital hypertrophy of retinal pigment epithelium	2 (4)
Idiopathic choroiditis	1 (2)
Retinopathy of prematurity	2 (4)
Histoplasmosis	1 (2)
Total	56

Abbreviation: VPT, vasoproliferative retinal tumor.
Source: Data from Shields CL, Kaliki S, Al-Daamash S, et al. Retinal vasoproliferative tumors. Comparative clinical features of primary versus secondary tumors in 334 cases. JAMA Ophthalmol 2013;131 (3):328–334.

monitoring for cerebellar hemangioblastoma, pheochromocytoma, renal cell carcinoma, and other associated neoplasms and cysts (▶ Table 96.2). Brain and abdominal MRI should be performed periodically as outlined in published protocols. Treatment depends on tumor size, location, and other features. VHL-related tumors are more aggressive and should be considered for treatment promptly, even when small. Those in the macular, perimacular, or juxtapapillary region are often observed until vision is directly affected. Treatment for small (<3 mm) tumors involves laser photocoagulation or photodynamic therapy; for medium (3–6 mm) tumors treatment involves photodynamic therapy or cryotherapy; and large (>6 mm) tumors require photodynamic therapy, plaque radiotherapy, or internal resection by pars plana vitrectomy route. For hemangioblastoma unassociated with VHL disease, asymptomatic tumors without subretinal fluid are often observed, particularly if they are in the perimacular or juxtapapillary region. Some anecdotal cases have responded to oral propranolol, Diamox, and prednisone, but large studies have not been performed. Intravitreal anti-vascular endothelial growth factor (anti-VEGF) can assist with resolution of edema, but the tumor does not respond.

Retinal Cavernous Hemangioma

Most retinal cavernous hemangiomas require no treatment. This tumor rarely progresses and rarely produces visual symptoms. Vitreous hemorrhage can occur and is managed with observation or vitrectomy. Repetitive hemorrhage can be controlled with low-dose plaque radiotherapy. Systemic evaluation with brain MRI for related cerebral cavernomas and genetic testing for the CCM genes is advised, especially if there is a positive family history.

Racemose Hemangioma

Management includes both systemic and ophthalmic monitoring. The patient should be evaluated for Wyburn-Mason syndrome with brain imaging studies for similar vascular abnormalities. The retinal lesion usually remains stable and treatment is rarely needed.

Vasoproliferative Tumor

Small peripheral tumors can be cautiously observed if there is no leakage, but they can slowly progress and potentially lead to profound visual loss; thus, we generally treat peripheral lesions with laser photocoagulation or cryotherapy, even if they are not leaking. Active leakage requires therapy including laser photocoagulation, thermotherapy, indocyanine green-enhanced thermoablation, photodynamic therapy, cryotherapy, or plaque radiotherapy. Cryotherapy often leads to tumor control and can induce release of epiretinal membrane in 63% of cases. Plaque radiotherapy is employed for tumors greater than 3 or 4 mm thickness. Intravitreal anti-VEGF can assist in reducing remote macular edema, and sub-Tenon's triamcinolone can minimize inflammatory response to treatment.

Suggested Reading

[1] Shields JA, Shields CL. Intraocular Tumors. An Atlas and Textbook. 3rd ed. Philadelphia, PA: Lippincott Williams & Wilkins; 2016;389–426
[2] Shields CL, Douglass A, Higgins T, et al. Retinal hemangiomas: understanding clinical features, imaging, and therapies. Retina Today. 2015; 10:61–67
[3] Singh AD, Shields CL, Shields JA. von Hippel-Lindau disease. Surv Ophthalmol. 2001; 46(2):117–142
[4] Wong WT, Chew EY. Ocular von Hippel-Lindau disease: clinical update and emerging treatments. Curr Opin Ophthalmol. 2008; 19(3):213–217
[5] Maher ER, Neumann HP, Richard S. von Hippel-Lindau disease: a clinical and scientific review. Eur J Hum Genet. 2011; 19(6):617–623

97 Retinoblastoma

Victor M. Villegas and Timothy G. Murray

Summary

Historically, retinoblastoma (RB) has been associated with poor survival and visual outcomes. Currently, survival in industrialized countries is close to 100%. Developing nations continue to report significant mortality associated with this disease entity mainly due to late diagnosis. The most common presenting signs are leukocoria, strabismus, and decreased visual acuity. Early diagnosis and treatment are the most important factors in minimizing morbidity and mortality. Referral to a tertiary center could significantly reduce the mortality discrepancy. Globe-sparing treatments have replaced primary enucleation in the management of this rare condition mostly because new diagnostic and therapeutic options are available at tertiary centers that have allowed improved anatomical and visual outcomes in the most advanced stages. External beam radiation therapy was used prior to newer chemoreduction strategies. Several advanced chemotherapeutic treatments are currently available, including selective intra-arterial, periocular, and intravitreal in combination with focal ablation. Combination chemoreduction is currently being used during primary treatment at most large centers. Brachytherapy has been used as adjuvant treatment in select cases. Current clinical research with the most advanced diagnostic technologies and available treatment modalities may revolutionize the anatomic and visual outcomes associated with this condition.

Keywords: leukocoria, retinoblastoma, strabismus

97.1 Features

Retinoblastoma (RB) is the most common primary intraocular malignancy with an incidence of approximately 1:15,000 births. The tumor suppressor *RB1* gene is known to be key in the development of the disease. Most cases (60%) result from a somatic nonhereditary mutation; however, 40% arise from germline hereditary mutations that may occur spontaneously. There is no gender or racial predilection. Most RBs are diagnosed in children younger than 5 years; because of the lack of early symptoms, most children are diagnosed late in the disease process. The mean time of diagnosis in bilateral RB is 11 months. Solitary RB typically is diagnosed after 2 years of age. However, RB has been described in adults. Special attention to prior family history should be undertaken during the initial encounter. Historically, RB has been associated with poor survival and visual outcomes. Currently, survival in industrialized countries is close to 100%. Developing nations continue to report significant mortality associated with this disease entity mainly due to late diagnosis. The most common presenting signs are leukocoria, strabismus, and decreased visual acuity. Early diagnosis and treatment is the most important limitation associated with morbidity and mortality. Referral to a tertiary center could significantly reduce the mortality discrepancy.

Differential diagnoses include Coat's disease, persistent fetal vasculature (PFV), familial exudative vitreoretinopathy, retinal astrocytoma, osteoma, pediatric cataracts, retinopathy of prematurity, coloboma of the choroid, uveitis, vitreous hemorrhage, retinal dysplasia, retinal detachment, corneal opacities, myelinated nerve fiber, and parasitic infections. Expertise in the complete RB differential diagnosis is critically important at the time of diagnosis.

97.1.1 Common Symptoms

Mostly asymptomatic; pain may be present in advanced cases.

97.1.2 Exam Findings

RB is characterized by a creamy white retinal mass, unilateral or bilateral (▶ Fig. 97.1). In unilateral cases, it is important to determine if multifocal tumor burden is present. Different growth patterns may be present. Endophytic tumors grow toward the vitreous and develop vitreous seeding. Exophytic tumors grow toward the subretinal, choroidal, and scleral space and are associated with exudative retinal detachments. Diffuse tumors may thicken the retina and might be confused with other etiologies.

The most common physical exam finding is leukocoria, especially in large or macular tumors (▶ Fig. 97.2). However, in early or peripheral posterior segment disease, leukocoria might not be present. Strabismus secondary to central visual loss is the second most common sign at initial presentation. Less common presentations include uveitis, orbital cellulitis, hyphema, vitreous hemorrhage, cataract, glaucoma, pseudo-hypopyon, and proptosis. Any child younger than 5 years with a white or yellow posterior segment lesion should be evaluated under anesthesia for RB.

97.2 Key Diagnostic Tests and Findings

97.2.1 Optical Coherence Tomography

Most recently, spectral domain optical coherence tomography (SD-OCT) has become available in the operating room. It can help detect microscopic changes that are not clearly visible during indirect ophthalmoscopy such as intraretinal and subretinal fluid. It can be used to guide management decisions; however, lack of fixation during examination under anesthesia (EUA) may limit the comparison of images over time. OCT may also help with prognostication based on evaluation of foveal anatomic structure and may potentially have a role in the identification of subclinical tumors that manifest as retinal layer alterations (e.g., thickening of the middle retinal layers).

97.2.2 Fluorescein Angiography or Ultra-Widefield Fluorescein Angiography

Fluorescein angiography (FA) or near ultra-widefield fluorescein angiography (UWFA) during EUA has become available to

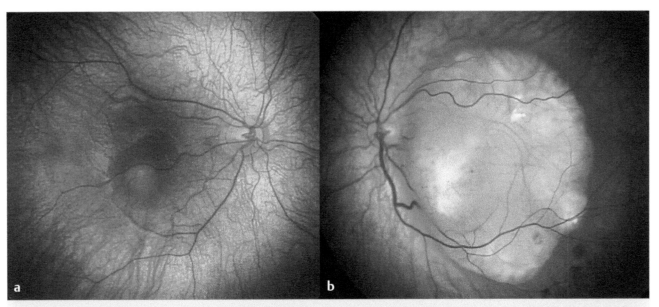

Fig. 97.1 Bilateral retinoblastoma. **(a)** Fundus photograph demonstrating small macular retinoblastoma. **(b)** Fundus photography of large macular retinoblastoma with associated epiretinal hemorrhage.

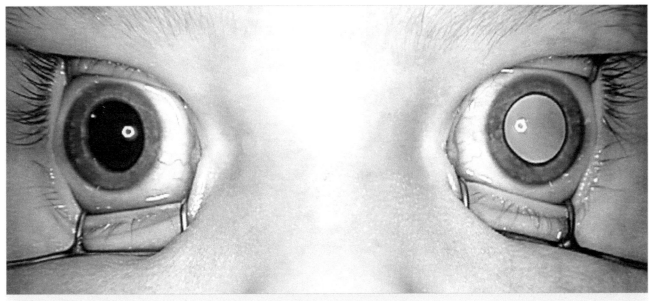

Fig. 97.2 Child with bilateral asymmetrical retinoblastoma with obvious leukocoria in the left eye.

large centers during the last decade. UWFA allows localization areas of vascular ectasia, capillary drop-off, and/or compromised vascular permeability that may be associated with tumoral activity. It may also aid in differentiation from other retinovascular diseases.

97.2.3 Fundus Autofluorescence

Autofluorescence may help detect intraocular calcifications. Autofluorescence of RB generally shows bright hyper-autofluorescence of the calcified portion and variable autofluorescence of the noncalcified portion. The presence, location, and

progression of intraocular calcifications facilitate in the diagnosis and management of RB.

97.2.4 Fundus Photography

Widefield fundus photography is extremely important during evaluation and follow-up of RB. Although it does not aid in diagnosis, it remains a vital tool for follow-up to detect subtle changes in time that may otherwise be unrecognized (▶ Fig. 97.3). These images can be tracked longitudinally over time to assess progression or arrest of RB. New ultra-widefield photography technologies allow documentation of the retinal periphery and better assessment during management.

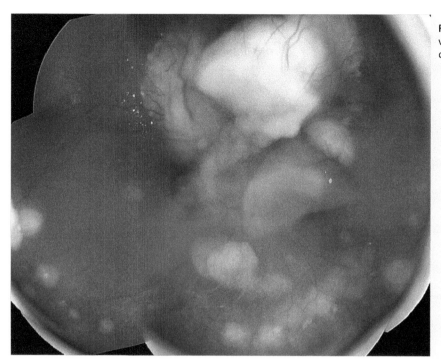

Fig. 97.3 Fundus photography demonstrates vitreous seeding, an ominous sign of advanced disease.

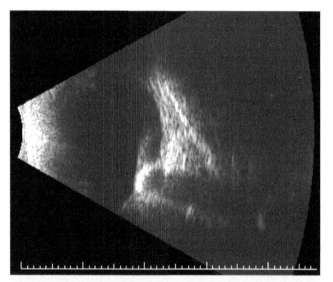

Fig. 97.4 Ultrasonography shows intraocular calcification in most cases with retinoblastoma.

97.2.5 Ultrasonography

A/B ultrasonography remains the imaging modality of choice to differentiate RB from other diseases. Calcification is found in most RB tumors at diagnosis. However, other disease entities in the RB differential diagnosis may also develop calcification. Ultrasonography allows the clinician to objectively follow RB regression over time. This technology is also important in the follow-up of vitreous seeds (▶ Fig. 97.4).

97.3 Critical Work-up

RB remains a clinical diagnosis. Fine needle aspiration biopsy should be avoided due to high risk of dissemination. Brain and orbit MRI with and without gadolinium should be performed under sedation in all children with RB to evaluate optic nerve invasion, extraorbital, and intracranial extension. Since children with germline RB are at risk for development of trilateral RB (i.e., bilateral RB and pineoblastoma), it is important to perform follow-up brain imaging for early diagnosis. MRI is the gold standard for intracranial involvement. CT scans should be avoided in all children with suspected RB because they may increase the secondary risk of malignancy in patients with germline mutations.

Unless extraocular extension is suspected or other neurological deficits are found on evaluation, lumbar puncture and bone marrow biopsy are not indicated. However, if extrascleral extension is suspected, additional studies should be performed since survival has been reported in association with high-dose alkylating agents and concomitant bone marrow transplant.

97.4 Management

RB management is mostly guided by the extent of the disease. Reese-Ellsworth (R-E) classification was originally developed in the late 1960s to predict visual prognosis in eyes treated with external beam radiation. Both tumor size and location were used in the classification system. However, the recent widespread use of chemotherapy for RB has led researchers to develop a new classification system since tumor size and location is less important than intraocular dissemination in this treatment modality. As a result, the International Classification

Table 97.1 International classification of retinoblastoma

Group	Subgroup	Clinical characteristics	Specific features
A	A	Small tumor	Retinoblastoma ≤ 3 mm
B	B	Larger tumor	Retinoblastoma > 3 mm
		Macula	≤ 3 mm to foveola
		Juxtapapillary	≤ 1.5 mm to disc
		Subretinal fluid	Clear subretinal fluid ≤ 3 mm from margin
C		Focal seeds	Retinoblastoma with:
	C1		Subretinal seeds ≤ 3 mm from retinoblastoma
	C2		Vitreous seeds ≤ 3 mm from retinoblastoma
	C3		Both subretinal and vitreous seeds ≤ 3 mm from retinoblastoma
D		Diffuse seeds	Retinoblastoma with:
	D1		Subretinal seeds > 3 mm from retinoblastoma
	D2		Vitreous seeds > 3 mm from retinoblastoma
	D3		Both subretinal and vitreous seeds > 3 mm from retinoblastoma
E	E	Extensive retinoblastoma	Extensive retinoblastoma occupying > 50% globe or
			Neovascular glaucoma
			Opaque media from hemorrhage in anterior chamber, vitreous, or subretinal space
			Invasion of postlaminar optic nerve, choroid (> 2 mm), sclera, orbit, anterior chamber

of Retinoblastoma was developed, placing special emphasis on intraocular seeding (▶ Table 97.1).

Management of RB tumors requires a multidisciplinary approach that may include an ocular oncologist, pediatric oncologist, pediatric ophthalmologist, pediatrician, interventional radiologist, and ocular pathologist. RB treatment is aimed at child survival. Globe salvage and preservation of vision are secondary goals. Early diagnosis remains the most crucial step in decreasing morbidity and mortality.

97.4.1 Treatment Options

Small Tumors

Tumors of ≤ 3 mm in vertical and horizontal diameter may be amenable to local ablative therapy if greater than 3 mm from the fovea and greater than 1 disc diameter from the optic disc. Multiple modalities may be used for tumor ablation. Laser treatments may be repeated monthly until complete tumor regression is documented. Indirect ophthalmoscopy and other diagnostic tools may determine tumor activity.

Large Tumors

Require multidrug intravenous and/or selective intra-arterial chemotherapeutic agents and focal consolidation (▶ Fig. 97.5). Currently, multiple chemotherapeutic options are available and no consensus among ocular oncologists exists on agents, delivery, cycles, or dose.

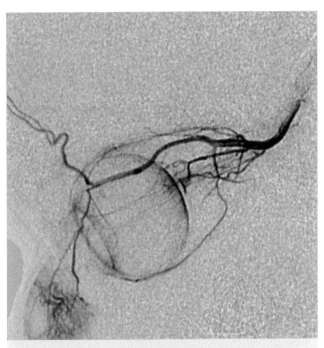

Fig. 97.5 Ophthalmic artery cannulation and angiography. Intra-arterial chemotherapy is performed after visual confirmation of selective catheterization of the ophthalmic artery with contrast.

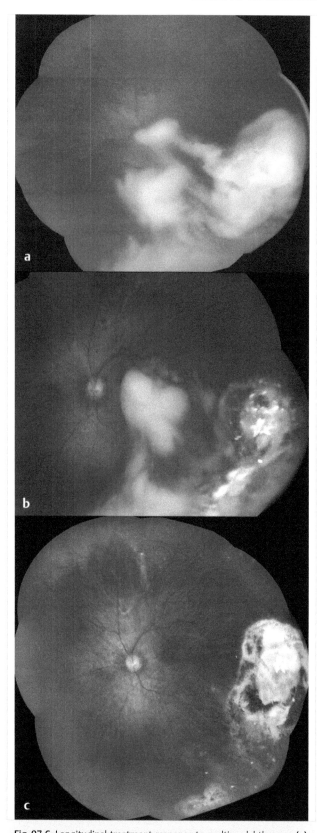

Seeding

When seeding is present, intravitreal chemotherapeutic agents have been reported to improve outcomes (▶ Fig. 97.6). Agents, dosing, and long-term outcomes associated with intravitreal agents are still under research.

97.4.2 Follow-up

Patients with RB need close follow-up. No standard guidelines are available. Monthly follow-up for patients with active RB should be considered. Children with inactive RB may be evaluated three to four times per year under anesthesia until the child can fully cooperate for a complete peripheral exam with indirect ophthalmoscopy.

Suggested Reading

[1] Villegas VM, Hess DJ, Wildner A, Gold AS, Murray TG. Retinoblastoma. Curr Opin Ophthalmol. 2013; 24(6):581–588
[2] Schefler AC, Cicciarelli N, Feuer W, Toledano S, Murray TG. Macular retinoblastoma: evaluation of tumor control, local complications, and visual outcomes for eyes treated with chemotherapy and repetitive foveal laser ablation. Ophthalmology. 2007; 114(1):162–169
[3] Francis JH, Brodie SE, Marr B, Zabor EC, Mondesire-Crump I, Abramson DH. Efficacy and toxicity of intravitreous chemotherapy for retinoblastoma: four-year experience. Ophthalmology. 2017; 124(4):488–495

Fig. 97.6 Longitudinal treatment response to multimodal therapy. **(a)** Fundus photograph of temporal group D2 retinoblastoma with globular seeding. **(b)** Fundus photograph demonstrating significant improvement after two treatments with intra-arterial chemotherapy, laser consolidation, and intravitreal chemotherapy. **(c)** Fundus photograph after four treatments with intra-arterial chemotherapy, laser consolidation, and intravitreal chemotherapy demonstrating significant improvement with associated atrophic changes.

98 Hamartomas of the Retina: Astrocytic and Retina/Retinal Pigment Epithelium

Mary E. Aronow and Arun D. Singh

Summary

Hamartomas are benign, focal malformations that resemble a neoplasm from the tissue of its origin. They can develop throughout the body in many organs such as the skin, brain, eye, kidney, and heart. Symptoms vary widely depending on the location and size of the growths. In the retina, they can take multiple forms: astrocytic hamartoma, solitary congenital hypertrophy of the retinal pigment epithelium (CHRPE), multifocal or grouped CHRPE, and combined hamartoma of the retina and retinal pigment epithelium.

Keywords: hamartomas, retinal pigment epithelium, focal malformations

98.1 Features

Hamartomas are benign, focal malformations that resemble neoplasms from the tissue of its origin. They can develop throughout the body in many organs such as the skin, brain, eye, kidney, and heart. Symptoms vary widely depending on the location and size of the growths. In the retina, they can take multiple forms: astrocytic hamartoma, solitary congenital hypertrophy of the retinal pigment epithelium (CHRPE), multifocal or grouped CHRPE, and combined hamartoma of the retina and retinal pigment epithelium (RPE).

98.1.1 Common Symptoms

Astrocytic Hamartoma

Typically asymptomatic.

CHRPE

Typically asymptomatic.

Multifocal/Grouped CHRPE

Typically asymptomatic.

Congenital Hamartoma of the Retina and RPE

Variable vision loss, metamorphopsia, or strabismus depending on severity.

98.1.2 Exam Findings

Astrocytic Hamartoma

Flat to minimally elevated, semitranslucent to white, lesion(s) arising from the retinal nerve fiber layer (▶ Fig. 98.1a). These are often subtle, and may be single or multiple. Some have glistening, yellow, nodular calcification ("mulberry" appearance).

CHRPE

Darkly pigmented (or depigmented), flat, round lesions at the level of the RPE with sharply demarcated, smooth, or scalloped borders (▶ Fig. 98.2). Some have a surrounding hyperpigmented or hypopigmented halo. The overlying retina and retinal vessels are normal. CHRPE frequently demonstrate central, "punched-out" lacunae.

Multifocal/Grouped CHRPE

These appear as multiple, circumscribed, flat areas of deep retinal pigmentation arranged in clusters. Lesions are

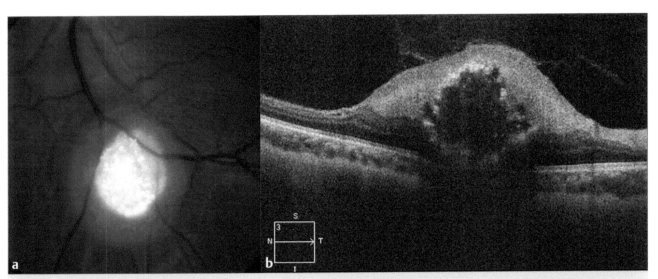

Fig. 98.1 Typical retinal astrocytic hamartoma associated with tuberous sclerosis complex. **(a)** Fundus photo demonstrating white retinal lesion. **(b)** Optical coherence tomography (OCT) demonstrating internal "moth-eaten" optically empty spaces primarily associated with the inner retina.

characteristically localized within a sector of the fundus (usually unilateral) with smaller areas surrounding larger ones, giving rise to a "bear track" appearance (▶ Fig. 98.3**a**). Occasionally, lesions may be amelanotic and are termed "polar bear tracks." In contrast to solitary CHRPE, lacunae are generally absent.

Congenital Hamartoma of the Retina and RPE

Lesions are most commonly unilateral and are frequently juxta-papillary and involving the macula. Epiretinal membrane for-

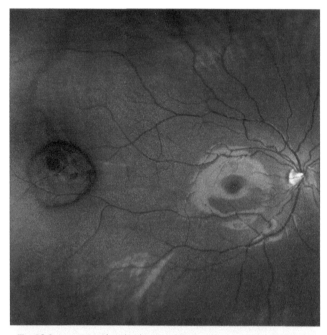

Fig. 98.2 Large peripheral solitary congenital hypertrophy of the retinal pigment epithelium (CHRPE). Ultra-widefield fundus photograph demonstrating temporal CHRPE with scalloped borders and lacunae.

mation is common. These hamartomas tend to have ill-defined borders, gray to black hyperpigmentation, and tortuosity of the large retinal vessels surrounding the optic nerve; this finding may be accentuated by contraction of fibroglial tissue (▶ Fig. 98.4**a**, ▶ Fig. 98.5**a**). When peripheral in location, dragging of the retinal vessels is common. Prominent capillary network formation and choroidal neovascularization can result in exudation.

98.2 Key Diagnostic Tests and Findings

98.2.1 Optical Coherence Tomography

Astrocytic Hamartoma

Confirms location within the retinal nerve fiber layer and may demonstrate internal "moth-eaten" optically empty spaces (▶ Fig. 98.1**b**).

CHRPE

Thickened or irregular RPE with thinning of the overlying outer retina due to loss of photoreceptors, and increased transmission through lacunae.

Multifocal/Grouped CHRPE

Retinal thinning with photoreceptor disruption.

Congenital Hamartoma of the Retina and RPE

An associated epiretinal membrane with corrugated retinal folds, and predominantly horizontal traction is common (▶ Fig. 98.4**b**, ▶ Fig. 98.5**b**). The membrane is usually epiretinal, but may have partial retinal interconnection, and less frequently communication with deeper aspects of the hamartoma (RPE).

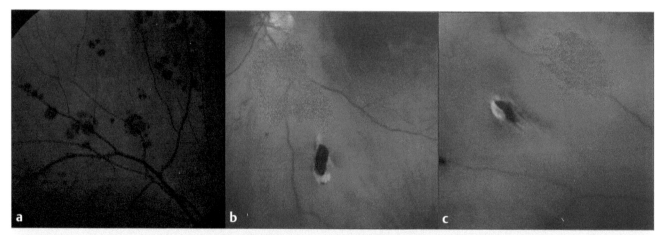

Fig. 98.3 **(a)** Grouped congenital hypertrophy of the retinal pigment epithelium or "bear tracks" with circular pigmentation without halos. **(b,c)** In contrast, pigmented ocular fundus lesions in patient with a known history of familial adenomatous polyposis demonstrate fewer lesions with an ovoid shape and surrounding halo.

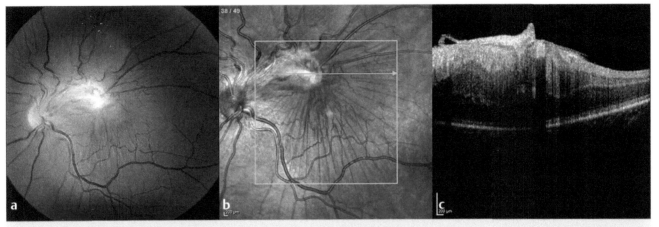

Fig. 98.4 **(a)** Fundus photograph of a combined hamartoma of the retina and RPE. **(b,c)** Optical coherence tomography through the central focus of the hamartoma demonstrates a thick preretinal membrane with deeper retinal involvement and apparent fold. (Courtesy of Emmanuel Y. Chang, MD, PhD, FACS, Retina and Vitreous of Texas, Houston, TX.)

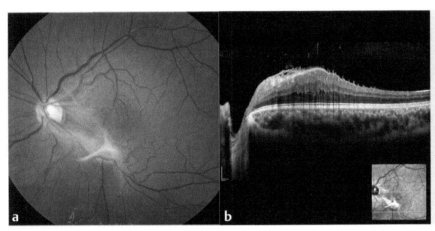

Fig. 98.5 **(a)** Combined hamartoma of the retina and retinal pigment epithelium. **(b)** Optical coherence tomography demonstrates thickened disorganized retina, epiretinal membrane, and fine overlying retinal traction peaks noted even off-center of the main foci of the hamartoma. (Courtesy of Henry Wiley, MD, National Eye Institute, National Institutes of Health, Bethesda, MD.)

98.2.2 Fluorescein Angiography or Ultra-Widefield Fluorescein Angiography

Astrocytic Hamartoma

Usually demonstrates filling of the hamartoma with variable leakage in later frames of the angiogram.

CHRPE

Retinal vascular changes, such as retinal capillary attenuation and overlying microaneurysms.

Multifocal/Grouped CHRPE

Early and stable hyperfluorescence within lesions without leakage.

Congenital Hamartoma of the Retina and RPE

Early hypofluorescence due to blockage corresponding to the pigmented region of the hamartoma. In the early phases,

microaneurysms and fine networks of capillaries may be seen. Late staining and leakage may be observed in later frames. Nonperfusion may be present in some cases.

98.2.3 Fundus Autofluorescence

Astrocytic Hamartoma

Calcium will demonstrate autofluorescence if present.

CHRPE

Generally hypo-autofluorescent.

Multifocal/Grouped CHRPE

Generally hypo-autofluorescent.

98.2.4 Ultrasonography

Astrocytic Hamartoma

B-scan ultrasonography confirms calcification if present.

Table 98.1 Systemic manifestations of tuberous sclerosis complex and neurofibromatosis

TSC		NF1	NF2
Major criteria		Café-au-lait spots	Vestibular schwannoma
Hypomelanotic macules		Axillary/inguinal freckles	Meningioma
Angiofibromas		Neurofibromas	Schwannoma
Ungal fibromas		**Optic nerve glioma**	**Glioma**
Shagreen patches		**Lisch nodules**	Neurofibroma
Astrocytic hamartomas		Sphenoid dysplasia	**PSC cataract**
Cortical dysplasias			
Subependymal nodules			
Subependymal giant cell astrocytoma			
Cardiac rhabdomyoma			
Lymphangioleiomyomatosis			
Angiomyolipomas			
Minor criteria			
"Confetti" skin lesions			
Dental enamel pits			
Intraoral fibromas			
Retinal achromic patches			
Multiple renal cysts			
Nonrenal hamartomas			

Abbreviations: TSC, tuberous sclerosis complex; NF, neurofibromatosis; PSC, posterior subcapsular.
Source: Adapted from the 2012 International TSC Consensus Conference.

98.2.5 Critical Work-up

Astrocytic Hamartoma

Can occur sporadically, or in association with tuberous sclerosis complex or neurofibromatosis. Referral for further work-up and genetic testing should be considered in individuals with other systemic features (▶ Table 98.1).

CHRPE

Congenital and have no known genetic predisposition or systemic associations.

Multifocal/Grouped CHRPE

Should be distinguished from the pigmented ocular fundus lesions (POFLs) associated with familial colon cancer syndromes (familial adenomatous polyposis [FAP]/Gardner syndrome and Turcot syndrome). POFLs are small (< 0.1 disc diameter), ovoid in shape, pigmented lesions located in the midperipheral and peripheral fundus (▶ Fig. 98.3**b,c**). POFLs may be surrounded by a hypopigmented halo and have a "comet-like" tail. They can be distinguished clinically from grouped CHRPE, as they are smaller, fewer in number, and more oval in shape compared to CHRPE. POFLs tend to occur bilaterally, while CHRPEs are frequently unilateral.

Congenital Hamartoma of the Retina and RPE

While this hamartoma occurs sporadically in most cases, there is an association with neurofibromatosis type 2 (and to a lesser extent neurofibromatosis type 1). There is a possible association with branchio-oculo-facial syndrome, brachio-oto-renal syndrome, juvenile nasopharyngeal angiofibroma, Gorlin Goltz syndrome, and ipsilateral Poland anomaly.

98.3 Management

98.3.1 Treatment Options

Astrocytic Hamartoma

Observation is warranted for asymptomatic lesions. For larger tumors (with visually significant fluid or exudation), photodynamic therapy may be helpful. There is a potential role for mammalian target of rapamycin inhibitors in more aggressive tumors; however, further investigation in this area is needed.

CHRPE

Observation warranted.

Multifocal/Grouped CHRPE

Observation warranted.

Congenital Hamartoma of the Retina and RPE

Visual symptoms result from membrane formation, progressive retinal traction, retinoschisis, accumulation lipid/fluid, retinal hemorrhage, vitreous hemorrhage, and rarely choroidal neovascularization. The role of membrane peeling and vitrectomy is controversial, but may be helpful in cases with preretinal gliosis or vitreous hemorrhage. Amblyopic therapy may benefit younger patients in some cases.

98.3.2 Follow-up

Astrocytic Hamartoma

Annual dilated examination with fundus photography for smaller, asymptomatic lesions. Astrocytic hamartoma may grow slowly over time.

CHRPE

Annual dilated examination with fundus photography. CHRPE may expand slowly over time. Rare cases of RPE adenoma (or adenocarcinoma) arising from CHRPE have been reported.

Multifocal/Grouped CHRPE

Annual dilated examination with fundus photography. Referral for colonoscopy/gastroenterology work-up when POFLs are observed. Four or more POFLs are a highly specific and sensitive marker for FAP.

Congenital Hamartoma of the Retina and RPE

Variable depending on the location and degree of symptoms.

Suggested Reading

[1] Shields CL, Say EAT, Fuller T, Arora S, Samara WA, Shields JA. Retinal astrocytic hamartoma arises in nerve fiber layer and shows "moth-eaten" optically empty spaces on optical coherence tomography. Ophthalmology. 2016; 123 (8):1809–1816

[2] Aronow ME, Nakagawa JA, Gupta A, Traboulsi EI, Singh AD. Tuberous sclerosis complex: genotype/phenotype correlation of retinal findings. Ophthalmology. 2012; 119(9):1917–1923

[3] Turell ME, Leonardy NJ, Singh AD. A unique presentation of grouped congenital hypertrophy of the retinal pigment epithelium. Ophthalmic Genet. 2011; 32(3):162–164

[4] Shields JA, Shields CL. Tumors and related lesions of the pigmented epithelium. Asia Pac J Ophthalmol (Phila). 2017; 6(2):215–223

Part X

Pediatric Vitreoretinal Disease

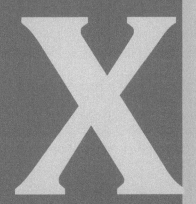

99 Coats Disease

Audina M. Berrocal and Linda A. Cernichiaro-Espinosa

Summary

Coats disease is within the differential diagnosis of exudative retinal detachments in children. Pathological vessels exist with aneurysmatic dilations and telangiectasia, which exudate over time resulting in retinal detachment. Classification of the disease is based on the severity of exudation that ranges from only vascular telangiectasia (stage 1) to phthisis bulbi (stage 5). Despite being a clinical diagnosis, it can be difficult to make a definitive diagnosis without the aid of ancillary testing in Coats such as fluorescein angiography, optical coherence tomography (OCT), and OCT angiography, and ultrasonography is crucial to avoid misdiagnosis. The objective of treatment is to diminish vascular endothelial growth factor (VEGF) and inflammatory mediators within the eye by ablative therapy, anti-VEGF intravitreal drugs, and/or surgery.

Keywords: Coats disease, telangiectasia, vascular disorder, children, exudative retinal detachment, external drainage, vitrectomy, VEGF, anti-VEGF

99.1 Features

Coats disease, first described in 1908, is a sporadic vascular disorder of the retina. The mean age of presentation is 5 years and is most commonly seen unilaterally in males. No direct genetic or racial association has been found in idiopathic Coats disease. A retinal–blood barrier disruption exists in pathological vessels. Inflammatory mediators are released, including vascular endothelial growth factor (VEGF), increasing vascular permeability that leads to exudative retinal detachment. As the disease progresses, hypoperfusion, ischemia, vitreoretinal pathological organization (preretinal fibrosis, subretinal fibrosis, or a combination), and retinoschisis or "retinal macrocysts" occur. It was classified in 2001 into the following stages depending on the severity.

- Stage 1: Retinal telangiectasia.
- Stage 2: Retinal telangiectasia and exudates (*2A* extrafoveal, *2B* foveal).
- Stage 3: Exudative retinal detachment (*3A* partial [extrafoveal or fovea] or *3B* total).
- Stage 4: Total retinal detachment and neovascular glaucoma.
- Stage 5: End-stage disease with or without phthisis bulbi.

99.1.1 Common Symptoms

Photopsia, and floaters common; decreased vision; disease progression can result in severe vision loss.

99.1.2 Exam Findings

Retinal vascular telangiectatic vessels, mild to extensive exudates, and "light bulb" aneurysms may be present (▶ Fig. 99.1, ▶ Fig. 99.2). In more severe cases, exudative retinal detachments may be seen (▶ Fig. 99.3). Deprivational strabismus can

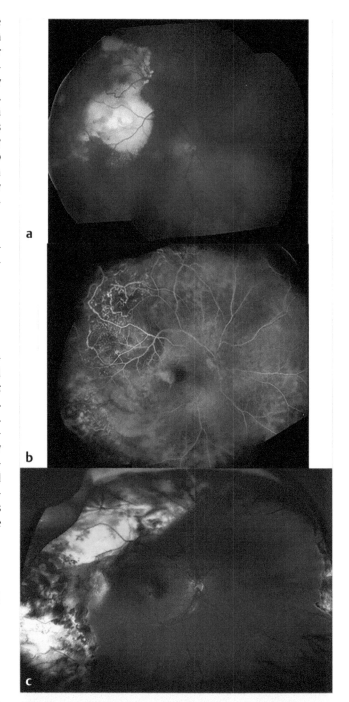

Fig. 99.1 (a) Widefield fundus photograph demonstrating yellow exudates that resemble a mass with overlying vascular abnormalities. (b) Widefield fluorescein angiography reveals vascular filling abnormalities and pooling. (c) Following 2 years of therapy and quiescence, widefield fundus photography document reactivation is noted as a yellow lesion posterior to the laser scars and temporal to the fovea.

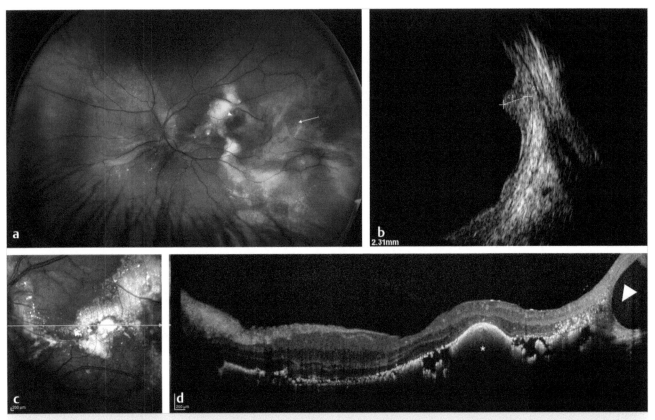

Fig. 99.2 Coats disease with extensive macular involvement. **(a)** Ultra-widefield fundus photograph reveals a subfoveal nodule (*), retinoschisis (*arrowhead*), and temporal extrafoveal fibrosis (*white arrow*). **(b)** B-scan ultrasonography demonstrates a highly reflective lesion in the equator without vascularization nor calcifications that correspond to the temporal extrafoveal fibrosis. **(c,d)** Optical coherence tomography facilitates visualization of extensive hyperreflective foci in the subretinal space and within the retina consistent with exudate. The subfoveal hyperreflective nodules are identified (*asterisk*). In addition, there is a temporal hyporeflective cyst (*arrowhead*).

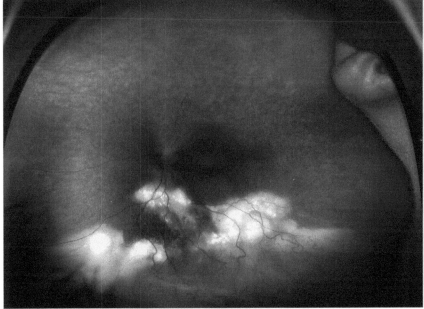

Fig. 99.3 Ultra-widefield photograph shows inferior Coats-like response in a patient with retinitis pigmentosa.

occur in early life. Leukocoria can be seen with a total retinal detachment, cataract, and/or cholesterol in anterior chamber. Less frequent, retinoschisis (retinal "macrocyst"), or vasoproliferative tumors (retinal angiomas or pseudoangiomatous retinal gliosis) can appear.

99.2 Key Diagnostic Tests and Findings

99.2.1 Optical Coherence Tomography

Hyperreflective cystic changes consistent with cystoid macular edema or schisis-like changes in the retina may be present. Subretinal fluid may be present. Hyperreflective lesions are exudates, subretinal fibrosis, sub-RPE fibrosis, and preretinal membranes. Optical coherence tomography is useful to guide treatment of cystoid macular edema, retinal detachments, and for surgical planning.

99.2.2 Fluorescein Angiography or Ultra-Widefield Fluorescein Angiography

Ultra-widefield fluorescein angiography is often instrumental for diagnosis and guiding treatment. Telangiectatic/aneurysmal hyperfluorescent lesions are typically present. Vascular leakage, pooling in the subretinal space, staining of fibrosis or scarring tissue, and leakage from neovascularization may all be present. Hypofluorescence indicative of capillary nonperfusion and retinal hemorrhages may be present. The fellow eye can present also vascular anomalies (e.g., aneurysms, peripheral avascular retina; ▶ Fig. 99.1, ▶ Fig. 99.2, ▶ Fig. 99.3).

99.2.3 Optical Coherence Tomography Angiography

Optical coherence tomography angiography is an emerging technology with preliminary findings in Coats disease that include nonperfusion, telangiectatic capillaries, vascularized fibrosis, and chorioretinal anastomosis.

99.2.4 Ultrasonography

If posterior pole visualization is obscured, ultrasonography helps characterize posterior pathologies, including retinal detachment. Crystals can be seen as hyperechoic multiple dots in the subretinal space. It is also a diagnostic tool to discern whether an intraocular mass or calcifications are found to help differentiate from retinoblastoma.

99.3 Critical Work-up

Depending on age and level of cooperation, examination under anesthesia should be considered to enable comprehensive evaluation. In severe Coats disease, one critical component to evaluation is rule-out retinoblastoma. In diffuse retinoblastoma, the fluorescein angiography (FA) may demonstrate a double image

of tortuous vessels. Other disorders that may be considered include retinopathy of prematurity, familial exudative vitreoretinopathy, Norrie disease, congenital cataract, persistent fetal vasculature. Secondary causes of Coats-like response should be considered, including retinitis pigmentosa, retinal vasculitis, Eales disease, infectious diseases, dyskeratosis congenita, among others.

99.4 Management

99.4.1 Treatment Options

Ablative Therapy

Treatment to the abnormal vasculature and hypoperfused areas guided by FA may be considered. Cryotherapy and laser photocoagulation have been advocated to be useful. Combination treatment with intravitreal pharmacotherapy is often used.

Intravitreal Pharmacotherapy

Both anti-VEGF agents and steroids can lower VEGF and inflammation and reduce the risk of progressive exudation. Initial treatment is often every 4 to 6 weeks.

Periocular and Systemic Steroids

Sub-Tenon triamcinolone provides an additional alternative for therapy to reduce the inflammatory burden. Oral steroids can serve as rescue therapy in refractory or postsurgical cases.

Surgery

Indications for surgical intervention include total retinal detachment (stage 3B) or a partial retinal detachment (3A) with poor response to previous therapies and/or organized vitreous that precludes intravitreal injection.

- *External drainage*: External drainage through a sclerotomy with an anterior chamber infusion is the option for bullous total retinal detachments. Subretinal fluid should be evaluated for the presence of malignant cells. Ablative therapy is typically performed to reduce the risk of recurrence.
- *Pars plana vitrectomy*: In select cases, vitrectomy may be utilized to remove tractional membranes, repair the retinal detachment, and apply endolaser. Silicone oil is often used as a long-acting tamponade. In these severe cases, the objective of treatment is globe salvage rather than vision improvement.
- *Scleral buckle*: Remains controversial in the management of Coats disease. May be considered in eyes with extensive circumferential traction. Caution must be taken to avoid anterior segment ischemia.
- *Enucleation*: Primarily considered for cases of blind painful eyes or in rare cases of blind where the diagnosis is in doubt and retinoblastoma is not able to be ruled out.

99.4.2 Follow-up

While undergoing therapy, follow-up is fairly frequent (e.g., every 4–8 weeks). Once stabilized, the follow-up interval is extended. Depending on the age of the patient and visual potential of the eye, amblyopia management should also be coordinated with a pediatric ophthalmologist.

Suggested Reading

[1] Daruich AL, Moulin AP, Tran HV, Matet A, Munier FL. Subfoveal nodule in Coats' disease: toward an updated classification predicting visual prognosis. Retina. 2017; 37(8):1591–1598

[2] Suzani M, Moore AT. Intraoperative fluorescein angiography-guided treatment in children with early Coats' disease. Ophthalmology. 2015; 122(6): 1195–1202

[3] Sein J, Tzu JH, Murray TG, Berrocal AM. Treatment of Coats' disease with combination therapy of intravitreal bevacizumab, laser, photocoagulation, and Sub-Tenon corticosteroids. Ophthalmic Surg Lasers Imaging Retina. 2016; 47 (5):443–449

[4] Ong SS, Buckley EG, McCuen BW, II, et al. Comparison of visual outcomes in Coats' disease. A 20-year experience. Ophthalmology. 2017; 124(9):1368–1376

100 Retinopathy of Prematurity

Avery E. Sears and Jonathan E. Sears

Summary

Retinopathy of prematurity (ROP) is a vasoproliferative disorder of premature infants. Although the pathogenesis of ROP is naturally specific to severely premature infants, ROP is at the nexus of a progressive understanding of angiogenesis and retinal development that has led to the two-step hypothesis of neovascularization applicable to other neovascular disorders of the eye. The eye normally has a 40-week gestation to complete retinovascular development, but premature birth separates the fetus from the maternal circulation, thus requiring oxygen supplementation to prevent infant death. Unfortunately, the decrease in mortality is accompanied by oxygen-induced toxicity to susceptible premature developing tissues, such as the retina. This chapter reviews the clinically relevant history, epidemiology, oxygen-based mechanism of disease, and current diagnosis and management of ROP.

Keywords: cryotherapy for ROP, early treatment for ROP, hyperoxia, neovascularization

100.1 Features

Retinopathy of prematurity (ROP) is a vasoproliferative disorder of premature infants. The retina begins to develop at age 16 weeks in utero and typically completes development from the optic nerve to the nasal and temporal ora serrata by 36 and 40 weeks of gestational age (GA), respectively. There are 13 million premature births worldwide annually, leading to 150,000 new cases of infant blindness per year. The survival of premature infants is continually increasing as developed and undeveloped countries improve premature infants' chance of survival.

First reported in 1942, as retrolental fibroplasia (RLF) in an infant weighing less than 3 pounds at birth, ROP and associated neovascularization is thought to occur from an initial ischemic insult followed by reactive proliferation of blood vessels. The causal relationship with oxygen has been demonstrated through the first phase which is characterized by retinovascular growth attenuation and vascular obliteration during hyperoxia (at this point hyperoxic and ischemic) which results in the second phase of vasoproliferation from the same ischemic areas that were hypoxic and ischemic. A key stimulator of vasoproliferation, vascular endothelial growth factor (VEGF), is induced by hypoxia-inducible factor (HIF), a transcription factor that is suppressed by hyperoxia of phase 1. The fetus is normally subject to "normoxic hypoxia," a state in which oxygen concentrations rarely reach 20 mm Hg oxygen, in contrast to an adult who has 50% higher oxygen concentrations in arterioles. For example, oxygen saturation in utero may be closer to 80 to 85% in comparison to ex utero saturations of 91 to 95% in at-risk neonates receiving oxygen supplementation. In addition, fetal hemoglobin is designed to deliver oxygen in low oxygen tensions unlike the saturations seen after birth.

100.1.1 Common Symptoms

Infants are asymptomatic and must be screened; children whose ROP has subsided are at greater risk of developing myopia, strabismus, and amblyopia.

100.1.2 Exam Findings

A critical clinical sign of active ROP is plus disease, first defined as venous engorgement at the disc, but vascular tortuosity can be seen posterior to the ridge, in midperipheral retina and can affect tortuosity and engorgement of arterioles as well. Aggressive posterior retinopathy of prematurity (AP-ROP), a relatively new term, is recognized in children who have very active early disease (typically in corrected GA [CGA] of 34 weeks or less). This is primarily zone 1 disease with massive PLUS and quite often flat neovascularization. It is not unusual for AP-ROP to be accompanied by dilated iris vessels in a circular pattern, the pupillary margin simulating neovascularization of the iris.

ROP is described by zone and by stage. Zone 1 is described as vascularized retina that has the peripheral circumference less than or equal to a diameter twice the radius of the disc to the fovea, whereas zone 2 is described as having a circumference anterior to zone 1 and nearly adjacent to the nasal ora serrata. Zone 3 is the temporal crescent anterior to zone 2 temporally (▶ Fig. 100.1). Practically, this means that if the disc and the edge of vascularized retina can be seen with a single image using a 28D lens anywhere, the infant is zone 1. If scleral depression nasally shows any avascular retina outside of zone 1, the infant is zone 2. Analogously, if the retina is avascular temporally but vascularized nasally, the infant is zone 3. Concerning staging, stage 0 is immature normally developing retina; stage 1 is a sharp border between vascular and avascular tissue, with or without a flat white demarcation line; stage 2 is where the demarcation line is elevated; stage 3 is neovascularization on the ridge, accompanied or not by a fibrovascular membrane; stage 4a is retinal detachment sparing the fovea, 4b with fovea involved; and stage 5 is total retinal detachment (▶ Fig. 100.2).

100.2 Key Diagnostic Tests and Findings

100.2.1 Optical Coherence Tomography

May help distinguish 4a detachments from tractional schisis. OCT may also identify foveal developmental abnormalities, including intraretinal fluid.

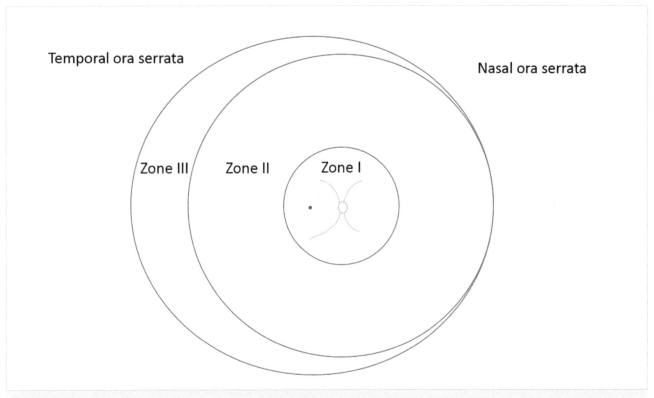

Fig. 100.1 Zones of retinopathy of prematurity denote area of vascularized retina. Note that zone 1 is a circle of radius twice the distance of the nerve to the fovea, zone 2 includes zone 1 and retina posterior to the nasal ora serrata, whereas zone 3 eyes are described as vascularized nasally but remaining avascular temporally.

100.2.2 Fluorescein Angiography or Ultra-Widefield Fluorescein Angiography

Remains the most revealing diagnostic test for ROP severity but is labor intensive and might expose the infant to unnecessary risk. However, diagnostic imaging will reduce overtreatment and/or the risk of missing a child that requires treatment. FA/ UWFA demonstrates the extent of nonperfusion and areas of leakage (▶ Fig. 100.3).

100.2.3 Telemedicine

A promising alternative to ROP examinations; although the specificity and sensitivity of fundus photos is not as accurate as a physical exam, telemedicine can prevent blindness because fundus photos can gauge which infants require referral for a dilated exam, termed "referral-warranted" ROP with sensitivities and specificities of 100 and 99%, respectively. This remote imaging solves the logistical problems of NICUs not served by competent screeners, as nonophthalmic personnel can obtain the pictures for electronic viewing by a specialist. As cameras become less expensive and in-house photographers more experienced,

telemedicine also offers the chance to quantify features of ROP such as extent of PLUS disease.

100.3 Critical Work-up

The consensus in western countries is that any child weighing less than 1,500 g at birth, less than 32 weeks of CGA at birth, or considered at risk by the NICU staff requires an exam. The first exam should be performed at 4 to 6 weeks after birth. Generally, this is a safe practice in countries that provide access to oxygen blenders and accurate oxygen saturation monitors. However, in underdeveloped countries there is a phenomenon of very large, older babies who develop disease, presumably because their NICUs unfortunately have only very high oxygen delivery systems that are unable to dilute oxygen from 100%. The ROP exam is usually performed after dilation with Cyclomydril (1.0% phenylephrine and 0.5% cylogyl mixture), a drop of tetracaine, 28D lens, scleral depressor, and lid speculum. The importance of serial exams cannot be minimized, as often it is not the exact findings but rather the cadence of disease that predicts the need for treatment. For example, most children develop ROP at 30 weeks, regardless of their CGA at birth, and will reach treatable ROP at 35 to 37 weeks. Oxygen setting and sepsis can affect the clinical course of ROP.

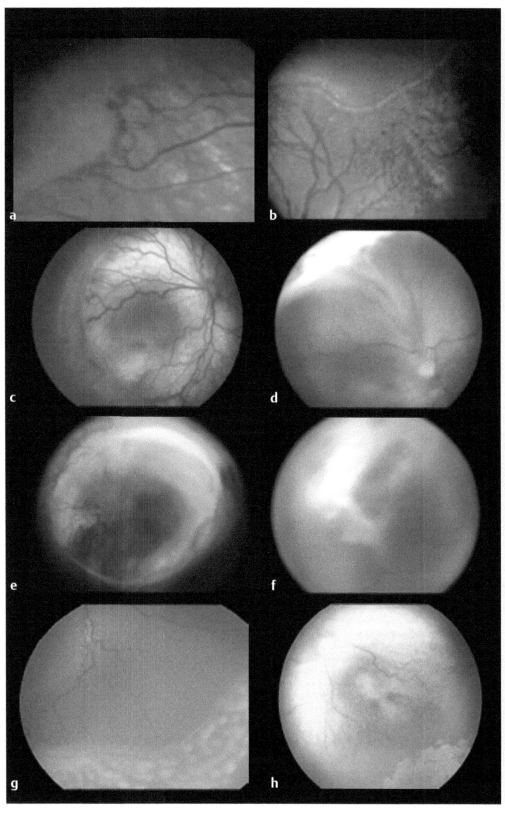

Fig. 100.2 Retinopathy of prematurity is also classified into stages: **(a)** stage 1, **(b)** stage 2, **(c)** stage 3, **(d)** stage 4a, **(e,f)** stage 5. **(g)** Type 1 disease just after laser therapy and **(h)** 2 weeks post–laser therapy. Note the regression of stage 3 disease, here with fibrovascular membrane present, and PLUS disease.

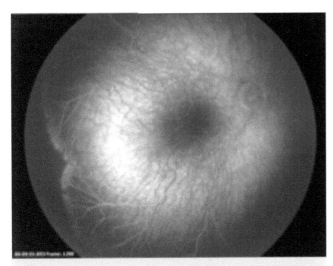

Fig. 100.3 Vascular arrest 2 months after bevacizumab injection for type 1 zone 1 disease.

The ETROP classification for treat versus watch (i.e., 1-week follow-up). Note the emphasis on zone 1 disease accounts for the increase in zone 1 eyes as a consequence of infants with lower CGA surviving premature birth.

- Type 1 (treat):
  - Zone I any stage ROP with plus.
  - Zone I stage 3 with or without plus.
  - Zone II stage 2 or 3 with plus.
- Type II (watch):
  - Zone I stage 1 or 2 no plus.
  - Zone II stage 2 or 3 no plus.

100.4 Management

100.4.1 Treatment Options

Cryotherapy

The Cryotherapy for ROP (Cryo-ROP) study was the first to demonstrate the relationship of low birth weight and low CGA to ROP. Cryo-ROP found that cryotherapy of the peripheral avascular retina decreased the risk of unfavorable outcome twofold from 43 to 21.8%. It also definitively demonstrated that prevention of retinal detachment could be achieved by ablating the avascular retina because it is the substrate for disease. Cryo is currently used less frequently than laser, if at all.

Laser

The Early Treatment for ROP (ETROP) study used laser rather than cryotherapy. ETROP differed from Cryo-ROP most importantly because it distinguished the difference between eyes with posterior disease, in zone 1, from eyes with zone 2 disease. This randomized prospective trial tested whether the use of laser in eyes that were less severe than the standard threshold criteria might increase the chance of preventing retinal detachment or fold and has provided the clearest and most up to date guidelines regarding the treatment of ROP with laser (Box 100.1 (p.407)). Early laser reduced the risk of unfavorable outcome by 6% from 15 to 9.6%. Especially valuable is the concept of type II (watch and wait, reassess in 1 week) disease versus type I (treat within 24 hours) disease (Box 100.1 (p.407)). Laser can be performed under conscious sedation. Typically, a midperipheral zone 2 eye requires 1,200 laser spots using a diode laser with power that ranges from 140 to 180 mW, near confluent-to-confluent laser (▶ Fig. 100.2). Care should be taken to avoid ablating the long posterior ciliary artery, inducing hypotony, or the iris, which can transfer energy to the lens and induce phacolytic glaucoma and phthisis bulbi. Post-laser prednisolone acetate drops QID and cylogyl 0.5 to 1.0% drops BID should be continued for 7 days.

Anti-VEGF

The use of anti-VEGF therapy was first examined in a randomized prospective trial to test bevacizumab for the treatment of ROP (BEAT-ROP). Despite initial concerns regarding the choice of dose, the primary outcome measure, the lack of long-term ocular and systemic follow-up, and the disregard for any harmful developmental features of anti-VEGF therapy in this patient population, this trial set guidelines showing for the first time that anti-VEGF improved the anatomical outcomes of zone 1 disease compared to laser. Minimizing the dose is important and no more than 0.5 mg bevacizumab (0.02 mL of 2.5 mg/mL bevacizumab). Recent trials have shown efficacy using 0.03 mg bevacizumab.

Oxygen

Oxygen itself is a drug, and the judicious use of it in older children (increasing oxygen at CGA > 34 weeks) can decrease the neovascular drive and leakiness of retinal vessels. The supplemental oxygen to treat ROP (STOP-ROP) clearly showed that increasing oxygen when stage 3 disease is manifest can reduce PLUS disease and decrease neovascularization. Often increasing oxygen saturations in babies older than 34 weeks can reduce the need for treatment. Although a biphasic approach to oxygen administration (85–91% targets less than 34 weeks of CGA and > 95% saturation older than 34 weeks of CGA) prevents ROP, this has not been tested in a randomized prospective trial and hence oxygen standards remain at static 91 to 95%.

Surgical Management of ROP

Surgical management of ROP was revolutionized by the advent of lens-sparing vitrectomy. It successfully demonstrated that entering the eye through pars plana 1.5 mm posterior to the surgical limbus could save most 4a and the majority of 4b eyes without immediate cataract formation or iatrogenic tears. The principle goals of stage 4 surgery are to not make a retinal break, to induce a PVD if possible, and to release the anteroposterior vitreoretinal traction from the ridge to the lens. Hemostasis is critical. Stage 5 surgery requires lensectomy and has limited success anatomically and functionally. There is ongoing debate as to the merits of what is considered a futile but heroic attempt to prevent blindness. The visual outcomes of stage 5 are not near the visual outcomes of stage 4 surgery. The former often averages Hand Motion/Light Perception acuity, whereas the latter is generally between 20/40 and 20/200.

100.4.2 Follow-up

As discussed, close follow-up and serial exams are critical in these at-risk eyes. Once the disease is stabilized, ongoing follow-up is important to manage sequelae that may develop and to provide early intervention as needed for amblyopic management.

Suggested Reading

[1] Hartnett ME, Lane RH. Effects of oxygen on the development and severity of retinopathy of prematurity. J AAPOS. 2013; 17(3):229–234

[2] Sears JE, Hoppe G, Ebrahem Q, Anand-Apte B. Prolyl hydroxylase inhibition during hyperoxia prevents oxygen-induced retinopathy. Proc Natl Acad Sci U S A. 2008; 105(50):19898–19903

[3] Palmer EA, Hardy RJ, Dobson V, et al. Cryotherapy for Retinopathy of Prematurity Cooperative Group. 15-year outcomes following threshold retinopathy of prematurity: final results from the multicenter trial of cryotherapy for retinopathy of prematurity. Arch Ophthalmol. 2005; 123(3):311–318

[4] Good WV, Early Treatment for Retinopathy of Prematurity Cooperative Group. Final results of the Early Treatment for Retinopathy of Prematurity (ETROP) randomized trial. Trans Am Ophthalmol Soc. 2004; 102:233–248, discussion 248–250

[5] Mintz-Hittner HA, Kennedy KA, Chuang AZ, BEAT-ROP Cooperative Group. Efficacy of intravitreal bevacizumab for stage 3 + retinopathy of prematurity. N Engl J Med. 2011; 364(7):603–615

101 Familial Exudative Vitreoretinopathy

Edward H. Wood, Prethy Rao, and Kimberly A. Drenser

Summary

Familial exudative vitreoretinopathy (FEVR) is an inherited vitreoretinal disease characterized by abnormal retinal vascular development. Potential features include progressive retinal capillary dropout, vessel dragging, retinal folds, exudation, hemorrhage, neovascularization, vitreoretinal interface changes, and retinal detachment. The most prominent feature on fundus photography is peripheral avascular retina, which is highlighted with ultra-widefield fluorescein angiography also reveal prominent features. FEVR requires long-term follow-up with frequent exams and intervention as warranted.

Keywords: LAPPEL, retinopathy of prematurity, vitreoretinal disease

101.1 Features

Familial exudative vitreoretinopathy (FEVR) is an inherited vitreoretinal disease characterized by abnormal retinal vascular development. FEVR is a lifelong disease that often shows progression with periods of quiescence and exacerbation and has been linked to the Wnt pathway. Wnt signaling is an evolutionarily conserved signal transduction pathway that controls the fate of cells during animal development and functions in the process of maintenance, repair, and self-renewal of adult tissues. Genetic associations of FEVR have been identified, roughly 50% of which can be linked to four causative genes (FZD4, LRP5, TSPAN12, and NDP) pertaining to the Wnt-signaling pathway. The expressivity and inheritance patterns (autosomal dominant, autosomal recessive, and X-linked recessive) are variable. Genetic testing is useful in guiding prognostication, family planning, and potential future therapeutic intervention.

101.1.1 Common Symptoms

Usually asymptomatic, possible decreased visual acuity, strabismus (typically esotropia) and strabismic amblyopia, latent nystagmus (as a consequence of binocularity disruption), and/or leukocoria.

101.1.2 Exam Findings

Bilateral (85%) but asymmetric exam findings which correspond to clinical staging (▶ Table 101.1). Peripheral avascular retina is the most prominent feature. Clinical features may include progressive retinal vascular dropout, vessel dragging, exudation, hemorrhage, and neovascularization. Also possible are retinal arterial tortuosity and dragging, supernumerary retinal vessels emerging from the optic nerve head, and aberrant circumferential retinal vessels with loops and/or shunts. Radial and/or circumferential retinal folds appearing as knife-like folds extending anteriorly from the optic nerve are typical (▶ Fig. 101.1). Preretinal vitreous organization; subretinal

exudation; and serous, tractional, and/or combined retinal detachment are possible.

101.2 Key Diagnostic Tests and Findings

101.2.1 Optical Coherence Tomography

Optical coherence tomography may reveal various forms of posterior hyaloid organization including vitreomacular traction, vitreopapillary traction, vitreoretinal fold, and vitreous laser scar adhesion. Other possible findings include blunted foveal contour, persistent fetal foveal architecture, cystoid macular edema, intraretinal exudates, subretinal lipid deposition, dry or edematous retinal folds, and disruption of the ellipsoid zone (EZ).

101.2.2 Fluorescein Angiography or Ultra-Widefield Fluorescein Angiography

Fluorescein angiography and/or ultra-widefield fluorescein angiography (UWFA) are used in cases where FEVR is suspected but not confirmed and also for screening of asymptomatic patient relatives. UWFA is particularly useful for assessing clinically normal FEVR patients who routinely show prominent angiographic changes such as retinal nonperfusion, delayed arteriovenous transit, venous–venous shunts (and a lack of arterial-venous shunts as seen in retinopathy of prematurity [ROP]), blunting of perifoveal capillaries, and fine bulbous vascular endings in a fern-like branching pattern at the juncture of vascularized and avascularized retina (▶ Fig. 101.2). LAPPEL (Late phase Angiographic Posterior and PEripheral vascular Leakage) characterized by fuzzy retinal vessel margins associated with leakage peaking around 3-minute transit time

Table 101.1 Stages and clinical features of familial exudative vitreoretinopathy (FEVR)

FEVR stage	Clinical features
Subclinical	Mild straightening of vessels Mild peripheral nonperfusion
Stage 1	Avascular peripheral retina without extraretinal vessels
Stage 2	Avascular peripheral retina with extraretinal vessels 2a. No exudate 2b. Exudate
Stage 3	Partial retinal detachment—fovea spared 2a. No exudate 2b. Exudate
Stage 4	Partial retinal detachment—fovea spared 2a. No exudate 2b. Exudate
Stage 5	Total retinal detachment 2a. No exudate 2b. Exudate

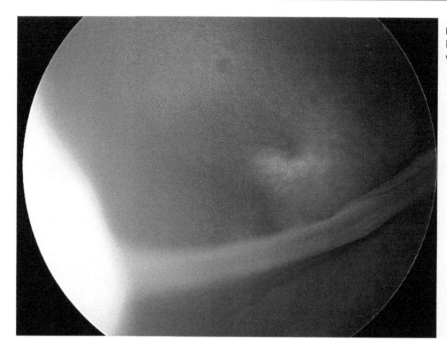

Fig. 101.1 Fundus photograph demonstrating knife-like dry fold in familial exudative vitreoretinopathy.

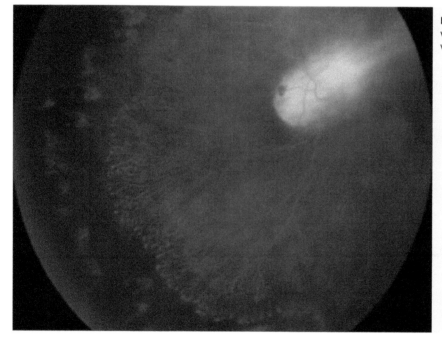

Fig. 101.2 Fluorescein angiography shows fine vascular bulbous endings in this familial exudative vitreoretinopathy example.

predicts future areas of retinal capillary dropout, and retinal neovascularization is possible (▶ Fig. 101.3).

101.2.3 Fundus Photography

Fundus photography, particularly ultra-widefield photography, is useful for documenting pathology and monitoring progression.

101.3 Critical Work-up

ROP should be considered as a differential diagnosis. In addition to conventional ROP, a subset of premature patients have been identified to have Wnt-signaling abnormalities and features consistent with FEVR and has been referred to as fROP. This should be considered in a minimally premature patient with an aggressive retinopathy associated with the following characteristics: lack of prominent ridge tissue, with more prominent arborization of vessels; lack of arterial-venous shunts, with the presence of venous–venous shunts; more relative exudation and vessel pruning than seen in ROP alone; and gestational age greater than 26 weeks with lower than predicted birth weight. Other disorders to consider based on clinical features include Norrie disease (X-linked, sensorineural hearing loss, and NDP positive), incontinentia pigmenti, persistent fetal vasculature, Coats disease, and retinoblastoma.

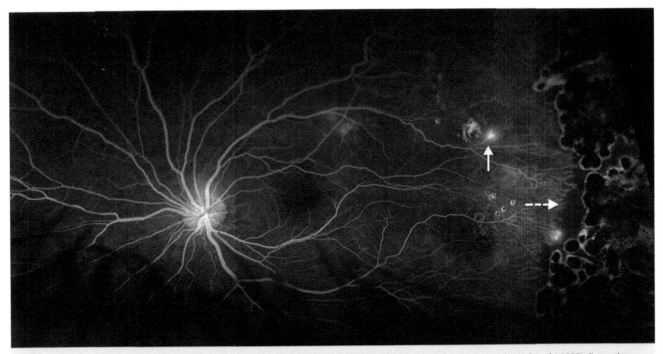

Fig. 101.3 Ultra-widefield fluorescein angiography in familial exudative vitreoretinopathy with neovascularization (*arrow*) and LAPPEL (Late phase Angiographic Posterior and PEripheral vascular Leakage) with fine vascular bulbous endings (*dashed arrow*).

101.4 Management

101.4.1 Treatment Options

LAPPEL

Topical therapy such as prednisolone acetate and topical non-steroidal anti-inflammatory drug may improve LAPPEL and potentially decrease the progression of capillary dropout.

FEVR Stage 2 or Higher

For avascular retina with neovascularization, targeted laser photocoagulation to avascular retina and/or beds of capillary drop-out is utilized. UWFA may help identify the border between vascular and avascular retina. Anti-VEGF agents may be particularly useful in cases where adequate laser uptake is not possible (e.g., prominent exudation or exudative-related detachments). A potential future therapeutic agent is the administration of the Norrin protein, which activates Wnt-signaling pathways that have a protective effect on human retinal endothelial cells.

FEVR Stage 3 or Higher

Decisions around surgical management in FEVR are complex. Various anatomic features may be predictive of feasibility of surgical repair. "Wet" retinal folds are amenable to surgery, whereas "dry" knife-like folds (i.e., photoreceptor-to-photoreceptor apposition) are not. When surgical management is chosen, typically pars plana/plicata vitrectomy is performed. Some groups elect to also utilize plasmin enzyme to facilitate the surgical dissection.

101.4.2 Follow-up

Patients must be informed that this is a lifelong disease that will require regular monitoring of disease activity and progression as well as assessment of response to treatment. Patients need follow-up for life often with fundus photography and wide-field angiography every 6 to 12 months.

Suggested Reading

[1] Clevers H. Eyeing up new Wnt pathway players. Cell. 2009; 139(2):227–229

[2] Wu W-C, Drenser K, Trese M, Capone A, Jr, Dailey W. Retinal phenotype-genotype correlation of pediatric patients expressing mutations in the Norrie disease gene. Arch Ophthalmol. 2007; 125(2):225–230

[3] Yonekawa Y, Thomas BJ, Drenser KA, Trese MT, Capone A, Jr. Familial exudative vitreoretinopathy: spectral-domain optical coherence tomography of the vitreoretinal interface, retina, and choroid. Ophthalmology. 2015; 122(11): 2270–2277

[4] Drenser KA, Dailey W, Vinekar A, Dalal K, Capone A, Jr, Trese MT. Clinical presentation and genetic correlation of patients with mutations affecting the FZD4 gene. Arch Ophthalmol. 2009; 127(12):1649–1654

102 Persistent Fetal Vasculature

Suruchi Bhardwaj Bhui, Vaidehi S. Dedania, and Yasha S. Modi

Summary

Persistent fetal vasculature (PFV) occurs when the fetal vasculature of the eye fails to undergo the normal involution process. While PFV may have a predominant anterior or posterior manifestation, the majority of cases have a combination of both anterior and posterior features. This results in several ocular sequelae including microphthalmos, cataracts, secondary angle-closure glaucoma, tractional retinal detachment, and vitreous hemorrhage. The majority of PFV cases are idiopathic, unilateral, and have no systemic associations. PFV, when bilateral, however, is often associated with systemic syndromes. Anterior PFV is often associated with the following findings: elongated ciliary processes, cataracts, or presence of a retrolental opacity. Patients with posterior PFV may have elevated vitreous membranes extending from the optic nerve, retinal folds and/or dysplasia, tractional retinal detachments, or optic nerve hypoplasia. For mild cases, observation is often appropriate. Treatment is directed at clearing the visual axis (removal of the cataract and retrolental space) and alleviating traction on the retina induced by the persistent hyaloid stalk. Outcomes are highly contingent on the extent of ocular involvement at presentation. Anterior PFV patients have better outcomes relative to combined or posterior PFV patients. Additionally, aggressive amblyopia management is imperative to achieve a functional visual outcome.

Keywords: hyaloid artery, leukocoria, persistent fetal vasculature, persistent hyperplastic primary vitreous, stalk

102.1 Features

Persistent fetal vasculature (PFV) occurs when the fetal vasculature of the eye fails to undergo the normal involution process. The cause of this incomplete regression of the fetal vasculature remains unknown. Formerly referred to as persistent hyperplastic primary vitreous (PHPV), PFV has become the preferred nomenclature as it includes all components of the fetal intraocular vasculature. During fetal development, the hyaloid artery and other blood vessels proliferate from the posterior to the anterior pole of the eye. They form a network of vessels that extend to cover the anterior and posterior surface of the lens (i.e., anterior and posterior tunica vasculosa lentis) and the iris (i.e., pupillary membranes), providing nutrition to the intraocular structures in the setting of an immature anterior chamber and absent aqueous humor. Persistence of these structures *ex utero* may result in several ocular sequelae, including microphthalmos, cataract, secondary angle-closure glaucoma, tractional retinal detachment, and vitreous hemorrhage. PFV is mostly idiopathic, unilateral, and have no other systemic associations; when bilateral, however, it is often associated with systemic syndromes such as Trisomy 13, Walker-Warburg syndrome, anencephaly, Norrie disease, oculo-dento osseous disease, and oculopalatal cerebral dwarfism.

102.1.1 Common Symptoms

Decreased vision may be present.

102.1.2 Exam Findings

Ocular findings associated with PFV include morning glory anomaly, Peter anomaly, macular hypoplasia, microcornea, and microphthalmos. On presentation, the patient may have a predominant anterior or posterior involvement. The majority, however, have a combination of both anterior and posterior features. While there is likely some overlap in terminology between anterior and posterior PFV, the features of each are listed below.

Anterior PFV

- *Persistent pupillary membranes*: Filamentary remnants of the anterior tunica vasculosa lentis; may rarely cause complications including spontaneous hyphema or corneal clouding when attached to the endothelium.
- *Retrolental opacification*: Due to persistent posterior tunica vasculosa lentis; may be centrally located and small or may extend to the ciliary processes.
- *Cataract*: A common feature associated with retrolental opacification.
- *Elongated ciliary processes*: Can occasionally be seen behind the lens and extending into the retrolental opacity.
- *Presence of iridohyaloid vessels*: Radially oriented blood vessels in the iris stroma act as a connection between the posterior and anterior tunica vasculosa lentis; when persistent can lead to notching in the pupillary sphincter or frank entropion or ectropion uveae.
- *Shallow anterior chamber angle*: May be secondary to an intumescent, cataractous lens or rotation of the ciliary body and lens.

Posterior PFV

- *Persistent hyaloid artery*: The most common remnant of the hyaloid artery is observed as an indistinct vessel in Cloquet's canal that may extend from the optic nerve to the posterior lens surface (▶ Fig. 102.1, ▶ Fig. 102.2); commonly referred to as the "stalk" in PFV that is visualized on ultrasound. The hyaloid artery may have persistent perfusion, which can be visualized on fluorescein angiography.
- *Congenital retina nonattachment*: Strong adherence of the fetal vasculature to the retinal may induce a tractional retinal detachment; there may also be elevated vitreous membranes emanating from the optic nerve; retina may be drawn up into the stalk in more severe cases.
- *Retinal folds*: May be due to persistent traction from the stalk.
- *Retinal dysplasia*: May manifest as disruption of the retinal laminations or "microscopic" dysplasia with grossly normal macular anatomy; both may limit vision despite adequate surgical and amblyopia therapy.

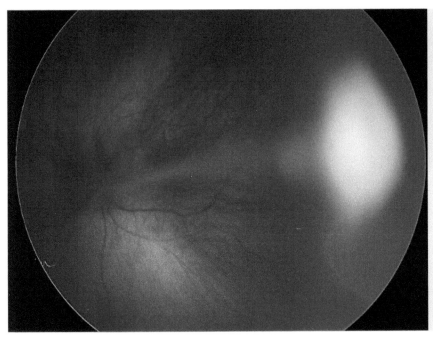

Fig. 102.1 Fundus photograph of a persistent hyaloid artery or "stalk" extending from the optic nerve to the posterior surface of the lens. (Image courtesy of Maxwell Stem and Michael T. Trese.)

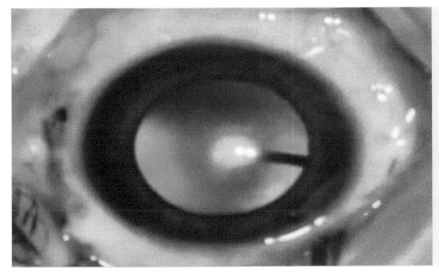

Fig. 102.2 Anterior segment intraoperative image demonstrating a persistent hyaloid artery attaching slightly nasally on the posterior surface of the lens.

- *Macular abnormalities*: Typically results from traction from the vascular stalk and may include macular schisis, cystoid spaces, and an absent foveal pit. In severe cases, there may be a macular fold.
- *Optic nerve head hypoplasia or dysplasia*: Both will inevitably limit long-term visual prognosis.

Combined PFV

Combination of anterior and posterior forms. Frequently occur together.

Incomplete Regression of Fetal Vasculature in Otherwise Normal Eyes

- *Mittendorf dot*: Represents the insertion of the hyaloid artery at the posterior lens; a common benign congenital anomaly found inferonasal to the center of the lens and is seen with a prevalence of 0.7 to 2.0%; frequently discovered on routine exam as it rarely affects vision.
- *Bergmeister papilla*: A fibrovascular tissue remnant of the hyaloid artery overlying the optic nerve. Not visually significant.

102.2 Key Diagnostic Tests and Findings

102.2.1 Fluorescein Angiography or Ultra-Widefield Fluorescein Angiography

Anterior segment fluorescein angiography (FA) may show abnormal vasculature including straight radial vessels within the iris or highlight the ciliary processes or a vascularized retrolental membrane. FA of the posterior segment after cataract extraction or in the setting of a clear lens may demonstrate loss of the foveal avascular zone or dragging of retinal vessels from retinal traction induced by the stalk.

102.2.2 Ultrasonography

B-scan can reliably identify a hyperechoic band extending from the posterior pole to the retrolental space, a hyperechoic lens, and tractional retinal detachment (▶ Fig. 102.3).

The axial length in eyes with PFV may be shorter than the contralateral eye in cases of microphthalmia on an A-scan.

102.2.3 Magnetic Resonance Imaging

Magnetic resonance imaging of the brain and orbits may be performed if there is ambivalence in the diagnosis and the B-scan is not confirmatory. This may require sedation in infants and toddlers but can demonstrate a shorter axial length and the hyaloid stalk (▶ Fig. 102.4); can also be helpful in differentiating PFV from Coats disease or retinoblastoma in the setting of leukocoria.

102.3 Critical Work-up

Differential diagnoses include retinoblastoma (usually not associated with microphthalmos and ultrasonography may reveal mass lesions with hyperechoic foci consistent with calcifica-

tions); severe Coats disease (a massive exudative retinal detachment may be present behind the lens which is usually clear and there is no stalk); retinopathy of prematurity (distinguished by bilaterality and absence of a true stalk); familial exudative vitreoretinopathy (distinguished by bilaterality and absence of a stalk); and systemic syndrome (bilaterality should raise suspicion for a genetic syndrome, especially Norrie disease, and a complete work-up is necessary).

102.4 Management

102.4.1 Treatment Options

It is important to assess risks and benefits of surgical intervention and consider the impact of any related congenital macular or optic nerve anomalies. In addition, with normal vision in the unaffected eye, successfully treated patients may still have limited vision secondary to amblyopia or retinal dysplasia. Visual outcomes are largely dependent on the extent of disease at presentation and aggressive amblyopia management in the postoperative course, although retinal dysplasia may be a vision-limiting factor. Positive prognostic factors include primarily anterior PFV and earlier age of diagnosis (with earlier treatment, as this minimizes the duration of deprivation amblyopia). Poor prognostic factors include microphthalmia, preoperative tractional retinal detachment, retinal folds, or optic nerve hypoplasia. In some cases, the macular anatomy may appear normal, and despite adequate treatment, including amblyopia therapy, vision may be limited secondary to retinal dysplasia. It is

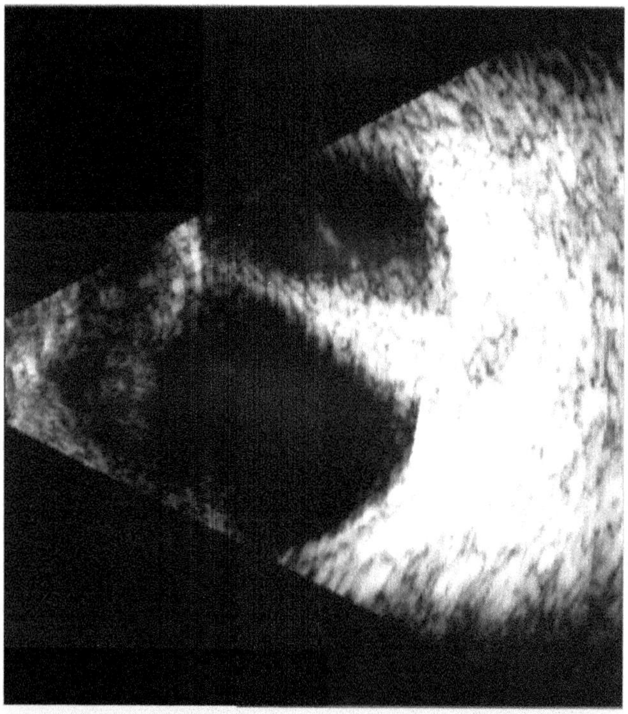

Fig. 102.3 B-scan ultrasonography demonstrating a hyperechoic band (stalk) extending from the optic nerve to the posterior surface of the lens. This appearance is consistent with a persistent hyaloid vessel in Cloquet's canal. The posterior surface of the lens is mildly hyperechoic as well.

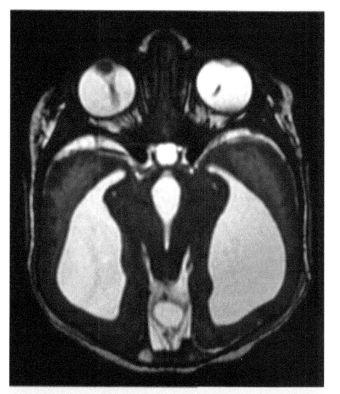

Fig. 102.4 T2-weighted MRI of the brain and orbits of a patient with bilateral persistent fetal vasculature demonstrating bilateral hypointense stalks. The anterior chamber of both eyes (most evident on the right eye in this axial slice) is shallow.

essential that this is discussed with the patient's family or guardian prior to surgery as vision may not improve.

Anterior PFV

Surgical decision making involves removing opacities in the visual axis accomplished by removal of the cataract and retrolental membrane. This may also be combined with anterior severing of the stalk to alleviate any posterior traction. Additionally, removal of the lens may be considered to prevent secondary angle-closure from an intumescent lens or anteriorly rotated ciliary processes.

Posterior PFV

Vitrectomy may be necessary for severe vitreous hemorrhage, progressive retinal detachment, vitreous bands causing traction, or centrally dragged ciliary processes causing shallowing of the anterior chamber. This may be accompanied by severing the stalk. Care must be taken to ensure there is no retina dragged into the stalk prior to severing it.

102.4.2 Follow-up

Follow-up frequency is dictated by severity of disease process and ongoing management strategies. Coordination with pediatric ophthalmology for amblyopia management is an important aspect of follow-up.

Suggested Reading

[1] Goldberg MF. Persistent fetal vasculature (PFV): an integrated interpretation of signs and symptoms associated with persistent hyperplastic primary vitreous (PHPV). LIV Edward Jackson Memorial Lecture. Am J Ophthalmol. 1997; 124(5):587–626

[2] Alexandrakis G, Scott IU, Flynn HW, Jr, Murray TG, Feuer WJ. Visual acuity outcomes with and without surgery in patients with persistent fetal vasculature. Ophthalmology. 2000; 107(6):1068–1072

[3] Dass AB, Trese MT. Surgical results of persistent hyperplastic primary vitreous. Ophthalmology. 1999; 106(2):280–284

Index

Note: Page numbers in **bold** or *italic* indicate headings or figures, respectively.